Complementary to this volume:

SIDE EFFECTS OF DRUGS ANNUALS 1—19 (1977—1995)
Edited by M.N.G. Dukes (Annuals 1—15) and J.K. Aronson (Annuals 16—19)

MEYLER'S SIDE EFFECTS OF DRUGS, 13th EDITION (1996)
Edited by M.N.G. Dukes

SEDBASE—The Side Effects of Drugs Database

DRUG-INDUCED DISORDERS
Edited by M.N.G. Dukes

Vol. 1 Drug-Induced Hepatic Injury, 2nd Edition (1992)
B.H.Ch. Stricker and P. Spoelstra

Vol. 2 Drug-Induced Diseases in the Elderly (1986)
F.I. Caird and P.J.W. Scott

Vol. 3 Treatment-Induced Respiratory Disorders (1989)
G.M. Akoun and J.P. White

Vol. 4 Drug-Induced Immune Diseases (1990)
J. Descotes

UNWANTED EFFECTS OF COSMETICS AND DRUGS USED IN
DERMATOLOGY, 3rd EDITION (1994)
A.C. de Groot, J.W. Weyland and J.P. Nater

IMMUNOTOXICOLOGY OF DRUGS AND CHEMICALS, 2nd EDITION (1986)
J. Descotes

DRUGS AND HUMAN LACTATION, 2nd Edition (1996)
P.N. Bennett

DRUG SAFETY IN PREGNANCY (1990)
P.I. Folb

RESPONSIBILITY FOR DRUG-INDUCED INJURY (1988)
M.N.G. Dukes and B. Swartz

THE INTERNATIONAL JOURNAL OF RISK AND SAFETY IN MEDICINE
Edited by M.N.G. Dukes

A MANUAL OF ADVERSE DRUG INTERACTIONS, 5th Edition (1997)
J.P. Griffin and P.F. D'Arcy

SIDE EFFECTS OF DRUGS ANNUAL 20

A worldwide yearly survey of new
data and trends

EDITOR

J.K. ARONSON M.A., D.PHIL., M.B., F.R.C.P.

Clinical Reader in Clinical Pharmacology
University Department of Clinical Pharmacology
Radcliffe Infirmary, Oxford, United Kingdom

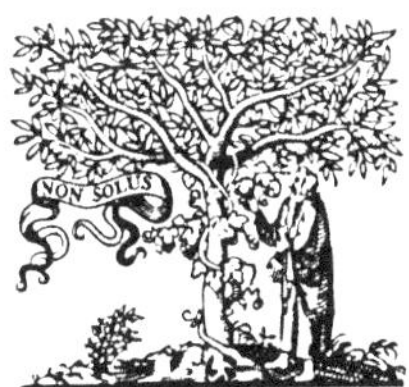

1997

ELSEVIER
Amsterdam – Lausanne – New York – Oxford – Shannon – Singapore – Tokyo

ISBN 0-444-82532-0
ISSN 0378-6080

Library of Congress Cataloging Card Number: 78-644057(ISSN 0378-6080))

This book is printed on acid free paper.

Published by:
Elsevier Science B.V.
P.O. Box 211
1000 AE Amsterdam
The Netherlands

Printed in The Netherlands

Contributors

J.K. ARONSON, M.A., M.B.CH.B., D. PHIL., M.B., F.R.C.P.
  Department of Clinical Pharmacology, Radcliffe Infirmary, University of Oxford,
  Woodstock Road, Oxford OX2 6HE, U.K.

I. AURSNES, M.D.
  Department of Pharmacotherapeutics, University of Oslo, P.O. Box 1065 Blindern,
  0316 Oslo 3, Norway

A.G.C. BAUER, M.D.
  Havenziekenhuis, Haringvliet 2, 3011 TD Rotterdam, The Netherlands

G. BOMAN, M.D., PH.D.
  Department of Lung Medicine, Uppsala University, S-751 85 Uppsala, Sweden

A. BUITENHUIS, M.D.
  Department of Clinical Pharmacology, Academisch Medisch Centrum, Meibergdreef 15,
  1105 AZ Amsterdam, The Netherlands

W. BURN
  Academic Unit of Psychiatry, St. James University Hospital, Clinical Science Building,
  Leeds LS9 7TF, U.K.

A. CARVAJAL
  Facultad de Medicina, Sistems Espanol de Farmacovigilancia, Avda. Ramon y Cajal 7,
  47005 Valladolid, Spain

N.H. CHOULIS, M.D., PH.D.
  School of Pharmacy, University of Athens, P.O. Box 4315, 102 10 Athens, Greece

J. COSTA, M.D.
  Clinical Pharmacology Department, Hospital Universitari, Cintra de Canyet s/n,
  08916 Badalona, Spain

P.J. COWEN, M.D.
  Department of Psychiatry, University of Oxford, MRC Clinical Pharm Unit, Oxford
  OX4 4XN, U.K.

S. CURRAN
  Academic Unit of Psychiatry, St. James University Hospital, Clinical Science Building,
  Leeds LS9 7TF, U.K.

P. DAWSON
  Department of Diagnostic Radiology, Hammersmith Hospital, Du Cane Road, London
  W12 0NN, U.K.

M.J. DEDICOAT
  Birmingham Heartlands Hospital, Bordesley Green East, Birmingham B9 5ST, U.K.

A.C. DE GROOT, M.D., PH.D.
  Department of Dermatology, Carolus-Liduina Hospital, P.O. Box 1101, 5200 BD
  Den Bosch, The Netherlands

M.D. DE JONG, M.D.
  Department of Infectious Diseases, National AIDS Therapy Evaluation Center,
  University of Amsterdam, P.O. Box 22700, 1100 DE Amsterdam, The Netherlands

A. DEL FAVERO, M.D.
  Istituto di Medicina Interna e Science Oncologiche, Policlinico Monteluce, University
  Degli Studi di Perugia, via Brunamonti, 06 122 Perugia, Italy

J. DESCOTES
  Department of Pharmacology & Med. Tox., Fac. de Médecine Alexis Carrel, INSERM
  U80, F 69008 Lyon, France

F.A. DE WOLFF, M.D.
  Academic Medical Center, University of Amsterdam, P.O. Box 22700, 1100 DE
  Amsterdam, The Netherlands

S. DITTMANN, M.D., D.SC.MED.
  a.i. Integrated Programme on Communicable Diseases, World Health Organisation,
  8 Scherfigsvej, 2100 Copenhagen O, Denmark

R.E. EDWARDS, M.B.B.S., F.R.C.A.
  Division of Addictive Behaviour, St. George's Hospital Medical School, Cranmer
  Terrace, London SW17 0RE, U.K.

H.W. EIJKHOUT, M.D.
  Bloodtransfusie Dienst, Central Laboratory of the Netherlands, Plesmanlaan 125, 1066
  CX Amsterdam, The Netherlands

C.J. ELLIS, M.D., F.R.C.P.
  Department of Infection & Tropical Diseases, Birmingham Heartlands Hospital,
  Bordesley Green East, Birmingham B9 5ST, U.K.

E. ERNST
  Center for Complementary Health Studies, University of Exeter, 25 Victoria Park Road,
  Exeter EX2 4NT, U.K.

M. FARRÉ
  Clinical Pharmacology Department, Germans Trias i Pujol, Hospital Universitari, Cintra
  de Canyet s/n, 08916 Badalona, Spain

P.I. FOLB, M.D., F.R.C.P.
  Department of Pharmacology, Groote Schuur Hospital, K45 Old Main Building,
  Observatory, Cape Town, 7925 South Africa

J.A. FRANKLYN, M.D.
Department of Medicine, University of Birmingham, Edgbaston, Birmingham B15 2TH, U.K.

M.G. FRANZOSI, PH.D.
"Mario Negri", Istituto de Richerche Farmacologiche, Via Eritrea 62, 20157 Milano, Italy

A.H. GHODSE, M.D., PH.D., F.R.C.P., F.R.C.PSYCH.
Division of Addictive Behaviour, Hunter Wg, St. George's Hospital Medical School, Cranmer Terrace, Tooting, London SW17 0RE, U.K.

A.I. GREEN, M.D.
Massachusetts Mental Health Center, Harvard Medical School, 74 Fenwood Road, Boston, MA 02215, U.S.A.

S. KHOO
Department of Pharmacology and Therapeutics, University of Liverpool, Ashton Street, Liverpool L69 3BX, U.K.

H.M.J. KRANS, M.D.
Stofwisselingsziekten en Endocrinologie, Gebouw 1, C4-R, Academisch Ziekenhuis Leiden, Postbus 9600, 2300 RC Leiden, The Netherlands

R. LATINI, M.D.
"Mario Negri", Istituto di Ricerche Farmacologiche, Via Eritrea 62, 20157 Milano, Italy

M. LEUWER, M.D., PH.D.,
Abt. Anästhesiologie II, Zentrum Anästhesiologie, Medizin. Hochschule Hannover, Konstanty Gutschow Str. 8, 30625 Hannover, Germany

P. MAGEE, M.D.
Walsgrave Hospitals, NIIS TRUST, Clifford Bridge Road, Coventry CV2 2DX, U.K.

A.P. MAGGIONI, M.D.
"Mario Negri", Istituto de Ricerche Farmacologiche, Via Eritrea 62, 20157 Milano, Italy

L.H. MARTíN ARIAS
Fac. de Medicina, Instituto de Farmacoepidemiologia, Sistems Espanol de Farmacovigilancia, Avda. Ramon y Cajal 7, 47005 Valladolid, Spain

G.T. McINNES, B.SC., M.D., F.R.C.P.
Department of Medicine & Therapeutics, Gardiner Institute, Western Infirmary, University of Glasgow, Glasgow G11 6NT, U.K.

R.H.B. MEYBOOM, M.D.
Bremhoeven 1, 5244 GV Rosmalen, The Netherlands

T. MIDTVEDT, M.D., PH.D.
Laboratory of Medical Microbial Ecology, Karolinska Institute, Box 60 400, S-171 77 Stockholm, Sweden

J.K. PATEL, M.D.
Massachusetts Mental Health Center, Harvard Medical School, 74 Fenwood Road, Boston, MA 02215, U.S.A.

E. PERUCCA, M.D., PH.D.
Clinical Pharmacology Unit, University of Pavia, Piazza Botta 10, 27100 Pavia, Italy

J.R. PETERS, M.D.PH.D.
Department of Medicine, University Hospital of Wales, Heath Park, Cardiff CF4 4XW, U.K.

M. PIRMOHAMED, M.D.
New Medical Building, University of Liverpool, Ashton Street, Liverpool L69 3BX, U.K.

B.C.P. POLAK, M.D.
Department of Ophthalmology, VU Ziekenhuis, Postbus 7057, 1007 MB Amsterdam, The Netherlands

R.E. POUNDER, M.A., M.D., D.DC.(MED.), F.R.C.P.
Royal Free Hospital, Pond Street, Hampstead, London NW3 2QG, U.K.

P. REISS, M.D., PH.D.
National AIDS Therapy Evaluation Center, Academisch Medisch Centrum, Meibergdreef 9, 1105 AZ Amsterdam, The Netherlands

H.D. REUTER, PH.D.
Siebengebirgsallee 24, 50939 Köln, Germany

M. SCHACHTER, M.D.
Department of Clinical Pharmacology, Imperial College of Science and Technology, London W2 1NY, U.K.

M. SCHOU, M.D.
Psychiatric Hospital, 2 Skovagervej, 8240 Risskov, Denmark

S.A. SCHUG
Department of Pharmacology, School of Medicine, University of Auckland, Private Bag 92019, Auckland, New Zealand

R.P. SEQUEIRA, PH.D.
Department of Pharmacology, Arabian Gulf University, P.O. Box 22979, Manama, Bahrain

D. SIDEBOTHAM
Department of Psychiatry Addictive Behaviour, St. George's Hospital Medical School, Cranmer Terrace, London SW17 0RE, U.K.

A. STANLEY, PH.D., M.R.PHARM.S.
Birmingham Oncology Hospital, St. Chad's Unit, Dudley Road Hospital, Dudley Road, Birmingham B18 7QH, U.K.

L. TURNER, DIP.PHARM.
  Department of Pharmacology, Medical School, Health and Medicines Information
  Services, P.O. Box 21638, Kloof Street, 8008 South Africa

W.G. VAN AKEN, M.D.
  Bloodtransfusion Service, Central Laboratory of the Netherlands, Plesmanlaan 125,
  1066 CX Amsterdam, The Netherlands

C.J. VAN BOXTEL, M.D., PH.D.
  Afd. Inwendige Geneeskunde, Academisch Medisch Centrum, Meibergdreef 9, 1105 AZ
  Amsterdam, The Netherlands

G.B. VAN DER VOET, M.D.
  Laboratorium voor Toxicologie, Academisch Ziekenhuis Leiden, Postbus 9600, 2300 RC
  Leiden, The Netherlands

R. VERHAEGHE, M.D.
  Inwendige Geneeskunde, University Ziekenhuis Gasthuisberg, Herestraat 49,
  3000 Leuven, Belgium

J. VERMYLEN, M.D.
  Center for Molecular Biology, Katholieke Universiteit Leuven, Herestraat 49, B 3000
  Leuven, Belgium

T. VIAL, M.D.
  Centre Regional de Pharmacovigilance, Hôpital Edouard Herriot,
  5 Place d'Arsonval, 69347 Lyon Cédex 03, France

T. WALLEY
  Department of Pharmacology, University of Liverpool, Ashton Street, Liverpool
  L69 3BX, U.K.

P.A. WINSTANLEY, M.D.
  New Medical Building, Department of Pharmacology and Therapeutics, Ashton Street,
  Liverpool L69 3BX, U.K.

E. WONG, M.D.
  Psychiatry, Harvard Medical School, Massachusetts Mental Health Center, Boston,
  MA 02115, U.S.A.

F. ZANNAD, M.D.
  Cardiologie & Pharmacologie Clinique, Centre Hospitalier Reg. et Université,
  29, Avenue de Marechal de Lattre, 54035 Nancy Cédex, France

O. ZUZAN, M.D.
  Department of Anesthesiology, Medizin. Hochschule Hannover, Konstanty Gutschow
  Str. 8, 30625 Hannover, Germany

Contents

How to use this book

THE SCOPE OF THE 'ANNUAL'

The Side Effects of Drugs Annual has been published each year since 1977. It is designed to provide a critical and up-to-date account of new information relating to adverse drug reactions and interactions from the clinician's point of view. The *Annual* can be used independently or as a supplement to the standard encyclopedic work in this field, *Meyler's Side Effects of Drugs*, the 13th edition of which was published in December, 1996.

SPECIAL REVIEWS

As new data appear, older findings may be discredited and existing concepts may require revision. The 'special reviews' deal critically with such topics, interpreting conflicting evidence and providing the reader with clear guidance. Special reviews are identified by the traditional prescription symbol and are printed in italic type. Older papers cited in these reviews are either listed by name or via cross-references to previous Annuals or past editions of Meyler's Side Effects of Drugs, which can be found in most medical libraries.

SELECTION OF MATERIAL

In compiling the *Side Effects of Drugs Annual* particular attention is devoted to those publications which provide essentially new information or throw a new light on problems already recognized. In addition, some authoritative new reviews are listed. Publications which do not meet these criteria are omitted. Readers anxious to trace all references on a particular topic, including those which duplicate earlier work, are advised to consult *Adverse Reactions Titles*, a monthly bibliography of titles from approximately 3400 biomedical journals published throughout the world, compiled by the Excerpta Medica International Abstracting Service.

PERIOD COVERED

The present *Annual* reviews all reports presenting significant new information on adverse reactions to drugs from July 1995 to June 1996. During the production of this *Annual*, more recent papers have been included.

CLASSIFICATION

Drugs are classified according to their main field of application or the properties for which they are most generally recognized. In borderline cases, however, some supplementary discussion has been included in other chapters relating to secondary fields of application. Fixed combinations of drugs are dealt with according to their most characteristic component.

DRUG NAMES

Drug products are in general dealt with in the text under their most usual non-proprietary names; where these are not available, chemical names have been used; fixed combinations usually have no proprietary connotation and here trade names have been used as necessary.

SYSTEM OF REFERENCES

References in the text are coded as follows:
R: In the original paper, the point is *reviewed* in some detail with reference to other literature.
r: The original paper *refers* only briefly to the point, on the basis of evidence adduced by other writers.
C: The original paper presents *detailed original clinical evidence* on this point.
c: The original paper provides *clinical evidence*, but only *briefly or anecdotally*.
The code has not been applied to animal pharmacological papers.
The various Editions of *Meyler's Side Effects of Drugs* are cited in the text as SED-11, SED-12 etc.; *SED Annuals 1—18* are cited as SEDA-1, SEDA-2 etc.

INDEXES

Index of drugs: this index provides a complete listing of all references to a drug in this volume.

Index of side effects: this index is necessarily selective, since a particular side effect may be caused by very large numbers of compounds; the index is therefore mainly directed to those side effects which are particularly serious or frequent, or are discussed in special detail. Before assuming that a given drug does not have a particular side effect, one should consult the relevant chapters.

For *interactions*, the reader should refer to the *Index of drugs* where all interactions are listed under the drugs concerned, irrespective of the chapter in which they appear.

It should be borne in mind that American spelling has been used throughout, e.g. anemia, estrogen etc. (instead of anaemia, oestrogen etc.).

Complementary/alternative medicine: what should we do about it?

E. Ernst*

Complementary/alternative medicine is a booming business. Its prevalence is 50% in Australia, 33% in the US, and 25% in the UK (1—3). Sales of herbal and homoeopathic remedies are predicted to double within 5 years (4), and the numbers of practitioners in the US are predicted to grow by about 90% between 1994 and 2010 (5). Not a day passes without media reports on some (usually sensational) aspect, and the public's romance with complementary medicine seems to get more intense with every such report. The terminology is confusing: the words used almost interchangeably with complementary medicine range from paramedicine to unorthodox medicine. An inclusive definition, which has also been adopted by the Cochrane field in complementary medicine, is as follows: "Complementary medicine is diagnosis, treatment, and/or prevention which complements mainstream medicine by contributing to a common whole, by satisfying a demand not met by orthodoxy or by diversifying the conceptual frameworks of medicine" (6). In practical terms complementary medicine comprises a heterogeneous group of treatments, of which acupuncture, herbalism, homoeopathy, and spinal manipulation are currently the four most popular.

What should physicians do about this phenomenon?

Simply ignore it

Romances, we all know, may not last all that long. One might assume that if we ignore it for long enough, complementary medicine will one day have vanished into thin air. Whether this is a realistic prospect or mere wishful thinking, this strategy would almost certainly be ill-advised. If you contemplate negating complementary medicine altogether, presumably you are not taken by it. You probably have doubts about complementary medicine itself, its representatives, or both. Regardless of whether this stance is right or wrong, it is foremost not compatible with the physician's most fundamental task: to look after the best interests of the patient. Patients need informed advice here and now—after all they are likely to use complementary medicine today or try it tomorrow. Thus, to ignore complementary medicine seems utterly wrong; even if your advice would be "stay well clear", this advice still needs to be given and it needs to be based on some sort of knowledge or insight. Beware, if you do give recommendations; they had better be based on something better than intuition or prejudice.

I should stress that many who should know better seem thoroughly dedicated to the "let's ignore it all" strategy. Government officials frequently pay lip-service to complementary medicine, particularly when elections are looming, but there is ample evidence that this is done with profound insincerity for the obvious reason of attracting votes. Of the total medical research budget, for instance, the

*The Side Effects of Drugs Essay is written each year by a guest author. E. Ernst, MD PhD FRCP (Edin), is Professor in the Department of Complementary Medicine, Postgraduate Medical School, University of Exeter, 25 Victoria Park Road, Exeter EX2 4NT.

British NHS spends all of 0.08% on complementary medicine (7), which is overtly out of proportion with the current UK prevalence figure (3).

If you can't beat 'em, join 'em

No question, if you are convinced that complementary medicine does more good than harm, you should use it in your daily practice. The evidence that the benefits outweigh the risks is, however, far from compelling (8). This, of course, is a generalization, and one should look at the merits of each method separately. For instance, there are reports of more than 200 serious complications following spinal manipulation. In one of our own surveys, 12% of users of spinal manipulation reported (mostly mild) adverse effects (9). There are at least five documented deaths after acupuncture (10), and the adverse events associated with herbal remedies are uncountable (11). On the other side of the equation, the evidence that complementary therapies work is fragmentary in most cases. But you may believe that the practice of medicine need not rely totally on an evidence-based approach, or you may argue that the evidence base is shaky in many fields of (orthodox) medicine also. Thus, you may want to practise complementary medicine in spite of convincing evidence that the benefits outweigh the risks.

You may also want to join, because it is fashionable, different, or even profitable—yes, of course, it can be immensely profitable. If you play your cards right, patients (particularly private patients) will queue up. And remember: the more you pay, the more worthwhile it seems.

But again, beware! Some may call you a quack. Quackery is characterized by the promotion of false or unproven health schemes for profit (12). On second thoughts, therefore, you may want to consider a different strategy.

Declare war

In medicine, there is a long and solid tradition of being self-righteous and dogmatic. Never mind the data (if any)—what is not taught at Medical School cannot be worth knowing and most likely is even wrong. As physicians we must oppose what is wrong with our health-care systems. So why not fight complementary medicine where we can?

This strategy looks attractive to many and has been tried again and again. Yet it has one major flaw: it does not work. Patients are immune to it. They just carry on using complementary medicine as before. What is more, blind opposition can have obvious adverse effects. The patient who, driven by whatever motives, wants to try complementary medicine will be at best confused or at worst put off by the mainstream practitioner who denounces it. This will create a gap between complementary medicine on the one side and orthodoxy on the other. However successful you are at throwing hand grenades across the gap, the patient will be left in the middle and in acute danger of getting hurt.

And what about rigorous research?

There is an undeniable paucity of reliable data on complementary medicine. In particular, three fundamental questions are unanswered:
- is it efficacious?
- is it safe?
- does it save money?

In the absence of such information it is difficult, even impossible, rationally to adopt any of the above strategies. If you are against (or in favour of) complementary medicine, what are your reasons and on what data do you base your opinion? It doesn't require the mind of a genius to conclude that research could be the solution.

But hold on, there are arguments against even this approach. In order to decide whether or not to research complementary medicine, some argue that "we need to compare the prior probabilities of conventional therapy hypotheses . . . ." (13). Many of the theories of complementary medicine are overtly implausible; thus, the conclusion of such a comparison would usually be to confine research to areas in which a positive result is most promising, namely in orthodox medicine.

Although this argument sounds logical, it does not hold water. First, history tells us that valuable innovations (in medicine or other fields of research) have often come from the 'fringe'. Secondly, if so many people are using complementary medicine already, is it not irresponsible not to investigate whether all that time, money, and effort is being spent without some sort of benefit? Thirdly (and most importantly) it would be downright unethical (14) not to make sure that at least no major harm is being done by practitioners of complementary medicine—and this, of course, requires rigorous research.

The way ahead

Complementary medicine is popular and will almost certainly become even more so in the near future. We may love this or hate it. However, in order to have a rational attitude towards it, there seems only one way ahead—get on with well-focused, rigorous research.

This is fine as far as it goes, but how should we do this? In my view we need rigorous clinical trials to demonstrate efficacy. Never mind the implausibility of some of these therapies—if they are used by large proportions of the population we ought to know whether or not they work. Researching the underlying mechanisms could be tackled once efficacy has been demonstrated. In parallel we need to investigate the safety issue.

And which treatments represent a priority? It seems to me that those most popular should be investigated most urgently. Some people say that conventional trial designs are not applicable to complementary medicine. This is true only to some degree and only in some instances. But regardless of whether or not blinding is possible or a credible placebo can be found, randomized clinical trials are feasible in all cases.

Thus, the strategy should be to do randomized trials of the four major complementary treatments (see above) to test whether these treatments are more efficacious and safer than control treatments for defined conditions. It goes without saying that this strategy requires adequate funding, and this may well be the biggest obstacle of all.

REFERENCES

1. MacLennan AH, Wilson DH, Taylor AW. Prevalence and cost of alternative medicine in Australia. Lancet 1996;347:569−73.
2. Eisenberg DM, Kessler RC, Foster C, Norlock FE, Calkins DR, Delbanco TL. Unconventional medicine in the United States. New Engl J Med 1993;328:246−52.
3. Fisher P, Ward A. Complementary medicine in Europe. Br Med J 1994;309: 107−11.
4. Mintel. Report on complementary medicines. February 1997.
5. Cooper RA, Stoflet SJ. Trends in the education and practice of alternative medicine clinicians. Health Affairs 1996;15:226−38.
6. Ernst E, Resch KL, Mills S, Hill R, Mitchell A, Willoughby M, White A. Complementary medicine—a definition. Br J Gen Pract 1995; Sep:506.
7. Ernst E. Only 0.08% of funding for research in NHS goes to complementary medicine. Br Med J 1996;313:882.
8. Ernst E, editor. Complementary medicine: an objective appraisal. London: Butterworth, 1996.
9. Abbot NC, White AR, Ernst E. Complementary medicine. Nature 1996;381:361.
10. Ernst E, White A. Acupuncture: safety first. Training programmes should include basic medical knowledge and experience. Br Med J 1997;314:1362.
11. Ernst E, De Smet PAGM. Adverse effects of complementary therapies. In: Dukes MNG, editor. Meyler's Side Effects of Drugs, 13th Edn. Amsterdam: Elsevier, 1996:1427−54.
12. Jarvis W. Homeopathy. A position statement by the National Council Against Health Fraud. Skeptic 1994;3:50−7.
13. Stalker DF. Evidence and alternative medicine. Mount Sinai J Med 1995;62:132−43.
14. Ernst E. The ethics of complementary medicine. J Med Ethics 1996;22:197−8.

Reginald P. Sequeira

1 Central nervous system stimulants and drugs that suppress appetite

METHYLXANTHINES *(SED-13, 1; SEDA-17, 1; SEDA-18, 1; SEDA-19, 1)*

Caffeine

The ability of low-dose caffeine (less than 100 mg) to reinforce the coffee drinking habit, contributing to the development of dependence, has been investigated (1[C]). *Drowsiness, headache*, and *fatigue* were more severe with decaffeinated coffee than caffeinated coffee; the occurrence of greater drowsiness, fatigue, and headache with placebo predicted subsequent caffeine reinforcement. In everyday life, caffeine reinforcement can occur as a result of the alleviation by caffeine of the adverse effects of overnight caffeine abstinence (negative reinforcement) in adults (2[C])—(4[C]) and young adolescents (5[C]).

Theophylline

Although there is a relation between theophylline concentrations and symptoms associated with toxicity in acutely intoxicated or elderly patients, it may not be extrapolated to younger patients taking long-term theophylline. The predictive value and prevalence of symptoms in patients with high serum theophylline concentrations (over 20 mg/l or 110 µmol/l) have been retrospectively evaluated (6[C]). The results of 483 theophylline measurements in 450 asthmatic patients showed that although in 46 instances the theophylline concentration was over 20 mg/l, only three of these patients were symptomatic. Subse-quently, 113 theophylline measurements were made in 90 patients; 13 exceeded 20 mg/l. None of the symptoms, such as nausea or gastrointestinal upset, headache, palpitation or irregular heart beat, and tremor or shakiness was a sensitive predictor of a high theophylline concentration. Nevertheless, it was unclear whether there were cardiac or neurological electrophysiological abnormalities in the absence of symptoms in these adult asthmatics taking long-term theophylline therapy. Hence, conservative use of theophylline and regular monitoring of serum concentrations is prudent.

Cardiovascular The cardiotoxic potential of intravenous theophylline has been evaluated by measuring the cardiospecific isoenzyme component of creatine kinase (MB-CK) in 12 patients with bronchial asthma or spastic bronchitis (7[C]). They received theophylline by infusion on three days; twice on day 1 (400 mg in the morning and 300 mg in the evening, each over 30 min, at a rate of 10—15 mg/min) and once each on days 2 and 3 (400 mg). Enzyme activity and serum theophylline concentration were measured immediately after the infusion and at 1, 3, and 6 h. *Cardiac dysrhythmias* correlated with the time of theophylline administration and the serum theophylline concentration. In most patients heart rate increased during theophylline infusion and on the third day. Four patients developed clinically silent ventricular dysrhythmias, which correlated with increased MB-CK activity and theophylline concentrations. One patient had a bout of atrial fibrillation lasting 5 h and resolving spontaneously. The authors emphasized the need for carefully adjusting the dosage of intravenous theophylline, espe-

Side Effects of Drugs, Annual 20
J.K. Aronson, ed.

1

cially in patients with tissue hypoxia and in those treated with β-adrenoceptor agonists.

Nervous system   A hypothesis that adenosine release in the central nervous system is partly responsible for the neurotoxicity of methotrexate has prompted an investigation of the effectiveness of aminophylline, an adenosine receptor antagonist, in ameliorating this neurotoxicity (8[C]). Six patients who had methotrexate neurotoxicity unresponsive to standard treatment received aminophylline 2.5 mg/kg. Four of six patients with toxic signs and symptoms attributed to methotrexate and unrelieved by steroids, epidural blood patch, promethazine, 5HT-receptor antagonists, paracetamol, or narcotics, had complete resolution of neurotoxicity after or during a 1-h infusion of aminophylline; two others had pronounced improvement but persistent nausea. Concentrations of adenosine in the CSF of patients receiving methotrexate were greatly increased. Taken together, these results give fairly strong support to the view that subacute methotrexate neurotoxicity may be mediated by adenosine and relieved by aminophylline.

Interactions   *Grapefruit juice*, which contains narangin, inhibits the biotransformation of caffeine, which is metabolized by the cytochrome P450 isoform CYP1A2. Although CYP1A2 is also involved in theophylline biotransformation, no pharmacokinetic interaction of theophylline with grapefruit juice was found in a randomized crossover study in 12 young healthy male non-smokers (9[C]).

Grepafloxacin In five healthy men serum theophylline concentrations were increased by grepafloxacin, a quinolone antimicrobial (10[C]), suggesting that grepafloxacin is similar to ciprofloxacin in inhibiting the cytochrome P450 isoform CYP1A2.

Zileuton A pharmacokinetic interaction of theophylline with zileuton, causing theophylline toxicity, has been described (10[C]). Zileuton is a selective 5-lipoxygenase inhibitor, currently being used in mild to moderate bronchial asthma. In a double-blind crossover study in 16 non-smoking healthy men theophylline (Slophyllin; 200 mg every 6 h) and zileuton (800 mg bd) were given for 5 days. During co-administration, the mean theophyl-

line concentration increased, apparent plasma clearance fell, the time to peak concentration was delayed, and the elimination half-life was prolonged; 14 subjects reported 44 mild to moderately severe adverse effects, mainly headache (27 vs. 44%), nausea (6.7 vs. 25%), and dyspepsia (0 vs. 25%). The increased incidence of adverse events in patients taking theophylline and zileuton compared with those taking theophylline and placebo, was most probably due to theophylline toxicity resulting from a pharmacokinetic interaction rather than to zileuton itself. Consistent with this idea, the most common adverse events included the generally recognized adverse effects of theophylline. Although none of the adverse events was severe, three volunteers taking theophylline with zileuton withdrew from the study prematurely, and in these individuals the plasma concentrations of theophylline were 22, 14, and 21 mg/l, measured 5, 21, and about 12 h after withdrawal.

STIMULANT AND ANORECTIC AGENTS *(SED-13, 13; SEDA-17, 8; SEDA-18, 7; SEDA-19, 2)*

Fenfluramine and dexfenfluramine

The effect of dexfenfluramine 15 mg bd for 3 months in combination with a low-calorie diet has been investigated in a multicenter open trial (11[C]). The patients were suffering from obesity with either no complications ($n = 210$) or with the following complications: hypertension ($n = 59$), type II diabetes mellitus ($n = 86$), or an eating disorder ($n = 60$). Most of them were women (83%). The results of this study of the everyday care a large population of obese patients confirmed the efficacy and safety of dexfenfluramine, especially for complicated obesity. Adverse events were generally transient and moderate and occurred mainly at the start of treatment. They were *drowsiness* (6.3%), *dry mouth* (5.3%), and *headache* (5.3%). During the study 9.4% patients were withdrawn, because of adverse events in only 3.8% of cases.

Cardiovascular   An attempt to determine prior exposure to appetite suppressants, especially fenfluramine, in UK patients with *primary pulmonary hypertension* has been reported (12[C]). A total of 55 patients were identified; of these, three women had been exposed to appetite suppressants: fenfluramine (*n* = 2) or diethylpropion (*n* = 1). In each case, exposure was brief and apparently predated the development of symptoms by several years. Exposure of patients with severe primary pulmonary hypertension to fenfluramine and other appetite suppressants seems to be uncommon in the UK, unlike in France, whence most of the cases associating primary pulmonary hypertension with fenfluramine have originated.

Methylphenidate

Cardiovascular   There is increasing evidence to support anxiety as a determinant of cardiovascular adverse effects of stimulant medication in children with attention deficit hyperactivity disorder (ADHD). In a study of 63 children aged 6—12 years, baseline blood pressure and heart rate did not differ between anxious and non-anxious children with ADHD; however, there was an *exaggerated diastolic blood pressure response* to methylphenidate 60 min after ingestion in anxious-ADHD, a time corresponding to the peak effect (13[C]),(14[C]). The stimulant-related increases in heart rate and blood pressure were modest and generally of little clinical concern. However, these data on differential medication responses in anxious children with ADHD add to the growing evidence that anxious children with ADHD constitute a distinct subgroup (15[C]).

Nervous system   Stimulants are most often given in the morning and at noon to children with ADHD, a third administration in the late afternoon being avoided because of concern about insomnia. The effects on behavior and sleep of methylphenidate given at 16:00 h to 12 children with ADHD have been evaluated in a double-blind, crossover study. The children derived substantial symptom reduction from methylphenidate given in the late afternoon, with no untoward effects on sleep latency and sleep adequacy (16[C]). As expected, 10 of the children lost an average of 1.2 kg body weight during the 12-day study. These findings should encourage clinicians to consider thrice-daily stimulants for patients who show good day-time responses to a twice-daily

regimen but who are disruptive and overactive in the evening. Nevertheless, one needs to be alert to possible problems of *anorexia* and *insomnia* in out-patient pediatric practice. This conservative conclusion is reasonable, since the patients in this study were particularly disturbed and data were obtained in the context of in-patient treatment.

The use of methylphenidate to improve cognitive problems due to HIV infection has been reviewed (17[R]). Dosages of methylphenidate of 10—90 mg/day were used in two or three divided doses, with reported improvements in both affective and cognitive symptoms. Adverse effects were mild and no additional, unusual, or disease-specific adverse effects were reported. There are some important issues in relation to the use of methylphenidate in HIV infection. No studies have been carried out in the early stages of HIV disease, in which a significant minority of patients have similar complaints in the absence of clinically apparent immunosuppression. None of the studies has been placebo-controlled, nor has any study specifically investigated women with HIV disease and cognitive symptoms.

Yet another critical question is to dissociate the cognitive benefit due to zidovudine treatment from that of methylphenidate in HIV disease. It has been argued that although clinical treatment is justifiable on ethical and clinical grounds, it would be helpful to have data from a controlled prospective study of various dosages of methylphenidate at all stages of HIV disease in patients with documented neuropsychiatric deficits and in the absence of confounding factors such as depression and acute medical illnesses. An attempt in this direction has been made in a recent randomized, double-blind comparison of the efficacy and safety of methylphenidate and desimipramine in 20 HIV-antibody-positive patients with depressive symptoms (18[C]). Methylphenidate and desimipramine relieved depressive symptoms with similar efficacy. Adverse effects were more common with methylphenidate early in treatment, but more common with desimipramine later on; significant adverse effects (mainly *insomnia, anxiety, nervousness, dry mouth*, and *anorexia*) were reported by 22 and 16%, respectively. The patients were relatively free from severe cognitive impairment and had no significant changes in cognitive function quantified by neuropsychological testing. These results have to be interpreted cautiously since the sample size was small.

Metabolic   In a prospective 21-month, open-label, out-patient study, 23 boys with ADHD were treated with methylphenidate (0.55 mg/kg) and compared with 23 unmedicated boys with ADHD (19[C]). The patients were aged 7–12 years at entry, and there were no significant changes in weight, height, heart rate, or blood pressure at the end of the study. Considering the age of the patients the authors proposed that the weight gain associated with the pubertal growth spurt was larger than the putative weight loss due to methylphenidate. One of the limitations of this study was that data were gathered only at the beginning and end of the study; it is possible that transient changes during the study went unnoticed. Considering the variable findings of earlier studies (20[C]), (21[C]) addressing the same issue of whether methylphenidate affects growth in patients with ADHD, it is plausible that the effect of an extended period of treatment is determined by the dosage used and the ages of the patients studied.

Interactions   Concern has been raised, especially by the US media, about the safety of concomitant use of methylphenidate and *clonidine* for ADHD in children. A review of the FDA database uncovered four life-threatening or fatal cases; however, these cases were so confounded by other possible factors that it was difficult to attribute any of the three deaths to clonidine, methylphenidate, or their combination (22[Cr]). This concern is difficult to address, because of the sparsity of data. This drug combination has never been studied in randomized controlled trials in children, and so there is little chance of finding a good estimate of its safety or even efficacy. The author therefore emphasized the importance of post-marketing surveillance.

Pseudoephedrine

Several H_1-receptor antagonists have been evaluated in combination with oral decongestants for the management of allergic rhinitis. A modified-release formulation containing pseudoephedrine 240 mg and loratadine 10 mg (SCH-434QD) given once daily has been compared with loratadine 10 mg/day, pseudoephedrine sulfate 120 mg every 12 h, or placebo for seasonal allergic rhinitis in a total of 874 subjects (about 200 in each group) (23[C]). The study lasted 2 weeks. The modified-release formulation was superior to the other treatments in relieving symptoms. All the treatments were well tolerated, with no serious or unusual adverse events. *Insomnia* and *nervousness*, commonly associated with pseudoephedrine, were noted in significantly more patients who took SCH-434QD or pseudoephedrine than those treated with loratadine or placebo. *Hyperkinesia* was more frequently reported with pseudoephedrine.

In another study the effectiveness and safety of a solution of pseudoephedrine with astemizole was compared with a syrup of pseudoephedrine and loratadine for allergic rhinitis in 50 children (24[C]). While 84% of the children treated with pseudoephedrine plus astemizole had clinical improvement, 64% treated with pseudoephedrine plus loratadine improved. One of the former and two of the latter showed the usual adverse effects (*somnolence* and *irritability*).

OTHER CENTRALLY-ACTING DRUGS

Tacrine *(SED-13, 370; SEDA-17, 11; SEDA-18, 10; SEDA-19, 4, 148)*

Attempts have been made to understand *hepatotoxicity* in relation to the polymorphically expressed detoxification enzyme, glutathione-*S*-transferase (GSTMI gene). There were no differences in the frequency of this genotype in patients with tacrine-induced increases in transaminases compared with controls, suggesting that prospective determination of GSTMI status cannot be used to predict individual susceptibility to tacrine-induced liver damage (25[C]).

REFERENCES

1. Hughes JR, Oliveto AH, Bickel WK, Higgins ST, Badger GJ. The ability of low doses of caffeine to serve as reinforcers in humans: a replication. Exp Clin Psychopharmacol 1995;3:358—63.

2. Rogers PJ, Richardson NJ, Elliman NA. Overnight caffeine abstinence and negative reinforcement of preference for caffeine containing drinks. Psychopharmacology 1995;120:457—62.

3. Richardson NJ, Rogers PJ, Elliman NA, O'Dell RJ. Mood and performance effects of caffeine in relation to acute and chronic caffeine deprivation. Pharmacol Biochem Behav 1995; 52:313—20.

4. Michell SH, de Wit H, Zancy JP. Caffeine withdrawal symptoms and self administration following caffeine deprivation. Pharmacol Biochem Behav 1995;51:941—5.

5. Hale KL, Hughes JR, Oliveto AH, Higgins ST. Caffeine self administration and subjective effect in adolescents. Exp Clin Psychopharmacol 1995; 3:364—70.

6. Melamed J, Beaucher WN. Minor symptoms are not predictive of elevated theophylline levels in adults on chronic therapy. Ann Allergy Asthma Immunol 1995;75:516—20.

7. Chazan R, Karwat K, Tyminska K, Tadeusiak W, Droszcz W. Cardiac arrhythmias as a result of intravenous infusion of theophylline in patients with airway obstruction. Int J Clin Pharmacol Ther 1995;32:170—5.

8. Bernini JC, Fort DW, Greiner JC, Kane BJ, Chappell WB, Kamen BA. Aminophylline for methotrexate-induced neurotoxicity. Lancet 1995; 345;544—7.

9. Fuhr U, Meier A, Keller M, Steinijans VW, Sauter R, Staib AH. Lacking effects of grapefruit juice on theophylline pharmacokinetics. Int J Clin Pharmacol Ther 1995;33:311—14.

10. Granneman GR, Braekman RA, Locke CS, Cavanaugh JII, Dube LM, Awni WM. Effect of zileuton on theophylline pharmacokinetics. Clin Pharmacokinet 1995;29 Suppl 2:77—83.

11. Enzi G and DIMOS (Dexfenfluramin Italian Multicentre Open Study) Group. Efficacy and safety of dexfenfluramine in the treatment of patients with simple or complicated obesity. Drug Invest 1995;10:249—56.

12. Thomas SHL, Butt AY, Corris PA, Egan JJ, Higenbottam TW, Madden BP, Waller PC. Appetite suppressants and primary pulmonary hypertension in the United Kingdom. Br Heart J 1995;74:660—3.

13. Urman RU, Ickowicz A, Fulford P, Tannock R. An exaggerated cardiovascular response to methylphenidate in ADHD children with anxiety. J Child Adolesc Psychopharmacol 1995;5:29—37.

14. Tannok R, Schachar R, Logan G. Methylphenidate and cognitive flexibility: dissociated dose effects in hyperactive children. J Abnorm Child Psychol 1995;23:235—66.

15. Pliska SR. Comorbidity of attention-deficit hyperactive disorder and over-anxious disorder. J Am Acad Child Adolesc Psychiatry 1995;31:197—203.

16. Kent JD, Blader JC, Koplewicz HS, Abikoff H, Foley CA. Effects of late afternoon methylphenidate administration on behavior and sleep in attention-deficit hyperactivity disorder. Pediatrics 1995;96:320—5.

17. Brown GR. The use of methylphenidate for cognitive decline associated with HIV disease. Int J Psychiatry Med 1995;25:21—37.

18. Fernadez F, Levy JK, Samley HR, Pirozzollo FJ, Lachar D, Crowley J, Adams S, Ross B, Ruiz P. Effects of methylphenidate in HIV-related depression: a comparative trial with desimipramine. Int J Psychiatry Med 1995;25:53—67.

19. Zeiner P. Body growth and cardiovascular function after extended treatment (1.75 years) with methylphenidate in boys with attention-deficit hyperactivity disorder. J Child Adolesc Psychopharmacol 1995;5:129—38.

20. Kalachnik JE, Sprague RL, Sleator EK, Cohen M, Ullmann RK. Effect of methylphenidate hydrochloride on stature of hyperactive children. Dev Med Child Neurol 1982;24:586—95.

21. Mattes JA, Gittelman R. Growth of hyperactive children on maintenance regimen of methylphenidate. Arch Gen Psychiatry 1983;40:317—21.

22. Fenichel RR. Combining methylphenidate and clonidine: the role of post-marketing surveillance. J Child Adolesc Psychopharmacol 1995; 5:155—6.

23. Bronsky E, Boggs P, Findlay S, Gawchik S, Georgitis J, Mansmann H, Sholler L, Wolfe J, Meltzer E, Morris R, Munk Z, Paull B, Pleskow W, Ratner P, Danzig M, Harrison J, Lorber R. Comparative efficacy and safety of once-daily loratadine-pseudoephedrine combination versus its components alone and placebo in the management of seasonal allergic rhinitis. J Allergy Clin Immunol 1995;96:139—47.

24. Martinez DP, Parra ER. Evaluation comparativa del astemizole-pseudoefedrina y loratadina-pseudoefedrina en ninos con rhinitis alergia. Rev Allergia Mex 1995;42:105—9.

25. Green VJ, Pirmohamed M, Kitteringham NR, Knapp MJ, Park BK. Glutathione S-transferase (genotype (GSTMI + 0) in Alzheimer's patients with tacrine transaminitis. Br J Clin Pharmacol 1995;39:411—15.

2   Antidepressant drugs

MONOAMINE OXIDASE INHIBITORS (MAOIs) *(SED-13, 35; SEDA-17, 16; SEDA-18, 14; SEDA-19, 7)*

Interactions People who take selective MAO inhibitors, such the MAO-A inhibitor *moclobemide* and the MAO-B inhibitor *selegiline*, can usually also take foods that contain tyramine, without concern about hypertensive reactions. When selegiline was combined with moclobemide there was some potentiation the pharmacodynamic effects of each, but this was not considered clinically important (1[C]). However, the combination did potentiate the pressor effects of tyramine (presumably because of simultaneous inhibition of both MAO-A and MAO-B). Therefore, if the two drugs are to be used together, a tyramine-free diet is needed.

The combination of non-selective irreversible MAOIs with drugs that potentiate serotonin function, particularly *selective serotonin re-uptake inhibitors* (SSRIs), can cause a serotonin syndrome, with an occasionally fatal outcome (SEDA-18, 14). In small series of healthy subjects and depressed patients SSRIs have been safely combined with moclobemide. However, overdosage of moclobemide and SSRIs can be fatal.

A woman was given a single dose of moclobemide (150 mg) 1 day after stopping fluoxetine 20 mg daily (2[C]). Within a few hours she developed shivering, tremor, restlessness, confusion, and incoordination, symptoms compatible with serotonin toxicity. The symptoms settled within 24 h of withdrawal of moclobemide. The same adverse effect occurred on rechallenge.

This report suggests that the combination of moclobemide and SSRIs in therapeutic dosages can provoke a serotonin syndrome. The combination, if used at all, should be used only with great caution and with close monitoring.

TRICYCLIC ANTIDEPRESSANTS *(SED-13, 42; SEDA-17, 17; SEDA-18, 16; SEDA-19, 7)*

GENERAL

Conventional tricyclic antidepressants are widely used for the treatment of depression in primary care. Consensus guidelines on the use of tricyclic antidepressants have emphasized that low dosages of tricyclic antidepressants (75 mg daily and under) seem to be no better than placebo in relieving major depression. Over 80 000 prescriptions for tricyclic antidepressants in primary care have been reviewed, using data from three separate sources (3[r]). Over 85% of these prescriptions were for dosages below those recommended by the consensus guidelines. In contrast, SSRIs and the second generation tricyclic antidepressant lofepramine were prescribed in appropriate dosages. These data suggest that tricyclic antidepressants are widely prescribed in ineffective doses in primary care, presumably because of concern about their adverse effects. It is, however, uncertain what proportion of patients in primary care for whom tricyclic antidepressants are prescribed would meet the criteria for major depression. For example, some of these prescriptions would have been for patients with mild anxiety and depression and/or sleep difficulties.

Cardiovascular The use of tricyclic antidepressants for the treatment of major depression in children and adolescents is problematic, because antidepressant efficacy in this population has not been proven, although this may be because of lack of high quality studies with adequate power (4[c]). Another concern is that the administration to children of tricyclic antidepressants, particularly desipramine, may cause *abnormalities of cardiac conduction* and even sudden death (SEDA-19, 7). Electrocardiograms have been recorded in 47 patients (mean age 13.5 years) who had been treated with desipramine and clomipramine as part of a 5-week, double-blind, crossover study for the treatment of obsessive compulsive disorder (5[C]). Both desipramine and clomipramine increased heart rate and prolonged the PR, QRS, and QTc intervals. Desipramine caused incomplete intraventricular conduction delay more than clomipramine (23 vs. 2%), but clomipramine increased the QTc interval more. During longer-term clomipramine treatment in 25 of these subjects some of the cardiographic abnormalities resolved but others appeared. The authors concluded that treatment with tricyclic antidepressants in children and adolescents should be accompanied by cardiographic monitoring.

INDIVIDUAL DRUGS

Desipramine

Interactions *Carbamazepine* induces hepatic cytochrome P450 drug metabolizing enzymes. After 3 weeks of treatment with carbamazepine in six healthy volunteers there was a 30% increase in the plasma clearance of desipramine and a similar increase in the urinary excretion of 2 hydroxydesipramine (6[C]). These data suggest that carbamazepine can increase the hydroxylation of desipramine (and probably other tricyclic antidepressants) enough to impair antidepressant efficacy.

Nortriptyline

Risk factors It is often believed that elderly people do not tolerate treatment with tricyclic antidepressants well because of the risks of anticholinergic toxicity and orthostatic hypotension. Such adverse effects occur less often with secondary amines, such as nortriptyline, than with tertiary amines, such as amitriptyline and imipramine. In a 12-month placebo-controlled study 40 elderly depressed patients (mean age 66.5 years) took nortriptyline maintenance treatment (7[C]). Dosing of nortriptyline was determined by plasma concentration measurement. Relative to placebo, nortriptyline caused an *increased pulse rate* and higher frequencies of *dry mouth* and *constipation*. However, these symptoms were judged to be clinically mild, and the overall burden of adverse effects was not significantly greater in the nortriptyline-treated patients. Maintenance nortriptyline did not cause orthostatic hypotension, weight gain, tiredness, or sleep disturbance; when tiredness and sleep disturbance occurred, they were influenced strongly by depression rating scores, whether the subjects were taking nortriptyline or placebo. The results of this study suggest that, in the absence of contraindications, nortriptyline is well tolerated in elderly depressed patients. However, the age range of the group was at the younger end of elderly depressed patients seen in clinical practice.

SELECTIVE SEROTONIN RE-UPTAKE INHIBITORS (SSRIs)

(SED-13, 65; SEDA-17, 19; SEDA-18, 19; SEDA-19, 9)

Nervous system Animal studies have suggested that aggressive behaviour can be attenuated by drugs that increase brain serotonin function, such as SSRIs. However, in some patients SSRIs has been associated with *behavioral activation* and *increased aggression* (SEDA-19, 9). The effect of treatment with fluoxetine (20 mg daily for 8 weeks) on aggressive behaviour has been studied in 19 adult in-patients with epilepsy and learning difficulties (8[C]). Fluoxetine was associated with a statistically significant increase in verbal and self-directed aggression. There was a reduction in the amount of aggressive behavior when fluoxetine was withdrawn. This study suggests that SSRIs can increase aggression in some patients. Of relevance here may be the presence of pre-existing organic brain disease and concomitant treatment with anticonvulsants, including barbiturates, benzodiazepines, and carbamazepine.

SSRIs are being increasingly used to treat depression in children and adolescents. The charts of 33 patients (mean age 13 years) with major depression who had received sole therapy with sertraline (mean dose 100 mg daily) for periods ranging from a few days to 10 weeks have been reviewed (9[C]). There was behavioral activation (irritability, agitation, and aggression) in seven patients, two of whom had symptoms of mania. In three subjects this adverse effect occurred in the first 2 weeks of treatment, while in the remainder it occurred after 12 weeks of therapy. Although the distinction between behavioral activation and mania may be difficult in young people, these data suggest that SSRIs are more likely to cause aggression and irritability in children and adolescents than in adults. The onset of this effect may be acute or delayed for several weeks.

Skin and appendages *Photosensitivity reactions* are common in patients taking phenothiazines, but rare in patients taking antidepressants. A 39-year-old woman was treated with fluoxetine (20 mg daily), with good relief of depressive symptoms but an unusual increase in her sensitivity to sunlight (10[C]). When possible she limited her exposure to the sun, but after being in bright sunlight for 2 h without protection she experienced painful burning, persistent erythema, and blisters on exposed areas. The photosensitivity reaction was probably due to the fluoxetine, because she was not taking any other medications. This reaction must be rare. It is noteworthy that the patient had experienced a photosensitivity reaction previously in response to tetracycline, suggesting a predisposition to this reaction.

Withdrawal effects Evidence continues to accumulate that abrupt withdrawal of SSRI treatment is associated with *withdrawal symptoms*, notably *nausea, diarrhea, light-headedness*, and *fatigue* (SEDA-19, 10). Paroxetine (20−60 mg/day) was given for 12 weeks in a double-blind, placebo-controlled design to 120 patients with panic disorder (11[c]). Following double-blind withdrawal significantly more paroxetine-treated patients experienced adverse effects than those taking placebo (35 vs. 15%). Withdrawal effects may be more common after withdrawal of SSRIs with shorter half-lives, such as fluvoxamine and paroxetine, but have also been rarely reported after withdrawal of fluoxetine (12[R]).

Overdosage SSRIs are generally safer in overdose than tricyclic antidepressants. However, six patients who committed suicide by taking an overdose of citalopram have been reported (13[C]). As is common in such cases, five of the six subjects had taken other substances, such as ethanol and minor tranquilizers; however, these were not thought to have contributed significantly to the fatal outcome. These findings raise the possibility that citalopram may be more toxic than other SSRIs in overdosage. Citalopram may do this by *prolonging the QTc interval*.

Overdosage of fluoxetine has been implicated in the development of *seizures*, but usually only when it is taken with other substances. A 15-year-old girl had a tonic-clonic seizure after overdosage of fluoxetine alone (14[c]). Recovery was uneventful. This report suggests that fluoxetine can indeed cause seizures in overdose. However, in contrast to tricyclic antidepressants, this effect is rare.

Interactions SSRIs can inhibit a number of the cytochrome P450 isoenzymes, causing clinically significant drug interactions. The growing awareness of this problem has been highlighted by several reviews of this topic in the psychiatric literature (15[R])−(17[R]). Fluoxetine, paroxetine, and to a lesser extent sertraline inhibit CYP2D6 activity. This can give rise to significant interactions with *secondary tricyclic antidepressants, antipsychotic drugs*, some *β-adrenoceptor antagonists*, and *Class IC antidysrhythmic drugs*. While fluvoxamine is a weak inhibitor of CYP2D6 activity, it is a potent inhibitor of CYP1A2, and increases plasma concentrations of theophylline, tertiary tricyclic antidepressants, haloperidol, and clozapine.

SSRIs, particularly fluvoxamine and fluoxetine, also inhibit the activity of CYP3A4, which metabolizes numerous drugs, including *carbamazepine, alprazolam, triazolam, terfenadine, astemizole, cisapride*, and *quinidine*. Interactions between SSRIs and drugs such as terfenadine, astemizole, and cisapride, which can result in cardiac dysrhythmias, are of particular concern.

SSRIs also appear to inhibit the activity of the CYP2C subfamily, and this has been reported to give rise to increased plasma concentrations of *diazepam, tolbutamide*, and *warfarin* (17[R]).

Knowledge about the substrates of particular P450 enzymes and the inhibitory effects of

SSRIs and other antidepressants is still incomplete, and great caution is needed, particularly if high concentrations of the co-administered drug can cause serious toxicity. From current evidence, citalopram seems to be the SSRI least likely to cause pharmacokinetic interactions with other drugs.

OTHER ANTIDEPRESSANTS

Nefazodone *(SED-13, 61)*

Nefazodone is a recently introduced antidepressant. It is related to trazodone but has less α_1-adrenoceptor antagonist activity and is therefore less sedative. It is generally well-tolerated. Characteristic adverse effects observed in placebo-controlled trials include (in decreasing order of frequency) *dry mouth, somnolence, nausea, dizziness, constipation, weakness, light-headedness,* and *blurred vision* (18[R]). The incidence of adverse sexual effects, for example delayed orgasm, seems to be less with nefazodone than with SSRIs (19r).

Interactions Nefazodone is a potent inhibitor of the CYP3A4 enzyme system, and increases plasma concentrations of *alprazolam* and *triazolam* (16[R]), (17[R]). Combined administration with *terfenadine* and *astemizole* should be avoided.

Nefazodone may increase serum concentrations of *carbamazepine* (20[C]).

A 35-year-old woman with bipolar mood disorder was maintained on carbamazepine 1 g daily, with serum concentrations between 5 and 6 µg/ml. She started to take nefazodone 100 mg bd, increasing to 150 mg bd after 1 week. Two weeks later she complained of perceptual disturbances, sedation, slurred speech, and hypersomnia. The serum carbamazepine concentrations had risen to 15 µg/ml. Nefazodone was discontinued and the carbamazepine dosage educed to 600 mg/day. Within 5 days her carbamazepine concentration had fallen to 6 µg/ml.

The concentrations of nefazodone and its metabolites may be increased by *fluoxetine* and *paroxetine* (18[R]).

Venlafaxine *(SED-13, 64)*

Venlafaxine is a potent inhibitor of the re-uptake of serotonin, but unlike the SSRIs it also inhibits the re-uptake of noradrenaline. In placebo-controlled trials the reported adverse effects of venlafaxine were (in decreasing frequency) *nausea, somnolence, dry mouth, insomnia, dizziness, constipation, weakness, nervousness,* and *sweating. Adverse sexual effects* occurred with a frequency similar to that of the SSRIs (21[R]).

In a small proportion of patients, venlafaxine causes *increased blood pressure.* This presumably reflects its ability to facilitate noradrenaline neurotransmission in the absence of postsynaptic α_1-adrenoceptor blockade. In placebo-controlled trials, clinically significant increases in blood pressure (an increase in diastolic blood pressure of at least 15 mmHg) were seen in 5.5% of patients treated with dosages of venlafaxine over 200 mg/day (22[R]). The increase in blood pressure with venlafaxine appears to be dose-related. Presumably subjects with pre-existing hypertension (whether treated or not) would be at greater risk of this adverse reaction, although this question has not been specifically addressed.

Interactions As with other drugs that potentiate brain serotonin function, venlafaxine can cause a serotonin syndrome when co-administered with *MAOIs* (23[c]).

A 43-year-old man with recurrent depression had partially responded to isocarboxazid, 30 mg/day. Venlafaxine (75 mg) was added, and after the second dose he developed agitation, hypomania, shivering, sweating, and dilated pupils. These symptoms rapidly subsided after venlafaxine was withdrawn. Subsequently he received the same combination, and developed serious serotonin toxicity, with myoclonic jerking, visual hallucinations and stupor. He was treated with benzodiazepines and the serotonin antagonist, cyproheptadine, but still took 6 days to recover fully.

A case of serotonin toxicity has also been reported in association with phenelzine and venlafaxine (24[c]). These reports suggest that, as with SSRIs, the combination of venlafaxine with non-selective MAOIs is contraindicated.

Current evidence suggests that venlafaxine has less of an inhibitory effect on P450 enzyme activity than SSRIs (16[R]), (17[R]). *Cisapride*

(5—10 mg twice daily) has been reported to produce good relief of venlafaxine-induced nausea in six patients (25[c]). Tolerance of cisa-pride in this small case series appeared to have been good but plasma drug monitoring was not carried out.

REFERENCES

1.   Dingemanse J, Kneer, J, Wallnöfer A, Kettler R, ZHrcher G, Koulu M, Korn A. Pharmacokinetic—pharmacodynamic interactions between two selective monoamine oxidase inhibitors: moclobemide and selegiline. Clin Neuropharmacol 1996; 19:399—414.

2.   Benazzi F. Serotonin syndrome with moclobemide—fluoxetine combination. Pharmacopsychiatry 1996;29:162.

3.   Donoghue JM, Tylee A. The treatment of depression: prescribing patterns of antidepressants in primary care in the UK. Br J Psychiatry 1996;168:164—8.

4.   Hazell P, O'Connell D, Heathcote D, Robertson J, Henry D. Efficacy of tricyclic drugs in treating child and adolescent depression: a meta-analysis. Br Med J 1991;310:897—900.

5.   Leonard HL, Meyer MC, Swedo SE, Richter D, Hamburger SD, Allen AJ, Rapoport JL, Tucker E. Electrocardiographic changes during desipramine and clomipramine treatment in children and adolescents. J Am Acad Child Adolesc Psychiatry 1995;34:1460—8.

6.   Spina E, Avenoso A, Campo GM, Caputi AP, Perucca E. The effect of carbamazepine on the 2-hydroxylation of desipramine. Psychopharmacology 1995;117:413—16.

7.   Reynolds CF, Frank E, Perel JM, Miller MD, Paradis CF, Stack JA, Pollock BG, Rifai AH, Cornes C, George CJ, Mazumdar S, Kupfer DJ. Nortriptyline side effects during double-blind, randomized, placebo-controlled maintenance therapy in older depressed patients. Am J Geriatr Psychiatry 1995;3:170—5.

8.   Troisi A, Vicario E, Nuccetelli F, Ciani N Pasini A. Effects of fluoxetine on aggressive behavior of adult inpatients with mental retardation and epilepsy. Pharmacopsychiatry 1995;28:73—6.

9.   Tierney E, Joshi PT, Llinas JF, Rosenberg LA, Riddle MA. Sertraline for major depression in children and adolescents: preliminary clinical experience. J Child Adolesc Psychopharmacol 1995; 5:13—27.

10.   Gaufberg E, Ellison JM. Photosensitivity reaction to fluoxetine. J Clin Psychiatry 1995;56: 486.

11.   Oehrberg S, Christiansen PE, Behnke K, Borup AL, Severin B, Soegaard J, Calberg H, Judge R, Ohrstrom JK, Manniche PM. Paroxetine in the treatment of panic disorder: a randomised, double-blind, placebo-controlled study. Br J Psychiatry 1995;167:374—9.

12.   Lane RM. Withdrawal symptoms after discontinuation of selective serotonin reuptake inhibitors (SSRIs). J Serotonin Res 1996;3:75—83.

13.   Öström M, Eriksson A, Thorson J, Spigset O. Fatal overdose with citalopram. Lancet 1996;348:339—40.

14.   Braitberg G, Curry SC. Seizure after isolated fluoxetine overdose. Ann Emerg Med 1995;26: 234—7.

15.   Taylor D, Lader M. Cytochromes and psychotropic drug interactions. Br J Psychiatry 1996; 168:529—32.

16.   Ereshefsky L, Riesenman C, Francis YW. Serotonin selective reuptake inhibitor drug interactions and the cytochrome P450 system. J Clin Psychiatry 1996;57:17—25.

17.   Nemeroff CB, DeVane L, Pollock BG. Newer antidepressants and the cytochrome P450 system. Am J Psychiatry 1996;153:311—20.

18.   Marcus RN. Safety and tolerability profile of nefazodone. J Psychopharmacol 1996;10:11—17.

19.   Baldwin DS. Depression and sexual function. J Psychopharmacol 1996;10:30—4.

20.   Ashton AK, Wolin RE. Nefazodone-induced carbamazepine toxicity. Am J Psychiatry 1996; 153:733.

21.   Danjou P, Hackett D. Safety and tolerance profile of venlafaxine. Int Clin Psychopharmacol 1995;10:15—20.

22.   Feighner JP. Cardiovascular safety in depressed patients: focus on venlafaxine. J Clin Psychiatry 1995;56:574—9.

23.   Klysner R, Larsen JK, Sørensen P, Hyllested M, Dyrlund Pedersen B. Toxic interaction of venlafaxine and isocarboxazide. Lancet 1995;346: 1298—9.

24.   Phillips SD, Ringo P. Phenelzine and venlafaxine interaction. Am J Psychiatry 1995;152: 1400—1.

25.   Russell JL. Relatively low doses of cisapride in the treatment of nausea in patients treated with venlafaxine for treatment-refractory depression. J Clin Psychopharmacol 1996;16:35—7.

3

Lithium

LITHIUM *(SED-13, 81; SEDA-17, 26; SEDA-18, 25; SEDA-19, 14)*

GENERAL

Formulations Adverse effects with lithium can sometimes occur because of problems with formulations.

Serum lithium concentrations, and hence adverse effects, may not be the same after administration of lithium carbonate tablets and liquid lithium citrate (1[c]).

A 9-year-old aggressive boy was treated with lithium carbonate 900 mg/day and had serum lithium concentrations around 0.8 mmol/l. Because he continued to have behavioral problems the dosage of lithium carbonate was increased to 1050 mg/day. His serum lithium concentration was now 1.20 mmol/l, and he started to vomit. He was switched to liquid lithium citrate but still vomited. The vomiting did not stop until the dosage of lithium citrate was reduced to 750 mg lithium carbonate equivalent; at that time the serum lithium concentration was 0.82 mmol/l.

The authors recommended that on switching from lithium carbonate to lithium citrate, one should start by reducing the dosage of lithium ion by at least 20%.

A woman was switched from the lithium formulation Priadel to another unidentified formulation which contained gluten, after which she developed gastrointestinal symptoms and her mood became less well controlled (2[c]). As a youth she had suffered from a malabsorption syndrome that had disappeared when she avoided wheat starch, of which the active ingredient is gluten. When she switched to a gluten-free lithium formulation her mood again became stabilized, and the gastrointestinal symptoms disappeared.

Permanent cerebellar sequelae developed in a patient who by mistake in the pharmacy was given lithium carbonate instead of calcium carbonate (3[c]).

Dosage schedules Daily and alternate-day dosing schedules for lithium maintenance treatment have been compared in 50 patients. There were no differences between the two procedures as regards either adverse effect profiles (4[C]) or 12-h brain lithium concentrations measured by ^{7}Li magnetic resonance spectroscopy (5[C]).

EFFECTS ON ORGANS AND SYSTEMS

Cardiovascular Three recently observed cases of lithium-induced *sinus node dysfunction* manifesting primarily as *sinus bradycardia* have been reviewed, together with 13 similar cases from the literature (6[Cr]). Psychiatrists who treat patients with lithium are advised to have a low threshold for seeking cardiological evaluation when cardiovascular symptoms occur. This has been emphasized by the report of a 56-year-old woman with *syncope* and *sinus node dysfunction* after long-term lithium therapy (7[c]). Following withdrawal of lithium, the sinus node dysfunction recovered completely, but on resumption of lithium in a low dosage sinus node dysfunction recurred and did not recover, despite further withdrawal of lithium. A permanent pacemaker was implanted.

Nervous system Lithium may exacerbate the vulnerability of patients with affective disorder to dyskinesias (8[c]). Among 130 stable outpatients, 110 were taking lithium at the time of evaluation, 37 in combination with antidepressants, and 19 in combination with neuroleptic drugs; in addition, 40 had a history of neuroleptic drug treatment during the previous 6 months. Assessment with a rating scale for parkinsonism, akathisia, dystonia, and tardive dyskinesia showed that the combination of lithium and a neuroleptic drug was

Side Effects of Drugs, Annual 20
J.K. Aronson, ed.

associated with a high prevalence of extra-pyramidal symptoms.

A 34-year-old man suffered from lithium-induced acute akathisia. Mianserin, 15 mg/day, ameliorated it (9[c]).

Ten women, all but one over 50 years of age, were treated with lithium (serum concentration over 2 mmol/l in only two patients) and developed dementia, increased CSF protein, and abnormal electroencephalograms (10[C]). Several of them had co-morbid neurological conditions, and the role played by lithium was unclear.

In 19 patients taking lithium there was no correlation between the total general adverse effects score and serum, erythrocyte, or brain lithium concentrations, the latter being determined by ^{7}Li magnetic resonance spectroscopy (11[C]). Patients with hand tremor had significantly higher brain lithium concentrations than patients without tremor.

Psychological Neuropsychological adverse effects of lithium may include slowed information processing, a sense of lethargy, and memory disturbance; they resemble symptoms seen in hypothyroidism. To test a possible connection, neuropsychological functioning was assessed in 16 psychiatric patients taking lithium. Eight subclinically hypothyroid patients performed significantly worse on measures of *verbal learning* and *memory* than did their eight euthyroid counterparts, and performance was more highly correlated with thyrotropin concentrations than with serum lithium concentrations (12[C]), (13[C]). I might add that I personally know of a few lithium-treated patients who, although clinically and biochemically euthyroid, derived large benefit from the co-administration of small doses of thyroxine, with improved mental function and a subjective feeling of improved alertness.

Endocrine, metabolic *Thyroid* A cohort of 61 patients at various stages of lithium treatment was followed up for 6 years in order to evaluate the course of thyroid abnormalities (14[C]). Ultrasonography confirmed that lithium can increase thyroid size, especially in cigarette smokers, and that it can affect the texture of the gland. However, the incidence of clinical *hypothyroidism* or *specific thyroid autoimmunity* did not exceed that found in the general population. The addition of carbamazepine to lithium may counteract lithium-induced subclinical hypothyroidism.

Case reports on the effect of lithium on thyroid function continue to appear. A 48-year-old woman treated with lithium for 2 years developed *thyrotoxicosis* and a *diffuse goiter*; fine-needle aspiration biopsy suggested Hashimoto's disease (15[c]). A 26-year-old woman developed reversible thyrotoxicosis during lithium treatment for 2 years; large-needle biopsy showed extensive follicular cell disruption with no lymphocytic infiltration (16[c]). A 59-year-old woman took lithium for 10 years; she developed hyperthyroidism 3 months after lithium withdrawal; five similar cases have been described previously; the causal role played by discontinuation of lithium is uncertain but suggestive (17[C]).

Pituitary diabetes insipidus Lithium-induced *diabetes insipidus* is usually nephrogenic, but a 70-year-old woman has been described who suffered in addition from central diabetes insipidus (18[c]).

Weight Advice about healthy eating was given to 25 patients before the start of lithium treatment and no such advice was given to another 25 patients, alternate patients being allocated to one or other group (19[c]). The patients given dietary advice gained significantly less weight than those in the control group, and the mean weight gain in those who gained weight was significantly less in the former than in the latter. Dietary advice before the start of lithium treatment is recommended.

Mineral and fluid balance *Calcium* The serum concentration of *ionized calcium* was significantly higher among 13 patients taking lithium than among 19 healthy controls. There was no significant difference between the serum parathyroid hormone concentrations in the two groups (20[C]).

Urinary system After 18 years (range 15—24) on lithium, 18 patients discontinued treatment and were re-examined after a further 4—16 weeks. They were compared with 18 patients with affective disorder not taking lithium and matched for age and sex (21[C]). *Glomerular filtration rate* was reduced in two of the patients who had discontinued lithium and in none of the controls. *Maximal urinary concentrating capacity* remained reduced during the period off lithium, on average 637 mOsm/kg compared with 856 mOsm/kg in the controls.

Urinary excretion of albumin and transferrin was determined in 40 patients before and after 6 months of either daily or alternate-day lithium carbonate treatment (22[C]). Excretion of these two indicators of glomerular permeability was higher in the lithium-treated patients than in a control group, but there was no difference between the two treatment groups.

Lithium treatment rarely leads to more pronounced proteinuria, but two lithium-treated women developed heavy *proteinuria* and *acute renal insufficiency* attributable to acute tubular necrosis (23[C]). The symptoms resolved on withdrawal.

A 48-year-old man taking lithium developed *polyuria*, with a daily urine output of around 4—5 l. It did not respond to indomethacin, but reduced dramatically with intravenous ketorolac, 30 mg every 6 h. After discontinuation of ketorolac on day 22 the urine volume began to increase, but without reaching polyuric values (24[c]).

Skin and appendages *Lichenoid lesions of the buccal mucosa* developed during lithium treatment in two cases; drug withdrawal caused resolution (25[c]).

A review (26[C]) and an experimental study (27) have addressed the possible modes of action of lithium in the pathogenesis of *psoriasis*. The hypotheses include effects on cyclic AMP, the protein kinase C/phosphoinositide pathway, and cytokines.

Sexual function Patients taking long-term lithium sometimes complain about *sexual dysfunction*, but a systematic comparison of sexual function in 24 manic-depressive patients taking lithium and in 42 surgical patients without psychiatric illness and not taking lithium showed no significant difference (28[C]). A case has nevertheless been reported in which repeated courses of lithium treatment were associated with *erectile impotence* that disappeared when the patient was given neuroleptic drugs alone or was off medication altogether (29[c]).

Risk factors Factors associated with an increased risk of lithium intoxication, apart from the administration of too high a dosage, include fever, vomiting, and diarrhea, prolonged unconsciousness, major surgery, a low salt diet, a drastic slimming diet, treatment with diuretics, treatment with non-steroidal anti-inflammatory drugs, and treatment with angiotensin-converting enzyme inhibitors (30[R]).

Risk factors are not always known or remembered. In a 45-year-old lithium-treated woman, who had chronic constipation, an ileorectal anastomosis was established. Lithium treatment was interrupted during the operation, but resumed 2 days later, and no serum lithium determinations were carried out. The patient died 6 days after the operation with 'cardiac' (presumably ventricular) fibrillation in association with fluid and electrolyte deficiency. The patient's husband took the case to the national 'liability council', but the physicians pleaded ignorance of the risk involved in operating on patients taking lithium and were acquitted, because the council considered the risk to be 'very little known' (31[c]).

This case caused another journal to restate the following precautions (32[r]):

- the recommended serum lithium concentration in blood samples drawn about 12 h after the last dose of lithium intake is 0.5—0.8 mmol/l; or 0.4—1.0 mmol/l if particularly sensitive and particularly resistant patients are included;
- physicians are advised to record and justify higher or lower concentrations in the case notes;
- lithium treatment should be discontinued or the dosage reduced before major (nonacute) surgery and should not be resumed until fluid and salt balance have become normal;
- if lithium treatment is continued in a reduced dosage, serum lithium concentrations should be determined at frequent intervals (preferably every two or three days during the acute illness);
- during lithium treatment, the administra-

tion of intravenous glucose and intravenous saline may be indicated in cases of dehydration and salt deficiency, respectively, but none of these procedures 'wash lithium out of the body';

- hemodialysis may be considered when the serum lithium concentration is higher than 1.5 mmol/l and/or falls with a half-life longer than 24 h and/or the patient's clinical condition is poor;
- hemodialysis with bicarbonate solution seems to be more effective than with acetate solution; continuous hemodiafiltration may be better than intermittent hemodialysis, because rebound of the serum lithium concentration is avoided.

Effects in children A study of adverse effects in 20 lithium-treated children aged 4—6 years has shown that adverse effects occur frequently in such children during the initial phase of lithium treatment, possibly related to higher lithium dosages per kg body weight, higher serum lithium concentrations, and possibly concurrent medical illness (33[C]).

Second-generation effects A 17-year-old woman who continued lithium treatment during pregnancy gave birth to an infant at 37 weeks gestational age (34[c]). The mother's serum lithium concentration several hours before delivery was 2.6 mmol/l. The infant's initial serum lithium concentration was 2.1 mmol/l; on day 3 it had fallen to 1.4 mmol/l. During the first 4 days of life the infant was lethargic.

A 29-year-old pregnant woman taking lithium developed lithium intoxication, with a serum lithium concentration that was higher than 4 mmol/l but fell rapidly after hemodialysis (35[c]). An infant was delivered by cesarean section before hemodialysis (time of gestation not given); both the amniotic fluid and the umbilical vein at delivery had lithium concentrations over 4 mmol/l. Apgar scores were 4 and 7 at 1 and 5 min after delivery.

A 25-year-old woman taking lithium became pregnant (36[c]). A prenatal check revealed *Potter's syndrome* (agenesis of the kidneys, clubfeet, deep-seated ears), a non-specified *vascular transposition*, and a non-specified *cardiac abnormality*. Pregnancy was terminated during the 22nd week.

Two reviews have dealt with the possible *teratogenic effects* of lithium treatment (37[R]), (38[R]), but none has matched the detail and balance of advice given in a review published 2 years ago (39[R]).

Records from the International Register of Lithium Babies and from a cohort of manic-depressive pregnant women have been analyzed. More than one-third of infants reported to the register were *born prematurely*, and 37% of the premature infants were *large for gestational age* (40[C]).

Electroconvulsive shock In yet another case-control study of 31 patients treated with lithium and electroconvulsive shock and 135 sex- and age-matched controls, the combination of lithium with electroconvulsive shock was not associated with increased frequency of adverse effects (41[C]). This is in accordance with most previous findings.

Overdosage and intoxication Delayed and secondary peak lithium concentrations have been reported in a 42-year-old man following an overdose with an unidentified modified-release formulation (42[c]).

A 34-year-old man took an overdose of lithium (serum lithium concentration 11.5 mmol/l) and developed shock and hypoxemia resistant to vasoactive drugs. Despite hemodialysis he died 72 h after admission to hospital (43[c]).

The pharmacokinetics of lithium have been shown to differ in acutely intoxicated patients ($n = 4$) and chronically intoxicated patient ($n = 10$), the latter having longer terminal plasma half-lives (36—79 vs. 19—29 h) and lower rates of renal clearance (0.16 vs. 0.38 ml/min/kg) than the former (44[C]).

Two opposing procedures in the treatment of lithium intoxication are currently under debate. Whereas traditionally one seeks to remove lithium from the body as quickly and effectively as possible, during the last 3 years it has been claimed that procedures that increase the rate of removal do more harm to the brain than a more gradual lowering of the lithium concentration (45[C]), (46[C]); both single cases and series of patients have been presented to support this view (47[C]), (48[C]). In last year's review (SEDA-19, p. 18) and elsewhere (49[r]) I have drawn attention to this non-traditional view and have suggested the following alternative interpretation: since in cases of lithium intoxication the choice of dialysis or conservative procedures has not been made randomly, hemodialysis may have been used in sicker patients with a poor prognosis, and conservative treatment in less ill patients with a better prognosis. It is to be hoped that this debate will instigate a systematic inquiry into this important and controversial matter.

To achieve the rapid removal of lithium aimed for according to the traditional procedure, intermittent hemodialysis is usually the preferred method (50[R]). A hemodialysis prediction scheme based on pharmacokinetic analysis has been proposed (51). Continuous arteriovenous and venovenous hemodiafiltration seem to offer advantages, because rebound of the serum lithium concentration is avoided; in a series of seven patients treated with these methods lithium clearances were 60—85 l/day (52[C]).

Interactions   Drug interactions with lithium have been extensively reviewed (53[R]).

Neuroleptic drugs Prolonged neurological sequelae, primarily dysarthria and ataxia, developed in a patient taking a combination of lithium and neuroleptic drugs (*haloperidol* and *chlorpromazine*); the serum lithium concentration was not determined (54[c]). Long-lasting cerebellar sequelae after lithium intoxication have been reviewed, and it has been suggested that lithium, cytokines, and neuroleptic drugs may synergize to disrupt calcium homeostasis and elicit calcium-mediated neurotoxicity (55[R]).

Amiodarone Two patients developed sudden hypothyroidism within 2—3 weeks of concomitant administration of lithium and the anti-anginal agent amiodarone, 400 mg/day in both cases (56[C]). In no case had there been evidence of thyroid dysfunction before the combined administration of lithium and amiodarone. The authors suggested that amiodarone had precipitated subclinical lithium-induced hypothyroidism.

Angiotensin-converting enzyme inhibitors The potential interaction between lithium and the angiotensin-converting enzyme inhibitors cap-topril, enalapril, and lisinopril (dosages not stated) has been investigated in a retrospective study of 20 hypertensive patients previously stabilized on lithium (57[C]). During treatment with the combination, steady-state serum lithium concentrations increased by 36% and lithium clearance fell by 26%. Four patients had symptoms of lithium toxicity. ACE inhibitors facilitate the reabsorption of sodium and water in the proximal renal tubule and this may cause retention of lithium.

Antidepressants The neuroleptic malignant syndrome developed in a 61-year-old man treated with a combination of lithium carbonate 900 mg/day and *amitriptyline* 75 mg/day (58[C]). Intestinal pseudo-obstruction was a prominent feature in this patient.

In a review of the combined use of lithium and *selective serotonin reuptake inhibitors* (SSRIs) it was concluded that "despite reports of some single case studies of severe adverse events, the combination of SSRIs and lithium must generally be considered an effective and safe procedure" (59[R]). The same conclusion was reached in two studies in patients (60[C]), (61[C]). A patient developed long-lasting cerebellar symptoms after heat stroke during concomitant treatment with lithium and fluoxetine; however, the serum lithium concentration was not determined (62[c]). A study in healthy subjects showed that the reported occurrence of neurotoxic symptoms after lithium augmentation of unsuccessful treatment with *fluoxetine* is not due to a pharmacokinetic interaction resulting in modified lithium kinetics (63[C]).

In a study of the effects of the serotonin and noradrenaline reuptake inhibitor venlafaxine (50 mg 8-hourly for 7 days) on the pharmacokinetics of a single dose of lithium carbonate (600 mg) and of a single dose of lithium on the disposition of venlafaxine, there was no clinically significant pharmacokinetic interaction (64[C]).

Carbamazepine A 53-year-old woman developed tiredness, tremors, stumbling, unsteadiness, and slumping in her chair 2 weeks after carbamazepine (serum concentration 3.3 mg/l) had been added to lithium (serum concentration 0.72 mmol/l); the symptoms disappeared after withdrawal of carbamazepine (65[C]).

Clozapine A 46-year-old African-American man developed diabetic ketoacidosis during treatment with lithium (0.8 mmol/l) and clozapine 500 mg/day (66[c]). This case bears a close resemblance to one reported 2 years ago, also dealing with an African-American patient (67[c]). Another patient, a 34-year-old man, did well while lithium (0.8 mmol/l) and clozapine 300 mg/day were given in combination, but developed an organic brain syndrome with initial illusory misperceptions and a confusional state, and lapsed into pre-coma 3 days after clozapine therapy had been tapered off (and 7 days after the start of concomitant haloperidol treatment, 15 mg/day) (68[c]).

Olanzapine There was no pharmacokinetic in-teraction between lithium (in a single dose of 32.4 mmol) and the 5HT$_2$ receptor antagonist olanzapine (10 mg/day for 8 days) in healthy volunteers (69[C]).

Sodium valproate Lithium carbonate (300 mg/day) and sodium valproate (1500 mg/day) were co-administered for 12 days to 16 healthy volunteers without any significant increase in adverse effects over valproate alone (70[C]).

A case of suspected dietary interference with lithium treatment seems dubious. In a 56-year-old woman who used to have serum lithium concentrations of 0.5—0.6 mmol/l there was a fall from this concentration to values of 0.1 mmol/l after she drank an "effervescent and digestive dinner water", which contained sodium bicarbonate plus malic and tartaric acids. No attempt was made to test whether this combination increases the renal clearance of lithium (71[c]).

REFERENCES

1.   Reischer H, Pfeffer CR. Lithium pharmacokinetics. J Am Acad Child Adolesc Psychiatry 1996;35:130—1.
2.   Lumley F. Lithium carbonate-gluten intolerance. Aust NZ J Psychiatry 1995;29:520—1.
3.   Lal LS, Anassi EO. Misadventure. Pharmacist 1995;20:H8—10.
4.   Jensen HV, Davidsen K, Toftegaard L, Mellerup ET, Plenge P, Aggernæs H, Bjørum N. Double-blind comparison of the side-effect profiles of daily versus alternate-day dosing schedules in lithium maintenance treatment of manic-depressive disorder. J Affect Disord 1996;36:89—93.
5.   Jensen HV, Plenge P, Stensgaard A, Mellerup ET, Thomsen C, Aggernæs H, Henriksen O. Twelve-hour brain lithium concentration in lithium maintenance treatment of manic-depressive disorder: daily versus alternate-day dosing schedule. Psychopharmacology 1996;124:275—8.
6.   Joseph M, Vieweg V. Electrocardiographic changes of sinus bradycardia and sinus node dysfunction among patients with therapeutic levels of lithium. Depression 1995;2:226—31.
7.   Terao T, Abe H, Abe K. Irreversible sinus node dysfunction induced by resumption of lithium therapy. Acta Psychiatr Scand 1996;93:407—8.
8.   Ghadirian AM, Annable L, Bélanger MC, Chouinard G. A cross-sectional study of parkinsonism and tardive dyskinesia in lithium-treated affective disordered patients. J Clin Psychiatry 1996;57:22—8.
9.   Poyurovsky M, Kreinin A, Modai I, Weizman A. Lithium-induced akathisia responds to low-dose mianserin: case report. Int Clin Psychopharmacol 1995;10:261—3.
10.   Crapanzano KA, Casanova MF, Mannheim G. Association between lithium, gender, abnormal EEG's, dementia, and increased CSF protein. Neurol Psychiatry Brain Res 1995;3:17—20.
11.   Kato T, Fujii K, Shiori T, Inubushi T, Takahashi S. Lithium side effects in relation to brain lithium concentration measured with lithium^7 magnetic resonance spectroscopy. Prog Neuro-Psychopharmacol Biol Psychiatry 1996;20:87—97.
12.   Prohaska ML, Stern RA, Steketee MC, Prange AJ. Lithium-thyroid interactive hypothesis of neuropsychological deficits: a review and proposal. Depression 1995;2:241—51.
13.   Prohaska ML, Stern RA, Nevels CT, Mason GA Prange AJ. The relationship between thyroid status and neuropsychological performance in psychiatric outpatients maintained on lithium. Neuropsychiatry Neuropsychol Behav Neurol 1996; 9:30—4.
14.   Bocchetta A, Cherchi A, Loviselli A, Mossa P, Velluzzi F, Derai R, Del Zompo M. Six-year follow-up of thyroid function during lithium treatment. Acta Psychiatr Scand 1996;94:45—8.
15.   Becerra-Fernández A. Autoimmune thyrotoxicosis during lithium therapy in a patient with manic-depressive illness. Am J Med 1995;99:575.
16.   Mizukami Y, Michigishi T, Nonomura A, Nakamura S, Noguchi M, Takazakura E. Histological features of the thyroid gland in a patient with lithium induced thyrotoxicosis. J Clin Pathol 1995;48:582—4.

17. Weber E, Coche E. Hyperthyroïdie après arrêt du lithium: coïncidence ou non? Rev Méd Interne 1995;16:437—9.

18. Posner L, Mokrzycki MH. Transient central diabetes insipidus in the setting of underlying chronic nephrogenic diabetes insipidus associated with lithium use. Am J Nephrol 1996;16:339—43.

19. Holt RA, Maunder EMW. Is lithium-induced weight gain prevented by providing healthy eating advice at the commencement of lithium therapy? J Hum Nutr Diet 1996;9:127—33.

20. Komatsu M, Shimizu H, Tsuruta T, Kato M, Fushimi T, Inoue K, Kobayashi S, Kuroda T. Effect of lithium on serum calcium level and parathyroid function in manic-depressive patients. Endocr J 1995;42:691—5.

21. Bendz H, Sjödin I, Aurell M. Renal function on and off lithium in patients treated with lithium for 15 years or more: a controlled, prospective lithium-withdrawal study. Nephrol Dial Transplant 1996;11:457—60.

22. Jensen HV, Holm J, Davidsen K, Toftegaard L, Aggernæs H, Bjørum N. Urinary excretion of albumin and transferrin in lithium maintenance treatment: daily versus alternate-day lithium dosing schedule. Psychopharmacology 1995;122:317—20.

23. Tam VKK, Green J, Schwieger J, Cohen AH. Nephrotic syndrome and renal insufficiency associated with lithium therapy. Am J Kidney Dis 1996;27:715—20.

24. Burke C, Fulda GJ, Castellano J. Lithium-induced nephrogenic diabetes insipidus treated with intravenous ketorolac. Crit Care Med 1995;23:1924—7.

25. Menni S, Barbareschi M, Fargetti G, Hendrickx I. Éruptions lichénoïdes de la muqueuse buccale induites par le carbonate de lithium. Ann Dermatol Venéréol 1995;122:91—3.

26. Paduart O, Heenen M. Pharmacological action of lithium in the pathogenesis of psoriasis. Eur J Dermatol 1995;5:413—15.

27. Ockenfels HM, Wagner SN, Keim-Maas C, Funk R, Nussbaum G, Goos M. Lithium and psoriasis: cytokine modulation of cultured lymphocytes and psoriatic keratinocytes by lithium. Arch Dermatol Res 1996;288:173—8.

28. Kristensen E, Jørgensen P. Sexual function in lithium-treated manic-depressive patients. Pharmacopsychiatry 1987;20:165—7.

29. Livianos L, Luengo MA, Rodrigo G. Impotencia coeundi induced by lithium salts. Eur Psychiatry 1995;10:266—7.

30. Schou M. Lithium treatment of manic-depressive illness: a practical guide. 5th rev. ed. Basel, Freiburg, Paris, London, New York, New Delhi, Singapore, Tokyo, Sydney: Karger, 1993.

31. Anonymous. Dåligt känd litiumbiverkning vid operation orsakade kvinnas död. Läkartidningen 1995;92:3924.

32. Schou M. Kirurgi, anæstesi og litiumbehandling. Ugeskr Læg 1996;158:435.

33. Hagino OR, Weller EB, Weller RA, Washing D, Fristad MA, Kontras SB. Untoward effects of lithium treatment in children aged four through six years. Am Acad Child Adolesc Psychiatry 1995;34:1584—90.

34. Flaherty B, Dean BS, Krenzelok EP. Neonatal lithium toxicity as a result of maternal toxicity. J Toxicol Clin Toxicol 1995;33:555.

35. Nishiwaki T, Tanaka K, Sekiya S. Acute lithium intoxication in pregnancy. Int J Gynecol Obstet 1996;52:191—2.

36. Eikmeier G. Potter-syndrome under lithium-treatment. Pharmacopsychiatry 1995;28:174.

37. Léonard A, Hantson P, Gerber GB. Mutagenicity, carcinogenicity and teratogenicity of lithium compounds. Mutat Res 1995;339:131—7.

38. Altschuler LL, Cohen L, Szuba MP, Burt VK, Gitlin M, Mintz J. Pharmacologic management of psychiatric illness during pregnancy: dilemmas and guidelines. Am J Psychiatry 1996;153:592—606.

39. Cohen LS, Friedman JM, Jefferson JW, Johnson EM, Weiner ML. A reevaluation of risk of in utero exposure to lithium. J Am Med Assoc 1993;271:146—50.

40. Troyer WA, Pereira GR, Lannon RA, Belik J, Yoder MC. Association of maternal lithium exposure and premature delivery. J Perinatol 1993;13:123—7.

41. Jha AK, Stein GS, Fenwick P. Negative interaction between lithium and electroconvulsive therapy: a case-control study. Br J Psychiatry 1996;168:241—3.

42. Dupuis RE, Cooper AA, Rosamond LL, Campbell-Bright S. Multiple delayed peak lithium concentrations following acute intoxication with an extended-release product. Ann Pharmacol 1996;30:356—60.

43. Camacho Pulido JA, Rucabado Aguilar L, Estecha Foncea MA, Quesada Blanca JL, Jurado Lara B, Jiménez Sánchez JM. Shock e hipoxemia severa en intoxicación por litio. Farm Clin 1995;12:509—10.

44. Ferron G, Debray M, Buneaux F, Baud FJ, Scherrmann JM. Pharmacokinetics of lithium in plasma and red blood cells in acute and chronic intoxicated patients. Int J Clin Pharmacol Ther 1995;33:351—5.

45. Swartz CM, Jones P. Hyperlithemia correction and persistent delirium. J Clin Pharmacol 1994;34:865—70.

46. Swartz CM, Jones CM. Hyperlithemia correction: an untraditional view. Reply to Schou. J Clin Psychiatry 1996;57:42—3.

47. Swartz CM, Dolinar LJ. Encephalopathy associated with rapid decrease of high levels of lithium. Ann Clin Psychiatry 1995;7:207—9.

48. Swartz CM. Lithium levels in brain and serum. J Clin Psychopharmacol 1995;15:375.

49. Schou M. Hyperlithemia correction: an untraditional view. J Clin Psychiatry 1996;57:42.

50. Voiculescu A, Hefter H, Falck M, Kutkuhn B, Grabensee B. Therapie der schweren Lithium-

intoxikation mittels Hämodialyse. Intensivmedizin 1995;32:433—7.

51. LeGatt DF, Mock T. Lithium overdose: prediction of hemodialysis treatment using a pharmacokinetic model. Ther Drug Monit 1995;17:426.

52. Leblanc M, Raymond M, Bonnardeaux A, Isenring P, Pichette V, Geadah D, Quimet D, Ethier J, Cardinal J. Lithium poisoning treated by high—performance continuous arteriovenous and venovenous hemodiafiltration. Am J Kidney Dis 1996;27:365—2.

53. Finley PR, Warner MD, Peabody CA. Clinical relevance of drug interactions with lithium. Clin Pharmacokin 1995;29:172—91.

54. Mani J, Tandel SV, Shah PU, Karnad DR. Prolonged neurological sequelae after combination treatment with lithium and antipsychotic drugs. J Neurol Neurosurg Psychiatry 1996;60:350—1.

55. Grignon S, Bruguerolle B. Cerebellar lithium toxicity: a review of recent literature and tentative pathophysiology. Thérapie 1996;51:101—6.

56. Ahmad S. Sudden hypothyroidism and amidarone-lithium combination: an interaction. Cardiovasc Drugs Ther 1995;9:827—8.

57. Finley PR, O'Brien JG, Coleman RW. Lithium and angiotensin-converting enzyme inhibitors: evaluation of a potential interaction. J Clin Psychopharmacol 1996;16:68—71.

58. Fava S, Galizia AC. Neuroleptic malignant syndrome and lithium carbonate. J Psychiatry Neurosci 1995;20:305—6.

59. Bauer M. The combined use of lithium and SSRIs. J Serotonin Res 1995;2:69—76.

60. Bhaumik S, Collacott RA, Gandhi D, Duggirala C, Wildgust HJ. A naturalistic study in the use of antidepressants in adults with learning disabilities and affective disorders. Hum Psychopharmacol 1995;10:283—8.

61. Bauer M, Linden M, Schaaf B, Weber HJ. Adverse events and tolerability of the combination of fluoxetine/lithium compared with fluoxetine. J Clin Psychopharmacol 1996;16:130—4.

62. Albukrek D, Moran DS, Epstein Y. A depressed workman with heatstroke. Lancet 1996;347:1016.

63. Breuel HP, Müller-Oerlinghausen B, Nickelsen T, Heine PR. Pharmacokinetic interactions between lithium and fluoxetine after single and repeated fluoxetine administration in young healthy volunteers. Int J Clin Pharmacol Ther 1995;33:415—19.

64. Troy SM, Parker VD, Hicks DR, Boudino FD, Chiang ST. Pharmacokinetic interaction between multiple-dose venlafaxine and single-dose lithium. J Clin Pharmacol 1996;36:175—81.

65. Marcoux AW. Carbamazepine-lithium drug interaction. Ann Pharmacother 1996;30:547.

66. Peterson GA, Byrd SL. Diabetic ketoacidosis from clozapine and lithium cotreatment. Am J Psychiatry 1996;153:737—8.

67. Koval MS, Rames LJ, Christie S. Diabetic ketoacidosis associated with clozapine treatment. Am J Psychiatry 1994;151:1520—1.

68. Hellwig B, Hesslinger B, Walden J. Acute brain syndrome after tapering off clozapine in clozapine-lithium combination. Prog Neuro-Psychopharmacol Biol Psychiatry 1996;20:179—83.

69. Müller-Oerlinghausen B, Demolle D, Onkelinx C. Pharmacokinetic interaction between olanzapine and lithium in healthy male volunteers. Pharmacopsychiatry 1995;28:201.

70. Granneman GR, Schneck DW, Cavanaugh JH, Witt GF. Pharmacokinetic interactions and side effects resulting from concomitant administration of lithium and divalproex sodium. J Clin Psychiatry 1996;57:204—6.

71. Castrogiovanni P, Pieraccini F. Dietary interferences with lithium therapy. Eur Psychiatry 1996;11:53—4.

Jayendra K. Patel, Eileen Wong and Alan I. Green

4

Drugs of abuse

AMPHETAMINES *(SED-13, 16; SEDA-17, 35; SEDA-18, 35; SEDA-19, 24)*

Although amphetamine and its derivatives have clear medical indications (for example, attention deficit disorder with hyperactivity, narcolepsy, and obesity), reports on the adverse effects associated with abuse of this drug group continue to appear.

Ecstasy, or 3,4-methylenedioxymethamphetamine (MDMA), is a synthetic amphetamine analog originally developed as an appetite suppressant. The use of ecstasy at 'raves' (dancing parties) in the UK, and its association with serious outcomes such as *seizures, hyperthermic reactions, hepatic dysfunction, acute renal failure*, and even *death*, has been discussed in previous Annuals. The acute renal failure reported after the use of Ecstasy usually involves rhabdomyolysis and disseminated intravascular coagulation as the underlying causes. However, a new report has described the development of acute renal failure secondary to severe *hypertension* after the use of Ecstasy (1[c]).

A 37-year-old man was seen 2 days after having used ecstasy at a rave. He was unconscious secondary to hypertensive encephalopathy (blood pressure of 220/140 mmHg), had microangiopathic hemolytic anemia, and suffered rapid-onset acute renal failure. Under medical management, he regained consciousness as his blood pressure stabilized. His renal function, however, deteriorated over the next 7 days and he required intermittent hemodialysis. Renal biopsy showed evidence of accelerated hypertension. Four months after his initial presentation, the patient remained dialysis-dependent.

The authors reviewed how a transient rise in blood pressure and tachycardia is common after ingestion of Ecstasy, peaking at 1 h, the most likely mechanism being an amphetamine-like sympathomimetic effect. In this patient, there were neither fundoscopic nor electrocardiographic changes suggestive of chronic hypertension. The authors proposed that the persistent severe hypertension may have been due to renal or vascular changes secondary to accelerated hypertension following the use of Ecstasy.

In the older literature, few urological complications (with the exception of *urgency*) have been described secondary to Ecstasy (2[c]). Over the past year, however, a case has been described of a 19-year-old man who developed *acute retention of urine* 12 h after taking 15 ecstasy tablets (3[c]). He had a 1-year history of using Ecstasy, taking one to two tablets once or twice a week. The examination was unremarkable except for a painful palpable bladder. Therapy included catheterization over 36 h; there were no sequelae. The authors suggested that methamphetamine, a potent α-adrenoceptor agonist, can stimulate α-adrenergic fibers supplying the trigone and the bladder neck, and produce bladder neck dysfunction or closure, leading to acute urinary retention.

The smokable form of methamphetamine known as 'ice' or 'crystal', the free-based form of the drug, increased in popularity in the late 1980s (4[r]). When smoked, 'ice' is rapidly absorbed from the lungs, resulting in immediate clinical effects similar to those of intravenous drugs. Users report that the 'high' occurs in about 30 min. The average 'hit' is one-tenth of a gram, with effects lasting up to 15 h. Animal studies suggest that methamphetamine may be more toxic than amphetamine (5[R]). The clinical effects of 'ice' are similar to other stimulants and include psychiatric, cardiovascular, metabolic, and neuromuscular changes.

COCAINE *(SED-13, 14; SEDA-17, 35; SEDA-18, 36; SEDA-19, 26)*

There has been considerable interest in

Side Effects of Drugs, Annual 20
J.K. Aronson, ed.

evaluating drugs such as diethylpropion for attenuating the negative emotional state induced by craving for cocaine, in the hope of finding a drug for long-term treatment of cocaine dependence (6[C]). However, a study of 50 cocaine-dependent patients has shown a lack of therapeutic efficacy and significant adverse effects. Of the patients who took 25—75 mg/day of diethylpropion, 12% were withdrawn from the study: one developed coronary vasospasm and a second atrial fibrillation. These poor results are comparable to those of an earlier study with methylphenidate in cocaine addicts (7[C]). Thus an effective pharmacological intervention for treating cocaine dependence has yet to emerge.

Deaths that occurred from acute reactions to opiates/cocaine have been evaluated in six of the seven largest cities in Spain during the years 1983—1991 (8[C]). The number of deaths increased greatly between 1983 and 1991 and affected both sexes, but the relative increase in mortality was smaller for women (5.6 times) than men (7.3 times). Mortality increased in all age groups, but the largest relative increases were among those aged 30—34 and 40—44. Most of those who died were male (6:2 ratio of men to women).

Cardiovascular Several recent studies have provided valuable information on the cardiac adverse effects of cocaine. In a study of 51 patients with *chest pain* who had used both cocaine and tobacco within 12 h before presentation, the time of onset of the chest pain following cocaine was shorter in patients who used tobacco close to the time of the cocaine use (9[C]). The authors speculated that this may suggest a combined vasoconstrictor effect of both drugs. In a second study, a prospective multicenter investigation of 359 patients with chest pain, 60 (17%) patients had cocaine or its metabolites in the urine (10[C]). The cocaine-using patients were younger than the others. The authors suggested that cocaine may significantly increase the risk of chest pain in the young, and so recent use of cocaine is an important question to be asked of young patients with chest pain.

In another multicenter prospective study by the same author, 203 patients with cocaine-associated chest pain (when compared with other patients with chest pain) were not at a higher risk of cocaine-related myocardial infarction or death over the ensuing year, even though the majority of them continued to use cocaine after discharge (11[C]). Recurrent chest pain occurred in 74 of the 136 cocaine users during follow-up. Six patients died during the follow-up, but five of the six died of non-cardiac events that had been known at the time of index evaluation. The sixth patient had cardiomyopathy secondary to alcoholism.

A 34-year-old woman presented with 16 h of non-radiating substernal chest pain after a 1-day binge of smoking crack and snorting cocaine (12[c]). The pain, which started 2 h after the last dose of cocaine, was followed by sweating and nausea. Her physical and neurological examinations were non-focal, but she had a reduced level of consciousness, continuously falling asleep in the middle of the interview. Her electrocardiogram showed sinus tachycardia. She fell asleep on a hospital trolley for a few hours. When aroused, she complained of chest pain (resolved by glyceryl trinitrate ointment) that was puzzling, as she appeared very comfortable. Her cardiac enzymes were increased. She subsequently developed Q waves and inverted T waves. Echocardiography showed a dyskinetic posterior wall extending inferolaterally.

The authors speculated that the patient slept through her infarct, probably because of depletion of central dopamine, noradrenaline, and serotonin, a phenomenon also known as 'cocaine washed-out syndrome.'

Further adverse events due to the use of cocaine as a local anesthetic when combined with a sympathomimetic agent have been reported. This combination is often used by otorhinolaryngologists for operations on the nose.

A 23-year-old woman had a successful elective nasal septoplasty using 4% cocaine hydrochloride solution as a local anesthetic (13[c]). Phenylephrine 0.25% packing was placed in the nose before extubation to control bleeding and further nasal congestion; 15 min later, she developed a cardiac arrest after an acute increase in blood pressure and heart rate. She went from sinus tachycardia to ventricular bigeminy to ventricular tachycardia and fibrillation. She had a non-Q-wave myocardial infarction and a stunned myocardium that reversed in 2 weeks.

Three more cases of cardiac complications from using similar drug combinations have also been reported (12[c]).

A 9-year-old girl was given oral atropine, thiopentone anesthesia, and suxamethonium. Soon after a cocaine and epinephrine paste was put in her nose, she had ventricular fibrillation that reverted to normal with two precordial thumps. A 10-year-old boy was given the same anesthesia along with papaveretum. A paste of cocaine and epinephrine was placed in his nose and within 30 s ventricular fibrillation occurred. Sinus rhythm was regained with a direct current of 100 J. A 30-year-old woman was given temazepam, and anesthesia was induced with thiopentone and fentanyl. Intubation was facilitated using atracurium. A cocaine and epinephrine paste was placed in her nose 25 min after induction, and within seconds she developed tachycardia, multifocal ventricular extra beats, sustained hypertension, and ST segment depression. She responded to lidocaine and labetalol.

The authors cautioned against the use of cocaine and epinephrine paste for non-life-threatening surgery. However, this report generated criticism from others regarding the authors' inference and caution (14)—(17). Although the others agreed that the combination should be used cautiously, they suggested that the authors of the initial report had used higher than recommended doses of cocaine and poor techniques and had not followed standard procedures.

Respiratory system Reported pulmonary complications of crack cocaine range from acute symptoms (*coughing, chest pain, and palpitation*) to acute syndromes (*end-stage lung disease, eosinophilic infiltrates of the lung, and pulmonary infarction*). The single-breath diffusing capacity for carbon monoxide after the use of crack cocaine was reduced in three of six reports (18[R]). If confirmed, a *reduced CO-diffusing capacity* after crack use may signify damage to the alveolar capillary membrane or the pulmonary vasculature. It has been suggested that a well-designed controlled study to investigate the true impact of crack on the lung is necessary, since several confounding factors may account for the discrepancy in results (19[r]).

Dyspnea and *cough* have been reported after heavy crack cocaine smoking (20[c]).

A 28-year-old woman presented with dyspnea and cough. Sequential ventilation/perfusion scans suggested chronic airway disease or resolving pulmonary emboli. She recovered with anticoagulant therapy and bronchodilators. Two weeks later, she was readmitted with respiratory symptoms after having smoked cocaine 3—4 h earlier. She reported being compliant with anticoagulant therapy. A repeat ventilation/perfusion lung scan again showed diffuse air trapping with multiple segmental and subsegmental perfusion defects in a new distribution from the previous scans, suggesting recurrent pulmonary emboli, despite anticoagulant therapy. However, a pulmonary angiogram showed no evidence of pulmonary embolism and anticoagulant therapy was stopped. She recovered gradually over 3 days.

Apparently, the perfusion abnormalities occurred within hours of smoking cocaine and resolved within days. This provides the first in vivo evidence for pulmonary vasoconstriction or vasospasm secondary to cocaine as a pathogenic mechanism of these abnormalities.

Nervous system Many new cases of cocaine-associated *stroke* have been reported. The mechanism underlying these strokes, though not clear, is undoubtedly multifactorial, as discussed in SEDA-19 (p. 26). In three cases large-vessel vasospasm and clot formation may have occurred (21[c]).

In the first case, a 35-year-old woman had an abrupt onset of a left frontal supraorbital sharp piercing headache an hour after smoking crack. On arrival at the hospital she had a left lower facial weakness, dysarthria, and left hemiparesis. Cerebral angiography showed a large filling defect in the proximal right internal carotid artery. White fibrin clot obstructing the carotid artery was removed. However, echocardiography showed no thrombus, valve, or wall-motion abnormalities and the clot showed neither calcification nor micro-organisms. Her neurological function improved dramatically after surgery. In the second case, a 32-year-old woman, with a history of a convulsion several months earlier, was brought to the emergency room from a crack house, because she developed lethargy, dysarthria, and right-sided weakness. She was mute, had a systolic murmur, a right upper motor neurone facial weakness, and marked right hemiparesis. Her head CT scan showed a non-enhancing hypodensity in the left frontal and temporal lobes anteriorly with a left to right midline shift. She lapsed into coma and died 72 h after admission. On autopsy, she had a recent infarct in the distribution of the left anterior and middle cerebral arteries. The histopathological examination showed cerebral vessels with abnormal internal elastic lamina infolding and tunica media degeneration. The third case involved a 45-year-old man who developed left-sided weakness, throbbing bitemporal headache, nausea, vomiting, dysphagia, slurred speech, and urinary incontinence after drinking approximately a fifth of a gallon of vodka, 4 days after smoking 20 rocks of crack cocaine. He had marked left hemiparesis, secondary to a thrombus in the right carotid artery, with associated middle cerebral artery occlusion. Echocardiography also showed global left ventricular hypokinesis. Transesophageal echocardiography did not show thrombus.

The authors of this article suggested that some brain infarcts occurring in crack cocaine users may result from vasospasm of large arteries and secondary intravascular thrombus.

Two cases of intracerebral hemorrhage associated with cocaine use, with biopsy-proven cerebral vasculitis, have been reported (22[c]).

A 32-year-old right-handed man with a history of untreated hypertension presented with a right temporal headache and left-sided hemiparesis after using cocaine. His head CT scan initially showed a right putaminal hemorrhage with mass effect and a midline shift to the left; an echocardiogram showed left ventricular hypertrophy. An angiogram showed no evidence of an aneurysm, shunting, or vasculitis. A subsequent repeat CT scan showed extension of the hemorrhage into the right lateral ventricle. He underwent a craniotomy with evacuation of the hematoma, and the pathology report revealed a non-necrotizing leukocytoclastic angiitis. He recovered subsequently with residual neurological deficits. Another 20-year-old right-handed man presented with 2 days of headache, agitation, and speech difficulty. Although he had a normal CT scan, 48 h later he was acutely disoriented and dysphasic. A repeat CT scan showed a left temporoparietal hemorrhage. He had a history of daily marijuana and alcohol abuse, and had used cocaine within at least 6 months before admission. He had a fluent aphasia, a right hemianopia, and a positive Babinski response bilaterally. He underwent a left parietal craniotomy with evacuation of an intracerebral hematoma; in this case the pathology report noted small vessel vasculitis. His symptoms progressively improved.

The authors acknowledged that causes other than cocaine should be considered in the differential diagnosis.

An unusual case of cocaine-induced *cerebral vasculitis* has been reported, the diagnosis of which was suggested by magnetic resonance angiography (MRA) (23[c]).

A 42-year-old woman presented with a diffuse headache, persistent fever, lethargy, and meningism. Although a lumber puncture suggested bacterial infection, all CSF cultures were negative, and a trial of antibiotics was ineffective. An MRI scan showed a subacute infarct of the right caudate nucleus, and MRA showed that the anterior, middle and posterior cerebral arteries were diffusely irregular, with a beaded proximal segment of the right

middle cerebral artery. She became comatose and died.

The authors noted that cocaine-induced vasculitis can mimic bacterial meningitis.

A case of benign cocaine-induced *cerebral angiopathy* has been reported (24[c]).

A 44-year-old man, known to be a chronic cocaine user, whose last use had been 3 days before symptoms began, presented with a 2-day history of dysarthria, left-sided homonymous hemianopia, right-sided facial numbness, and weakness of the right arm and leg. He had high blood pressure with hypertensive retinopathy. An MRI showed lesions in the deep white matter (pons and right temporal lobe), consistent with vascular pathology or demyelination, and cerebral angiography showed multifocal areas of segmental stenosis and dilatation thought to represent vasculitis. Since a trial of steroids was not helpful, he underwent biopsy of the temporal lobe and leptomeninges that showed normal brain parenchyma. Further studies showed no vasculitis or indication of prior vascular injury. Without continued cocaine use, he slowly and steadily improved.

The authors concluded that this patient's condition was benign and thus did not warrant aggressive treatment.

Among other reports of neurological adverse effects, a case of cocaine-induced *chronic tics* has been reported (25[c]).

A 35-year-old woman had been using crack for 3 years while intermittently bingeing on alcohol. Her tic symptoms included flaring of her nostrils, arm jerks, grimaces, shoulder shrugging, grunting, and head jerks. The tics were complex with co-ordinated abnormal movements involving her entire body, including eye deviation, rolling facial contortions, and plaintive vocal sounds.

The authors suggested that this movement disorder was probably related to cocaine's effect on the dopaminergic system.

Hematological　At a prenatal clinic, 709 inner city women (who had at least one platelet count) were screened for cocaine-associated thrombocytopenia; 331 (47%) were considered not to be substance users (26[C]). One hundred and fifteen (16%) women reported or tested positive for cocaine use, 11 of whom reported also using heroin; 2.5% were positive for opiates and 33% used other drugs. Nineteen (2.6%) had *thrombocytopenia*; two of these cases were excluded because of a known underlying medical condition. The rate of thrombocytopenia in the non-drug-abusing group was 1.5%, whereas the rate in the cocaine group was 6.7%. Even after adjustments for HIV status, the cocaine-using group had a significantly higher rate of thrombocytopenia than the non-substance-using pregnant women. Thus, the authors concluded that cocaine use may be an independent risk factor for thrombocytopenia in an inner-city parturient population.

Gastrointestinal   Five cases of gastric perforation after cocaine use have previously been reported (SEDA-17, 37). In a retrospective review of 63 patients with *bowel perforation*, three of the cases appeared to be related to cocaine use (27[c]).

In the first case, a 31-year-old woman, with a 2-week history of progressive left quadrant abdominal pain associated with urinary frequency, constipation, fever, chills, and a sensation of pressure on standing, had a single sigmoid colon perforation with surrounding abscess and an enterocutaneous fistula. In the second case, a 25-year-old man electively admitted for a repair of a left ventricular wall aneurysm developed acute severe abdominal pain associated with sweating. He had a small jejunal perforation with purulent fluid throughout the peritoneal cavity requiring segmental jejunal resection and primary anastomosis. In the third case, a 38-year-old man developed acute abdominal pain related to a small prepyloric perforation.

Special senses   Cocaine abuse has been associated with ophthalmic complications, including *ulceration of the cornea, vasoconstrictor effects on the retinal vasculature, irregularities in oculomotor performance*, and *secondary optic neuropathy*. There has been a new report of retinal changes in 60 users of freebasing 'crack' cocaine (28[c]). *Microtalc retinopathy* and *retinal nerve fiber layer 'rake' or 'slit' defects* were detected by threshold visual field testing and fundus photographs. Some of these patients had visual field changes that mimicked glaucoma. Microtalc, a sparkling white dust that is used as crack's inert adulterant, was found in minute crystalline deposits in the retinal microcirculation and the inner retinal layers. Retinal nerve fiber layer defects resulted from focal areas of death along the optic nerve with subsequent retrograde retinal

ganglion cell degeneration. In most of the 60 patients with 'rake' or 'slit' defects, there were no detectable visual field defects. It is likely that, as in early glaucoma, visual function remains generally intact following the use of crack. However, with more prolonged use, it is possible that extensive neuronal death may take place and result in visual field defects.

Infections   There has been an interesting report of a study involving 415 patients, aged 16—85 years, 55 of whom were parenteral drug abusers, evaluating *soft tissue infection* over an 18-month period (29[c]). Ninety percent of the abscesses at an injection site occurred in the 55 parenteral drug abusers, 45 of whom were HIV-positive; 89% of the 55 drug users with abscesses required surgical treatment, indicating the advanced nature of the disease in these young, often immunocompromised addicts. The authors noted that a major problem in the care of parenteral drug abusers is their poor compliance. The mean delay in presentation after first signs of an abscess was 4 days. Skin and oropharyngeal pathogens were recovered from soft tissue abscesses associated with the use of illicit drugs.

The possible association of *syphilis* and *chancroid* with crack cocaine use in the US has recently been reviewed (30[R]). The incidence of syphilis and chancroid began to increase in the US among heterosexuals in the late 1980s. Although the incidence rates of primary and secondary syphilis peaked in the US overall, specific geographic areas continue to face problems. Based on their review of the available data, the authors reported that women who used crack cocaine constitute a core transmitter group for both diseases. Although the details of the relations among crack, sexual behavior, and the size and the nature of core transmitter groups are not known, the authors suggested that crack cocaine abuse may be a driving force behind the recent syphilis and chancroid epidemics in the US. They raised a concern about the possible co-transmission of HIV along with the chancroid lesion.

Effects on pregnancy   In a retrospective, case-control study, 76 pregnant women in labor (with positive urine drug screens for cocaine) were compared with 134 women in labor (with negative drug screens) to determine maternal infectious morbidity (31[C]). Women testing positive for cocaine had a significantly shorter second stage of labor. Interestingly, 9% of the control patients had fever compared with 1.3% of the cocaine-positive women. The rate of intra-amniotic infection and endometritis was comparable in both groups. Thus, in this study, cocaine did not appear to increase the risk of peripartum infection after controlling for well-established risk factors.

℞ *Second-generation effects of cocaine*

Cocaine use by a pregnant woman may have adverse effects on the fetus.

The effects of prenatal cocaine exposure have been assessed in a prospective study of 217 infants, 95 (44%) of whom had benzoylecgonine, a cocaine metabolite in their meconium (32[C]). Among these infants, benzoylecgonine concentration was inversely related to fetal growth (birth weight, length, and head circumference), whereas maternal self report of days of cocaine use did not correlate with either fetal growth or meconium benzoylecgonine concentration. The report suggested a dose-response relation between the magnitude of prenatal cocaine exposure and impaired fetal growth.

A prospective study to assess the effect of maternal cocaine use on infant outcome has been conducted in 224 women, of whom 105 were cocaine users and 119 were control subjects (33[C]). The infants were of gestational age 34 weeks or more and non-asphyxiated. The infants exposed to cocaine were more likely to be admitted to the newborn intensive care unit, to be treated for congenital syphilis or presumed sepsis, to have a greater length of stay, to have lower birth weight and head circumference, and to be discharged to a person other than the mother. The two groups, however, were similar in the incidence of abnormal cranial and renal ultrasonographic findings and abnormal pneumocardiograms. Moreover, when controlled for cigarette use and other confounders, there were no significant differences in the groups on growth retardation factors.

In a study of 39 cocaine-exposed infants and 39 control infants 35 weeks or older, head size

was smaller and birth weight tended to be lower in the cocaine-exposed infants (34[C]). Moreover, the head circumference of the cocaine-exposed infants was significantly smaller at any given birth weight than in the control infants. The behavioral scores were significantly higher (on days 1 and 2) in the cocaine-exposed infants; the higher scores were most frequently attributed to increased jitteriness, a hyperactive Moro response, and excessive sucking. Lastly, cocaine-exposed infants had an increase in flow velocity in the anterior cerebral arteries between days 1 and 2; however, there was no increased propensity to ischemic and/or hemorrhagic cerebral injury in the infants exposed to cocaine. The blood flow changes on the second day may have reflected falling infant cocaine concentrations after birth.

The effect of prenatal cocaine exposure on information processing and developmental assessment has been studied in 108 3-month-old infants, 61 of whom had been cocaine-exposed, and 47 controls using an infant-control habituation and novelty responsiveness procedure in a developmental assessment using the Bayley Scales of Infant Development (35[C]). Infants exposed to cocaine prenatally were significantly more likely than controls to fail to start the habituation procedure, and those who did were significantly more likely than controls to react with irritability early in the procedure. Cocaine-exposed infants had a comparatively depressed performance on the motor but not the mental scales of the Bayley. This information was obtained by raters blind to the history and controlled for both perinatal and sociodemographic factors. The majority of infants in both groups reached the habituation criteria, and among those who did there were no significant differences between cocaine-exposed and non-exposed infants in habituation or in recovery to a novel stimulus. Thus, differences in reactivity to novelty but not in information processing between cocaine-exposed and non-cocaine-exposed infants suggested that the effects of prenatal cocaine exposure may be on arousal and attention regulation rather than on early cognitive processes.

Developmental correlates have been assessed in three groups of children aged 4—6 (36[C]). In one group of 18 children there had been prenatal exposure to cocaine and the mothers had continued to use crack. The second group included 28 children without prenatal exposure but whose mothers used crack after the children were born. The third (control) group consisted of 28 children whose mothers had never used cocaine. Prenatally exposed children performed significantly worse than the others in tests of receptive language and visual motor drawing. Prenatal crack exposure was associated with poor visual motor performance, even after controlling for intrauterine alcohol and marijuana exposure, age, birth weight, and duration of maternal crack use.

Cardiovascular   *In a retrospective review of all dysrhythmia consultation records of children with prenatal cocaine exposure, 18 cases were detected in 554 infants who had positive urine screens for cocaine (37^C). Thirteen neonates had a dysrhythmia beyond the period of direct cocaine exposure. Six of the children had dysrhythmias after the neonatal period. Most of the dysrhythmias were supraventricular extra beats. Overall, the rate of consultations for dysrhythmias was higher among cocaine-exposed neonates than expected. Some cocaine-exposed children had symptomatic dysrhythmias that were persistent or recurrent and required treatment to maintain cardiac output and restore normal cardiac rhythm. Children who were exposed prenatally to cocaine appeared to remain at increased risk for abnormal responses to stress manifested by symptomatic dysrhythmia beyond the period of cocaine exposure. One child, at 12 months of age, presented with status epilepticus, sustained ventricular tachycardia, and a positive urine screen for cocaine. At 22 months he returned with a cardiac arrest, history of a fall, head injury, and a positive test for cocaine in the urine. He soon died.*

There has been a recent report of a myocardial infarct in a full-term infant born to a 28-year-old woman who had used cocaine two to three times per week and 40 mg of methadone daily (38^c).

The infant's Apgar score was 9/9 after 1 and 5 min. A few hours later, however, the infant became irritable and jittery, was diagnosed as having a neonatal abstinence syndrome, and started on a weaning schedule of paregoric. At 24 h the infant became ashen, tachypneic, and hypotensive, and soon developed ventricular tachycardia. The MB fraction of

creatine kinase activity was increased. The electrocardiogram showed 3 mm ST depression, and an echocardiogram showed a dilated left atrium and ventricle, with lateral and posterior left ventricular wall dyskinesia. Urine samples from both the mother and infant were positive for cocaine metabolites. The infant responded to treatment and survived.

Respiratory   *Apnea has been reported (39^c).*

A 36-day-old girl presented to the emergency room after having multiple episodes of apnea on that day, each requiring stimulation. Some spells were associated with vomiting, eye rolling, and limpness. She had also had self-limited apneic spells at 6 and 15 days of age. The product of a full-term pregnancy complicated by polyhydramnios and delivered by cesarean section for fetal bradycardia, she had missing middle phalanges on both index fingers and syndactyly of the second and third toes bilaterally (probably related to in utero cocaine exposure). Her urine drug screen was positive for cocaine metabolites and her mother's urine was positive for cocaine and tetrahydrocannabinol. The infant recovered. The source of cocaine was apparently passive inhalation of cocaine smoke from the mother.

Gastrointestinal   *Maternal use of cocaine during pregnancy may predispose a newborn infant to necrotizing enterocolitis (SEDA-17, 38). To investigate the hypothesis that necrotizing enterocolitis occurs at a younger age in cocaine-exposed infants than in infants not exposed to cocaine, the authors retrospectively reviewed over 1200 neonatal intensive care admissions to an inner city hospital (40^C). Infants with necrotizing enterocolitis were divided into cocaine-exposed and non-exposed groups, each subdivided into two birth-weight groups, using 1500 g as the cut-off weight. Of the cocaine-exposed infants 12% (28/231) developed necrotizing enterocolitis stage II or III compared with 3% (34/1053) in the non-exposed group. 8% of cocaine-exposed and 2% of non-exposed infants had necrotizing enterocolitis by day 7 compared with 20 and 5%, respectively, by day 28 after birth. Infants weighing more than 1500 g were at risk of necrotizing enterocolitis until day 8 only, whereas infants weighing less than 1500 g had both an early and continuing risk for necrotizing enterocolitis with a biphasic pattern of onset. In general, infants exposed to prenatal cocaine had a risk of necrotizing enterocolitis 3.8 times greater than the non-exposed group. The authors suggested that this effect of cocaine may be related to its vasoconstrictor action. Interestingly, the* *cocaine-exposed group with necrotizing enterocolitis contained more small-for-gestational-age infants than any of the other groups.*

Urinary system *Second-generation adverse effects involving the renal system have previously been reported (SEDA-19, 27). There has now been a study involving the collection of urine samples (to detect infection) from 110 cocaine-exposed infants and 98 controls, whose ages ranged from birth to 40 weeks of age (mean = 5 weeks) (41^C). Fifteen (14%) infants had urinary tract infection, but only four (4%) of the control infants had infections. The reported incidence of urinary tract abnormalities in this study was significantly higher than reported in other studies: of the 89 infants given ultrasonography, 16% had abnormal evaluations. There was no association between the presence of identifiable urinary tract abnormalities and urinary tract infections. The authors suggested that urine culture screening should be done for these infants routinely. Additionally, renal ultrasonography screening also may be indicated.*

HEROIN *(SED-13, 175; SEDA-18, 40; SEDA-19, 29)*

Deaths have been reported in users of a purer form of heroin. In Glasgow, Scotland, an increase in heroin overdoses was responsible for a significant rise in drug-related deaths in 1991 (42^C). Between 1991 and 1992, drug deaths increased from 10–15 per annum to over 50. A similar increase did not occur elsewhere in Britain. The increase continued through 1993 (101 deaths) and 1994. Concomitantly, there was an absence of a proportional increase in the population of drug injectors and no increased deaths from AIDS. The authors were able to clarify that Scottish heroin users differed from their English counterparts. Most Scottish users injected heroin; they were also more diversified in what they injected. In the mid-1980s they were injecting buprenorphine, a synthetic opioid partial agonist, and temazepam, a benzodiazepine. From 1990 on, as the purity of heroin increased, the Scottish users tended to inject heroin (not buprenorphine) with the other

drugs. Many cases in 1991 and 1992 involved fatal drug overdoses of drug combinations. The most common mixtures were heroin plus one or more of temazepam, diazepam and alcohol.

Nervous system Neurological symptoms (*myoclonus, tremor, rigidity, catalepsy,* and *akathisia*) often associated with the use of neuroleptic drugs, are occasionally reported to occur with opioid exposure. A recent report of an increased risk of akathisia occurring in terminally ill patients given morphine is noteworthy (43^C). Opioids, like neuroleptic drugs, also trigger prolactin secretion, apparently secondary to an effect on the hypothalamic–hypophyseal axis. It has been postulated that opioids may act on neurotransmitter pathways (dopamine and serotonin) that are thought to be prime sites of action of the neuroleptic drugs (44^r).

Urinary system The adverse outcome of acute renal failure associated with heroin abuse has previously been described (SEDA-18, 40). Heroin-related *nephropathy* typically presents as the nephrotic syndrome, with hypertension, azotemia, reduced organ size, and anemia. Renal biopsy shows glomerular and tubular damage. Progression to end-stage renal disease may occur within months to 2–3 years. It has recently been reported that there has been a sharp fall in the incidence of heroin-associated nephropathy in New York City in recent years (45^C). Retrospective analysis spanning 1981–93 showed that there had been no new cases of end-stage renal disease during 1991–93. The authors proposed that a possible cause for the decreased frequency of end-stage renal disease due to heroin-associated nephropathy could be in increased purity of street heroin.

Immunological and hypersensitivity reactions Some of the current knowledge of heroin and its possible adverse effects on the immunological system is based on research conducted on work-place exposure to opiates. The National Institute for Occupational Safety and Health (NIOSH) Health Hazard Evaluation (HHE) investigation was done on workers in a factory that makes opiate-containing drugs. Eight non-exposed controls and

33 opiate-exposed workers were studied. Common health complaints among the workers included *dyspnea, wheezing, tiredness, headache,* and *skin reactions.* Ten were diagnosed as having new-onset adult *asthma* after beginning work. In an initial article (46[C]), the authors reported finding opiate-specific IgG antibodies, positive epicutaneous tests, and reductions in pulmonary function in the opiate-exposed workers, but not in the controls. In a subsequent NIOSH paper, the results of immunological analysis of peripheral leukocytes were presented (47[C]). Lymphocyte subpopulation absolute numbers were measured and percentages were derived. The authors reported that occupational opiate exposure may either change the number and types of circulating peripheral blood leukocytes or alter the expression of receptors on the surface of these cells. Specifically, the sensitivity of B cells to pokeweed mitogen stimulation appeared to be reduced. The authors proposed that these cellular changes in lymphocytes may be important in the as yet unclear pathogenesis of occupational opiate-induced asthma.

MARIJUANA *(SEDA-17, 35)*

Smoking marijuana, the chopped flowering tops of the plant *Cannabis sativa*, results in immediate effects of a pleasant dreamy state with impaired attention, cognition, and psychomotor performance. The controversy continues about whether products extracted from cannabis should be used for their possible therapeutic benefits and what the possible long-term adverse effects of maintenance use are (48[r]), (49[r]), (50).

The possible role of marijuana in the pathogenesis of *lung cancer* has been examined (51[C]). DNA damage was measured in pulmonary alveolar macrophages retrieved by bronchial lavage from six subjects including non-smokers and smokers of marijuana, tobacco, or cocaine, either alone or in combination. By means of the alkaline unwinding method, DNA single-strand breaks in alveolar macrophages related to superoxide anion (O^2-) production were determined. The authors discussed that alveolar macrophages recovered from the marijuana smokers (both those who were tobacco smokers and those who were not) showed a trend toward DNA damage.

Cannabis ingestion in an unsuspecting user can have some serious consequences (52[c]). The Netherlands has a liberal policy on the use of marijuana; hashish, the plant's resin, is sold in 'coffee shops.' One such shop-offering is 'space cake', prepared with butter, which is enriched with the cannabis extract tetrahydrocannabinol. The color and taste of the extract are often masked with chocolate and a coloring agent. Ingestion of 'space cake' by people who seldom use or have never used cannabis before can result in mental status changes including *confusion, anxiety, loss of logical thinking, fits of laughter, hallucinations, hypertension,* and/or *paranoid psychosis,* which can last as long as 8 h.

REFERENCES

1. Woodrow G, Harnden P, Turney J. Acute renal failure due to accelerated hypertension following ingestion of 3,4-methylenedioxymethamphetamine ('ecstasy'). Nephrol Dial Transplant 1995;10:399—400.

2. Worsey J, Goble N, Stott M, Smith J. Bladder outflow obstruction secondary to intravenous amphetamine abuse. Br J Urol 1989;64:320.

3. Bryden A, Rothwell P, O'Reilly P. Urinary retention with misuse of 'ecstasy.' Br Med J 1995;310:504.

4. Beebe D, Walley E. Smokable methamphetamine ('ice'): an old drug in a different form. Am Fam Phys 1995;2:449—53.

5. Derlet R, Heischober B. Methamphetamine: stimulant of the 1990's? West J Med 1990; 153:625—8.

6. Alim TN, Rosse RB, Vocci Jr. FJ, Linquist L, Deutsch SI. Diethylpropion pharmacotherapeutic adjuvant therapy for inpatient treatment of cocaine dependence: a test for cocaine agonist hypothesis. Clin Neuropharmacol 1995;18:183—95.

7. Gawin F, Riordan C, Kleber H. Methylphenidate treatment of cocaine abusers without attention deficit disorder: a negative report. Am J Drug Alcohol Abuse 1985;11:193—7.

8. Sanchez J, Rodriguez B, Fuente LDL, Barrio G, Vicente J, Roca J, Royuela L, and the State Information System on Drug Abuse (SEIT)

Working Group. Opiates or cocaine: mortality from acute reactions in six major Spanish cities. J Epidemiol Commun Health 1995;49:54−60.

9. Hollander JE, Thode HC Jr, Hoffman RS. Chest discomfort, cocaine and tobacco. Acad Emerg Med 1995;2:238.

10. Hollander JE, Todd KH, Green G, Heilpern KL, Karras DJ, Singer AJ, Brogan GX, Funk JP, Strahan JB. Chest pain associated with cocaine: an assessment of prevalence in suburban and urban emergency departments. Ann Emerg Med 1995;26:671−6.

11. Hollander JE, Hoffman RS, Gennis P, Fairweather P, Feldman JA, Fish SS, DiSano MJ, Schumb DA, Dyer S. Cocaine-associated chest pain: one-year follow-up. Acad Emerg Med 1995;2:179−84.

12. Trabulsy ME. Cocaine washed out syndrome in a patient with acute myocardial infarction. Am J Emerg Med 1995;13:538−9.

13. Ashchi M, Wiedemann HP, James KB. Cardiac complication from use of cocaine and phenylephrine in nasal septoplasty. Arch Otolaryngol Head Neck Surg 1995;121:681−4.

14. Nicholson RA, Rogers JEG. Cocaine and adrenaline paste: a fatal combination? Br Med J 1995;311:250−1.

15. Burton M, Marks R. Dangers of cocaine and adrenaline paste. Exceeding the recommended dose may have serious sequelae. Br Med J 1995;311:1089−90.

16. Williamson P, Slack R. Accurate measurement of dose and patience are important. Br Med J 1995;311:1089.

17. Ellis PDM, Wilkey BR. Other aspects of anaesthetic technique may have added to danger. Br Med J 1995;311:1089.

18. Haim D, Lippmann M, Goldberg S, Walkenstein M. The pulmonary complications of crack cocaine: a comprehensive review. Chest 1995; 1:233−40.

19. Tashkin D. What is the true impact of crack on the lung? Chest 1995;108:1180−1.

20. Smith G, McClaughry P, Purkey J, Thompson W. Crack cocaine mimicking pulmonary embolism on pulmonary ventilation/perfusion lung scan: a case report. Clin Nucl Med 1995;1:65−8.

21. Konzen JP, Levine SR, Garcia JH. Vasospasm and thrombus formation as possible mechanisms of stroke related to alkaloidal cocaine. Stroke 1995;26:1114−18.

22. Merkel PA. Koroshetz WJ, Irizarry MC, Cudkowicz ME. Cocaine-associated cerebral vasculitis. Semin Arthritis Rheum 1995;25:172−83.

23. Gradon JD, Wityk R. Diagnosis of probable cocaine-induced cerebral vasculitis by magnetic resonance angiography. South Med J 1995; 88:1264−6.

24. Martin K, Rogers T, Kavanaugh A. Central nervous system angiopathy associated with cocaine abuse. J Rheumatol 1995;22:780−2.

25. Attig E, Amyot R, Botez T. Cocaine induced chronic tics. Br Med J 1143−4.

26. Kain ZN, Mayes LC, Pakes J, Rosenbaum SH, Schottenfeld R. Thrombocytopenia in pregnant women who use cocaine. Am J Obstet Gynecol 1995;173:885−90.

27. Pugh CM, Mezghebe HM, Leffall, LD Jr. Spontaneous bowel perforation in drug abusers. Am J Emerg Med 1995;13:113−14.

28. Rofsky J, Townsend J, Ilsen P, Bright D. Retinal nerve fiber layer defects and microtalc retinopathy secondary to free-basing 'crack' cocaine. J Am Optom Assoc 1995;66;712−20.

29. Simmen HP, Giovanoli P, Battaglia H, Wust J, Meyer VE. Soft tissue infections of the upper extremities with special consideration of abscesses in parenteral drug abusers, a prospective study. J Hand Surg 1995;20:797−800.

30. Martin D, DiCarlo RP. Recent changes in the epidemiology of genital ulcer disease in the United States: the crack cocaine connection. STD 1994:March−April Suppl:S76−S80.

31. Burkhead JM, Eriksen NL, Blanco JD. Cocaine use in pregnancy and risk of intraamniotic infection. J Reprod Med 1995;40:198−200.

32. Mirochnick M, Frank DA, Cabral H, Turner A, Zuckerman B. Relation between meconium concentration of the cocaine metabolite benzoylecgonine and fetal growth. J Pediatr 1995; 126:636−8.

33. Hurt H, Brodsky NL, Braitman LE, Giannetta J. Natal status of infants of cocaine users and control subjects: a prospective comparison. J Perinatol 1995;15:297−304

34. King TA, Perlman JM, Laptook AR, Rollins N, Jackson G, Little B. Neurologic manifestations of in utero cocaine exposure in near-term and term infants. Pediatrics 1995;96:259−64.

35. Mayes LC, Bornstein MH, Chawarska K, Granger RH. Information processing and developmental assessments in 3-month-old infants exposed prenatally to cocaine. Pediatrics 1995; 95:539−45.

36. Bender SL, Word CO, DiClemente RJ, Crittenden MR, Persaud NA, Ponton LE. The developmental implications of prenatal and/or postnatal crack cocaine exposure in preschool children: a preliminary report. J Dev Behav Pediatr 1995;16: 418−24.

37. Frassica JJ, Orav J, Walsh EP, Lipshultz SE. Arrhythmias in children prenatally exposed to cocaine. Arch Pediatr Adolesc Med 1994;148: 1163−9.

38. Bulbul ZR, Rosenthal DN, Klienman CS. Myocardial infarction in the perinatal period secondary to maternal cocaine abuse. Arch Pediatr Adolesc Med 1994;148:1092−6.

39. Okoruwa E, Shah R, Gerdes K. Apnea and vomiting in an infant due to cocaine exposure. J Iowa Med Soc 1995;85:449−50.

40. Lopez SL, Taeusch HW, Findlay RD, Walther FJ. Time of onset of necrotizing enterocolitis in newborn infants with known prenatal cocaine exposure. Clin Paed 1995;August:424−9.

41. Gottbrath-Flaherty EK, Agrawal R, Thaker V, Patel D, Ghai K. Urinary tract infections in cocaine-exposed infants. J Perinatol 1995; 15:203−7.

42. Hammersley R, Cassidy M, Oliver J. Drugs associated with drug-related deaths in Edinburgh and Glasgow, November 1990 to October 1992. Addiction 1995;90:959—65.

43. Gattera, J, Charles B, Williams G. A retrospective study of risk factors of akathisia in terminally ill patients. J Pain Symptom Manage 1994;9:454—61.

44. Mercadante S. Opioids and akathisia. J Pain Symptom Manage 1995;10:415.

45. Friedman E, Rao T. Disappearance of uremia due to heroin-associated nephropathy. Am J Kidney Dis 1995;25:689—93.

46. Biagini R, Klincewicz S, Henningsen G, MacKenzie B, Gallagher J, Bernstein D, Bernstein I. Antibodies to morphine in workers occupationally exposed to opiates at a narcotics manufacturing facility and evidence for similar antibodies in heroin abusers. Life Sci 1990;47:897.

47. Biagini R, Henningsen G, Klincewicz S. Immunologic analyses of peripheral leukocytes from workers at an ethical narcotics manufacturing facility. Arch Environ Health 1995;50:1.

48. Nahas G, Latour C. The human toxicity of marijuana. Med J Aust 1992;156:495—7.

49. Christie M, Chesher G. The human toxicity of marijuana. Med J Aust 1994;161:338—9.

50. Consroe P. The human toxicity of marijuana. Med J Aust 1995;162:54—5.

51. Sherman M, Aeberhard E, Wong V. Effects of smoking marijuana, tobacco or cocaine alone or in combination on DNA damage in human alveolar macrophages. Life Sci 1995;56:2201—7.

52. Uges D. Unintended toxicity (intoxication) by cannabis ingestion of space cake. J Forens Sci 1994;40:927—8.

Stephen Curran and Wendy Burn

5   Hypnotics and sedatives

℞ *Use of hypnotics*

Despite the development of non-benzodiazepine hypnotics, clinicians continue to be reluctant to prescribe hypnotic drugs. This may be partly because of worries about litigation and the effects such drugs have on daily activities, but it has been suggested that this 'perceived risk' is generally misplaced (1[R]). However, concerns about 'dependence and addiction' ensure that clinicians remain very cautious. There is also a view amongst some clinicians that insomnia is a 'benign' disorder and often little time is devoted to the assessment of patients with insomnia. This is surprising, considering that as many as 35% of adults suffer from insomnia (2[R]). Assessment should include a full history and physical examination, as well as appropriate laboratory investigations, in order to exclude both physical and psychiatric causes of insomnia. It is also useful to ask the patient to keep a sleep diary and to seek additional information from other sources to corroborate the patient's account (there is often little correlation between the subjective experience of sleep and objective measures). Although there are many classifications of sleep disorders, insomnia can be divided into transient, short-term, and chronic; it is the transient group for which hypnotics, especially benzodiazepines, are most appropriate. Hypnotic drugs do not provide a long-term solution to the problem of insomnia and the risk of dependence increases with both the dose and length of treatment. In addition, there is currently no hypnotic that is entirely free from adverse effects.

It is also important to note that a number of drugs may cause insomnia, including non-prescription medications (such as decongestants, caffeine, nicotine, and alcohol) and prescribed drugs (including α-agonists, aminophylline,

β-blockers, corticosteroids, calcium antagonists, diuretics, and various CNS stimulants). The most common benzodiazepines used to induce sleep include triazolam (short-acting), temazepam and estazolam (intermediate-acting), and flurazepam (long-acting). Non-benzodiazepine hypnotics include zolpidem and zopiclone.

The main adverse effects of hypnotics are residual sedative effects, rebound insomnia, physical dependence, tolerance, drug interactions (especially with CNS depressants), memory impairment, and respiratory depression (3[R]). Mixing benzodiazepines with other CNS depressants such as alcohol can lead to severe intoxication, and adverse reactions are more common in elderly people. In addition, elderly people with withdrawal symptoms may present with acute confusional states. Triazolam does not cause day-time sleepiness, but it may be associated with rebound insomnia, tolerance, and memory disturbance. Temazepam has a good adverse effects profile, but although it is good for sleep maintenance, it is less useful for sleep induction. Estazolam is also associated with rebound insomnia and memory difficulties. The longer acting benzodiazepines cause considerable day-time drowsiness and thus have limited value. Zolpidem and zopiclone produce hypnotic effects similar to triazolam and are not associated with next-day sedation, psychomotor impairment, or rebound insomnia (1[R]).

Sedative drugs, particularly benzodiazepines, are also commonly used in medically ill patients. These are particularly useful in intensive care because of their anxiolytic, sedative, hypnotic, and anterograde amnestic properties. Although these drugs have high therapeutic/toxic ratios, they can nevertheless be associated with serious complications in such settings, including airway obstruction, respiratory depression, hypotension, and pain at injection sites (for example with diazepam and chlordiazepoxide). A commonly used benzo-

Side Effects of Drugs, Annual 20
J.K. Aronson, ed.

diazepine in this context is midazolam (see below), which is a short-acting water-soluble benzodiazepine that can be given by intravenous injection but has a number of active metabolites. In general, benzodiazepines are metabolized by hepatic microsomal enzymes either by oxidation (for example diazepam) or glucuronide conjugation (for example lorazepam); the oxidation process is particularly susceptible to the effect of a number of drugs, for example, erythromycin significantly reduces the metabolism of midazolam (4[R]).

Benzodiazepines remain extremely useful drugs in a variety of clinical settings. Patients with insomnia for which there is no physical or psychiatric cause can be treated for a short period with either a short-acting benzodiazepine or one of the newer drugs, such as zolpidem. Sedatives and hypnotics should only be given for short periods and smaller dosages will be needed in elderly people. In addition, these drugs have a number of important interactions, especially with CNS depressants. They should therefore be used with caution in elderly people and in patients in medical settings.

An excellent review of short-acting hypnotics, including a discussion of their pharmacology, pharmacokinetics, clinical efficacy, and adverse reactions has recently been published (3[R]).

INDIVIDUAL BENZODIAZEPINES *(SED-13, 109; SEDA-17, 44; SEDA-18, 44; SEDA-19, 33)*

Benzodiazepines are characterized by a considerable amount of inter-individual variability in response to a given dose. This is due to a variety of factors, including individual sensitivities, age, underlying medical conditions, and concurrent drug administration (5[R]). The ability to reverse the effects of benzodiazepines is important and this can be achieved with flumazenil.

Alprazolam

High-potency benzodiazepines, such as alprazolam and clonazepam, are generally regarded as clinically effective in the treatment of panic disorder, but one of the major ad-

verse effects in this context is sedation (6[R]). Although relief of symptoms is rapid, problems with cognitive clouding, dependence, and withdrawal symptoms seriously limits their longer-term clinical usefulness.

Chlordiazepoxide

Various management strategies for alcohol dependence syndrome have been evaluated in 102 patients, 46% of whom were treated with more than one benzodiazepine (7[C]). Delirium tremens occurred in 12% of patients, suggesting that the management of this common problem was poor in a large proportion of patients. Lorazepam 1—2 mg tds or chlordiazepoxide 25—50 mg tds are effective at controlling withdrawal symptoms (fits, anxiety, etc.) and are well tolerated with minimal adverse effects. Benzodiazepines remain the treatment of choice for patients with alcohol withdrawal symptoms who do not respond to supportive care (8[R]).

Clobazam

The clinical efficacy of clobazam (a 1,5-benzodiazepine derivative) in the short-term treatment of anxiety disorders, particularly generalised anxiety disorder has been reviewed (9[R]). Clobazam 30—80 mg/day was as effective as equipotent doses of diazepam, lorazepam, dipotassium clorazepate, chlordiazepoxide, bromazepam, and alprazolam, with maximum anxiolytic effect at 7—14 days after the start of treatment. Clobazam was very well tolerated, with less sedation, impaired psychomotor performance, and memory impairment compared with other benzodiazepines. The author suggested that clobazam may be particularly useful for the short-term management of out-patient anxiety disorders, although it is more commonly regarded as a treatment for myoclonic seizures (10[R]), (11[R]).

Diazepam

It has been reported that drowsiness associated with diazepam and chlordiazepoxide is more likely in non-smokers than smokers (12[R]) for which there may be two explanations. First, nicotine enhances the metabolism of diazepam and chlordiazepoxide by inducing liver enzymes. Secondly, the psychostimulant action of nicotine may contribute to the reversal of drowsiness. Nevertheless, this effect should be borne in mind when prescribing diazepam, and smaller dosages may be needed in smokers. Recently the pharmacokinetic and pharmacodynamic interaction between venlafaxine (a new serotonin and noradrenaline re-uptake inhibitor for the treatment of depression) and diazepam has been investigated in a randomised, double-blind, placebo-controlled study in 18 men (13[C]). Venlafaxine had no effect on the pharmacokinetics of desmethyldiazepam (a metabolite of diazepam), but there was a slight increase in sedation, identified by critical flicker fusion threshold (a sensitive measure of CNS arousal/sedation). However, the authors concluded that this interaction was not clinically significant.

Lorazepam

Lorazepam has recently been recommended for the control of agitated behaviour/physical aggression in patients with dementia in the absence of psychosis in doses of 0.25—1 mg (orally, intramuscularly, or intravenously) every 1—2 h. It is important to control such behaviour rapidly in demented patients on general medical wards, where there are likely to be many vulnerable patients. However, lorazepam is known to be addictive and it should therefore be used with extreme caution and for short periods. Alternatively, oxazepam 10—15 mg every 3—4 h as needed can be used (14[R]). Neuroleptic drugs are more commonly used in the management of behaviorally disturbed demented patients, and benzodiazepines may lead to a worsening of such behaviour.

Midazolam

Midazolam is a short-acting benzodiazepine routinely used for sedation in intensive care. One of its main metabolites, β-hydroxymidazolam, has recently been reported to accumulate in patients with renal failure, leading to prolonged sedative effects, and five cases in which this occurred have been described (15[c]). However, this can be reversed by flumazenil, a benzodiazepine receptor antagonist. Sedation may also be greater in patients with hepatic failure (4[R]).

Midazolam is an effective premedicant for children undergoing surgery. It minimizes the emotional trauma and facilitates smooth induction. In one double-blind study, the preoperative sedative effects of two premedicants (midazolam 0.5 mg/kg and diazepam 0.6 mg/kg) and postoperative recovery were studied in 102 children (16[C]). Both drugs produced good separation and induction but midazolam was significantly better. In addition, no serious adverse effects were noted with midazolam. Reports continue to appear indicating that intravenous midazolam is a safe and well-tolerated treatment in young children who need sedation before surgery (17[C]). Recent guidelines have been published for the use of intravenous midazolam in a variety of clinical settings for sedation and anxiety control. This includes a loading dose of 25—100 μg/kg (depending on the severity of symptoms) and a maintenance dose of 0.25—2.5 μg/kg/min, depending on the severity of symptoms (18[R]).

Temazepam

In a recent study, 30 subjects were randomly assigned to receive either 10 or 20 mg of temazepam in a double-blind, placebo-controlled design. They were asked to maintain their normal daily routines as much as possible. Both drugs significantly impaired daily activities the following morning owing to 'fatigue' and 'slowing' and there were no significant differences between the two (19[C]), i.e. temazepam 10 mg caused as much next-day sedation as 20 mg.

Abecarnil

Abecarnil is a mixed/partial agonist at benzodiazepine receptors. It has shown to have anxiolytic activity in phase III trials (20[C]). It has been hypothesized that partial agonists at benzodiazepine receptor may have advantages over classical benzodiazepines, including a lower propensity for producing sedation, tolerance, and withdrawal effects. Animal data suggest that abecarnil may have some or all of these advantages, but clinical data are very limited. One trial in 129 patients with DSM-III-R diagnostic criteria for generalized anxiety disorder were given abecarnil in doses of 3—30 mg/day for 3 weeks. Adverse effects were correlated with dosage and the most common adverse effect was drowsiness (31%, 3—9 mg/day; 51%, 7.5—15 mg/day; and 71%, 15—30 mg/day) (20[C]). Other adverse effects included loss of equilibrium, confusion, depression, dizziness, lethargy, fatigue, amnesia, insomnia, and lack of concentration.

NON-BENZODIAZEPINE HYPNOTICS *(SED-13, 111; SEDA-17, 46; SEDA-18, 45; SEDA-19, 37)*

Zolpidem

The ideal hypnotic would induce sleep rapidly, have no residual sedation, and not impair memory. In addition, it would have no active metabolites and not be associated with tolerance, physical dependence, or respiratory depression. Zolpidem, a non-benzodiazepine, non-barbiturate hypnotic is an imidazopyridine. It has a rapid onset of action and a short half-life (1.5—2.4 h). It is generally very well tolerated and is efficacious in the treatment of insomnia (3[R]). It binds to the benzodiazepine binding site on the GABA receptor complex and has a high affinity for the central benzodiazepine-1 receptor subtype (which may be responsible for some of its hypnotic, myorelaxant, and anxiolytic effects) (21). In a double-blind, placebo-controlled, crossover trial, zolpidem (up to 20 mg) had a positive effect on sleep architecture in elderly subjects (22[C]). It has also been shown to have no effect on cognitive or psychomotor performance the following morning in elderly subjects (23[C]). It is rapidly absorbed. Although it has a relatively high first-pass metabolism none of its metabolites are pharmacologically active. It is efficacious in both young and elderly insomniacs and reduces sleep latency, without REM suppression or rebound insomnia. Adverse effects are relatively uncommon and not serious, but the most frequently reported include amnesia (2.6%), headache (2.4%), nau-

sea (2.4%), and vertigo (2.1%). Clinical trials data involving 2600 patients have shown that repeated doses of zolpidem 10 mg in young adults and of zolpidem 5 mg in elderly insomniacs are associated with minimal adverse effects the following day (24[C]). There have been conflicting reports regarding tolerance, but this appears to be considerably less than with benzodiazepine hypnotics, and the general consensus is that there is very little or no tolerance during the first 4 weeks. It is also relatively safe when taken in overdosage and no fatalities have been reported in doses up to 1400 mg (3[R]). No severe complications have been published after overdosage in elderly subjects (25[c]).

Zopiclone

Zopiclone belongs to the new class of sedative hypnotics known as the cyclopyrrolones. Although it is not available in the US, it is available in a number of other countries, including the UK. Zopiclone binds to a site related to the benzodiazepine binding site on the GABA receptor complex. It has a relatively short half-life (5—6 h). The systemic availability of zopiclone is slightly higher than that of zolpidem (80 and 67%, respectively), but zopiclone's N-oxide metabolite has hypnotic activity (but only about 10% of the dose). It has been well established as a hypnotic for elderly (26[C]) younger patients (27[C]). In a large study involving over 2000 patients taking therapeutic dosages of zopiclone for 21 days, the most common adverse effects included bitter taste (3.6%), dry mouth (1.6%), and early morning sedation (1.3%). The early morning sedation was much commoner with doses of 7.5 mg compared with 3.75 mg. There were eight falls in elderly patients but none was serious (28[C]). In healthy volunteers, zopiclone 7.5 mg is associated with some rebound insomnia, but this does not appear to be significantly greater than with triazolam (3[R]). Mild anterograde amnesia has also been reported with zopiclone 7.5 mg. In therapeutic dosages it does not appear to be associated with respiratory depression in healthy individuals, but it may cause mild respiratory depression in patients with chronic obstructive airways disease

(29^C). There are also several reports suggesting a lack tolerance in patients taking zopiclone for up to 17 weeks. There is currently no evidence for the development of physical dependence after 4 weeks of zopiclone. Zopiclone is also relatively safe in overdosage, the commonest problem being CNS depression. Withdrawal effects are less pronounced than with benzodiazepines, and it is claimed to be associated with considerably less physical dependence. However, there are a few reports of zopiclone dependency in patients with a history of alcohol and drug dependence. It has also been associated with occasional episodes of psychosis. Other adverse effects include dry mouth, nightmares, memory loss, and tremor. Zopiclone should be used with caution in patients with a psychiatric history, alcohol or drug dependence, respiratory disease, or severe liver impairment (30^R). It should only be used for the short-term management of insomnia, and a course should not normally last longer than 4 weeks. A more detailed review of zopiclone can be found elsewhere (3^R).

Azapirones

The azapirones modulate serotonergic neurotransmission via $5HT_{1A}$ receptors and appear to have potential in the treatment of some psychiatric disorders. Buspirone, the only azapirone so far available, is helpful in the management of anxiety, depression, panic disorder, and obsessive-compulsive disorder (31^R). Buspirone is well tolerated and has a number of advantages over traditional benzodiazepines. In particular, there is said to be no withdrawal syndrome after stopping the drug and it has a lower potential for dependence and fewer cognitive/psychomotor effects. There is also said to be a lower risk of potentiation of other CNS drugs with sedative properties and no respiratory depression. Adverse effects include gastric upset, dizziness, headache, insomnia, vomiting, and fatigue. In behaviorally disturbed demented patients, neuroleptic drugs remain the treatment of choice (32^R). Symptoms that appear to be most responsive include anxiety, fear, tension, and agitation. In addition, benzodiazepines may cause paradoxical agitation in some elderly demented patients. Buspirone may have some advantages and fewer adverse effects in this context, but further clinical work is needed (33^R). Another compound in a relatively advanced stage of development is tandospirone, which has a similar profile to buspirone, but clinical data are still awaited (34^R).

α_2-Adrenoceptor agonists

The best known example of this group of drugs is clonidine, which has a wide range of actions, including sedation, anxiolysis, and analgesia. It may be used as a premedication before surgery because of its sedative effects, and postoperatively in the management of post-operative pain. Its effect in anxiety disorders has been neglected and would benefit from further investigation (35^R).

REFERENCES

1.   Lahmeyer H. Hypnotics: a powerful tool for a serious problem. Pharmacol Ther 1995;July:438–55.
2.   Mellinger GD, Balter MH, Uhlenhuth EH. Insomnia and its treatment; prevalence and correlates. Arch Gen Psychiatry 1985;42:225–32.
3.   Mendelson WB, Jain B. An assessment of short-acting hypnotics. Drug Saf 1995;13:257–70.
4.   Prielipp RC, Coursin DB, Wood KE, Murray MJ. Complications associated with sedative and neuromuscular blocking drugs in critically ill patients. Crit Care Clin 1995;11:983–1003.
5.   Bertaccini E, Geller E. Benzodiazepine antagonists and their role in anaesthesia and critical care. Anaesth Pharmacol Rev 1995;3:74–81.
6.   Stahl SM, Soefje S. Panic attacks and panic disorder: the great neurologic imposters. Semin Neurol 1995;15:126–32.
7.   Newman JP, Terris DJ, Moore M. Trends in the management of alcohol withdrawal syndrome. Laryngoscope 1995;105:1–7.
8.   Erstad BL, Cotugno CL. Management of alcohol withdrawal. Am J Health Syst Pharmacol 1995;52:697–709.
9.   Beaumont G. Clobazam in the treatment of anxiety. Hum Psychopharmacol 1995;10:S27–S41.
10.   Robertson MM. The place of clobazam in the treatment of epilepsy; an update. Hum Psychopharmacol 1995;10:S43–S63.

11.   Trimble M (editor). New anticonvulsant drugs and the role of clobazam as adjunctive therapy. Hum Psychopharmacol 1995;10:S56—S79.

12.   Schein JR. Cigarette smoking and clinically significant drug interactions. Drug Interaction 1995;29:1139—48.

13.   Troy SM, Lucki I, Peirgies AA, Parker VD, Klockowski PA, Chiang ST. Pharmacokinetic and pharmacodynamic evaluation of the potential drug interaction between venlafaxine and diazepam. J Clin Pharmacol 1995;35:410—19.

14.   Tueth MJ. Dementia: diagnosis and emergency behavioural complications. J Emergency Med 1995;13:519—25.

15.   Bauer TM, Ritz R, Haberthur C, Ha HR, Hunkeler W, Sleight AJ, Scollo-Lavizzari G, Haefeli WE. Prolonged sedation due to accumulation of conjugated metabolites of midazolam. Lancet 1995;346:145—7.

16.   Pywell CA, Hung Y-J, Nagelhout J. Oral midazolam versus meperidine, atropine and diazepam: a comparison of premedicants in pediatric outpatients. J Am Assoc Nurse Anaesthetists 1995;63:124—30.

17.   Pruitt JW, Goldwasser MS, Sabol SR, Prstojevich SJ. Intramuscular ketamine, midazolam and glycopyrrolate for pediatric sedation in the emergency department. Am Assoc Oral Maxillofac Surgeons 1995;53:13—17.

18.   Woodward C. Criteria for the use of continuous midazolam infusion in adult inpatients. Am J Health Syst Pharmacol 1995;52:754—5.

19.   Aldenkamp AP, Baker G, Pieters MSM, Schoemaker HC, Cohen AF, Schwabe S. The neurotoxicity scale: the validity of a patient-based scale, assessing neurotoxicity. Epilepsy Res 1995;20:229—39.

20.   Onbekend C. Abecarnil shows promise in generalised anxiety disorder. Drugs Ther Perspect 1995;5:7—8.

21.   Blanchard JC, Boireau A, Garrett C. In vitro and in vivo inhibition by zopiclone of benzodiazepine binding to rodent brain receptors. Life Sci 1979;24:2417—20.

22.   Scharf MB, Mayleben DW, Kaffeman M. Dose response effects of zolpidem in normal geriatric subjects. J Clin Psychiatry 1991;52:77—83.

23.   Fairweather DB, Kerr JS, Hindmarch I. The effects of acute and repeated doses of zolpidem on subjective sleep, psychomotor performance and cognitive function in elderly volunteers. Eur J Clin Pharmacol 1992;43:597—601.

24.   Unden M, Schechter BR. Next day effects after night-time treatment with zolpidem; a review. Eur Psychiatry 1996;11(Suppl 1):21—30.

25.   Allain H, Monti J. General safety profile of zolpidem; safety in elderly, overdose and rebound effects. Eur Psychiatry 1995;10:1—9.

26.   Dehlin O, Rundgren A, Borjesson L. Zopiclone to geriatric patients; a parallel, double-blind, dose-response clinical trial of zopiclone as a hypnotic to geriatric patients; a study in a geriatric hospital. Pharmacology 1983;27 Suppl:173—8.

27.   Elie R, Prenay M, Le Morvan P. Efficacy and safety of zopiclone and triazolam in the treatment of geriatric insomniacs. Int Clin Psychopharmacol 1990;5 Suppl 2:39—46.

28.   Allain H, Delahaye C, Le Cox F. Postmarketing surveillance of zopiclone in insomniacs; analysis of 20,513 cases. Sleep 1991;14:408—13.

29.   Muir JF, DeFouilloy P, Broussier R. Comparative study of the effects of zopiclone and placebo on respiratory function in patients with chronic obstructive respiratory insufficiency. Int Clin Psychopharmacol 1990;5 Suppl:85—94.

30.   Schneiderman C. Zopiclone. Kino Comm Hosp News Lett 1995;5:410.

31.   Anonymous. Azapirones have potential in a wide variety of CNS disorders. Drugs Ther Perspect 1995;5:5—7.

32.   Jarrett PG, Rockwood K, Mallery L. Behavioural problems in nursing home patients. Postgrad Med 1995;97:189—96.

33.   Yeager BF, Farnett LE, Ruzicka SA. Management of the behavioural manifestations of dementia. Arch Intern Med 1995;155:250—60.

34.   Murasaki M. Overview of serotonin 1A receptor selective agents in anxiety disorders—the developmental situation in Japan. Int Rev Psychiatry 1995;7:105—13.

35.   Maze M, Poree L, Rabin, BC. Anesthetic and analgesic actions of α_2-adrenoceptor agonists. Pharmacol Commun 995;6:175—82.

Alfonso Carvajal and Luis H. Martín Arias

6 Antipsychotic drugs

GENERAL *(SED-13, 117; SEDA-17, 49; SEDA-18, 47; SEDA-19, 40)*

Antipsychotic drugs have many, sometimes incapacitating, adverse effects, the severity of the conditions for which they are prescribed being the only justification for their use.

Cardiovascular *Torsade de pointes* is a life-threatening ventricular tachycardia that is often associated with prolongation of the electrocardiographic QT interval (SED-13, 119; SEDA-18, 47). Two case series have further illustrated the possible relation between haloperidol and torsade de pointes (1[c]), (2[c]). In the first series, the dysrhythmia developed in three patients who were admitted to hospital with cirrhosis and bleeding varices but without prior cardiac disease (1[c]). All received intravenous vasopressin, glyceryl trinitrate, and sedation with haloperidol or droperidol; two had concurrent electrolyte abnormalities (hypokalemia and hypomagnesemia). The reactions were primarily attributed to the administration of neuroleptic drugs, which can prolong the QT interval, as was found in these cases. In the second series, three patients, who had been treated with high-dose intravenous haloperidol for sedation, developed torsade de pointes after prolongation of the QTc interval and immediately after an additional large intravenous bolus dose of haloperidol (2[c]). In one case there was no history of previous cardiac disease. There were no sequelae after withdrawal.

Many reports of sudden death associated with neuroleptic drugs preclude definitive conclusions, because of small sample sizes, sparse laboratory and historical data, and wide variation in dosage regimens (SED-13, 120). A recent report has underlined the difficulty in establishing a causal link between neuroleptic drug exposure and sudden death (3[cR]).

A psychiatric patient, after a sudden outburst of violent behavior, was given intramuscular haloperidol 20 mg and diazepam 10 mg; 20 min later he became cyanosed and limp. Attempts at resuscitation failed. At autopsy the pathologist concluded that the cause of death had been acute heart failure related to drug therapy.

In extremely agitated patients, neurally mediated sudden cardiac arrest can occur even in unmedicated patients. These fatal dysrhythmias are believed to be precipitated by increased release of catecholamines and glucocorticoids, or by excess vagal and adrenergic stimulation.

Nervous system There are many discrepant findings in regard to the effects of neuroleptic drugs on *cognitive functioning* in schizophrenics (SED-13, 120; SEDA-18, 48). These effects have recently been evaluated before and after neuroleptic drug therapy, using a test-retest design in 18 consecutive patients who met DSM-III-R criteria for schizophrenia, and who were included in the study if they had been off oral neuroleptic drugs for at least 4 weeks, and off depot neuroleptic drugs for at least 3 months (4[c]). The mean (SD) duration of illness was 11 (7) years. Healthy controls (n = 18) were drawn from among the hospital personnel or from the community and were matched with the schizophrenic patients for age, sex, and education. The patients, as expected, performed worse than the controls in tests of frontal and temporal lobe function. There was the same degree of impairment in patients off and on neuroleptic drugs. The authors concluded that neuroleptic drugs have no negative effects on cognitive function in schizophrenic patients.

Subjective *dysphoria* has been said to occur as an important adverse effect in the absence of objective signs of akathisia (SED-13, 121; SEDA-19, 44). Therefore, patients who are

Side Effects of Drugs, Annual 20
J.K. Aronson, ed.

irritable or who complain of tension or panic may be given excessive treatment rather than dosage reduction. When a single, oral dose of haloperidol (5 mg) was given on two separate days to two groups of healthy volunteers (26 and 25 subjects), dysphoria occurred in about 40% of the subjects on both occasions, but akathisia was detected in only 8% (first group) and 16% (second group) (5[C]). All adverse effects were transient and were abolished in nine of 10 subjects who developed dysphoria when given procyclidine.

Extrapyramidal signs The pathogenesis, prevention, and treatment of neuroleptic-induced movement disorders have been reviewed (6[R]).

In a population-based study, the prescription of anticholinergic antiparkinsonian drugs has been used as an indicator of extrapyramidal adverse effects (7[C]). The study lasted from January 1986 to December 1989 and was carried out in the province of Rome (3 750 000 inhabitants). All the subjects who had taken neuroleptic drugs for two or more consecutive months were selected. Out of 17 195 subjects treated with different neuroleptic drugs, 11% had taken anticholinergic drugs in the first 2 months. A logistic regression model relating the prescription of anticholinergic drugs to the type and dosage of neuroleptic drug and to the age and sex of the subjects showed that trifluperidol and haloperidol were more often associated with antiparkinsonian therapy. Similarly, the frequency of prescriptions for anticholinergic drugs increased with dosage, from 5% in those taking less than 675 mg of chlorpromazine equivalents per month to 16% in those taking more than 2250 mg of chlorpromazine equivalents per month. In a case-control study, 5479 elderly patients taking neuroleptic drugs were 5.4 times more likely to begin antiparkinsonian medication than 16 437 non-users (8[C]). There was a clear dose-response relation between oral neuroleptic drug dosages (mg of chlorpromazine equivalents) and the initiation of antiparkinsonian treatment. When the type of antiparkinsonian drugs was considered, the risk for anticholinergic drugs was 8.5 (95% CI, 4.8—6.1) and, surprisingly, 2.2 (1.9—2.7) for dopaminergic drugs. Dopaminergic drugs are generally contraindicated in this situation and their prescription may reflect mistaken diagnoses of idiopathic Parkinson's disease in a

substantial number of elderly patients with extrapyramidal signs.

Three cases of exacerbation of pre-existing postural tremor with the emergence of parkinsonism after treatment with neuroleptic drugs have been reported (9[c]).

Asymmetrical cogwheel rigidity has been reported in a 28-year-old Asian woman treated with neuroleptic drugs. The authors speculated that in spite of the suggestion that asymmetrical cogwheeling is related to idiopathic Parkinson's disease, right-sided asymmetrical cogwheeling is often noted in younger patients during the first 3 months of drug exposure (10[c]).

A new scale (the Yale Extrapyramidal Symptom Scale, YESS) has been proposed for the early assessment of extrapyramidal symptoms during neuroleptic drug treatment (11[C]). It is an eight-item scale, five items being devoted to the assessment of parkinsonian symptoms (rigidity, gait, arm swing, facial immobility, and tremor), two to akathisia (objective and subjective), and one to dystonia. These items were chosen to shorten and facilitate use of the scale in acutely ill patients. The scale was used in 41 consecutive patients who received neuroleptic drugs. The inter-rater agreement was good to excellent; there were also good correlations between the YESS rating and two other scales that were used to assess extrapyramidal signs. Other extrapyramidal adverse effects scales tend to focus on one dimension of extrapyramidal symptoms (for example, the Abnormal Involuntary Movement Scale, AIMS, for tardive dyskinesia and the Simpson-Angus Neurologic Rating Scale, SAS, for parkinsonian symptoms). The new scale (YESS) includes the extrapyramidal signs that are most likely to occur and that are relatively easy to assess during acute treatment.

A rare case of death attributed to benzhexol toxicity has been reported (12[c]).

A 48-year-old schizophrenic man was receiving fluphenazine decanoate, 37.5 mg every 3 weeks, and benzhexol hydrochloride, 6 mg/day in divided doses. He was addicted to Coca-Cola and was a heavy smoker. Two weeks before he died he was given erythromycin for a productive cough and 1 week later was treated with Granocol granules (sterculia and frangula bark) for constipation. He developed a mild patchy bronchopneumonia and an empyema. The most remarkable finding at post-mortem examination was that the concentrations of benzhexol in femoral artery blood (0.12 mg/l) and liver (0.5 mg/kg) were high, and 0.4 mg was found in the stomach.

The blood benzhexol concentration in this case was said to be at about the mid-point of the concentrations associated with death; self-poisoning was not suspected.

Akathisia has been associated with iron deficiency (SEDA-17, 49). However, the rationale for iron supplementation in the treatment of akathisia is poor, and there are potential long-term adverse consequences (13[R]). A similar conclusion has emerged from another review of the epidemiology of drug-induced akathisia (14[R]).

℞ Tardive dyskinesia

Occurrence Spontaneous dyskinesias are not rare, having been found in 5.8% of individuals in 18 population studies (15[R]). Even higher rates have been recorded, especially among elderly patients; in two studies of drug-free elderly subjects, senile dyskinesias were reported in 9 and 37%, respectively. The presence of baseline extrapyramidal signs (bradykinesia, rigidity, and cogwheel rigidity) and spontaneous dyskinesia has again been examined (16[C]). Of 89 neuroleptic drug-naive patients admitted to hospital, 17% had extrapyramidal signs, but only one had spontaneous dyskinesia at baseline.*

The point prevalence of tardive dyskinesia in numerous surveys averages 25% with wide variation from 0.5 up to 65% (SED-13, 121). Three of 17 patients, aged 16—21, hospitalized in a mental health center in Israel, had either pronounced or subtle signs of tardive dyskinesia (17[C]). In another study, 64 out-patients aged 40 or under, who had received neuroleptic drugs for at least 6 months, were surveyed to assess anamnestic and clinical factors associated with the presence of chronic dyskinesia (18[C]). There was tardive dyskinesia in 16 (25%), and 20 (31%) had mild choreiform dyskinesia either at rest or elicited by tests; this is a high incidence among young psychotic out-patients receiving moderate to low dosages of neuroleptic drugs. The proportion of patients with a positive history of early brain damage was significantly higher in the tardive

and mild dyskinesia groups. There was no significant difference in psychiatric diagnosis or handedness between tardive dyskinetic, mild dyskinetic, and non-dyskinetic groups, nor in sex or age. Age, however, cannot be dissociated from other confounding factors, such as life-long psychopathological disturbances, chronic in-patient status, long duration of exposure to neuroleptic drugs, and late development of neurological damage from degeneration, arteriosclerosis, or other causes. In fact, there was a trend suggesting that longer exposure to neuroleptic drugs is associated with the presence of dyskinesias.

The frequency of dyskinesia in elderly patients has also been surveyed in a follow-up study of 266 middle-aged and elderly out-patients with a median duration of 21 days of total lifetime neuroleptic exposure (19[C]). The incidence of tardive dyskinesia at 1 year was 26% (95% CI, 19—33). The cumulative proportion by the end of 24 months was 52% and by the end of 36 months 60%. In a cumulative multivariate analysis controlling for other confounding factors, five significant predictors emerged: fixed duration of prior neuroleptic drug use at baseline, time-dependent cumulative dose of high-potency neuroleptic drugs, a history of alcohol abuse/dependence (the only categorical predictor), time-dependent AIMS global score, and time-dependent tremor on instrumental assessment. Age, which has repeatedly been observed to be an important predictor of tardive dyskinesia, correlated significantly with the logarithm of the cumulative dose, and was a significant predictor of the incidence of tardive dyskinesia in univariate analysis but not in the final cumulative multivariate analysis. This strongly suggests that the apparent effects of age on the risk of tardive dyskinesia in the previous study (18[C]) was secondary to the effects of other significant predictors, such as the cumulative dose. The observation that a small but significant number of the patients developed tardive dyskinesia after less than 3 months of neuroleptic drug treatment made the authors suggest that in older subjects the current research criterion of the minimum length of treatment before a diagnosis of tardive dyskinesia should be changed from 3 months to 1 month. This has in fact been done for the clinical diagnosis of tardive dyskinesia in DSM-IV.

Mechanism MPTP (1-methyl-4-phenyl-1,2, 3,6-tetrahydropyridine) has been identified as the toxin responsible for an irreversible syndrome closely resembling Parkinson's disease. It is actively taken up by dopaminergic neurones in the striatum and selectively inhibits the first enzymatic step in the mitochondrial electron transport chain. Since the chemical structures and neurological effects of haloperidol and MPTP are similar, the effects of neuroleptic drugs on the mitochondrial electron transport chain have been studied in 25 patients with schizophrenia (20[C]). Impairment of the function of the electron transport chain will lead to accumulation of NADH and the secondary inhibition of Krebs cycle activity. Accordingly, different substrates of the Krebs cycle (alanine, aspartate, lactate, and pyruvate) could be affected. Seven patients were free of medication and 11 had tardive dyskinesia, eight of whom were currently taking medication and three were unmedicated. After controlling for tardive dyskinesia status, only CSF concentrations of alanine were significantly higher in the medicated patients than in the unmedicated, but were not significantly correlated with neuroleptic drug dosage. Controlling for medication status, the patients with tardive dyskinesia had significantly higher CSF concentrations of aspartate than those without tardive dyskinesia. The authors considered this to be preliminary evidence of an effect of neuroleptic drugs on oxidative phosphorylation and of a relation between aspartate concentrations in CSF and tardive dyskinesia. However, they pointed out that only two comparisons, out of a total of eight between four substrates and two forms of neurological adverse effects, had yielded significant differences between the groups.

Predisposing factors Predisposing factors are a topic of particular interest, to which much attention has been devoted (SED-13, 122). In an acute geriatric psychiatry in-patient unit, 386 subjects underwent assessment for medical, psychiatric, and treatment factors that might have contributed to tardive dyskinesia (21[C]). The risk of dyskinesia rose with duration of use: 10% of 152 patients with no history of neuroleptic drug use had spontaneous dyskinesia, 16% of 81 patients with less than 3 months use, 29% of 49 patients with 3−12 months

use, 31% of 59 patients with 1−10 years use, and 41% of 27 patients with more than 10 years use. The respective relative risks were 1.6 (95% CI, 0.8−3.2), 2.8 (1.5−5.5), 3.1 (1.7−5.7), and 4.1 (2.1−8.0). Duration of neuroleptic drug use was the strongest predictor of tardive dyskinesia. Increased age did not make an independent contribution to the risk. There was no association between a diagnosis of diabetes and an increased risk of tardive dyskinesia.

Organicity (neurodevelopmental/cognitive disturbances; SED-13, 122) has been proposed as another risk for tardive dyskinesia (SED-13, 122). It has been hypothesized that a small amplitude of the auditory evoked potential (P3 or P300) could be a marker of this subgroup of patients. In a 2-year follow-up study of 88 patients, those who developed tardive dyskinesia (eight patients) had a smaller P3 than matched controls (22[Cr]). Also, 12 of 16 patients with tardive dyskinesia at the time when the auditory evoked potentials were recorded were in the group with small P3 amplitudes. Indirect support for a link between P3 and tardive dyskinesia stems from the consistent finding in the literature that cognitive disturbances, which are associated with a small P3, indicate a higher risk of tardive dyskinesia.

The adverse effects of neuroleptic drugs, especially tardive dyskinesia, have been assessed in 73 elderly Japanese patients (mean age 76) with dementia compared with 74 patients with dementia who had never received neuroleptic drugs (23[C]). The most common adverse effect when first using neuroleptic drugs was constipation. A significantly higher proportion (44%) of patients had tardive dyskinesia among the neuroleptic drug-treated group compared with the non-treated group (14%). The only significant risk factors for tardive dyskinesia were the length of neuroleptic drug therapy and the duration of hospitalization. The authors concluded that despite the lower dosages of neuroleptic drugs used in elderly people in Japan, there is still a high risk of dyskinesia.

Adverse effects such as tardive dyskinesia might be reduced by optimizing the dosage of neuroleptic drugs (SEDA-18, 49). Impaired metabolism could account for increased plasma concentrations and a higher risk of toxicity. However, among 16 patients who had *developed tardive dyskinesia during neuroleptic treatment, there was no over-representation of subjects with impaired metabolism, although the study was too small to be sure (24[C]).*

Unusual presentations *Respiratory dyskinesia with tardive dyskinesias occurring during neuroleptic drug treatment has been previously reported (SEDA-19, 43); its clinical importance should be stressed, since sometimes the association with neuroleptic drugs is not appreciated and misdiagnosis is common. Laryngeal movement disorder was sought in six men and six women aged 35—70 years (25[C]). All had been receiving neuroleptic drug therapy for non-schizophrenic psychiatric illnesses for at least 6 months and none was taking anticholinergic or dopaminergic drugs at the time of examination. They all had classical tardive dyskinesia of the orobuccolingual region, which persisted for over 3 months; five patients had difficulty in swallowing, eight had speech disorders, and eight had breathing irregularities and polypnea as shown by endoscopy and electromyography. The results suggested involvement of the pharyngeal and laryngeal musculature by abnormal movements. An additional report of five patients with respiratory dyskinesia has further highlighted the important clinical features of the condition (26[cR]).*

There seems to be a diurnal variation in the severity of tardive dyskinesia, and this has been assessed in 10 patients with tardive dyskinesia for at least 6 months (27[C]). All were taking haloperidol (0.2 mg/kg bd). The total AIMS scores, subdivided into limb-trunk scores and rank order global impression scores, were all worse in the afternoon compared with the early morning. This suggests that rating sessions should be held at least several hours after the patient wakes, to ensure that the severity of the involuntary movements is maximal.

Rabbit syndrome has been previously described as a late-onset adverse effect associated with neuroleptic drugs (SED-13, 123). It can be difficult to differentiate between rabbit syndrome and tardive dyskinesia. In tardive dyskinesia, the movements of the mouth are usually irregular and slow, while in rabbit syndrome the movements are rapid and rhythmic, often associated with a sound produced by the lips, and no dyskinesia of the tongue. In rabbit

syndrome, the movements improve after treatment with anticholinergic drugs, which aggravates tardive dyskinesia. A new case has been published (28[cr]).

A 56-year-old woman was treated with haloperidol 50 mg/day and trihexyphenidyl 10 mg/day for an acute paranoid episode. Following improvement, the dosage of haloperidol was reduced to 30 mg/day. After 18 months she was treated with haloperidol alone in a low dosage. During this time hypothyroidism was detected and the patient took L-thyroxine 100 µg/day. Gradually, haloperidol was withdrawn. Because she complained of apathy, haloperidol was reintroduced, and a few months later she developed involuntary movements of the mouth (rapid movements of the jaw in a vertical axis without tongue involvement). An increased dosage of haloperidol was not effective, and neither was the addition of tiapride 300 mg/day. Rabbit syndrome was diagnosed, and oral trihexyphenidyl was started. Within a few days the movements diminished markedly, but 4 weeks later she developed tardive dyskinesia with involuntary movements of the trunk and arms. Haloperidol and trihexyphenidyl were gradually withdrawn and she was given sulpiride up to 400 mg/day. A few months later she had no signs of rabbit syndrome or tardive dyskinesia.

Treatment *To date there is no satisfactory treatment for tardive dyskinesia, but antiparkinsonian drugs are frequently used to treat neuroleptic-induced extrapyramidal adverse effects (SED-13, 122; SEDA-17, 50; SEDA-17, 55; SEDA-18, 49; SEDA-19, 41). In a double-blind crossover study the effects of biperiden and amantadine on neuroleptic-induced extrapyramidal symptoms and tardive dyskinesia have been compared in 26 of 32 schizophrenic patients on long-term stable antipsychotic and trihexyphenidil treatment who were initially randomly assigned to either amantadine 100 mg bd or biperiden 2 mg bd for 2 weeks and who completed the study (29[C]). Simpson-Angus and AIMS scores did not differ significantly between amantadine and biperiden, but were significantly lower than during placebo, 1 week before each of the two treatment phases. As the authors pointed out, the duration of treatment was short and the possibility that changes would have emerged over longer periods could not be excluded. Challenge and rechallenge with amantadine have demonstrated its efficacy in a 38-year-old man (30[c]).*

Changes in AIMS scores after challenge and repeated rechallenge with amantadine were seen in a 38-year-old man who developed tardive dyskinesia when treated with neuroleptic drugs. After a score of 19, amantadine (100 mg bd) was started and tardive dyskinesia noticeably decreased; when the amantadine was discontinued, the tardive dyskinesia worsened. Amantadine was restarted and the AIMS score fell to 3; on withdrawal for 3 days the movements reappeared (AIMS score of 17). Amantadine again was restarted, reducing the AIMS score to 5.

Tardive dystonia (SED-13, 123) In 200 consecutive in-patients admitted to a psychiatric emergency ward, tardive dystonia was present in eight (4%) and tardive dyskinesia in 44 (22%) (31^C). All had at least a 3-month history of total cumulative neuroleptic drug exposure. Patients with tardive dystonia were younger than those with tardive dyskinesia (38 vs. 50 years) and fewer years had passed since their first neuroleptic drug treatment (7 vs. 15 years). As this was an uncontrolled study, no firm conclusion can be reached. It is possible that the older the patient the longer exposure time to treatment. Indeed, in this study the differences between age and years of exposure were not significant.

R꙼ *Neuroleptic malignant syndrome*

Neuroleptic malignant syndrome and malignant hyperthermia have been compared in a recent thorough review, with emphasis on the different pathogenesis of the two syndromes (32^R).

Occurrence Neuroleptic malignant syndrome is a rare, idiosyncratic, and potentially lethal adverse effect that occurs in 0.5–1% of all patients receiving neuroleptic drugs (SED-13, 124; SEDA-17, 51; SEDA-18, 50; SEDA-19, 46).

Presentation The characteristic signs and symptoms include mental changes and increased muscle rigidity leading to hyperthermia. Sustained muscle contraction can cause breakdown of muscle, resulting in increased creatine kinase activity and rhabdomyolysis.

Several cases have further illustrated the fea-

tures of neuroleptic malignant syndrome. For instance, in a series of 11 cases, symptoms occurred within 4 weeks of drug exposure, high potency drugs being involved in most cases (33^C). Three patients (27%) died of necrotic bed sores, septicemia, and respiratory failure. Complications were renal infection in four patients, gastrointestinal bleeding in one, and pneumonia in another.

Hyperventilation alternating with apnea has been reported as the main feature of a case of neuroleptic malignant syndrome associated with metoclopramide and cisapride (34^c).

A 77-year-old dentist had been well and working in his office until March 1991. He had been given metoclopramide (30 mg/day) and cisapride (7.5 mg/day) for gastroparesis, nausea, and poor appetite. A week later he noticed stiffness of the legs. Over the next week, he became increasingly immobile and tremulous and had difficulty in swallowing and speaking. A few days later, he was admitted with fever, leukocytosis, lethargy, muscle rigidity, tachycardia, and alternate hyperventilation and apnea. Neuroleptic malignant syndrome was diagnosed and metoclopramide and cisapride were discontinued; 13 days later he had recovered, but after 45 days he died of suffocation after vomiting.

Only a few previous cases of metoclopramide-induced neuroleptic malignant syndrome have been reported (SED-13, 1079).

Mechanism Dysfunction of the dopaminergic system has been suggested as a pathogenic mechanism in neuroleptic malignant syndrome (35^C). In a recent study, the complete coding sequences of the dopamine D$_2$ receptor gene was examined for structural abnormalities. The sample comprised 10 unrelated individuals with histories of sporadic neuroleptic malignant syndrome and two cases of familial neuroleptic malignant syndrome, a mother and her daughter. There was no statistical association, as only one patient was found with a mis-sense variation in the dopamine D$_2$ receptor gene.

Risk factors Lithium salts have been proposed as a risk factor for neuroleptic malignant syndrome, but in a recent case report lithium itself seems to have been responsible for the syndrome (36^c). In a 61-year-old man, neuroleptic malignant syndrome occurred 7 days after stopping neuroleptic drugs and starting lithium, 300 mg tds, in combination with ami-

triptyline tds; no depot formulations of neuroleptic drugs had been used and liver function was not altered.

Trauma may also be a risk factor for neuroleptic malignant syndrome (37[c]), (38[c]).

Diagnosis *The criteria required for the diagnosis of neuroleptic malignant syndrome, listed in appendix B of DSM-IV, include severe muscle rigidity and increased temperature, as well as at least two symptoms or signs from a list of 10. However, neuroleptic malignant syndrome sometimes presents without increased body temperature (39[cr]). In one case diagnosis and treatment were delayed because fever did not occur until several days after the onset of other symptoms (40[c]). The physicians felt that neuroleptic malignant syndrome was not a tenable diagnosis because of the absence of fever. A marked increase in temperature (rectal temperature 38.3°C) occurred for the first time about 84 h after the onset of rigidity.*

A case of neuroleptic malignant syndrome following the appearance of lethal catatonia has previously been reported (SEDA-19, 47), and a new case, in which a catatonic syndrome seemed to precede and follow neuroleptic malignant syndrome, has underlined the difficulty in differentiating the two syndromes (41[c]). In fact, they may be the same syndrome over a continuum of severity, the most severe example being lethal catatonia.

A 52-year-old Caucasian with a mild learning disability was thought to be predisposed to catatonic symptoms. Although there was no evidence of schizophrenia, he was given neuroleptic drugs and after a few days developed neuroleptic malignant syndrome, following recovery from two different episodes of catatonia, which appeared without any drug exposure. On each occasion he was successfully treated with diazepam.

Other case reports (42[c])—(44[c]) have drawn attention to the possibility of misdiagnosis of lethal catatonia: anyone who presents to a psychiatrist with agitation and altered sensorium is likely to be given a neuroleptic drug, to which are then attributed such signs of lethal catatonia as pyrexia and rigidity, and another diagnosis of neuroleptic malignant syndrome is made.

Treatment *The management and outcome of neuroleptic malignant syndrome may be improved by avoidance of suspected risk factors, early recognition of developing signs, education of staff, discontinuation of neuroleptic drugs, and supportive care. Recognition and investigation of neuroleptic malignant syndrome has led to a probable fall in mortality and morbidity.*

Dantrolene sodium has been very effective in rapidly reversing the effects of anesthesia-induced malignant hyperthermia, and case reports have described its success in the treatment of neuroleptic malignant syndrome (SED-13, 125); the ideal dose is questionable and varies enormously from case to case. Successful treatment with dantrolene has been reported (38[c]).

A haloperidol drip (5 mg/h) was used to treat severe agitation in a 38-year-old trauma patient; 2 days after admission, he remained agitated and the haloperidol dosage was increased to 10 mg/h, with a good result. After 4 days, the haloperidol was tapered off and a propofol drip was begun but, because of an increased serum triglyceride concentration, propofol was discontinued after 5 days. Haloperidol (2—5 mg intravenously every 2—4 h as necessary) was given again. Three days later the patient was in moderate respiratory distress, non-responsive to verbal stimuli, and catatonic. His temperature was 41.7°C, the pulse 140/min, and the systolic blood pressure 80 mmHg. When the temperature rose to 42.1°C dantrolene sodium (2 mg/kg intravenously) was given and the temperature fell to 38.5°C within 3 h. After 4 days (six doses) of dantrolene sodium, the patient remained afebrile and his creatine kinase activity fell to 1350 IU/l. The creatine kinase activity peaked at 10 316 IU/l on the second day and fell to within the reference range by the 11th day.

Sequelae *Sequelae have been reported after neuroleptic malignant syndrome (SEDA-16, 50; SEDA-19, 48), and new cases of neurological damage have been reported.*

A 27-year-old man treated for neuroleptic malignant syndrome with dantrolene sodium (80 mg intravenously), bromocriptine (5 mg/12 h), and fluid replacement developed leg myalgia, impaired motility, and loss of vision a few days later (45[c]). Electromyography showed signs of axonotmesis in the tibialis anterior, triceps brachii, and forearm flexor muscles; 8 months later the condition persisted.

A 42-year-old woman with a bipolar psychiatric disorder developed neuroleptic malignant syndrome and died (46[c]). Autopsy showed widespread rhabdomyolysis and myoglobin-induced renal tubular necrosis. Diagnosis and treatment with dantrolene 2 mg/kg were delayed by 8 and 10 days, respectively.

Endocrine, metabolic   The *syndrome of inappropriate antidiuretic hormone secretion* (SIADH; SED-13, 125) is characterized by sustained release of antidiuretic hormone from the posterior pituitary. This causes a reduced ability to excrete a dilute urine, fluid retention, and expansion of the extracellular fluid volume with hypo-osmolarity. One of the cardinal sins is hyponatremia. Psychotropic drug-induced SIADH has been reviewed (47[R]).

Neuroleptic drugs may cause *galactorrhea* by increasing pituitary prolactin release (SED-13, 125; SEDA-17, 56; SEDA-18, 50). The individuality and complexity of this reaction can lead to underestimation of its frequency. The occurrence of galactorrhea has been studied in 150 hospitalized schizophrenic women (20–42 years old) treated with different dosages of neuroleptic drugs (48[C]). In 21 cases galactorrhea occurred between the 7th and 75th days after the start of neuroleptic therapy; seven other women reported that it had occurred during early neuroleptic drug treatment before hospitalization. Surprisingly, 12 of the 28 affected patients welcomed this effect, six saw the effect as reinforcing their feminine identity, and four as an expression of their ability to conceive children. Only eight (of the 28) mentioned the effect on their own initiative and/or had spoken to their doctor about it.

Weight gain has long been a well-known adverse effect of antipsychotic drugs (SED-13, 125). The authors of a review concluded that controlling weight gain could improve compliance and patients' physical health, and also increase social acceptance of the mentally ill (49[R]).

Liver   In a recent review of the hepatotoxicity of different psychotropic agents, the specific features of neuroleptic-induced liver damage have been discussed (50[R]). Likewise, the estimated prevalence of increased liver enzyme during treatment with neuroleptic drugs is said to be relatively high, yet the incidence of clinical *jaundice* in patients receiving chlor-

promazine, for instance, has been reported to be lower (0.5–1%).

Gastrointestinal   *Ischemic colitis* (SEDA-17, 57) and *acute necrotizing colitis* (SED-13, 127; SEDA-19, 50) have been associated with neuroleptic drugs, and a new case has been reported (51[C]).

A 32-year-old man treated for several years with phenothiazine for chronic psychosis developed acute necrotizing colitis. He was taking no other drugs. He required emergency total colectomy and was discharged after 7 weeks of hospitalization in the intensive care unit.

The pathophysiological mechanism of the syndrome has been related to the anticholinergic effect of neuroleptic drugs, which can be reinforced by the concomitant administration of anticholinergic drugs, resulting in a reduction in intestinal peristalsis and subsequent distension.

Skin and appendages   Complications at the site of injection of depot neuroleptic drugs may occur more often than has previously been documented, according to the results of a prospective study of the prevalence and types of complications in 217 patients who received 2354 injections (52[C]). There were 31 episodes of unusual *pain*, 21 of *bleeding* or *hematoma*, 19 of clinically important *leakage of drug* from the injection site, 11 of *acute inflammatory induration*, and two of *transient nodules*. Higher concentrations were associated with a higher risk of complications.

Nicolau syndrome (embolia cutis medicamentosa) is local, aseptic, cutaneous, and sometimes muscular necrosis at an intramuscular injection site. A recent case report (53[cr]) has further emphasized the importance of taking precautions like back-aspirating before giving an intramuscular injection and stopping the procedure if pain occurs.

A sedative mixture (meperidine, 12.5 mg, promethazine, 3.25 mg, and chlorpromazine, 3.25 mg in a total of 1.5 ml) was injected into the upper anterolateral aspect of the left thigh of a 2-year-old boy about to undergo renal biopsy for nephrotic syndrome. There was intense pain with an immediate pale macula at the injection site, followed by erythema, which within hours became a stellate, livedoid, violaceous patch, painful to the touch. Six days later the lesion was well-defined, reticulate, violaceous to blackish, measuring 2—6 cm, the center of which corresponded to the injection site. Gradually, a black eschar appeared; it fell off after 3 months, leaving a pink, atrophic scar with loss of adnexa.

An *ulcerative skin reaction* resulting from a subcutaneous infusion of methotrimeprazine (a phenothiazine) and diamorphine has also been reported (54[c]). These types of infusions are frequently used, especially in patients who require sedation or an antiemetic. They require careful medical supervision.

Musculoskeletal Case reports of psychotropic drug-related *rhabdomyolysis* have been previously dealt with in these Annuals (SEDA-17, 58; SEDA-19, 50). A new case of rhabdomyolysis with acute renal failure after large doses of haloperidol has been published (55[c]). The main feature was the lack of high temperature and rigidity, which classically characterize the neuroleptic malignant syndrome.

Sexual function Most antipsychotic agents affect sexual function, although it is not clear to what extent the psychiatric disorder and/or the pharmacological treatment are responsible. Sexual function has been compared in treated ($n = 51$) and untreated ($n = 20$) schizophrenic men and healthy subjects ($n = 51$) (56[c]) using a published questionnaire (57[Cr]). All the participants were aged 21—45 years and were married or had been living in a stable relationship with a female sexual partner for at least 6 months. Alcohol and/or drug abusers were excluded as were subjects with physical illness. The strength of coital erection was significantly reduced in the schizophrenic population, and more so in the treated than in the untreated patients. The strength of masturbatory erection was also reduced in the treated schizophrenic patients but unaltered in the untreated. Ease of sexual arousal was significantly reduced only in the treated patients.

Miscellaneous In a double-blind crossover study (2×8 weeks; $n = 34$) the efficacy of zuclopenthixol and haloperidol have been compared in learning-disabled patients (58[c]). There were no differences in either the

number or severity of adverse effects. The adverse effects most frequently cited were *fatigue* ($n = 8$) and *increased duration of sleep* ($n = 7$).

Risk factors Psychiatric patients are often smokers, and schizophrenics are said to have a higher frequency of smoking than healthy people. *Cigarette smoking* has been surveyed in all patients hospitalized at a state hospital in Pennsylvania ($n = 360$) (59[C]); most ($n = 325$, 90%) were taking neuroleptic drugs. The overall frequency of smoking in the population was 79%; more men (88%) than women (63%) and more schizophrenic (85%) than non-schizophrenic patients (67%) were smokers. High dosages of neuroleptic drugs (over 1000 mg/day chlorpromazine equivalents) were associated with smoking in a univariate analysis, the odds ratio being 3.3 (95% CI 1.3—7.9), but multivariate logistic regression analysis showed no relation.

Cytochrome P450 CYP2D6 is responsible for the metabolism of several neuroleptic drugs. Up to 10% of the population are slow metabolizers (60[C]), and many drugs commonly used by older patients competitively or non-competitively inhibit CYP2D6. The role of *phenotypic variation in CP2D6* has been examined in relation to the adverse effects of perphenazine (0.1 mg/kg for 2 weeks) in 45 in-patients with dementia (81 ± 8 years of age), all of whom were being treated for the first time (61[C]). By debrisoquine phenotyping 40 were extensive metabolizers. Adverse effects, which were predominantly extrapyramidal and sedative, scored significantly higher in the five poor metabolizers.

Withdrawal effects The risks associated with neuroleptic drug withdrawal in schizophrenic patients have been estimated by meta-analysis of 66 studies involving a total of 4365 subjects (3141 subjects withdrawn from neuroleptic therapy and 1224 comparison subjects maintained on neuroleptic drug therapy) (62[Cr]). The mean rates of relapse for the withdrawal and maintenance groups were 52 and 16%, respectively, over a mean follow-up period of 9.7 months. No specific predictors of relapse were found, except for average length of follow-up. The authors raised a possible clinical and medicolegal dilemma, since a physician may be held liable either for withdrawing neuroleptic therapy and 'precipitating' a relapse or for maintaining neuroleptic therapy and 'predisposing' to tardive dyskinesia. The optimal solution in a substantial proportion of cases would probably be to taper neuroleptic drug therapy slowly to the lowest dosage that would satisfactorily control the symptoms of schizophrenia.

Abrupt discontinuation of therapy (suspension therapy) has been tried in a study of 22 schizophrenic patients in whom haloperidol has produced a partial remission (defined by a reduction in the Brief Psychiatric Rating Scale total score by 50% or less) (63[C]). After 3 weeks of treatment at a mean daily dose of about 30 mg, abrupt discontinuation had a favorable effect on depression and lack of drive; extrapyramidal adverse effects underwent remission. However, the effects of discontinuation were extremely variable, and three types were distinguished in one-third of the cases: no improvement; partial, substantial remission, yet neuroleptic medication was resumed for therapeutic reasons; and favorable, almost complete remission, neuroleptic medication being resumed for prophylactic reasons.

Second-generation effects An infant girl developed *psychomotor disturbances* at the age of 2 weeks (64[c]). Her mother had received perphenazine decanoate 108 mg by intramuscular injection four times during the second and third trimesters of pregnancy. The signs resembled those of tardive dyskinesia, and periodically the baby was restless and uttered high-pitched cries.

Interactions The pharmacokinetic and pharmacodynamic interactions of antipsychotic drugs with antihypertensive drugs have been reviewed (65[R]). Some *β-blockers*, such as propranolol or pindolol, increase plasma concentrations of thioridazine or chlorpromazine. Accordingly, the combination of a β-blocker with a phenothiazine should be avoided if possible.

In a randomized, double-blind 6-week study in 41 patients, of the effects of adding fluoxetine to neuroleptic drugs in schizophrenia, *fluoxetine* significantly increased the serum concentrations of the neuroleptic drugs (66[C]). All of the patients had received a stable dose of a depot neuroleptic for at least 6 months and were randomly assigned to fluoxetine 20 mg/day (n = 20) or placebo (n = 21). Serum concentrations of fluphenazine increased by 65% from baseline to week six in the 15 patients who took fluoxetine compared with 11% in the 11 patients in the placebo group. Fluoxetine increased serum haloperidol concentrations at week four by 20% in three patients, compared with a mean fall of 13% in five patients in the placebo group. Surprisingly, the percentage change in serum neuroleptic drug concentrations from baseline to week six did not correlate with changes in SAS scores, the akathisia item of the SAS, or AIMS in 17 patients in the fluoxetine group.

Thioridazine seems to inhibit the metabolism of *trazodone*. When thioridazine 40 mg/day was given for 1 week to 11 depressed patients who had taken trazodone for 1—18 weeks, mean plasma trazodone concentrations increased significantly (from 713 to 969 ng/ml) (67[C]). The clinical significance of this is not clear.

Two patients, aged 86 and 89, became agitated after being given a preoperative injection of 50 mg of *pethidine* (*meperidine*) and 25 mg of promethazine, and surgery had to be cancelled (68[c]). Promethazine potentiates the effects of opiates, but the mechanism is unknown.

Monitoring adverse effects Scales for measuring the adverse effects neuroleptic drugs have appeared in the last few years (SEDA-19, 42), and a new scale (the Liverpool University Neuroleptic Side Effect Rating Scale, LUNSERS) has been validated (69[C]). While new scales may improve the assessment of adverse effects, the fact that there are many of them precludes homogeneity.

Whether the dosage or plasma concentration of a neuroleptic drug predict clinical improvement or adverse effects during treatment has been controversial (SED-13, 117; SEDA-19, 41). The authors of two different studies, in the light of their results, have strongly advocated the use of neuroleptic drug plasma concentrations as a guide to optimizing dosages (70[C]), (71[C]); nevertheless, in clinical practice, the dosing of antipsychotic drugs depends on trial and error. In the first study, fluphenazine was given in fixed, randomized, double-blind dosages (10, 20, or 30 mg/day) for 4 weeks to 72 in-patients with acute schizophrenic exacerbations (70[C]). Neither dosage nor plasma concentration predicted response. However, among the responders both dosage and plasma concentration were significant predictors of the magnitude of response. Akathisia was more common and extrapyramidal symptoms more severe at higher plasma concentrations. By means of multivariate analysis, akathisia was predicted by the log dose/kg and the log plasma concentration. When dosage and plasma concentration were analysed separately, only log plasma concentration predicted akathisia. Therefore, plasma concentration was more useful in predicting akathisia. In the second study haloperidol oral dosages and blood concentrations were compared in 43 consecutive chronic schizophrenics identified as 'non-responsive patients' (71[C]). All medications were given three times a day. None of the 15 individuals with maximum blood concentrations below 30 ng/ml had evidence of adverse effects; three (19%) of 16 with maximum concentrations between 30 and 50 ng/ml had evidence of toxicity; and 10 (91%) of 11 were toxic with blood concentrations over 50 ng/ml. Adverse effects abated or disappeared when the blood concentration was reduced. The oral dosage of haloperidol needed to achieve a blood concentration of 10 ng/ml, considered as optimum in most of the cases, was 6.5—100 mg/day, a 15-fold difference. Four of the eight patients with the highest dosage to blood concentration ratios were also taking anticonvulsants, which may have contributed (SED-13, 130).

INDIVIDUAL DRUGS

Clotiapine

Clotiapine is an atypical antipsychotic agent which shares with clozapine strong antiserotonergic properties. It was introduced in Europe in the 1960s, at the same time as clozapine. *Compulsive behavior* in relation to washing and cleaning has been reported during treatment with clotiapine in an 8-year-old schizophrenic child (72[cr]). The symptoms

appeared within 2 days of the start of treatment, lasted unchanged for 2 weeks, and with behavioral treatment gradually subsided over the next 2 weeks, despite continuation of clotiapine. When the dosage of clotiapine was later increased, the compulsive symptoms also increased. The authors suggest that antagonistic activity at postsynaptic serotonin receptors might have been responsible for the development of obsessive-compulsive symptoms, according to a hyposerotonergic hypothesis of obsessive-compulsive disorder.

Clozapine *(SED-13, 118; SEDA-17, 59; SEDA-18, 52; SEDA-19, 51)*

The efficacy and safety of clozapine treatment have been comprehensively reviewed (73[R]). MEDLINE, MEDLARS, and PSYCLIT databases were searched back to 1966 and references in the articles obtained were checked to ensure that relevant articles not otherwise identified were included. The analysis showed that the most significant adverse effects of clozapine therapy include: *agranulocytosis*, the risk of developing agranulocytosis with clozapine is 10 times greater than that with traditional neuroleptic drugs, with a cumulative incidence ranging from 0.05 to 2%; *seizures*, the rate of occurrence being 1—10%; *weight gain* (13—23%); *hypotension* (8—13%); *tachycardia* (12—25%); *sedation*, the most common adverse effect (20—50%); perhaps *rebound psychosis* (with abrupt discontinuation of medication). Clozapine-induced agranulocytosis is most likely to occur within the first 6 months of treatment, and 75—80% of all cases occur within the first 4—18 weeks. The authors concluded that there is substantial evidence that clozapine is associated with increased risks of agranulocytosis and seizures, and is also associated with a reduced likelihood of extrapyramidal adverse effects (incidence 4—7%). Clozapine is said to have a lower risk of neuroleptic malignant syndrome and tardive dyskinesia. On the other hand, most of the studies analysed showed that clozapine is at least as effective as traditional neuroleptic drugs.

In an Oregon state psychiatric hospital, 287 patients received clozapine, 5% of all those treated from May 1991 to January 1994 (74[C]). Most of the patients (83%) continued clozapine therapy and 17% discontinued it because of lack of clinical improvement, refusal to comply with therapeutic criteria, or adverse reactions. Furthermore, 61% of the patients who took clozapine were discharged to the community while still taking the drug, and 55% were discharged from hospital less than 6 months after starting clozapine. Of the in-patients who were taking clozapine at the end of the study, 45% had been taking it for at least 1 year. Only 1% of the patients had clozapine withdrawn because of leukopenia; one of these patients had agranulocytosis.

Older patients may be more prone to the adverse effects of clozapine. Clozapine was prescribed for four patients over the age of 65, in two of whom psychotic symptoms were eventually relieved (75^c). All four experienced events after starting to take clozapine, including falls (two patients), symptomatic bradycardia (two patients) and delirium (one patient). All of these adverse effects occurred with dosages ranging from 6.25 to 37.5 mg/day, and the three patients with moderate to severe dementia experienced these severe adverse effects after administration of the first dose.

Clozapine, in low dosages, effectively suppressed psychotic symptoms in Parkinsonian patients taking dopaminergic drugs (76^c). There was no motor deterioration and neutropenia did not occur. In some patients in whom clozapine was withdrawn the psychiatric symptoms returned.

Cardiovascular During the period from December 1991 to November 1993, in a series of 70 patients who received clozapine, six patients, all aged between 25 and 54, died (77^{cr}). At autopsy pulmonary embolism was found to be the cause of death in two. Obesity, prolonged bed rest, and left and right ventricular failure are conditions that have been associated with a higher risk of venous thromboembolism. Other fatal cases have been reported (78^c), (79^{cr}). The immediate cause of death was said to be an embolus in the central pulmonary artery in the first report (78^c); the second report details two patients who died suddenly on the 63rd and 86th days of treatment with clozapine (79^{cr}). Although autopsies were not carried out, deaths were

attributed to myocardial infarction and pulmonary embolism, respectively.

Dose-dependent *electrocardiographic changes* are relatively common during treatment with antipsychotic drugs (SED-13, 119). Findings comparable to those seen with other neuroleptic drugs have been observed with clozapine, and the rate of occurrence has been estimated at 10% (SEDA-17, 60). There has since been a case of ventricular extra beats in a 44-year-old man who took clozapine 350 mg/day (80^c).

Clozapine-induced *hypotension* (SED-13, 119; SEDA-18, 55) has been successfully treated with a combination of moclobemide (a reversible inhibitor of monoamine oxidase A) and tyramine contained in Bovril (81^c).

Nervous system *Extrapyramidal adverse effects* of clozapine and haloperidol have been compared in an open study of 92 patients treated with clozapine for the first time, and 59 patients treated with haloperidol (82^c). Anticholinergic medication was used by 24% of those taking clozapine compared with 62% of those taking haloperidol. The 12-week cumulative incidence rates of extrapyramidal effects were (clonidine vs. haloperidol): tremor 24 vs. 39%; bradykinesia 21 vs. 48%; akathisia 5.6 vs. 32%. Thus, clozapine is not entirely free of extrapyramidal symptoms, but they are less common and usually less severe than those due to typical antipsychotic drugs.

Cases of *obsessive-compulsive symptoms* during clozapine treatment have been described (SEDA-17, 62; SEDA-19, 51), but their incidence and significance are still unclear. The hospital records of 142 randomly selected in-patients who started taking clozapine before July 1992 have been reviewed retrospectively (83^c). No de novo obsessive-compulsive symptoms were found that could be attributed to clozapine. However, the authors pointed out that retrospective analysis carries a significant risk of under-reporting bias.

Three cases of a *tic-like syndrome* associated with clozapine have been reported, purportedly the first reported cases (84^c). Dosage reduction resulted in gradual improvement in two cases. In the third case, a 26-year-old man who took clozapine 800 mg/day for 2 months developed tic-like facial movements. Obsessive-compulsive thinking was noticed at about the same time and clomipramine 25 mg/day was added. He gradually improved.

Seizures due to neuroleptic drugs are rare. However, clozapine is apparently associated with a higher prevalence than average, ranging from 1 to 5%, and the effect is dose dependent (SED-13, 120; SEDA-18, 53). Since a previous report of four cases of myoclonic jerks and drop attacks (SEDA-17, 62), there has been a report of five patients with clozapine-induced dose-dependent myoclonus (85[c]). All developed episodes of predominantly orofacial myoclonus that alternated between the two sides of the face and never occurred bilaterally. The symptoms were aggravated by psychological stress. There were no changes in consciousness nor any signs of sensory impairment during the episodes. The symptoms improved after reduction in clozapine dosage and subsided completely after withdrawal.

Dystonia has previously been associated with clozapine (SEDA-19, 52), and a new case has been reported in a 30-year-old woman (86[c]). Five days after starting clozapine 125 mg/day she had an oculogyric crisis that resolved rapidly with benztropine. Two more crises occurred 8 days later (clozapine dosage 250 mg/day), and they also responded to intramuscular benztropine. Regular oral procyclidine was prescribed and no further dystonias occurred.

Neuroleptic malignant syndrome It has been postulated that clozapine is unlike to cause the neuroleptic malignant syndrome, and that it can even be used with patients who have recovered or are recovering from this syndrome. Nevertheless, there have been some reports of the syndrome during clozapine therapy (SEDA-18, 52; SEDA-19, 53). Ten new cases associated with the use of clozapine (87[CR]) and another new case in a 33-year-old man, who also developed *disseminated intravascular coagulation* (88[c]), have been reported. Furthermore, a review of the literature from 1966 revealed 11 published case reports of neuroleptic malignant syndrome related to clozapine. The authors of this review added three new cases seen in Australia occurring in an estimated 1500 patients exposed to the drug (89[CR]). It seems

therefore that neuroleptic malignant syndrome does occur with clozapine and that its incidence may be as common as with the classic neuroleptic drugs. Nevertheless, the features of clozapine-induced neuroleptic malignant syndrome may be somewhat different, with fewer extrapyramidal adverse effects and a smaller rise in creatine kinase activity. However, two cases of extremely high serum creatine kinase activities (34 360 and 47 195 U/l, reference range 40—210) have been reported in asymptomatic out-patients treated with clozapine (90[c]). These patients were among approximately 28 members of a clozapine clinic in whom creatine kinase was monitored intermittently. It is possible that subclinical muscle injury also occurred.

Fever while taking clozapine may be considered as a sign of either neuroleptic malignant syndrome or agranulocytosis with an associated infection. In a retrospective review of the first 51 patients admitted to a Massachusetts hospital in 1990, 13 patients (26%) developed a fever; clozapine was withdrawn briefly and then restarted safely (91[C]). Two of the 51 patients had had a previous episode of neuroleptic malignant syndrome, but neither had fever during treatment with clozapine. There were no cases of agranulocytosis.

Hematological Recombinant granulocyte colony-stimulating factor (filgrastim) is currently being used to treat clozapine-induced *agranulocytosis* (SEDA-17, 63; SEDA-18, 55; SEDA-19, 54). Three additional cases of patients who developed clozapine-induced agranulocytosis and were successfully treated with filgrastim have been reported (92[cr]). White blood count and absolute neutrophil count returned to within the reference ranges in each patient after treatment with filgrastim 300 µg/day subcutaneously for 5—8 days. There were no adverse effects of filgrastim.

An association between some haplotypes and agranulocytosis has been reported (SED-13; 126). The selective vulnerability of patients to agranulocytosis and its association with human leukocyte antigen (HLA) haplotypes suggest a genetic basis for this hematological reaction to clozapine. HLA alleles and haplotypes of 31 patients with clozapine-induced agranulocytosis, 10 Ashkenazi Jews and 21 of non-Jewish ancestry, were compared with those of 52 patients (33 Ashkenazi Jews, 19 non-Jewish) (93[C]). The HLA haplotype was a marker for a risk of agranulocytosis in the Ashkenazi patients. The authors hypothesized that genes of the major histocompatibility complex, other than class I and class II, are responsible for clozapine-induced agranulocytosis; among them are variants of loci for the heat-shock proteins 70 and tumor necrosis factor.

Intermittent leukocytosis in an afebrile patient with intervening periods of normal white blood cell counts has been reported purportedly for the first time (94[cr]). It was suspected to have been related to pretreatment splenectomy.

A 50-year-old man with chronic schizophrenia was taking clozapine 350 mg/day, atenolol 50 mg/day for hypertension, and loxapine 50 mg at bedtime, the last being gradually discontinued. He had had a head injury and splenectomy at age 17 following a motor vehicle accident. There was no history of any blood dyscrasia. During the first 14 weeks of treatment, his white blood cell count remained in the range $5.2-12.2 \times 10^9$/l. During week 16 he developed a white cell count of 15.0×10^9/l, in the absence of a sore throat, a rash, or influenza-like symptoms. Subsequently, during weeks 16—23, he had intermittent leukocytosis alternating with normal white cell counts. All episodes of leukocytosis were due to neutrophilia, with normal lymphocyte, monocyte, and eosinophil counts.

Liver Patients taking clozapine often have increased liver enzymes (SEDA-17, 59), with no further consequences in most cases. The rate of liver dysfunction has been estimated at 1% (SEDA-15, 51). Two cases of *hepatitis* have been reported.

A 30-year-old woman who had been an intravenous opiate abuser several years earlier developed increased transaminase activities after 9 days of treatment with clozapine 250 mg/day, peaking after 14 days (133 U/l for aspartate aminotransferase and 424 U/l for alanine aminotransferase; reference ranges 9—32 and 7—55, respectively) (86[c]). There was no evidence of viral infection and no other drugs had been prescribed. With dosage reduction to 150 mg/day, her transaminase activities gradually fell over 4 weeks. After a second graduated dosage increase to 400 mg/day, liver function test results continued to normalize 8 weeks after peak activities. After 2 weeks at this dosage, however, a further transaminase increase occurred. This resolved with a dosage reduction to 200 mg/day.

A 35-year-old man with schizoaffective disorders

was given clozapine 300 mg/day (95[c]). On days 25—31, he complained intermittently of various symptoms, including joint pain, chills, nausea, fatigue, emesis, abdominal pain, and diarrhea. On day 32, he developed a pruritic rash on the backs of both hands and on his upper back. He also experienced angioedema, with a swollen lower lip and right lower cheek. Clozapine was discontinued on day 32. On day 33 he was febrile and disoriented; his alanine transferase was 719 U/l and his aspartate transferase 200 U/l. Serological tests for hepatitis A, B, and C were negative. Laboratory results normalized within 4—5 weeks.

Gastrointestinal Clozapine has been associated with nocturnal *hypersalivation* (SED-12, 113). Sialorrhea has been estimated to occur in 10 (96[Cr]) to 23% (97[Cr]) of patients. This phenomenon is poorly understood, since clozapine has a potent anticholinergic action. Transient *salivary gland swelling* has been retrospectively reviewed in four of 27 patients started on clozapine during a 6-month period (97[Cr]). None of these patients complained of hypersalivation. In three cases, serum amylase activity was increased in the presence of a normal serum lipase, indicating inflammation of the parotid gland. In all cases, the swelling resolved within days. It was concluded that, although it was not clearly related to sialorrhea, this phenomenon may share a similar pathophysiology and that the cause may be the formation of a calculus that blocks the duct and causes swelling. Another case of salivary gland swelling associated with clozapine has been reported (98[c]). The patient, a 43-year-old man, developed bilateral swelling and tenderness over both temporomandibular areas; his symptoms included dysphagia, anorexia, and sluggishness.

Although hypersalivation can be considered as a mild reaction, for some patients it is annoying and even socially stigmatizing. Anticholinergic drugs recommended to counteract sialorrhea may cause cardiovascular impairment and delirium. In a recent report, pirenzepine, a selective M1/4 muscarinic receptor antagonist, is said to have been successful in treating about 120 patients with clozapine-induced hypersalivation (96[Cr]). There were no adverse events, except mild diarrhea.

In addition to the muscarinic receptor blockade, clozapine also blocks α_2-adrenoceptors. Antagonism of α_2-adrenoceptors is related to reduced salivary secretion, and so this mechanism may underlie clozapine-induced hypersalivation. To test this hypothesis, the α_2-receptor agonist lofexidine was given to one patient in whom hypersalivation was particularly distressing (99[c]). With the addition of lofexidine 0.2 mg bd, there was significant improvement.

Three cases of diarrhea in patients with no infective cause have been previously reported (SEDA-17, 63). Four new cases of *eosinophilic colitis* have been associated with clozapine therapy (100[cr]). The authors proposed that clozapine should be added to the list of agents that may be associated with isolated allergic eosinophilic colitis. In contrast, it is known that clozapine often causes *constipation*. The Sandoz package insert mentions a 14% prevalence of this adverse effect; severe constipation has been estimated as occurring in 7.3% of cases (SEDA-17, 60). The authors of a recent study of 53 patients taking clozapine found a 60% prevalence of constipation (101[c]). The data were collected through a combination of chart reviews, patient interviews, and staff reports. One severe case of constipation resulted in death from aspiration of vomit secondary to obstruction of the transverse colon. In addition, a case of a prolonged postoperative paralytic ileus in a 42-year-old man taking long-term clozapine has been reported (102[cr]).

Urinary system   *Enuresis* has been described during clozapine therapy (SEDA-15, 53; SEDA-19, 54). Clozapine-induced enuresis has been successfully treated with intranasal desmopressin in a 32-year-old man (103[c]).

Skin and appendages   Dermatological adverse effects with clozapine have an estimated incidence of 1.2% (SEDA-17, 60). *Photosensitivity* occurred in a 56-year-old man after he had sat in the sun for several hours (104[c]). He had had a similar reaction with chlorpromazine.

Risk factors   A patient with chronic schizophrenia and peptic ulcer disease, developed agranulocytosis in the course of clozapine therapy, but this adverse effect disappeared within 7 days after withdrawal; the patient died 3 months later because of perforation of a duodenal ulcer (105[c]). Although peptic ulcer disease was suggested as a risk factor for agranulocytosis in this case, the relation was not clear.

Interactions   Caution has been recommended when starting clozapine in patients taking *benzodiazepines* (SEDA-19, 55). Three cases of delirium associated with clozapine and benzodiazepine combinations have been reported (106[c]).

The possible interaction of clozapine with *caffeine*, with subsequent psychotic exacerbation, may be due not only to a pharmacodynamic adenosine A_2 receptor-dopamine D_2 receptor mechanism in postsynaptic striatal membranes but also to a kinetic metabolic one (107[r]). Although most neuroleptic drugs are metabolized by the cytochrome P450 CYP2D6, clozapine and caffeine are both metabolized by CYP1A2.

Uncontrollable spasms that were diagnosed as myoclonic jerks were seen 79 days after *fluoxetine* had been given to a patient taking clozapine and lorazepam (108[c]). It was subsequently pointed out that other unidentified variables may have been involved in the reaction, since there was a long interval between the start of fluoxetine treatment and the appearance of myoclonus (109). Special caution is required in the use of clozapine with agents known or suspected to increase serum concentrations of other drugs, including fluoxetine and perhaps other serotonin reuptake inhibitors.

Lithium is often used in combination with neuroleptic drugs, and a major clinical concern is that lithium-induced leukocytosis may mask an impending drop in granulocyte count. In one case lithium given to a patient taking clozapine apparently caused an increase in both total leukocyte count and granulocyte count (110[c]).

The combination of clozapine with *valproate* in a 37-year-old man with schizoaffective disorder, bipolar type, resulted in significant sedation, confusion, functional impairment, and slurred speech (111[c]).

Droperidol *(SEDA-17, 64; SEDA-18, 55; SEDA-19, 55)*

Extrapyramidal adverse effects have been reported with droperidol, particularly *dys-*

tonia, akathisia, and *rigidity/akinesia*. A case of *neuroleptic malignant syndrome* has been published in a previously healthy 6-year-old girl who received droperidol 2.5 mg orally as premedication on induction of anesthesia (112[cr]).

Risperidone *(SEDA-17, 57; SEDA-18, 56; SEDA-19, 55)*

Risperidone is an atypical antipsychotic drug, which is a dopamine (D_2) and serotonin ($5\text{-}HT_2$) receptor antagonist. It was approved by the FDA (in 1994) and is only the second antipsychotic drug to have been introduced into the US since 1975. Some authors have suggested that risperidone has a low incidence of adverse effects, and although its reputation for efficacy and low toxicity is based mainly on pre-marketing studies, it has resulted in a rapid increase in its use.

A risk-benefit assessment of risperidone in schizophrenia has recently appeared (113[R]). The analysis showed that the most commonly reported adverse events are insomnia, agitation, anxiety, and headache. *Weight gain* is a feature of long-term risperidone treatment, and in one study the average weight gain was 2.3 kg. Less commonly reported are *somnolence, fatigue, dizziness, impaired concentration, constipation, dyspepsia, nausea, abdominal pain, blurred vision, erectile dysfunction, ejaculatory dysfunction, orgasmic dysfunction, rhinitis*, and *rash. Epileptic seizures* are rare. Risperidone also causes a dose-dependent increase in plasma prolactin concentration and this may lead to *galactorrhea, menstrual disturbances*, and *amenorrhea* in women and *infertility* in men. Risperidone may cause *neuroleptic malignant syndrome*, and there have been rare reports of water intoxication with hyponatremia, due either to *polydipsia* or the *syndrome of inappropriate secretion of antidiuretic hormone*.

Clinical trials data published between 1991 and 1994 have been reviewed (114[R]). The overall conclusion was that the data accumulated to date consistently suggest that risperidone is at least as effective as standard treatments for the positive symptoms of schizophrenia and is probably more effective for the negative symptoms; although the incidence of extrapyramidal effects with risperi-

done is lower than with haloperidol, it is also true that the absolute incidence of extrapyramidal effects is low with both drugs.

In a multinational, parallel-group, double-blind study in 110 centers in 15 countries, 1362 patients with chronic schizophrenia have been evaluated (115[C]). The patients were randomly assigned to risperidone 1, 4, 8, 12, or 16 mg/day or to haloperidol 10 mg/day for 8 weeks. The optimum risperidone dosages were 4 and 8 mg/day, with no differences in efficacy with haloperidol. Safety was primarily assessed by the Extrapyramidal Symptom Rating Scale (ESRS). Mean shifts in the maximum total ESRS scores versus baseline were significantly greater in haloperidol-treated patients (5.1, 95% CI 4.0–6.2) than in the risperidone 1-, 4-, 8-, and 12-mg/day groups (1.1, 0.3–1.9; 1.8, 0.9–2.7; 2.7, 1.8–3.6; and 3.2, 2.3–4.1, respectively). Risperidone was less likely to cause dystonic symptoms and akathisia.

The long-term effects of risperidone have been studied in 32 Swedish patients, all of whom took risperidone for at least 1 year and 19 for 2 years (116[C]). Risperidone produced significant improvement in the symptoms of schizophrenia, improved social functioning, and a reduction in the number of days spent in hospital. *Extrapyramidal effects* were assessed by the ESRS; there were significant reductions at 1 and 2 years on the questionnaire items, symptoms of parkinsonism, and parkinsonism plus dystonia plus dyskinesia. There was a slight increase in dyskinesia scores.

The efficacy and safety of risperidone versus clozapine have been compared in a randomized, double-blind, controlled trial in 59 patients, 20 of whom were treated with risperidone 4 mg/day, 19 with risperidone 8 mg/day, and 20 with clozapine 400 mg/day for 28 days (117[C]). Overall tolerability was significantly better with risperidone than clozapine. Adverse effects occurred in 47% with risperidone 4 mg, 53% with risperidone 8 mg, and 75% with clozapine. The most frequent spontaneously reported adverse effects were *dizziness, fatigue, disturbance of visual accommodation*, and *extrapyramidal adverse effects* in all treatment groups, and *increased salivation*, mainly in the clozapine-treated patients. There were no changes in vital signs during risperidone treatment, but clozapine was associated with a mean *reduction in heart rate* of 10 beats per minute.

Risk factors The effects of risperidone have been studied in seven children, mean age 12 years, with Tourette's syndrome or chronic motor tic disorder have been studied in an 11-week open trial (118[C]). The most frequent adverse effect was *weight gain*, ranging from 3.6 to 6.3 kg. In another open study, four patients with schizophrenia aged 12—17 years were treated with risperidone for 6 months without adverse effects (119[c]).

Risperidone has been used to treat 11 elderly hospitalized patients age 61—79 (120[C]). The most significant adverse effect that led to the withdrawal of risperidone was *hypotension*. Severe hypotensive episodes were noted in patients who had a history of hypertension and were taking either calcium antagonists or angiotensin-converting enzyme inhibitors; the *watery eyes* and '*heaviness of head*' reported by one patient have not been reported before.

Nervous system Risperidone is said to carry a reduced risk of extrapyramidal adverse effects. Five of six patients with psychosis and with akinetic-rigid syndromes experienced intolerable *exacerbation of parkinsonism* when they took risperidone (121[c]). Four subsequently did well with clozapine. The authors warned that risperidone is not a substitute for clozapine in treating psychosis in parkinsonian patients and hence should be used with caution.

A series of three cases of sensitivity to risperidone in Lewy body dementia has been published (122[c]).

A 63-year-old woman took risperidone for 2 days, then became rigid, mute, and unresponsive. An 88-year-old woman became stiff with extrapyramidal rigidity; she could not walk and needed to be fed until her physical and mental state began to return to pretreatment concentrations after 1 week. A 91-year-old man developed striking cogwheel rigidity and festinant and shuffling gait after 4 days of risperidone treatment; these extrapyramidal effects disappeared after risperidone was withdrawn.

In addition, risperidone-induced extrapyramidal adverse effects have been reported in a 30-year-old man with schizophrenia; he developed a parkinsonian tremor with risperi-

done 2 mg/day and the tremor worsened when the dosage was increased to 2 mg bd (123[c]).

The results of a monitoring program in 285 patients in a US psychiatric institution did not show a strong advantage of risperidone over better established antipsychotic agents with respect to extrapyramidal adverse effects (124[C]). The mean dosage of risperidone associated with extrapyramidal symptoms was 3.5 mg/day, considerably lower than that suggested by pre-marketing studies in a more selected patient group. The results of this study showed that the cost of using this drug are strikingly high. The profile of adverse reactions in this study suggests that risperidone produces rates of extrapyramidal adverse effects comparable to those seen with other antipsychotic drugs: perphenazine 1.7%, risperidone 2.1%, fluphenazine 1.8%, and haloperidol 1.8%. The authors warned that it is also possible that patients may have been selected for risperidone treatment because of a history of heightened sensitivity to extrapyramidal adverse effects, although the chart review suggested that this was the case in only one of six observed cases of risperidone-associated extrapyramidal adverse effects.

Since extrapyramidal adverse effects are related to the degree of D_2 receptor occupancy, a study has been conducted in nine patients taking risperidone 2—6 mg/day using ^{11}C-raclopride PET scanning in order to determine the in vivo D_2 receptor binding characteristics of risperidone (125[C]). The mean receptor occupancy was: 66% at 2 mg/day; 73% at 4 mg/day; and 79% at 6 mg/day. Three patients, those with the highest receptor occupancies, had mild extrapyramidal adverse effects, although none required antiparkinsonian drugs. The results of this study suggest that in vivo D_2 receptor occupancy by risperidone 4—6 mg/day is similar to that of typical neuroleptic drugs and higher than that of clozapine.

Two cases of *neuroleptic malignant syndrome* in elderly patients associated with risperidone have previously been reported (SEDA-19, 55) and now four new cases have been described (126[c])—(128[c]). In addition, a case of fever, confusion, and increased creatine phosphokinase in a 25-year-old man who took risperidone with lithium has also been reported (129[c]). The authors warned that lithium is thought to increase the risk of neurotoxicity and neuroleptic malignant syndrome during traditional therapy.

Dystonia has been reported to appear while changing from clozapine to risperidone in a 21-year-old man (130[c]).

Tardive dyskinesia during risperidone therapy has been reported, purportedly for the first time (131[c]).

A 28-year-old woman with a 6-year history of psychosis entered a 1-year double-blind comparison of haloperidol and risperidone. Four months later, her ESRS ratings showed moderate symptoms of tardive dyskinesia, predominantly affecting the jaw and tongue. She was taking risperidone 10 mg/day, and her dosage was reduced to 6 mg/day for 1 month without remission of tardive dyskinesia, but with a return of her psychotic symptoms.

Hypomania has been reported in a 31-year-old woman with chronic paranoid schizophrenia (132[c]). At the end of the first week on risperidone, she had hypomanic symptoms. She was elated, overactive, and disinhibited, and expressed grandiose ideation. The dosage was reduced and then the drug was withdrawn. She had had no previous manic episodes.

Four cases of *behavioral stimulation* characterized by anxiety, insomnia, and restlessness in the course of initiating risperidone treatment has been observed (133[c]).

Endocrine   Risperidone has previously been associated with increased *prolactin concentrations*. Three of five premenopausal women who were given risperidone developed galactorrhea, and all five developed amenorrhea (134[c]).

Sexual function   The package insert with risperidone states that priapism is a possible adverse effect. A case of a 41-year-old man with prolonged erection after 6 days of risperidone treatment has been reported (135[cr]).

Skin and appendages   A case of *angioedema* has been reported (136[c]).

Two weeks after starting risperidone 6 mg/day, a 30-year-old woman developed facial and periorbital edema. The dosage was halved and the edema subsequently subsided. Her mental state deteriorated, however, and risperidone was increased again to 6 mg/day. Within 3 days, her facial and periorbital edema recurred. Risperidone was withdrawn and the edema resolved completely over 2 weeks. She had had a similar reaction to lithium 1 year before.

Risk factors   Clinicians have been alerted to a potential cholinergic rebound (malaise, agitation, insomnia, restlessness, anorexia, nausea) that may occur when a potent antimuscarinic drug such as clozapine is abruptly replaced by another antipsychotic drug, such as risperidone, that does not have potent anticholinergic effects (137[r]).

REFERENCES

1. Faigel DO, Metz DC, Kochman ML. Torsade de pointes complicating the treatment of bleeding esophageal varices: association with neuroleptics, vasopressin, and electrolyte imbalance. Am J Gastroenterol 1995;90:822—4.
2. Di Salvo TG, O'Gara PT. Torsade de pointes caused by high-dose intravenous haloperidol in cardiac patients. Clin Cardiol 1995;18:285—90.
3. Dolan M, Boyd C, Shetty G. Neuroleptic induced sudden death a case report and critical review. Med Sci Law 1995;35:169—74.
4. Verdoux H, Magnin E, Bourgeois M. Neuroleptic effects on neuropsychological test performance in schizophrenia. Schizophr Res 1995; 14:133—9.
5. King DJ, Burke M, Lucas RA. Antipsychotic drug-induced dysphoria. Br J Psychiatry 1995; 167:480—2.
6. Ebadi M, Srinivasan SK. Pathogenesis, prevention, and treatment of neuroleptic-induced movement disorders. Pharmacol Rev 1995; 47:575—604.
7. Spila-Alegiani S, Diana G, Menniti-Ippolito F. Anticholinergic antiparkinsonian therapy in outpatients treated with neuroleptic drugs: a prescription survey. Eur J Clin Pharmacol 1995; 48:513—17.
8. Avorn J, Bohn RL, Mogun H, Gurwitz JH, Monane M, Everitt D, Walker A. Neuroleptic drug exposure and treatment of parkinsonism in the elderly: a case-control study. Am J Med 1995;99:48—54.
9. Playford ED, Britton TC, Thompson PD, Brooks DJ, Findley LJ, Marsden CD. Exacerbation of postural tremor with emergence of parkinsonism after treatment with neuroleptic drugs. J Neurol Neurosurg Psychiatry 1995;58:487—9.
10. Shader RI, Oesterheld JR. Case 5: the dextral dodder. J Clin Psychopharmacol 1995;15:232.
11. Mazure CM, Cellar JS, Bowers MB, Nelson

JC, Takeshita J, Zigun B. Assessment of extra-pyramidal symptoms during acute neuroleptic treatment. J Clin Psychiatry 1995;56:94—100.

12. Gall JAM, Drummer OH, Landgren AJ. Death due to benzhexol toxicity. Forensic Sci Int 1995;71:9—14.

13. Gold R, Lenox RH. Is there a rationale for iron supplementation in the treatment of akathisia? A review of the evidence. J Clin Psychiatry 1995;56:476—83.

14. Sachdev P. The epidemiology of drug-induced akathisia: Part I. Acute akathisia. Schizophr Bull 1995;21:431—49.

15. Baldessarini RJ. Clinical and epidemiologic aspects of tardive dyskinesia. J Clin Psychiatry 1985;46:8—13.

16. Chatterjee A, Chakos M, Koreen A, Geisler S, Sheitman B, Woerner M, Kane JM, Alvir J, Lieberman JA. Prevalence and clinical correlates of extrapyramidal signs and spontaneous dyskinesia in never-medicated schizophrenic patients. Am J Psychiatry 1995;152:1724—9.

17. Dorevitch A, Meretyk I, Umansky Y, Galili-Weisstub E. Antipsychotic drugs and tardive dyskinesia: preliminary results in an adolescent psychiatric ward. J Clin Pharmacol Ther 1995;20:63—5.

18. Pourcher E, Baruch P, Bouchard RH, Filteau MJ, Bergeron D. Neuroleptic associated tardive dyskinesias in young people with psychoses. Br J Psychiatry 1995;166:768—72.

19. Jeste DV, Caligiuri MP, Paulsen JS, Heaton RK, Lacro JP, Harris MJ, Bailey A, Fell RL, McAdams LA. Risk of tardive dyskinesia in older patients. Arch Gen Psychiatry 1995;52:756—65.

20. Goff DC, Tsai G, Beal MF, Coyle JT. Tardive dyskinesia and substrates of energy metabolism in CSF. Am J Psychiatry 1995;152:1730—6.

21. Sweet RA, Mulsant BH, Gupta B, Rifai AH, Pasternak RE, McEachram A, Zubenko GS. Duration of neuroleptic treatment and prevalence of tardive dyskinesia in late life. Arch Gen Psychiatry 1995;52:478—86.

22. Hegerl U, Juckel G, Müller-Schubert A, Pietzcker A, Gaebel W. Schizophrenics with small P300: a subgroup with a neurodevelopmental disturbance and a high risk for tardive dyskinesia? Acta Psychiatr Scand 1995;91:120—5.

23. Hayashi T, Yamawaki S, Nishikawa T, Jeste DV. Usage and side effects of neuroleptics in elderly Japanese patients. Am J Geriatr Psychiatry 1995;3:308—16.

24. Arthur H, Dahl ML, Siwers B, Sjöqvist F. Polymorphic drug metabolism in schizophrenic patients with tardive dyskinesia. J Clin Psychopharmacol 1995;15:211—16.

25. Fève A, Angelard B, Guily JL. Laryngeal tardive dyskinesia. J Neurol 1995;242:455—9.

26. Kruk J, Sachdev P, Singh S. Neuroleptic-induced respiratory dyskinesia. J Neuropsychiatry Clin Neurosci 1995;7:223—9.

27. Hyde TM, Egan MF, Brown RJ, Weinberger DR, Kleinman JE. Diurnal variation in tardive dyskinesia. Psychiatry Res 1995;56:53—7.

28. Schwarta M, Weller B, Erdreich M, Sharf B. Rabbit syndrome and tardive dyskinesia: two complications of chronic neuroleptic treatment. J Clin Psychiatry 1995;56:212.

29. Silver H, Geraisy N, Schwartz M. No difference in the effect of biperiden and amantadine on parkinsonian- and tardive dyskinesia-type invonluntary movements: a double-blind crossover, placebo-controlled study in medicated chronic schizophrenic patients. J Clin Psychiatry 1995;56:167—70.

30. Freudenreich O, McEvoy JP. Added amantadine may diminish tardive dyskinesia in patients requiring continued neuroleptics. J Clin Psychiatry 1995;56:173.

31. Raja M. Tardive dystonia. Prevalence, risk factors, and comparison with tardive dyskinesia in a population of 200 acute psychiatric inpatients. Eur Arch Psychiatry Clin Neurosci 1995;245:145—51.

32. Keck PE, Caroff SN, McElroy SL. Neuroleptic malignant syndrome and malignant hyperthermia: end of a controversy? J Neuropsychiatry Clin Neurosci 1995;7:135—44.

33. Arfai A, Pourafkary N. Experience with eleven cases of neuroleptic malignant syndrome. Iran J Med Sci 1995;20:38—41.

34. Shintani S, Shiigai T, Tsuchiya K, Kikuchi M. Hyperventilation alternating with apnea in neuroleptic malignant syndrome associated with metoclopramide and cisapride. J Neurol Sci 1995;128:232—3.

35. Ram A, Cao Q, Keck PE, Pope HG, Otani K, Addonizio G, McElroy SL, Kaneko S, Redlichova M, Gershon ES, Gejman PV. Structural change in dopamine D_2 receptor gene in a patient with neuroleptic malignant syndrome. Am J Med Genet Neuropsychiatry Genet 1995;60:228—30.

36. Fava S, Caruana Galizia A. Neuroleptic malignant syndrome and lithium carbonate. J Psychiatry Neurosci 1995;20:305—6.

37. Rother J, Jakob J, Bender HJ, Hewer W. Polytrauma und malignes neuroleptisches Syndrom. Kasuistische Darstellung diagnostischer Probleme. Anästhesiol Intensivmed Notf Med Schmerzther 1995;30:455—7.

38. Burke C, Fulda GJ, Castellano J. Neuroleptic malignant syndrome in a trauma patient. J Trauma 1995;39:796—8.

39. Velamoor VR, Swamy GN, Parmar L-RS, Williamson P, Caroff SN. Management of suspected neuroleptic malignant syndrome. Can J Psychiatry 1995;40:545—50.

40. Baker RW, Chengappa KNR. Further study of neuroleptic malignant syndrome. Am J Psychiatry 1995;152:1831.

41. Dent J. Catatonic syndrome following recovery from neuroleptic malignant syndrome. J Intell Disabil Res 1995;39:457—9.

42. Terlikowska M, Marzanski M. Roznicowanie miedzy ostra smiertelna katatonia i zlosliwym zespolem neuroleptycznym. Opis przypadku. Psychiatr Pol 1995;29:343—8.

43. Dammers S, Zeit T, Leonhardt M, Schar V, Agelink MW. Malignes neuroleptisches Syndrom. Dtsch Med Wochenschr 1995;120:1739—42.

44. Longhurst JG. Neuroleptic malignant syndrome. Br J Psychiatry 1995;166:537—8.

45. Mesejo A, Núñez C, Simó M, Blanquer J, Pérez PL, Ruiz F, Cuñat J. Síndrome neuroléptico maligno, fallo multiorgánico y polineuropatía periférica. Rev Neurol 1995;23:136—8.

46. Guadagnucci A, Tornaboni D, Vignali G, Mariotti M, Cincinelli A, Vignale L. Sindrome maligna da neurolettici. Minerva Med 1995;86:327—30.

47. Spigset O, Hedenmalm K. Hyponatraemia and the syndrome of inappropriate antidiuretic hormone secretion (SIADH) induced by psychotropic drugs. Drug Saf 1995;12:209—25.

48. Wesselmann U, Windgassen K. Galactorrhea: subjective response by schizophrenic patients. Acta Psychiatr Scand 1995;91:152—5.

49. Stanton JM. Weight gain associated with neuroleptic medication: a review. Schizophr Bull 1995;21:463—72.

50. Holt C, Csete M, Martin P. Hepatotoxicity of anesthetics and other central nervous system drugs. Gastroenterol Clin North Am 1995;24:853—74.

51. Ausseur A, Leroy C, Bazin B, Sarraz-Bournet B, Oureib J, Georges H. Entérocolite aiguë nécrosante au cours d'un traitement prolongé par neuroleptiques. Presse Méd 1995;24:577—9.

52. Hay J. Complications at site of injection of depot neuroleptics. Br Med J 1995;311:421.

53. Faucher L, Marcoux D. What syndrome is this? Nicolau syndrome. Pediatr Dermatol 1995;12:187—90.

54. Hatton MQF, McMurray A, Harnett AN. Ulcerative skin reaction from subcutaneous infusion of isotonic methotrimeprazine and diamorphine. Clin Oncol 1995;7:268—9.

55. Marsh SI, Dolson GM. Rhabdomyolysis and acute renal failure during high-dose haloperidol therapy. Renal Fail 1995; 17:475—8.

56. Aizenberg D, Zemishlany Z, Dorfman-Etrog P, Weizman A. Sexual dysfunction in male schizophrenic patients. J Clin Psychiatry 1995;56:137—41.

57. Schiavi RC, Schreiner-Engel P, Mandeli J, Schanzer H, Cohen E. Healthy aging and male sexual function. Am J Psychiatry 1990;147:766—71.

58. Malt UF, Nystad R, Bache T, Noren O, Sjaastad M, Solberg KO, Tonseth S, Zachariassen P, Mæhlum E. Effectiveness of zuclopenthixol compared with haloperidol in the treatment of behavioural disturbances in learning disabled patients. Br J Psychiatry 1995;166:374—7.

59. De Leon J, Dadvand M, Canuso C, White AO, Stanilla JK, Simpson GM. Schizophrenia and smoking: an epidemiological survery in a state hospital. Am J Psychiatry 1995;152:453—5.

60. Evans DAP, Maghoub A, Sloan TP, Idle JR, Smith RL. A family and population study of the genetic polymorphism of debrisoquin oxidation in a white British population. J Med Genet 1980; 17:102—5.

61. Pollock BG, Mulsant BH, Sweet RA, Rosen J, Altieri LP, Perel JM. Prospective cytochrome P450 phenotyping for neuroleptic treatment in dementia. Psychopharmacol Bull 1995;31:327—32.

62. Gilbert PL, Harris MJ, McAdams LA, Jeste DV. Neuroleptic withdrawal in schizophrenic patients. Arch Gen Psychiatry 1995;52:173—88.

63. Kuhs H, Folkerts H. Suspension therapy in acute schizophrenia. Neuropsychobiology 1995; 31:135—45.

64. Handal M, Matheson I, Bechensteen AG, Lindemann R. Antipsychotic agents and pregnant women. A case report. Tidsskr Nor Laegeforen 1995;115:2539—40.

65. Markowitz JS, Wells BG, Carson WH. Interactions between antipsychotic and antihypertensive drugs. Ann Pharmacother 1995;29:603—9.

66. Goff DC, Midha KK, Sarid-Segal O, Hubbard JW, Amico E. A placebo-controlled trial of fluoxetine added to neuroleptic in patients with schizophrenia. Psychopharmacology 1995;117:417—23.

67. Yasui N, Otani K, Kaneko S, Ohkubo T, Osanai T, Ishida M, Mihara K, Kondo T, Sugawara K, Fukushima Y. Inhibition of trazodone metabolism by thioridazine in humans. Ther Drug Monit 1995;17:333—5.

68. Irvin SM. Identification of potential problems for elderly outpatients after preoperative medication: a case study. J Post Anesth Nurs 1995;10:159—62.

69. Day JC, Wood G, Dewey M, Bentall RP. A self-rating scale for measuring neuroleptic side-effects. Br J Psychiatry 1995;166:650—3.

70. Levinson DF, Simpson GM, Cooper TB, Singh H, Yadalam K, Stephanos MJ. Fluphenazine plasma levels, dosage, efficacy, and side effects. Am J Psychiatry 1995;152:765—71.

71. Darby JK, Pasta DJ, Dabiri L, Clark L, Mosbacher D. Haloperidol dose and blood level variability: toxicity and interindividual and intraindividual variability in the nonresponder patient in the clinical practice setting. J Clin Psychopharmacol 1995;15:334—40.

72. Toren P, Samuel E, Weizman R, Golomb A, Eldar S, Laor N. Case study: emergence of transient compulsive symptoms during treatment with clothiapine. J Am Acad Child Adolesc Psychiatry 1995;34:1469—72.

73. Buchanan RW. Clozapine: efficacy and safety. Schizophr Bull 1995;21:579—91.

74. Love DJ, Woldemariam M. Clozapine use in an Oregon state psychiatric hospital. Am J Health-Syst Pharm 1995;52:508—10.

75. Pitner JK, Mintzer JE, Pennypacker LC, Jackson CW. Efficacy and adverse effects of clozapine in four elderly psychotic patients. J Clin Psychiatry 1995;56:180—5.

76. Rabey JM, Treves TA, Neufeld MY, Orlove E, Korczyn AD. Low dose clozapine in the treatment of levodopa-induced mental disturbances in Parkinson's disease. Neurology 1995;45:432—4.

77. Clardy J, Gale RH. Mortality risk and clozapine. Am J Psychiatry 1995;152:651.

78. Lilleng P, Morild I, Hope M. Clozapine and myocarditis. Tidsskr Nor Laegeforen 1995; 115:3026—7.

79. Diederich N, Keipes M, Graas M, Metz H. La clozapine dans le traitement des manifestations psychiatriques de la maladie de Parkinson. Rev Neurol 1995;151:251—7.

80. Aronowitz JS, Umbricht DSG, Safferman AZ. Clozapine and new-onset ECG abnormalities. Psychosomatics 1995;36:82—3.

81. Taylor D, Reveley A, Faivre F. Clozapine-induced hypotension treated with moclobemide and Bovril. Br J Psychiatry 1995;167:409—10.

82. Kurz M, Hummer M, Oberbauer H, Fleischhacker WW. Extrapyramidal side effects of clozapine and haloperidol. Psychopharmacology 1995; 118:52—6.

83. Ghaemi SN, Zarate CA, Popli AP, Pillay SS, Cole JO. Is there a relationship between clozapine and obsessive-compulsive disorder? A retrospective chart review. Compr Psychiatry 1995; 36:267—70.

84. Lindenmayer JP, Da Silva D, Buendia A, Zylberman I, Vital-Herne, M. Tic-like syndrome after treatment with clozapine. Am J Psychiatry 1995;152:649.

85. Bak TH, Bauer M, Schaub RT, Hellweg R, Reischies FM. Myoclonus in patients treated with clozapine: a case series. J Clin Psychiatry 1995;56:418—22.

86. Worrall R, Wilson A, Cullen M. Dystonia and drug-induced hepatitis in a patient treated with clozapine. Am J Psychiatry 1995;152:647—8.

87. Tsai G, Crisostomo G, Rosenblatt ML, Stern TA. Neuroleptic malignant syndrome associated with clozapine treatment. Ann Clin Psychiatry 1995;7:91—5.

88. Lowy A, Wilson A, Sachdev P, Lindeman R. Disseminated intravascular coagulopathy and thrombocytopenia associated with clozapine-induced neuroleptic malignant syndrome. Aust NZ J Med 1995;25:368.

89. Sachdev P, Kruk J, Kneebone M, Kissane D. Clozapine-induced neuroleptic malignant syndrome: review and report of new cases. J Clin Psychopharmacol 1995;15:365—71.

90. Kirson JI, McQuistion HL, Pierce DW. Severe elevations in serum creatine kinase associated with clozapine. J Clin Psychopharmacol 1995;15:287—8.

91. Nitenson NC, Kando JC, Frankenburg FR, Zanarini MC. Fever associated with clozapine administration. Am J Psychiatry 1995;152:1102.

92. Lamberti JS, Bellnier TJ, Schwarzkopf SB, Schneider E. Filgrastim treatment of three patients with clozapine-induced agranulocytosis. J Clin Psychiatry 1995;56:256—9.

93. Yunis JJ, Corzo D, Salazar M, Lieberman JA, Howard A, Yunis EJ. HLA associations in clozapine-induced agranulocytosis. Blood 1995;86: 1177—83.

94. Popli A, Pies R. Clozapine and leukocytosis. J Clin Psychopharmacol 1995;15:286—7.

95. Thatcher GW, Cates M, Bair B. Clozapine-induced toxic hepatitis. Am J Psychiatry 1995; 152:296—7.

96. Vasile JS, Steingard S. Clozapine and the development of salivary gland swelling: a case study. J Clin Psychiatry 1995;56:511—13.

97. Robinson D, Fenn H, Yesavage J. Possible association of parotitis with clozapine. Am J Psychiatry 1995;152:297—8.

98. Fritze J, Elliger T. Pirenzepine for clozapine-induced hypersalivation. Lancet 1995;346:1034.

99. Corrigan FM, MacDonald S, Reynolds GP. Clozapine-induced hypersalivation and the α_2 adrenoceptor. Br J Psychiatry 1995;167:412.

100. Friedberg JW, Frankenburg FR, Burk J, Johnson W. Clozapine-caused eosinophilic colitis. Ann Clin Psychiatry 1995;7:97—8.

101. Hayes G, Gibler B. Clozapine-induced constipation. Am J Psychiatry 1995;152:298.

102. Erickson B, Morris DM, Reeve A. Clozapine-associated postoperative ileus: case report and review of the literature. Arch Gen Psychiatry 1995;52:508—9.

103. Aronowitz JS, Safferman AZ, Lieberman JA. Management of clozapine-induced enuresis. Am J Psychiatry 1995;152:472.

104. Howanitz E, Pardo M, Losonczy M. Photosensitivity to clozapine. J Clin Psychiatry 1995; 56:589.

105. Zaluska M, Gajewska J. Agranulocytoza w trakcie stosowania kozapiny. Psychiatr Pol 1995;29:67—77.

106. Jackson CW, Markowitz JS, Brewerton TD. Delirium associated with clozapine and benzodiazepine combinations. Ann Clin Psychiatry 1995;7:139—41.

107. Carrillo JA, Jerling M, Bertilsson L. Comments to 'Interaction between caffeine and clozapine'. J Clin Psychopharmacol 1995;15:376—7.

108. Kingsbury SJ, Puckett KM. Effects of fluoxetine on serum clozapine levels. Am J Psychiatry 1995;152:473.

109. Baldessarini RJ, Centorrino F, Flood JG, Frankenburg FR, Kando J, Winkelman JW. Dr. Baldessarini and colleagues reply. Am J Psychiatry 1995;152:473—4.

110. Adityanjee. Modification of clozapine-induced leukopenia and neutropenia with lithium carbonate. Am J Psychiatry 1995;152:648—9.

111. Costello LE, Suppes T. A clinically significant interaction between clozapine and valproate. J Clin Psychopharmacol 1995;15:139—41.

112. Shaw A, Matthews EE. Postoperative neuroleptic malignant syndrome. Anaesthesia 1995; 50:246—7.

113. Curtis VA, Kerwin RW. A risk-benefit assessment of risperidone in schizophrenia. Drug Saf 1995;12:139—45.

114. Borinson RL. Clinical efficacy of serotonin-dopamine antagonists relative to classic neuroleptics. J Clin Psychopharmacol 1995;15 Suppl 1:24—9.

115. Peuskens J. Risperidone in the treatment of

patients with chronic schizophrenia: a multi-national, multi-centre, double-blind, parallel-group study versus haloperidol. Br J Psychiatry 1995;166:712—26.

116. Lindström E, Eriksson B, Hellgren A, von Knorring L, Eberhard G. Efficacy and safety of risperidone in the long-term treatment of patients with schizophrenia. Clin Ther 1995;17:402—11.

117. Klieser E, Lehmann E, Kinzler E, Wurthmann C, Heinrich K. Randomized, double-blind, controlled trial of risperidone versus clozapine in patients with chronic schizophrenia. J Clin Psychopharmacol 1995;15 Suppl 1:45—51.

118. Lombroso PJ, Scahill L, King RA, Lynch KA, Chappell PB, Peterson BS, McDougle CJ, Leckman JF. Risperidone treatment of children and adolescents with chronic tic disorders: a preliminary report. J Am Acad Child Adolesc Psychiatry 1995;34:1147—52.

119. Quintana H, Keshavan M. Case study: risperidone in children and adolescents with schizophrenia. J Am Acad Child Adolesc Psychiatry 1995;34:1292—6.

120. Madhusoodanan S, Brenner R, Araujo L, Abaza A. Efficacy of risperidone treatment for psychoses associated with schizophrenia, schizoaffective disorder, bipolar disorder, or senile dementia in 11 geriatric patients: a case series. J Clin Psychiatry 1995;56:514—18.

121. Rich SS, Friedman JH, Ott BR. Risperidone versus clozapine in the treatment of psychosis in six patients with parkinson's disease and other akinetic-rigid syndromes. J Clin Psychiatry 1995;56:556—9.

122. McKeith IG, Ballard CG, Harrison RWS. Neuroleptic sensitivity to risperidone in Lewy body dementia. Lancet 1995;346:699.

123. Mahmood T, Clothier EB, Bridgman R. Risperidone-induced extrapyramidal reactions. Lancet 1995;346:1226.

124. Carter CS, Mulsant BH, Sweet RA, Maxwell R, Coley K, Ganguli R, Branch R. Risperidone use in a teaching hospital during its first year after market approval: economic and clinical implications. Psychopharmacol Bull 1995;31: 719—25.

125. Kapur S, Remington G, Zipursky RB, Wilson AA, Houle S. The D_2 dopamine receptor occupancy of risperidone and its relationship to extrapyramidal symptoms: a pet study. Life Sci 1995;57:103—7.

126. Dave M, Singer S, Richards C, Boland RJ. Two cases of risperidone-induced neuroleptic malignant syndrome. Am J Psychiatry 1995; 152:1233—4.

127. Najara JE, Enikeev ID. Risperidone and neuroleptic malignant syndrome: a case report. J Clin Psychiatry 1995;56:534—5.

128. Murray S, Haller E. Risperidone and NMS? Psych Serv 1995;46:951.

129. Swanson CL, Price WA, McEvoy JP. Effects of concomitant risperidone and lithium treatment. Am J Psychiatry 1995;152:1096.

130. Radford JM, Brown TM, Borison RL. Unexpected dystonia while changing from clozapine to risperidone. J Clin Psychopharmacol 1995;15: 225—6.

131. Addington DE, Toews JA, Addington JM. Risperidone and tardive dyskinesia: a case report. J Clin Psychiatry 1995;56:484—5.

132. O'Croinin F, Zibin T, Holt L. Hypomania associated with risperidone. Can J Psychiatry 1995;40:51.

133. Byerly MJ, Greer RA, Evans DL. Behavioral stimulation associated with risperidone initiation. Am J Psychiatry 1995;152:1096—7.

134. Dickson RA, Dalby JT, Williams R, Edwards AL. Risperidone-induced prolactin elevations in premenopausal women with schizophrenia. Am J Psychiatry 1995;152:1102—3.

135. Tekell JL, Smith EA, Silva JA. Prolonged erection associated with risperidone treatment. Am J Psychiatry 1995;152:1097.

136. Cooney C, Nagy A. Angio-oedema associated with risperidone. Br Med J 1995;310:1204.

137. Gupta S, Daniel DG. Cautions in the clozapine-to-risperidone switch. Ann Clin Psychiatry 1995;7:149.

Emilio Perucca

7 Antiepileptic drugs

GENERAL TOPICS (SED-13, 136; SEDA-17, 72; SEDA-18, 61; SEDA-19, 61)

Nervous system *Drowsiness* is a common complaint in patients taking antiepileptic drugs, but it is difficult to document it objectively. Patients treated with phenytoin, phenobarbital, carbamazepine, and valproate ($n = 30$ in all) were less able to maintain wakefulness, measured by EEG, than healthy subjects ($n = 35$) and untreated epileptic patients ($n = 12$) (1[cr]). However, the untreated epileptic patients were not fully comparable in clinical characteristics to the drug-treated patients, and it is therefore unclear whether the impaired wakefulness was related to treatment or to the underlying disorder. Any inference about comparative sedative properties of the various drugs would be inappropriate from these data.

Endocrine, metabolic The incidence of *weight gain*, a complication of antiepileptic drug therapy, has been evaluated in a 12-year longitudinal study of 478 well-controlled patients taking monotherapy (2[c]). Of 180 patients taking valproic acid, 90 (50%) gained $1-11$ kg, with a mean weight gain of 2.7 kg in the 12 cases with self-imposed dietary restriction and 5.4 kg in the 78 cases without. Of 252 patients taking carbamazepine, 106 (42%) gained an average of 3.2 kg, while six of 16 patients (37%) taking other drugs gained on average 6.8 kg.

In 35 patients taking long-term phenytoin or carbamazepine, mean serum concentrations of *thyroid hormones* (T_4, FT_4, FT_3, and rT_3, but not T_3) were significantly lower than in 19 controls of similar age and sex (3[cr]). TSH concentrations were slightly higher in the patients, but the TSH response to TRH was not increased and other biochemical mea-

surements related to thyroid function were normal. Fourteen patients with subnormal FT_4 concentrations took part in a double-blind cross-over trial of thyroxine, without significant improvement in a clinical index of tissue hypothyroidism or systolic time intervals, although five subjects benefited subjectively. It was concluded that patients taking long-term anticonvulsant therapy do not need thyroxine supplementation.

Liver and pancreas A 26-year-old man with partial epilepsy had two episodes of acute *pancreatitis* separated by 16 months (4[c]). On the first occasion he was taking vigabatrin and valproic acid and the episode was ascribed to the latter, which was withdrawn. The second episode occurred while he was still taking vigabatrin (2.5 g/day), but lamotrigine (400 mg/day) had been introduced 5 months before. The pathogenic role of these drugs remains speculative. The second episode occurred 6 days after an attack of status epilepticus, which by itself may rarely be followed by pancreatitis.

Skin and appendages In a retrospective survey of 65 consecutive patients with malignant gliomas, prescription of anticonvulsants (mostly phenytoin) was associated with a *skin rash* in 26% of cases, and other clinically important toxic effects occurred in 14%, including three patients who developed an *encephalopathy* sufficient to require hospitalization (5[cr]). These data suggest that adverse effects of antiepileptic drugs are relatively common in these patients. Long-term seizure prophylaxis for patients with malignant glioma who are free of seizures at presentation was not clearly beneficial and should be studied prospectively.

Immunological and hypersensitivity reactions The *anticonvulsant hypersensitivity syndrome* is a potentially fatal reaction to anticonvulsants that produce arene oxide, such as phenytoin, carbamazepine, and phenobarbital (6^{cR}). It occurs in one in 1000—10 000 exposures and its main manifestations include fever, rash, and lymphadenopathy, accompanied by multiorgan system abnormalities. The reaction may be genetically determined, and siblings of affected patients may be at increased risk. Early identification is essential to ensure proper management, to avoid potentially fatal re-exposure, and to establish subsequent anticonvulsant treatment options.

Oncogenesis The possible influence of antiepileptic therapy on cancer risk has been assessed in a case-control study of 60 epileptic patients with hepatobiliary cancer or malignant lymphoma and 171 cancer-free controls (7^{Cr}). After exclusion of patients exposed to Thorotrast®, a known liver carcinogen, no association was found between phenobarbital treatment and cancer of the liver or the biliary tract, whereas there was a possible link between phenytoin and a risk of *non-Hodgkin's lymphoma* (odds ratio 1.8, 95% CI 0.5—6.6).

Second-generation effects *(SED-13, 136; SEDA-18, 61)* Compared with 80 healthy controls, adult epileptic patients treated with phenytoin ($n = 7$), carbamazepine ($n = 9$), or valproate ($n = 10$) had markedly reduced serum concentrations of all-*trans*-retinoic acid and 13-*cis*-retinoic acid (8^{C}). Since all-*trans*-retinoic acid deficiency has been implicated as a possible cause of malformations in the fetal alcohol syndrome, these observations might be relevant to teratogenicity.

Interactions *(SED-13, 141; SEDA-18, 62; SEDA-19, 63)* Carbamazepine and phenytoin are potent inducers of cytochrome CYP3A, and they stimulate the first-pass metabolism of high-clearance CYP3A substrates, such as *midazolam* (9^{Cr}). In six patients treated with these anticonvulsants, the AUC of oral midazolam (15 mg) was only 6% of that found in seven healthy controls, and the effects of midazolam on psychomotor function were markedly reduced. The same degree of interaction may not necessarily occur when midazolam is given parenterally, because after intravenous dosing the elimination of high clearance drugs depends more on liver blood flow than on metabolic enzyme activity.

Patients taking phenytoin and carbamazepine have a reduced response to non-depolarizing muscle relaxants (SEDA-18, 64). In a recent study, prolongation of the time to onset of action of *pipecuronium* was observed only in patients with plasma phenytoin and carbamazepine concentrations in the target range, but not in those with concentrations below the range. However, accelerated recovery from paralysis was seen whatever the plasma concentration of the anticonvulsant (10^{Cr}). Although a pharmacodynamic basis for the reduced response to non-depolarizing muscle relaxants cannot be excluded, the interaction appears to be at least in part pharmacokinetic. In 10 epileptic patients taking carbamazepine, plasma *vecuronium* clearance was more than twice that observed in 10 healthy controls (11^{Cr}).

INDIVIDUAL DRUGS

Benzodiazepines *(SED-13, 104; SEDA-17, 75; SEDA-18, 62 and 64; SEDA-19, 63)*

Respiratory system In an open prospective study of intravenous or rectal benzodiazepines in the management of acute convulsions and status epilepticus in 86 assessable children (mean ages 3.3—6.6 years in different groups), seizure control was achieved in 76% of patients given a single dose of lorazepam (0.05—0.1 mg/kg) and 51% of those given a single dose of diazepam (0.3—0.4 mg/kg) (12^{Cr}). In patients who did not respond to the initial dose, a second dose of the same drug was given. At the end of the study, 31% (17/53) of the diazepam-treated patients required additional anticonvulsants to terminate the seizure, compared with only 3% (1/33) of the lorazepam-treated patients. Respiratory depression occurred in 3% of the children treated with lorazepam and in 15% of those treated with diazepam. These data are consistent with evidence that lorazepam may be superior to diazepam in the management of acute seizure disorders.

Nervous system Among 63 children with refractory epilepsy treated with add-on clobazam (mean dosage 0.8 mg/kg/day) and followed for 15—64 months, 41% became seizure-free or had a greater than 90% reduction in seizure frequency (13[Cr]). In 35% of cases, however, clobazam had to be discontinued owing to adverse effects or loss of therapeutic benefit (seven patients). Adverse effects included severe *aggressive outbursts*, *hyperactivity*, *insomnia*, and *depression* with suicidal ideation.

Carbamazepine *(SED-13, 145; SEDA-17, 72; SEDA-18, 62; SEDA-19, 64)*

Nervous system A 32-year-old man with mental retardation and uncontrolled partial seizures treated with carbamazepine and divalproex sodium developed two episodes of *oculogyric crisis* (forced upward gaze), which resolved promptly after a reduction in the dosage of carbamazepine (14[Cr]). During each of the episodes he had other symptoms and signs of carbamazepine toxicity, such as anorexia, nausea, vomiting, and behavioral deterioration, which also improved after dosage reduction. Although dystonias are a known adverse effect of carbamazepine, there have been only four previous reports of oculogyric crisis.

Hematological Of 91 adult patients taking carbamazepine monotherapy for a mean duration of 85 months (mean dosage 1235 mg/day), nine (10%) had *hypofibrinogenemia* (1—1.5 g/l), seven (8%) had *reduced factor VIII, von Willebrandt factor antigen*, or *ristocetin co-factor*, and three (3%) had mild *thrombocytopenia* (15[c]). Of the 12 patients (13%) who reported evidence of bleeding (*petechiae*, spontaneous *hematomas*, prolonged *wound bleeding*), 10 had normal coagulation studies and only two had reduced factor VIII activity. Because of the lack of a control group, the suggestion that carbamazepine may alter coagulation should be interpreted with caution.

Among 131 adult patients taking carbamazepine, 21.4% had *leukopenia* (white cell count below 4.0×10^9/l) at some time during treatment, compared with 13.7% among 131 patients taking other anticonvulsants (16[Cr]). These data confirm that leukopenia may occur with all major anticonvulsants, but it is more common with carbamazepine. White cell count was inversely related to peak serum carbamazepine concentration. Persistent leukopenia was seen in only 17% of carbamazepine-treated patients with a low white cell count at any time. There were no clinical problems associated with the leukopenia.

Skin and appendages Skin rash is a common manifestation of carbamazepine hypersensitivity. Of 361 Japanese children started on carbamazepine monotherapy (10 mg/kg, increased 2 weeks later to 15 mg/kg if tolerated), 21 (5.8%) developed a rash, usually within 7—10 days of treatment (range 7—30 days). The manifestations were a *maculopapular erythema* in nine, *exfoliative dermatitis* in eight, and *Stevens-Johnson syndrome* in four (17[c]).

Interactions Since carbamazepine is being increasingly used in the management of psychiatric disorders, its interactions with psychotropic medications are being carefully studied.

A recent study has confirmed the evidence discussed in SEDA-19 (p. 66) that carbamazepine may lower serum *clozapine* concentrations by about 50% (18[Cr]). The ability of carbamazepine to reduce serum *haloperidol* concentrations has also recently been confirmed (19[Cr]). Plasma carbamazepine concentrations in patients not taking haloperidol were 30% lower than in patients co-medicated with haloperidol, despite a higher mean carbamazepine dosage in the former (8.2 vs. 6.1 mg/kg/day). This suggests that haloperidol may increase the serum concentration of carbamazepine, but these data should be interpreted cautiously because of lack of information about other co-medication.

Peak plasma *bupropion* concentrations and AUC after a single oral dose of 150 mg were about 90% lower in 12 patients with mood disorders stabilized on carbamazepine than in 17 control subjects treated with placebo (20[c]). Carbamazepine also reduced the plasma concentrations of the active metabolites threohydrobupropion and erythrohydrobupropion and increased those of hydroxybupropion, another active metabolite. In five patients, monotherapy with valproate was associated with increased hydroxybupropion concentrations but had no effect on the kinetics of the parent drug. It is not yet known how these interactions may affect the clinical response to bupropion.

Felbamate *(SED-13, 153; SEDA-17, 75; SEDA-18, 65; SEDA-19, 67)*

Because of the risk of aplastic anemia and hepatotoxicity (SEDA-19, 68), felbamate is restricted to patients with severe epilepsy refractory to other drugs. In most European countries, the approved indication is now limited to refractory Lennox-Gastaut syndrome.

Nervous system   Of 60 adult epileptic patients evaluated prospectively after starting felbamate, 20 (33%) experienced *headaches* considered to be drug-induced at least once a week (21[C]). The headaches had a steady or pounding quality, were mostly diffuse, and were rated as moderate or severe in almost all cases. Felbamate dosage in patients with headaches was 44 (SD 19) mg/kg/day, compared with 32 (15) mg/kg/day in patients without headaches. In many cases the headaches were controlled by non-steroidal analgesics and were relieved by a reduction in felbamate dosage in eight of 13 patients. Although this study was uncontrolled and a negative placebo effect cannot be excluded, the findings are consistent with previous reports. Other adverse effects recorded included *insomnia* (25%), *gastrointestinal symptoms* (27%), and *agitation* or *restlessness* (23%).

Involuntary movements are a rare complication of carbamazepine and phenytoin therapy. However, they may also occur with felbamate, as suggested by occasional reports in the manufacturer's data file and two published cases (22[c]). These included a 13-year-old child who developed akathisia and choreoathetosis and a 2-month-old boy who had an acute dystonic reaction with deviation of the eyes to the right. In both cases the symptoms occurred shortly after starting felbamate (41 mg/kg/day) and abated after withdrawal.

In 25 patients taken off felbamate (mean dose 2824 mg/day) over a period of 2.3 (range 1—4) weeks, mean seizure frequency compared with the pre-felbamate period increased by 41% during the taper month and by 113, 88, and 17% during the subsequent first, second, and third months, respectively (23[c]).

In 11 patients, seizure frequency more than doubled during one of the post-felbamate periods. These data suggest that withdrawal seizures may complicate rapid withdrawal of felbamate.

Rapid withdrawal of felbamate may also involve a risk of *status epilepticus*. Status epilepticus developed in a 41-year-old woman with refractory partial seizures when felbamate dosage was reduced from 3000 to 1200 mg/day at a rate of 600 mg every 5 days (24[C]). The patient was also taking phenobarbital 120 mg/day and no information was given on possible non-compliance as a potential contributory factor.

Immunological and hypersensitivity reactions   High titers of *antinuclear antibodies* were found in three of 35 patients taking felbamate; one had felbamate-induced aplastic anemia, one an unspecified systemic allergic reaction to felbamate, and one systemic lupus erythematosus secondary to phenytoin or carbamazepine (25[c]). Whether a high titer may allow prediction of susceptibility to felbamate-induced aplastic anemia remains to be determined.

Interactions   In 18 healthy subjects felbamate (1200—3600 mg/day for 14 days) inhibited the β-oxidation and enhanced the glucuronidation of *valproic acid* (26[C]). The former of these effects predominated, leading to dose-dependent and clinically relevant increases in serum valproic acid concentration.

In 16 women stabilized on an oral contraceptive, felbamate (2400 mg/day for 4 weeks) did not cause clinically significant changes in the kinetics of ethinylestradiol, but it reduced the AUC of *gestodene* by 42%; one subject reported intermenstrual bleeding (27[C]). In the same study, seven other subjects dropped out during felbamate treatment because of skin disorders (three), headache (two), or increased heart rate (two).

Gabapentin *(SED-13, 153; SEDA-17, 75; SEDA-18, 65; SEDA-19, 70)*

Gabapentin has a good tolerability profile, but efficacy results in patients refractory to other agents have not been impressive. Consequently, the value of using dosages above the hitherto upper recommended limit of 1800 mg/day is being explored.

Nervous system   Recent reports have suggested that gabapentin-induced *behavioral disturbances* may be more common than previously thought. In different retrospective surveys, aggressiveness, irritability, and/or dysphoric changes have been described in 15 out of 119 (13%) (28[c]), 19 out of 110 (16%) (29[c]), 24 out 120 (20%) (30[c]), and seven out of 32 (22%) (31[c]) patients. These effects sometimes occurred at gabapentin dosages as low as 1000—1300 mg/day (29[c]) and required withdrawal in 6—16% of treated cases. Unfortunately, none of these studies included a control group, which makes it difficult to ascertain the pathogenic role of the drug.

Both adults and children can be affected, but children may be at greater risk. In four reports which specifically addressed the problem of behavioral effects, aggressiveness, marked irritability and hyperactivity or oppositional behavior reversible after dosage reduction or withdrawal were described in a total of 16 children aged 1—16 years, most of whom had refractory partial seizures (32[C]), (33[C]), (34[c]), (35[c]). In most of these children, the behavioral problems occurred at relatively low dosages (500—900 mg/day). Many of the affected patients had mental retardation (28[c]), (29[c]), (35[c]) or a previous history of similar disorders (28[c]), (32[C]), suggesting that these may be important predisposing factors.

Endocrine, metabolic   *Weight gain* may be a significant complication of gabapentin therapy. In 57 patients treated for a mean of 7 months, body weight increased on average by 3.3 kg (4.9% of baseline); 11 patients gained 5—10% of their initial weight and 15 gained more than 10% (36[c]). In a retrospective survey (37[c]), 11 (16%) of 69 adult patients experienced weight gain (range 3.2—14.5 kg) after a mean of 3.5 months on gabapentin (mean daily dose 2464 mg/day). In another study, weight gain (mean 7, range 3—18 kg) occurred in 21 of 58 patients (36%), the effect being attributed to stimulation of appetite (38[c]).

Many antiepileptic drugs exacerbate acute intermittent porphyria, but gabapentin, which is not metabolized, may be safer. Two men with acute intermittent porphyria and partial epilepsy were treated with gabapentin 2100 and 900 mg/day for 10 and 12 months, respectively, without recurrence of porphyric attacks (39[C]). Another patient, a 60-year-old woman with epilepsy and porphyria cutanea tarda, was also treated successfully with gabapentin, 1200—1800 mg/day (40[C]).

Urinary system   Of 119 adults with partial seizures treated with gabapentin (900—5400 mg/day), five (4%) developed *urinary incontinence* that resolved after withdrawal (28[c]). Interestingly, four of the five patients had signs of spasticity, suggesting that this may be an important predisposing factor.

Lamotrigine *(SED-13, 153; SEDA-18, 65; SEDA-19, 70)*

Important skin rashes with lamotrigine

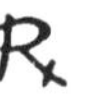

A skin rash is the most common reason for withdrawing lamotrigine. The incidence of rash can be minimized by slow dosage escalation, as discussed in SEDA-19 (p. 70). Lamotrigine-induced rashes are usually mild, but serious reactions, such as Stevens-Johnson syndrome, may also occur.

In a 6-month double-blind add-on multicenter study in 334 patients given lamotrigine in dosages up to 500 mg/day, rashes associated with lamotrigine were rated as serious in three patients, and one patient with Stevens-Johnson syndrome required hospitalization; all resolved on withdrawal (41[Cr]). Five additional cases of Stevens-Johnson syndrome have been described in two girls aged 8 and 12 years (42[c]), (43[c]), in an 18-year-old woman (44[c]), and in two men aged 29 and 40 years (45[c]), (46[C]). There has been one report suggesting that lamotrigine might have also been involved in a fatal case of toxic epidermal necrolysis in a 56-year-old man soon after switching from carbamazepine to a high initial dosage of lamotrigine (200 mg/day). The carbamazepine had caused a probable allergic reaction (swollen eyelids), and because of the temporal proximity of this reaction lamotrigine cannot be implicated with certainty (47[c]).

Of 68 children treated with lamotrigine, five

developed a rash, which in three cases required admission to hospital (two to the intensive care unit) (43[C]). One child who had recovered had a recurrence of the rash within 30 min of re-exposure to lamotrigine after 6 months. In another study, eight patients who had developed a rash were rechallenged with the drug, starting at a lower initial dosage (usually 25 mg/day or 12.5 mg daily or on alternate days) (48[C]). In six, the rash did not recur. Of the other two, one had a recurrence of a mild fluctuating and qualitatively different rash, while the other developed a dose-related rash that disappeared after dosage reduction, reappeared when the dosage was increased again, disappeared on further dosage reduction, and did not finally recur at the third attempt at increasing the dosage.

Taken alone, these data would suggest that patients who experience a mild rash but a good therapeutic response to lamotrigine might be considered for re-dosing under close supervision. However, this view should be reassessed in the light of more recent clinical data submitted to regulatory authorities, showing that in children potentially life-threatening lamotrigine-induced skin reactions (including Stevens-Johnson syndrome and more rarely toxic epidermal necrolysis) that require hospitalization are much more common than previously thought. According to Dear Doctor letters sent by the manufacturer in April 1997 to physicians in the US and UK, the risk of these reactions in children is between 1:50 and 1:100 (US) or 1:100 and 1:300 (UK), compared to a risk estimate of 1:1000 in adults. The age associated with increased risk is 12 years or under in the UK and under 16 years in the US. Almost all reactions occur during the first 2—8 weeks of starting therapy, although isolated cases have been reported after prolonged treatment, for example after 6 months. Although the majority of patients recover after drug withdrawal, some children experience irreversible scarring, and there have been rare cases associated with death. Concomitant use of valproate and high initial dosages of lamotrigine exceeding the recommended dosage escalation are recognized as important risk factors. The manufacturers have instructed doctors to discontinue lamotrigine at the first signs of a rash in all patients. Patients should also be warned to report immediately any sign of a rash or other signs of hypersensitivity, such as fever or lymphadenopathy, which may occur without evidence of a rash. Based on current assessment of the benefit-risk ratio, prescription of lamotrigine as initial monotherapy cannot be recommended, at least in children.

Nervous system   In a 6-month double-blind add-on multicenter study in 334 patients given lamotrigine in dosages up to 500 mg/day, *dizziness, diplopia, ataxia, blurred vision*, and *somnolence* occurred more commonly among patients taking lamotrigine ($n = 334$) than among those taking placebo ($n = 112$) (41[Cr]).

Serum lamotrigine concentrations in 18 patients with intolerable adverse effects (mostly headache, dizziness, and ataxia) ranged from 0.4 to 18.5 mg/l and overlapped widely with those associated with good control in other patients (49[Cr]). These data suggest that monitoring lamotrigine concentrations is unlikely to be useful in the prevention of adverse effects.

Psychotic symptoms have occasionally been reported after the start of lamotrigine therapy. A 44-year-old woman with partial epilepsy and no history of psychosis developed behavioral disturbances, agitation, confusion, and visual and acoustic hallucinations 40 days after lamotrigine, 100 mg/day, was added to carbamazepine therapy. Since she was seizure-free on lamotrigine, the reaction may have reflected forced normalization (a term describing the onset of psychotic symptoms when treatment causes disappearance of EEG abnormalities and seizures). Discontinuation of lamotrigine resulted in recurrence of seizures, but the psychotic symptoms disappeared after 16 weeks (45[c]).

Hematological   *Aplastic anemia* has been reported in a 42-year-old epileptic man after 9 months on an unspecified dose of lamotrigine (50[c]). The condition was diagnosed after repeated episodes of epistaxis, petechiae, and bruising, and was associated with a platelet count of 8×10^9/l, a white cell count of 3.1×10^9/l, a neutrophil count of 0.4×10^9/l, a hemoglobin of 6.3 g/dl and a bone marrow aspirate consistent with aplasia. Antinuclear antibodies were 'weakly positive' and various virology tests were negative. The condition improved after withdrawal and treatment with cyclosporin. The temporal relation in this case was consistent with a causative role of lamotrigine. However, the patient had recovered fully 7 years earlier from bone marrow aplasia ascribed to carbamazepine.

Severe acquired pure *red cell aplasia* (hemoglobin 2.8 g/dl) developed in a 32-year-old epileptic patient over 4 months after the addition of lamotrigine 200 mg/day to his previous carbamazepine therapy. Withdrawal of lamotrigine led to rapid recovery. The patient also had heterozygous β-thalassemia, and it is possible that lamotrigine, a weak inhibitor of dihydrofolate reductase, inhibited erythropoiesis already compromised by the thalassemic condition (51[c]). However, in another case lamotrigine up to 200 mg/day for 18 months did not adversely affect the blood in a 49-year-old woman with epilepsy and heterozygous β-thalassemia (52[c]).

A 35-year-old woman was admitted to hospital with septic shock secondary to *leukopenia* (white cell count 0.6×10^9/l) 10 days after starting add-on lamotrigine 25 mg daily for 7 days followed by 50 mg/day. She had an erythematous rash, nausea, vomiting, dizziness, sore throat, fever, and hypotension, and blood cultures were positive for *Staphylococcus aureus* and *Escherichia coli*. Lamotrigine was withdrawn, but recovery was complicated by two episodes of ventricular fibrillation associated with hypokalemia, hypomagnesemia, and hypocalcemia of unknown cause. Fifteen days later, her white cell count had risen to 5.1×10^9/l. At the time of this report, the Committee on Safety of Medicines had received four other reports of leukopenia and six of neutropenia associated with lamotrigine (53[c]).

Liver and pancreas A 22-year-old woman taking valproic acid and carbamazepine developed a *fever* and a *maculopapular rash* 3 weeks after starting lamotrigine (50 mg/day, increased to 100 mg bd), followed 3 days later by fulminant *hepatic failure* and *coma*. Despite subsequent improvement of liver function, she died unexpectedly with a pulmonary embolism 2 months later (54[c]). This seems to be the first report suggesting that lamotrigine may cause severe liver failure in the absence of major dysfunction of other organs, although multiorgan failure and disseminated intravascular coagulation have been described in a number of lamotrigine-treated patients (55[c]). Although it has been suggested that this was secondary to uncontrolled seizure activity and not to lamotrigine itself, in at least one case the drug was probably implicated because there was no history of seizure just before admission (56[c]).

Second-generation effects As of 30 September 1994, 53 pregnancies have been recorded among women exposed to lamotrigine in the first trimester (57[c]). There were four spontaneous abortions, 13 induced abortions (none because of a prenatally detected defect), 34 infants without birth defects, and two infants with unspecified defects. No data on concomitant medication were reported. However, the observed fetal malformation rate (2/36 live births or 5.5%) is within the range expected in women with epilepsy.

Phenobarbital *(SED-13, 154; SEDA-18, 67; SEDA-19, 72)*

Second-generation effects In two double-blind studies in a total of 114 subjects, adult men exposed prenatally to phenobarbital had lower *verbal intelligence scores* (approximately 0.5 SD) than predicted from data collected in 153 matched controls (58[Cr]). An exposure period that included the last trimester of pregnancy was the most detrimental. Lower socioeconomic status and being the offspring of an unwanted pregnancy increased the magnitude of the impairment. These data suggest that prenatal exposure to phenobarbital can have long-term deleterious effects on cognitive performance, which may be magnified by interaction with adverse environmental conditions.

Phenytoin *(SED-13, 141; SEDA-17, 73; SEDA-18, 67; SEDA-19, 72)*

Nervous system Adult epileptic patients randomly assigned to monotherapy with phenytoin ($n = 15$) or carbamazepine ($n = 16$) underwent a neuropsychological assessment after 6 and 24 months (59[c]). There were differential effects between the two drugs in only three of 32 measurements. Patients taking phenytoin did less well than those taking carbamazepine in visually guided motor speed of both hands and in a visual memory task. Mood scores were similar in the two groups. These results suggest that the long-term effects of phenytoin compared with those of carbamazepine are few and are restricted mainly to some *visually guided motor functions*.

Musculoskeletal Phenytoin in micromolar concentrations stimulates thymidine incorporation, and increases cell number, alkaline phosphatase specific activity, and collagen synthesis in normal human bone cells (60[Cr]). In 39 adult epileptic patients, phenytoin treatment was associated with increased serum concentrations of bone formation markers (osteocalcin, skeletal alkaline phosphatase, and procollagen peptide). These data suggest that phenytoin has an osteogenic action, which may explain its ability to cause *acromegaly-like facial features*.

Immunological and hypersensitivity reactions *Pseudolymphoma*, a rare complication of phenytoin, is usually characterized by lymphadenopathy, fever, and a diffuse erythematous macular skin eruption. A 17-year-old girl developed cervical and axillary enlarged lymph nodes without fever and rash after 1 year on phenytoin (200—300 mg/day) (61[Cr]). The condition cleared after withdrawal. Immunophenotypic immunoglobulin gene rearrangement and cytogenetic studies showed a polyclonal C-cell proliferation consistent with phenytoin-induced pseudolymphoma. The authors emphasized the importance of molecular biology and chromosome studies in making the differential diagnosis.

Interactions Phenytoin and *dexamethasone* are often used in combination, especially in patients with brain tumors. While phenytoin is known to stimulate dexamethasone metabolism and to increase its dosage requirements, the effect of dexamethasone on phenytoin kinetics is controversial. In a 48-year-old man with cerebral metastases receiving high-dosage dexamethasone (16—28 mg/day), unusually high dosages of phenytoin (600—1000 mg/day) were required to maintain serum phenytoin concentrations within the target range (40—80 μmol/l) (62[cr]). A similar case had been reported before (63[c]), but high phenytoin concentrations have been also described in dexamethasone-treated patients (64[c]). To minimize the consequences of possible interactions, phenytoin concentrations should be carefully monitored in these patients.

Remacemide *(SED-13, 155)*

The investigational antiepileptic drug remacemide is thought to act by sodium channel blockade and non-competitive antagonism of NMDA receptors. To date, 223 patients have entered blinded studies and many continue on open label treatment (65[c]). Thirteen patients have been treated for more than 1 year, 130 for 3—12 months, and 80 for under 3 months; 49 (22%) dropped out because of inefficacy (20), *gastric intolerance* (five), *increased seizure frequency* (four), *psychiatric/behavioral problems* (four), or other reasons (16). Major events were reported in 24 cases (11%). Ten events in nine patients (including eight withdrawals) were considered possibly related to treatment and included *exacerbated seizures* (four), *raised hepatic enzymes* (two), *gastric intolerance* (three), and *mood change* (one).

Tiagabine *(SEDA-19, 73)*

Among 1283 patients exposed to open-label tiagabine (up to 120 mg/day, median dose 44 mg/day) for up to 36 months in 118 centers in the US and Canada, 682 discontinued therapy because of adverse events (184), lack of efficacy (360), or other reasons (138). The most frequent adverse events were *dizziness, somnolence*, and *weakness* (66[c]).

In an open add-on trial of tiagabine (12—64 mg/day), 15 of 17 patients experienced adverse events (67[Cr]). The more common included *ataxia, tremor, drowsiness, dizziness, lethargy*, and *blurred vision*. Adverse events were mostly mild and transient, but in four cases (including one who developed *hallucinations* and *aggression*) they were sufficiently severe to require withdrawal.

Topiramate

In a double-blind add-on placebo-controlled trial of topiramate (titrated up to a maximum dosage of 800 mg/day), the most common adverse events were *fatigue* (79% of cases vs. 36% with placebo, $n = 28$/group), *impaired concentration* (25 vs. 0%), *weight loss* (25 vs. 0%), *dizziness* (21 vs. 4%), and *paresthesia* (18 vs. 4%) (68[Cr]). Adverse effects occurred mostly during the rapid titration phase or at high dosages and led to discontinuation in 21% of patients.

In a similar study in 60 patients given 600 mg/day topiramate or placebo, the most common effects were *headache* (27 vs. 10% on placebo), *somnolence* (23 vs. 13%), *dizziness* and *fatigue* (23 vs. 10%), *mental slowing* (20 vs. 0%), *depression*, and *weight loss* (17 vs. 7%) (69[Cr]).

Topiramate safety has been assessed from data based on 1244 subjects recruited in 39 separate trials (70[R]). These included 990 patients with epilepsy, 307 of whom took part in placebo-controlled double-blind add-on trials at dosages of 200—1000 mg/day. The duration of treatment was over 1 year in 336 patients and over 3 years in 116 patients. The most common adverse effects, which in double-blind studies occurred more than 10% more often than with placebo, were *dizziness*, *abnormalities of thought*, *somnolence*, *ataxia*, *fatigue*, *confusion*, *impaired concentration*, and *paresthesia* (70[R]), (71[c]). The event with the greatest difference in incidence versus placebo (cumulative incidence at 4 months 25 vs. 2.4%) was abnormal thinking, which refers to mental slowing but not psychosis. Most of the events were mild and transient, and there was a trend for the most severe episodes of a given event to be more common at higher dosages. Many events occurred early during therapy, and their incidence may have been artifactually high in double-blind studies, because of too rapid titration to either the target dose or the maximum tolerated dose. Across all studies, 13% of topiramate-treated patients were withdrawn because of adverse events, compared with 3% of those assigned to placebo. The withdrawal rate was greater at dosages over 600 mg/day. Of five serious adverse events in double-blind studies, three (accidental injury, agitation, presumptive cerebrovas-

cular accident) were considered to have been unrelated to the drug, and two (*abdominal pain*, *dyspnea*) were considered to be possibly related. *Falls in body weight* of 2—6% have been observed in double-blind trials. Topiramate is associated with a risk of *nephrolithiasis* of about 1.5%.

In an open long-term add-on study at dosages of 400—800 mg/day in 15 patients followed up for 14—21 months (72[c]), the most common adverse events were *somnolence*, *weight loss*, *mental slowing*, *fatigue*, *ataxia*, and *irritability*. Adverse events led to drug withdrawal in six cases (two with ataxia and one each with somnolence, metabolic acidosis, irritability, and psychotic symptoms). Many of the patients were taking two or three other anticonvulsants in combination, which may explain the high incidence of adverse effects in this study.

Nervous system Of 17 patients treated with topiramate for a mean of 29 months (1—60 months), the most common adverse events were *sedation* (59%), *headache* (41%), *impaired concentration* (35%), *word-finding difficulties* (35%), *impaired memory* (35%), and *ataxia* (35%) (73[c]). In a similar study in children treated for 6—30 months, adverse effects reported in nine of 15 patients included transient *weight loss* (four), *thirst* (three), *somnolence* (two), *reduced appetite* (two), *emotional lability* (two), and *ataxia*, *vomiting*, *cognitive problems*, and *reduced frequency of micturition* (one each) (74[c]). In both studies, the lack of a control group makes assessment difficult.

Endocrine, metabolic Like other carbonic anhydrase inhibitors, topiramate may cause *metabolic acidosis*. Of 15 adult epileptic patients who received add-on topiramate (400—800 mg/day) for up to 21 months, 11 had an increase in serum chloride and seven (out of nine assessed cases) had a fall in serum bicarbonate with raised arterial oxygen tension and reduced carbon dioxide tension (72[c]). Two patients had biochemical evidence of mild uncompensated metabolic acidosis, with a blood pH of 7.33 and 7.34, respectively. Of the two patients with uncompensated acidosis, one required drug discontinuation because of severe fatigue, lethargy, hypotonia, and hyperventilation. Whether the symptoms were partly related to acidosis is uncertain, but a relation was suggested by the observation that symptoms deteriorated with recurrent respiratory infections. Monitoring blood pH, blood gases, and serum bicarbonate is recommended in patients who develop symptoms consistent with acidosis.

Urinary system   By inhibiting carbonic anhydrase, topiramate reduces serum chloride and bicarbonate concentrations, reduces the urinary excretion of citrate, and increases urinary pH, leading to higher calcium phosphate saturation and a risk of *nephrolithiasis* (75[C]). During 1074 patient years of topiramate exposure in 1183 patients, 18 subjects (1.5%) had 21 episodes of definite renal calculi, suggesting an incidence of nephrolithiasis comparable to that reported for acetazolamide (76[C]).

Second-generation effects   Topiramate has teratogenic effects in mice and rats, similarly to other inhibitors of carbonic anhydrase (77[c]). However, there are too few data to assess possible teratogenic effects in humans.

Interactions   Enzyme-inducing anticonvulsants, such as *carbamazepine*, *phenytoin*, and *barbiturates*, enhance topiramate clearance and markedly reduce serum topiramate concentrations at steady state (78[R]), (79[C]), (80[C]), (81[c]), (82[c]), (83[c]). Adjustment in topiramate dosage may be required when enzyme-inducing anticonvulsants are added or withdrawn.

Withdrawal of *valproic acid* co-medication is associated with an increase in serum topiramate concentration by about 15% (84[C]). However, this interaction was considered to be of little or no clinical significance. Topiramate may slightly reduce serum valproic acid concentrations, the effect being associated with enhanced formation of the hepatotoxic metabolite 4-ene-valproic acid. The clinical relevance of this interaction is unknown.

Topiramate does not affect the serum concentrations of carbamazepine, carbamazepine-10,11-epoxide (76[R]), (77[C]), phenobarbital, primidone, and primidone-derived phenobarbital (82[c]). An increase in serum *phenytoin* concentration has occasionally been observed, possibly in relation to inhibition of cyto-

chrome CYP2C19 (80[C]), (85[c]), but in most cases the effect is small and of little clinical significance (78[R]), (80[C]).

Topiramate, in dosages of 200, 400, and 800 mg/day, dose-dependently reduced the plasma concentrations of *ethinylestradiol* by 18—30% in 12 women taking oral contraceptives. Although the concentrations of norethindrone were not affected, the reduced concentration of the estrogen may lead to reduced contraceptive efficacy (86[C]).

Topiramate inhibited the activity of cytochrome CYP2C19, but not the activity of cytochromes CYP1A2, CYP2A6, CYP2C9, CYP2D6, CYP2E1, and CYP3A4 in human liver microsomes (85[c]). These findings suggest that topiramate may reduce the clearance of substrates of CYP2C19, such as *mephenytoin*, *omeprazole*, and *diazepam*.

Valproate sodium *(SED-13, 149; SEDA-17, 73; SEDA-18, 69; SEDA-19, 73)*

The safety of intravenous sodium valproate has been assessed in 318 patients (mean age 34, range 2—87 years) hospitalized for seizure control or anticipated seizures (87[C]). Physicians were allowed to decide the number and duration of infusions as clinically indicated. Median dosage was 375 mg infused over 1 h, and the median number of doses was four over 2 days. Transient adverse effects were reported in 54 patients (17%) and included *headache*, *reactions at the injection site*, and *nausea* (2.2% each); *somnolence* (1.9%); *vomiting* (1.6%); *dizziness* and *taste abnormality* (1.3% each). These data suggest that at these dosages and rates of infusion intravenous valproate is generally well tolerated.

Nervous system   A possible association of valproic acid with reversible *dementia* and *pseudoatrophy of the brain* has been reported in two cases (88[c]). The first case was a 11-year-old boy with benign rolandic epilepsy whose full-scale IQ on the Wechsler Intelligence Scale for Children dropped from 96 (verbal 94, performance 101) to 74 (verbal 73, performance 79) after 3 years on divalproex sodium (625 mg tds). In addition to markedly deteriorated motor and verbal abilities, the child showed prominent inactivity, ataxia, intention tremor of the hands, mild dysmetria, and obesity. MRI showed cerebral and cerebellar atrophy, but laboratory investigations for a progressive degenerative disorder were negative. Substitution with felbamate and discontinuation of concurrent thioridazine (50 mg/day) and benztropine mesylate (2 mg/day) resulted in disappearance of all symptoms and signs within a few weeks. One year later his IQ on the Kaufmann Adolescents and Adults Intelligence scale was 92 and the MRI abnormalities had decreased substantially, with complete disappearance of brain atrophy over the next 12 months. The second case was a 9-year-old girl with benign rolandic epilepsy who developed drowsiness, emotional lability, and progressive apathy, with marked motor and intellectual deterioration, headaches, generalized tremor, hair loss, and nystagmus over a period between 3 weeks and 3 months after starting valproate (1000 mg/day, later reduced to 750 mg/day). At 3 months an MRI scan showed widespread cerebral and cerebellar atrophy. Phenobarbital was substituted and during the next 4 months the behavioral abnormalities, the intellectual impairment, tremor, ataxia, and nystagmus disappeared. A repeat MRI scan 6 months after withdrawal of valproate was normal. A third very similar case, previously reported, concerned a 17-year-old girl who developed marked cognitive impairment and other adverse effects (apathy, tremor, weight gain, and curly hair) within 3 weeks of starting valproate (2500 mg/day) (89[c]). A CT scan after 6 months showed shrinkage of the brain, which was rapidly reversible together with all symptoms on withdrawal.

These reports are very suggestive of a causative role of sodium valproate. All three patients had common features, such as high serum valproic acid concentrations (100—120 µg/ml), associated signs suggestive of toxicity, normal EEG background activity despite worsening of symptoms, and rapid improvement of clinical and imaging signs after drug withdrawal. In two cases the symptoms developed shortly after the introduction of valproate, while in the third there was a delay of over 2 years. A 2-year delay was also seen in a fourth case of valproate-induced dementia reported in a 21-year-old man, although there was no evidence of brain atrophy on CT scan (90[c]). The possibility of a drug-induced effect should be considered when brain atrophy and/or progressive intellectual deterioration occur in patients treated with valproate. There is clearly concern that the condition may be underdiagnosed. Although the presentation resembles a progressive degenerative disorder, normal background EEG activity should be useful in differentiating it from other conditions, including biochemical disturbances and epileptic states. The presentation also differs from valproate-induced stupor, in which consciousness is impaired and there may be clinical or EEG evidence of increased seizure activity.

Choreiform movements have been associated with various antiepileptic drugs, most notably phenytoin. Episodes of choreiform movements have now been reported in two girls aged 10 and 17 years and in a 36-year-old man, all with pre-existing severe brain damage, after 2—7 years of valproic acid therapy (91[c]). The disorder involved the head, mouth, tongue, trunk, and limbs, bilaterally in two cases and contralaterally in a third case with a unilateral vascular lesion in the caudate. The episodes occurred for several days, typically 1.5—4 h after each dose of valproate, and were followed by asymptomatic periods of several weeks. In one case the condition cleared after withdrawal of valproic acid, whereas in the other two cases replacement of valproic acid with divalproex sodium presumably reduced peak drug concentrations and resulted in no recurrence of the chorea. This seems to have been the first report suggesting an involvement of valproic acid in the development of chorea.

Endocrine, metabolic The use of valproate in young women has been associated with an increased incidence of *polycystic ovaries* and *hyperandrogenism*. A group of 10 women who had shown these abnormalities on valproate were switched to lamotrigine and reassessed 6 months later (92[c]). Serum testosterone concentration fell significantly from 3.1 (SD 0.9) to 2.5 (0.7) nmol/l and body weight from 82 (20) to 79 (19) kg. Fasting serum insulin concentrations and the number of ovarian follicles also tended to fall, but these changes were not significant. These data show that valproate-induced hyperandrogenism, weight gain, and possibly hyperinsulinemia and ovarian changes are reversible after switching to lamotrigine.

Patients with ornithine transcarbamylase deficiency are at special risk of developing symptomatic valproic acid-induced *hyperammonemia*. This has been confirmed in a mentally normal 7-year-old girl with generalized tonic-clonic seizures and an otherwise uneventful medical history (93[cr]). The introduction of valproate (20 mg/kg/day) resulted in irritability, alternating periods of drowsiness and agitation, visual and auditory hallucinations, headaches, and frequent vomiting. Investigations showed ammonium concentrations more than three times normal and other biochemical abnormalities suggestive of heterozygote ornithine transcarbamylase deficiency. All neurological symptoms cleared after withdrawal. This is at least the third published case of valproic acid-induced symptomatic hyperammonemia in previously normal heterozygotes for ornithine transcarbamylase deficiency. Valproate should be avoided whenever a disorder of the urea cycle is suspected.

Plasma carnitine concentrations are reduced by valproate and there is evidence that carnitine may alleviate valproate-induced hyperammonemia in some cases (94[R]). Although the best approach to symptomatic hyperammonemia is probably to reduce valproate dosage or to substitute another drug, a trial of carnitine may be considered, especially in patients with subnormal blood carnitine concentrations or known risk factors for carnitine deficiency. Carnitine treatment will probably be ineffective if the patient is asymptomatic, has few risk factors for carnitine deficiency, or has normal carnitine concentrations. There is no clear evidence that carnitine supplementation prevents valproate-induced hepatotoxicity.

Liver, pancreas, and gallbladder   Of 72 mentally retarded adults treated with valproate, five (7%) developed *pancreatitis* and one experienced *cholecystitis* (95[Cr]). All recovered fully. A literature search revealed a further 50 cases of pancreatitis associated with valproate. It was concluded that mentally retarded patients may be at increased risk of pancreatitis, and should be monitored carefully for this potentially fatal adverse effect.

Urinary system   A 13-year-old boy with isolated microhematuria of unknown origin and partial epilepsy developed frank *hematuria* and *acute renal failure* when given valproate (20 mg/kg). The condition cleared when carbamazepine was substituted, but hematuria and increased serum creatinine reappeared on rechallenge with valproate. This seems to have been the first report of acute renal failure with normal dosages of valproate and without other clinical or biochemical signs of valproate toxicity (96[c]).

Musculoskeletal   Compared with 27 healthy controls, 13 children with uncomplicated idiopathic epilepsy treated with valproate for more than 18 months (mean serum concentration 72 mg/l, 500 μmol/l) had 14 and 10% reductions in bone mineral density at axial and appendicular sites, respectively (97[Cr]). There was no significant reduction in bone density in 13 children treated with carbamazepine. These results are surprising, because valproate is not an enzyme inducer, and bone demineralization has been considered to be an adverse effect of enzyme induction. Whether the reported changes in bone mineral density predispose to an increased risk of fractures remains to be determined.

Immunological and hypersensitivity reactions   A 30-year-old woman with epilepsy and partial trisomy of chromosome 9 developed arthralgia, muscle weakness, fatigue, and fever after treatment with valproate for 1 year (1500 mg/day) and ethosuximide (750 mg/day) (98[Cr]). Laboratory investigations were suggestive of systemic lupus erythematosus. Discontinuation of valproate led to resolution of clinical, immunological, and hematological signs within 6 weeks. This appears to be the fourth reported case of valproate-induced *systemic lupus erythematosus*. A possible predisposing role of the chromosomal abnormality in the reaction remains speculative.

Overdose   A 15-month-old boy was admitted in coma after accidentally ingesting 4000 mg (400 mg/kg) of valproate, which had been prescribed for his mother (99[c]). His serum valproic acid concentration was 1316 mg/l (9125 μmol/l) and blood ammonia and liver function tests were normal, but analysis of urinary valproic acid metabolites showed abnormally low concentrations of β-oxidation products and increased concentrations of ω- and ω1-oxidation products. Administration of carnitine (100 mg/kg/day for 3 days) by nasogastric tube was associated with a rapid return of the metabolite pattern towards normal. The child regained consciousness after 3 days and was discharged on the eighth day. It was suggested that carnitine may be useful in valproate overdose.

Interactions Switching 11 epileptic patients from a regular to a modified-release formulation of valproate (800—2000 mg/day) resulted in an increased serum concentration of concomitantly administered *phenytoin* (from 58 to 75 µmol/l). The interaction was ascribed to reduced peak concentrations of valproic acid and consequent minimization of phenytoin displacement from plasma protein binding sites, although this would not explain the development of toxic symptoms in two patients (100[C]). Unbound serum phenytoin was not measured in this study.

The administration of valproic acid (mean serum concentration 62 mg/l, 430 µmol/l) to seven schizophrenic patients taking high-dosage *clozapine* (500—900 mg/day) reduced the steady-state serum concentrations of clozapine and norclozapine by 15 and 65%, respectively (101[C]). Norclozapine has been reported to be more toxic than clozapine on hemopoietic stem cells in vitro, but the suggestion that this interaction might reduce the risk of clozapine-induced agranulocytosis remains speculative.

Vigabatrin *(SED-13, 155; SEDA-17, 74; SEDA-18, 70; SEDA-19, 76)*

In a prospective open 1-year trial in 100 adults with newly diagnosed partial and/or generalized tonic-clonic seizures randomized to vigabatrin or carbamazepine monotherapy, no patient assigned to vigabatrin discontinued treatment because of adverse effects (102[C]). In contrast, 12 patients (24%) in the carbamazepine group were withdrawn because of skin rash (seven), hepatic toxicity (three), increased blood sugar (one), and confusion with personality changes (one). Compared with patients taking carbamazepine, those taking vi-

gabatrin reported less drowsiness (44 vs. 62%) and dizziness (7 vs. 20%), and more frequent *myoclonic jerks* (14 vs. 2%) and *visual scintillations* (16 vs. 0%). Vigabatrin had no detrimental effect on cognitive function, whereas performance in the tapping test deteriorated in the carbamazepine group. Seizure control was slightly better with carbamazepine. The suggestion from these findings that vigabatrin may be better tolerated (and possibly slightly less effective) than carbamazepine should be interpreted with caution, because the dosage of carbamazepine was increased up to intolerable toxicity, whereas the dosage of vigabatrin did not exceed 50—60 mg/kg irrespective of adverse effects. The study did confirm that skin rashes are far less common with vigabatrin than with carbamazepine.

Nervous system Vigabatrin may exacerbate myoclonic seizures, but the possible new appearance of myoclonus is not so widely recognized. In four patients with partial epilepsy (three adults and a 4-year-old child) vigabatrin caused de novo appearance of myoclonic jerks associated with paroxysmal EEG abnormalities (103[c]). This led to vigabatrin withdrawal in all cases.

Partial or generalized *status epilepticus* has been reported in patients with symptomatic generalized or partial epilepsy after a variable duration of vigabatrin therapy (104[C])—(106[C]). Although in some of these cases a causative role of vigabatrin could not be established or was questioned (107[C]), the possibility that vigabatrin may precipitate status should be considered. In two patients, complex partial status was associated with prominent psychiatric features, which made diagnosis more difficult (104[C]).

The association of vigabatrin with *psychiatric and behavioral disturbances* was discussed extensively in SEDA-18 (p. 71) and in a recent review (108[R]). In a retrospective study, 22 (16%) of 133 patients were withdrawn from vigabatrin because of psychiatric adverse reactions (109[Cr]). The same study did not support the view that a previous history of behavioral and psychiatric disorders increases the risk of such disturbances (relative risk 1.23, 95% CI 0.57—2.66), and there was also no evidence that the risk can be reduced by a low starting dosage. The risk of psychosis in vigabatrin-treated patients has been calculated from global safety data submitted to the FDA and the UK Post-Marketing Prescription Event Monitoring System, totalling about 10 000 patients (110[C]). The incidence of psychosis was 1.1% in the global safety data and 0.64% in the UK database. In US and Canadian trials in resistant partial seizures, eight of 279 vigabatrin-treated patients (2.9%) and none of 188 placebo-treated patients developed psychosis. Symptoms were typically transient and responded to withdrawal or antipsychotic drug treatment. Although most reported cases have occurred in adults, children may also be at risk. A 7-year-old boy with intractable epilepsy developed an acute psychosis 3 days after starting vigabatrin (111[c]). His symptoms resolved within 48 h of drug withdrawal, and reintroduction of vigabatrin with a slower dose escalation 2 months later was uneventful.

Depression is another significant psychiatric adverse effect of vigabatrin. In a retrospective survey, 43 of 162 patients (27%) with refractory epilepsy treated with vigabatrin developed depression and irritability (112[C]). Since these events may also be related to underlying disease or concurrent medication, the lack of a control group makes it difficult to assess the causative role of vigabatrin in these patients.

Skin and appendages   Skin reactions due to vigabatrin are extremely rare. Cutaneous manifestations consistent with *erythema multiforme* appeared 4 weeks after starting vigabatrin (unspecified dose) in a 38-year-old man with epilepsy, porphyria cutanea tarda, and liver disease secondary to hepatitis B, hepatitis C, and alcohol abuse (113[c]). The lesions disappeared 3 weeks after drug withdrawal. This is the first description of a bullous skin reaction associated with vigabatrin, but a causative role of the drug remains speculative.

Interference with laboratory tests   Vigabatrin acts primarily by inhibiting GABA transaminase. However, *alanine aminotransferase* (AlT) may also be inhibited. In nine adults, plasma AlT activity fell to very low values after 2 weeks on vigabatrin 23—42 mg/kg (114[Cr]). The magnitude of the change was greater than in previous studies and appeared to involve an in vivo effect, not simply in vitro interference with the assay. The effect was considered to be of no clinical concern, although surprisingly the authors did not discuss potential implications related to the use of AlT as a diagnostic test.

Vigabatrin increases concentrations of *α-aminoadipic acid*, an effect that has been ascribed to possible inhibition of α-aminoadipic acid transaminase (115[C]). Plasma and urinary α-aminoadipic acid concentrations were increased in each of eight children (ages 3 months to 5 years) treated with vigabatrin (24—100 mg/day); in three children assessed off therapy, α-aminoadipic acid concentrations were normal. Although there is no evidence that this effect causes any harm, it could lead to incorrect diagnosis of α-aminoadipicaciduria, a rare genetic metabolic disease. Even though plasma α-aminoadipic acid concentrations are generally higher in patients with α-aminoadipicaciduria, metabolic testing for this disease should be performed before starting vigabatrin.

In 13 healthy volunteers, antipyrine clearance, urinary 6-β-hydroxycortisol excretion, and γ-glutamyltransferase activity were not affected by vigabatrin (3000 mg/day for 28 days), suggesting that vigabatrin is devoid of enzyme inducing properties in therapeutic dosages (116[c]).

REFERENCES

1.   Salinsky MC, Oken BS, Binder LM. Assessment of drowsiness in epilepsy patients receiving chronic antiepileptic drug therapy. Epilepsia 1996;37:181—7.
2.   Dean JC, Penry JK. Weight gain patterns in patients with epilepsy: comparison of antiepileptic drugs. Epilepsia 1995;36 Suppl 4:72.
3.   Tiihonen M, Liewendahl K, Waltimo O, Ojala M, Valimaki M. Thyroid status of patients receiving long-term anticonvulsant therapy assessed by peripheral parameters: a placebo-controlled thyroxine therapy trial. Epilepsia 1995;36:1118—25.
4.   Jadresic DA. Acute pancreatitis associated with dual vigabatrin and lamotrigine therapy. Seizure 1994;3:319.
5.   Moots PL, Maciunas RJ, Eisert DR, Parker RA, Laporte K, Abou-Khalil B. The course of seizure disorders in patients with malignant gliomas. Arch Neurol 1995;52:717—24.
6.   Vittorio CC, Muglia JJ. Anticonvulsant hyper-

sensitivity syndrome. Arch Int Med 1995; 155:2285—90.

7.   Olsen JH, Schulgen G, Boice JD Jr, Whysner J, Travis LB, Williams GM, Johnson FB, McGee JO. Antiepileptic treatment and risk for hepatobiliary cancer and malignant lymphoma. Cancer Res 1995;55:294—7.

8.   Fex G, Larsson K, Andersson A, Berggren-Soderlund M. Low serum concentrations of all-trans and 13-cis retinoic acids in patients treated with phenytoin, carbamazepine and valproate. Possible relation to teratogenicity. Arch Toxicol 1995;669:572—4.

9.   Backman JT, Olkkola KT, Ojala M, Laaksovirta H, Neuvonen PJ. Concentrations and effects of oral midazolam are greatly reduced in patients on carbamazepine or phenytoin. Epilepsia 1996; 37:253—7.

10.   Hans P, Ledoux D, Bonhomme V, Brichant JF. Effect of plasma anticonvulsant level on pipecuronium-induced neuromuscular blockade: preliminary results. J Neurosurg Anesthesiol 1995; 7:254—8.

11.   Alloul K, Whalley DG, Shutway F, Ebrahim Z, Varin F. Pharmacokinetic origin of carbamazepine-induced resistance to vecuronium neuromuscular blockade in anaesthetized patients. Anesthesiology 1996;84:330—9.

12.   Appleton R, Sweeney A, Choonara I, Robson J, Molyneux E. Lorazepam versus diazepam in the acute treatment of epileptic seizures and status epilepticus. Dev Med Child Neurol 1995;37:682—8.

13.   Sheth RD, Ronen GM, Goulden KJ, Penney S, Bodensteiner JB. Clobazam for intractable pediatric epilepsy. J Child Neurol 1995;10:205—8.

14.   Gorman M, Barkley GL. Oculogyric crisis induced by carbamazepine. Epilepsia 1995;36: 1158—60.

15.   Lenders T, Bauer J, Elger CE. Does carbamazepine alter coagulation parameters? An investigation of 91 epileptic patients receiving carbamazepine monotherapy. Epilepsia 1995;36 Suppl 3:70.

16.   Hughes JR, DeTolve-Donoghue M. Chronic leukopenia associated with carbamazepine and other antiepileptic drugs. J Epilepsy 1995;8:282—8.

17.   Miura H, Takanashi S, Shirai H, Sunaoshi W, Hosoda N, Abo K, Katgiri T, Takei K. Skin rash caused by carbamazepine. Epilepsia 1995;36 Suppl 3:69.

18.   Tiihonen M, Vartiainen H, Hakola P. Carbamazepine-induced changes in plasma levels of neuroleptics. Pharmacopsychiatry 1995;28:26—8.

19.   Iwahashi K, Miyatake R, Suwaki H, Hosokawa K, Ichikawa Y. The drug-drug interaction effects of haloperidol on plasma carbamazepine levels. Clin Neuropharmacol 1995;18:233—6.

20.   Ketter TA, Jenkins JB, Schroeder DH, Pazzaglia PJ, Marangell LB, George MS, Callahan AM, Hinton ML, Chao J, Post RM. Carbamazepine but not valproate induced bupropion metabolism. J Clin Psychopharmacol 1995;15:327—33.

21.   Ettinger AB, Jandorf L, Berdia A, Andriola MR, Krupp LB, Weisbrot DM. Felbamate-induced headache. Epilepsia 1996;37:503—5.

22.   Kerrick JM, Kelley BJ, Maister BH, Graves NM, Leppik IE. Involuntary movement disorders associated with felbamate. Neurology 1995; 45:185—7.

23.   Welty TE, Privitera M. Increased seizure frequency during and immediately following felbamate withdrawal. Epilepsia 1995;36 Suppl 4:64.

24.   DeGiorgio CM, Lopez JE, Lekht Z, Rabinowicz AL. Status epilepticus induced by felbatol withdrawal. Neurology 1995;45:1021—2.

25.   Penovich PE, Korby B, Moriarty GL, Gates JR. Antinuclear antibodies in patients on Felbatol. Epilepsia 1995;36 Suppl 4:65.

26.   Hooper WD, Franklin ME, Glue P, Banfield CR, Radwanski E, McLaughlin DB, McIntyre ME, Dickinson RG, Eadie MJ. Effect of felbamate on valproic acid disposition in healthy volunteers: inhibition of β-oxidation. Epilepsia 1996; 37:91—7.

27.   Saano V, Glue P, Banfield R, Reidenberg P, Colucci RD, Meehan JW, Haring P, Radwanski E, Nomeir A, Lin CC, Jensen PK, Affrime MB. Effects of felbamate on the pharmacokinetics of a low-dose combination oral contraceptive. Clin Pharmacol Ther 1995;8:23—31.

28.   Doherty KP, Gates JR, Penovich PE, Moriarty MD. Gabapentin in a medically refractory epilepsy population: Seizure response and unusual side effects. Epilepsia 1995;36 Suppl 4:71.

29.   Litzinger MJ, Wiscombe N, Hanny A, Yau J, Green D. Increased seizures and aggression seen in persons with mental retardation and epilepsy treated with Neurontin. Epilepsia 1995;36 Suppl 4:71.

30.   Shantz D, Towbin JA, Spitz MC. Changes in mood and affect in patients on gabapentin. Epilepsia 1995;36 Suppl 4:73.

31.   Cugley AL, Swatz BE. Gabapentin-associated mood changes? Epilepsia 1995;36 Suppl 4:72.

32.   Lee DO, Steingard RJ, Cesena M, Helmers SL, Riviello JJ, Mikati MA. Behavioural side effects of gabapentin in children. Epilepsia 1996;37:87—90.

33.   Tallian KB, Nahata MC, Lo W, Tsao CY. Gabapentin associated with aggressive behavior in pediatric patients with seizures. Epilepsia 1996;37:501—2.

34.   Wolf S, Shinnar S, Kang H, Gil KB, Moshe SL. Gabapentin toxicity in children manifesting as behavioural changes. Epilepsia 1995;36:1203—5.

35.   Zupanc ML, Schroeder VM. Behavioural changes in children on gabapentin. Epilepsia 1995;36 Suppl 4:73.

36.   Asconape J, Collins T. Weight gain associated with the use of gabapentin. Epilepsia 1995;36 Suppl 4:72.

37.   Gidal BE, Maly MM, Nemire RE, Haley K. Weight gain and gabapentin therapy. Ann Pharmacother 1995;29:1048.

38.   King JA, Bayles RL. Weight gain during add-

on therapy using gabapentin. Epilepsia 1995;36 Suppl 4:72.

39.   Tatum WO, Zachariah SB. Gabapentin treatment of seizures in acute intermittent porphyria. Neurology 1995;45:1216—7.

40.   Krauss GL, Simmonds-O'Brien E, Campbell M. Successful treatment of seizures and porphyria with gabapentin. Neurology 1995;45:594—5.

41.   Schachter SC, Leppik IE, Matsuo F, Messenheimer JA, Faught E, Moore EL, Risner ME. Lamotrigine: a six-month, placebo controlled, safety and tolerance study. J Epilepsy 1995; 8:201—9.

42.   Duval X, Chosidow O, Semah F, Lipsker D, Frances C, Herson S. Lamotrigine vs carbamazepine in epilepsy. Lancet 1995;345:1300—2.

43.   Dooley J, Camfield P, Gordon K, Camfield C, Wirrell Z, Smith E. Lamotrigine-induced rash in children. Neurology 199;46:240—2.

44.   Campistol J, Geli M, Llistosella E, Molins J, Llobet M. Sindrome de Steven-Johnson tras la introduccion de lamotrigina. Rev Neurol 1995; 23:1236—8.

45.   Martin M, Munoz-Blanco JL, Lopez-Ariztegui N. Acute psychosis induced by lamotrigine. Epilepsia 1995;36 Suppl 3:118.

46.   Arnold ST. Bourgeois BFD, Montouris GD, Harden CL, Carson D, French DA, Rosenfeld WE, Schaefer P. Safety profile of lamotrigine in children. Epilepsia 1995;36 Suppl 4:67.

47.   Sterker M, Berrouschot J, Schneider D. Fatal course of toxic epidermal necrolysis under treatment with lamotrigine. Int J Clin Pharmacol Ther 1995;33:595—7.

48.   Tavenor SJ, Wong IC, Mewton R, Brown SW. Rechallenge with lamotrigine after initial rash. Seizure 1995;4:67—71.

49.   Kilpatrick ES, Forrest G, Borodie MJ. Concentration-effect and concentration-toxicity relations with lamotrigine: a prospective study. Epilepsia 1996;37:534—8

50.   Gonzalez Perez S, Perez Encinas M, Rabunal Martinez MJ, Bendana Lopez A, Lete Achirica I, Bello Lopez JL. Aplasia medular secundaria a lamotrigina. Sangre 1995;40 Suppl 4:296.

51.   Haedicke C, Angrick B, Hauswaldt. Lamotrigine vs carbamazepine in epilepsy. Lancet 1995;345:1300—2.

52.   Pavone A, Falsaperla A, Marino G, Di Virgilio R, Agrosi F. La lamotrigina in una paziente con beta-talassemia eterozigote. Boll Lega It Epil 1995;91—92:167—8.

53.   Nicholson RJ, Kelly KP, Grant IS. Leucopenia associated with lamotrigine. Br Med J 1995;310:504.

54.   Makin AJ, Fitt S, Williams R, Duncan JS. Fulminant hepatic failure induced by lamotrigine. Br Med J 1995;311:292.

55.   Yuen AWC, Bihari DJ. Multiorgan failure and disseminated intravascular coagulation in severe convulsive seizures. Lancet 1992;342:618.

56.   Schaub JEM, Williamson PJ, Barnes EW, Trewby PN. Multisystem adverse reaction to lamotrigine. Lancet 1994;344:481.

57.   Eldridge RR, Tennis P, and The Lamotrigine Pregnancy Registry Advisory Committee. Monitoring birth outcomes in the Lamotrigine Pregnancy Registry. Epilepsia 1995;36 Suppl 4:90.

58.   Reinisch JM, Sanders SA, Mortensen EL, Rubin DB. In utero exposure to phenobarbital and intelligence deficits in adult men. J Am Med Assoc 1995;274:1518—25.

59.   Pulliainen V, Jokelainen M. Comparing the cognitive effects of phenytoin and carbamazepine in long-term monotherapy: a two-year follow-up. Epilepsia 1995;36:1195—202.

60.   Lau KHW, Nakade O, Barr B, Taylor AK, Houchin K, Baylink DJ. Phenytoin increases markers of osteogenesis for the human species in vitro and in vivo. J Clin Endocrinol Metab 1995; 80:2347—53.

61.   Jeng YM, Tien HF, Su IJ. Phenytoin-induced pseudolymphoma: reevaluation using modern molecular biology techniques. Epilepsia 1996; 37:104—7.

62.   Recuenco I, Espinosa E, Garcia B, Carcas A. Effect of dexamethasone on the decrease of serum phenytoin concentrations. Ann Pharmacother 1995;29:935.

63.   Lackner TE. Interaction of dexamethasone with phenytoin. Pharmacotherapy 1991;11:344—7.

64.   Lawson LA, Bluoin RA, Smith RB, Rapp RP, Young AB. Phenytoin-dexamethasone interaction: a previously unreported observation. Surg Neurol 1981;16:23—4.

65.   Veloso F. Safety and tolerability of remacemide hydrochloride. Epilepsia 1995;36 Suppl 4:55.

66.   Sachdeo RC, Brunswick N, Biton V, Boellner SW, Schachter SC, Alto GH, Kaply CW, Phillips HB, Kardatzke, Pixton G, Sommerville KW. Long term safety of tiagabine HCl. Epilepsia 1995;36 Suppl 4:55.

67.   Bauer J, Stawowy B, Lenders T, Bettig U, Elger CE. Efficacy and tolerability of tiagabine: results of an add-on study in patients with refractory partial seizures. J Epilepsy 1995;8:83—6.

68.   Ben-Menachem E, Henriksen O, Dam M, Mikkelsen M, Schmidt D, Reid S, Reife R, Kramer L, Pledger G, Karim R. Double-blind, placebo-controlled trial of topiramate as add-on therapy in patients with refractory partial seizures. Epilepsia 1996;37:539—43.

69.   Tassinari CA, Michelucci R, Chauvel P, Chodkiewicz J, Shorvon, S, Henriksen, O, Dam, M, Reife R, Pledger G, Karim R. Double-blind, placebo-controlled trial of topiramate (600 mg daily) for the treatment of refractory partial epilepsy. Epilepsia 1996;37:763—8.

70.   Reife RA, Pledger G. Safety of topiramate in clinical use. Adv AED Ther 1995;1:24—9.

71.   Reife RA, Lim P, Pledger G. Topiramate: Side effect profile in double-blind studies. Epilepsia 1995;36 Suppl 4:34.

72.   Tartara A, Sartori I, Manni R, Galimberti CA, Di Fazio M, Perucca E. Efficacy and safety of topiramate in refractory epilepsy: a long-term prospective trial. Ital J Neurol (in press).

73. Pavkovic I, Sackellares C, Beydoun A. Efficacy and safety of topiramate in epilepsy. Epilepsia 1995;36 Suppl 4:55.

74. Espe-Lillo J, Ritter FJ, Frost M, Spiegel RH, Reife R. Topiramate in childhood epilepsy: titration, adverse events, and efficacy in multiple seizure types. Epilepsia 1995;36 Suppl 4:56.

75. Wasserstein AG, Rak I, Reife RA. Investigation of the mechanistic basis for topiramate-associated nephrolithiasis: examination of urine and serum constituents. Epilepsia 1995;36 Suppl 3:153.

76. Wasserstein AG, Rak I, Reife RA. Nephrolithiasis during treatment with topiramate. Epilepsia 1995;36 Suppl 3:153.

77. Ben-Menachem E. Potential antiepileptic drugs: Topiramate. In: Levy RH, Mattson RH, Meldrum BS, editors. New York: Raven Press, 1995:1063—70.

78. Doose DR. Gisclon LG, Liao S, Wu WN. Pharmacokinetics of topiramate. Adv AED Ther 1995;1:7—16.

79. Sachdeo RC, Sachdeo SK, Walker SA, Kramer LD, Nayak RK, Doose DR. Steady-state pharmacokinetics of topiramate and carbamazepine in patients with epilepsy during monotherapy and concomitant therapy. Epilepsia 1996; 37:774—80.

80. Sachdeo RC, Sachdeo SK, Levy RH, Nayak RK, Kramer LD, Gisclon LG. Topiramate and phenytoin pharmacokinetics in patients with epilepsy during monotherapy and combination therapy. Epilepsia (in press).

81. Doose DR, Walker SA, Sachdeo R, Kramer LD, Nayak RK. Steady-state pharmacokinetics of Tegretol (carbamazepine) and Topamax (topiramate) in patients with epilepsy on monotherapy and during combination therapy. Epilepsia 1994;35 Suppl 8:54.

82. Doose DR, Walker SA, Pledger G, Lim P, Reife RA. Evaluation of phenobarbital and primidone/phenobarbital (primidone's active metabolite) plasma concentrations during administration of add-on topiramate therapy in five multicenter, double-blind, placebo controlled trials in outpatients with partial seizures. Epilepsia 1995;36 Suppl 3:S158.

83. Gisclon LG, Curtin CR, Kramer LD, Sachdeo RC, Levy RH. Steady-state pharmacokinetics of phenytoin (Dilantin) and topiramate (Topamax) in epileptic patients on monotherapy and during combination therapy. Epilepsia 1994;35 Suppl 8:54.

84. Rosenfeld WE, Liao S, Kramer LD, Anderson G, Palmer M, Levy RH, Nayak RK. Comparison of the steady-state pharmacokinetics of topiramate and valproate in patients with epilepsy during monotherapy and concomitant therapy. Epilepsia 1997;38:324—33.

85. Levy RH, Bishop F, Streeter AJ, et al. Explanation and prediction of drug interactions with topiramate using a CYP450 inhibition spectrum. Epilepsia 1995;36 Suppl 4:47.

86. Rosenfeld WE, Doose DR, Walker SA, Nayak RK. Effect of topiramate on the pharmacokinetics of an oral contraceptive containing norethindrone and ethinyl estradiol in patients with epilepsy. Epilepsia 1997;38:317—23.

87. Devinsky O, Leppik I, Willmore LJ, Pellock JM, Dean C, Gates J, Ramsay RE, Abou-Khalil B, Ahmann P, Barkley G, Bogdanoff B, Brown L, Cahill W, Dean C, Devinsky O, Drinslane F, Eaton J, Ehle A, Faught R. Safety of intravenous valproate. Ann Neurol 1995;38:670—4.

88. Papazian O, Canizales E, Alfonso I, Archila R, Duchowny M, Aicardi J. Reversible dementia and apparent brain atrophy during valproate therapy. Ann Neurol 1995;38:687—91.

89. McLachlan RS. Pseudoatrophy of the brain with valproic acid monotherapy. Can J Neurol Sci 1987;14:294—6.

90. Zaret BS, Cohen RA. Reversible valproic acid-induced dementia: a case report. Epilepsia 1986;27:234—40.

91. Lancman ME, Asconape JJ, Penry JK. Choreiform movements associated with the use of valproate. Arch Neurol 1994;51:702—4.

92. Isojarvi JIT, Tapanainen J, Rattya J, Knip M, Pakarinen AJ, Tekay A, Myllyla VV. Changes in body weight, fasting serum insulin and testosterone levels and ovarian structure in women with epilepsy after substituting lamotrigine for valproate. Epilepsia 1995;36 Suppl 4:57.

93. Leao M. Valproate as a cause of hyperammonemia in heterozygotes with ornithine-transcarbamylase deficiency. Neurology 1995;45:593—4.

94. Coulter DL. Carnitine deficiency in epilepsy: Risk factors and treatment. J Child Neurol 1995;10 Suppl 2:2S32—9.

95. Buzan RD, Firestone D, Thomas M, Dubovsky SL. Valproate-associated pancreatitis and cholecystitis in six mentally retarded adults. J Clin Psychiatry 1995;56:529—32.

96. Benninger C, Freund M, Wuhl E, Mehls O. Reversible acute renal failure during valproate therapy. Epilepsia 1995;36 Suppl 3:S68.

97. Sheth RD, Wesolowski Ca, Jacob JC, Penney S, Hobbs GR, Riggs JE, Bodensteiner JB. Effect of carbamazepine and valproate on bone mineral density. J Pediatr 1995;127:256—62.

98. Gigli GL, Scalise A, Pauri F, Silvestri G, Diomedi M, Placidi F, Pomponi MG, Masala C. Valproate-induced systemic lupus erythematosus in a patient with partial trisomy of chromosome 9 and epilepsy. Epilepsia 1996;37:587—8.

99. Murakami K, Sugimoto T, Woo M, Nishida N, Muro H. Effect of l-carnitine supplementation on acute valproate intoxication. Epilepsia 1996;37:687—9.

100. Suzuki Y, Nagai T, Mano T, Arai H, Kodaka R, Matsuoka T, Itagaki Y, Ono J, Okada S. Interaction between valproate formulation and phenytoin concentrations. J Clin Pharmacol 1995; 48:61—3.

101. Longo LP, Salzman C. Valproic acid effects on serum concentrations of clozapine and norclozapine. Am J Psychiatry 1995;152:650.

102. Kalviainen R, Aikia M, Saukkonen AM, Mervaala E, Riekkinen PJ. Vigabatrin versus carbamazepine monotherapy in patients with newly diagnosed epilepsy: a randomized controlled study. Arch Neurol 1995;52:989—96.

103. Marciani MG, Gigli GL, Maschio MCE, Spanedda F, Curatolo P, Orlandi L, Bernardi G. Vigabatrin-induced myoclonus in four cases of partial epilepsy. Epilepsia 1995;36 Suppl 3:107.

104. Rogers D, Bird J, Eames P. Complex partial status after starting vigabatrin. Seizure 1993; 2:155—6.

105. Van der Zwan Jr A, Van der Zwan A. Vigabatrin: ervaringen met een nieuw anti-epilepticum bij 57 patienten in een algemene neurologische praktijk. Ned Tijd Geneesk 1994;138:1859—63.

106. De Krom MC, Verduin N, Visser E, Kleijer M, Scholtes F, De Groen JH. Status epilepticus during vigabatrin treatment: a report of three cases. Seizure 1995;4:159—62.

107. Arzimanoglou A. Vigabatrin and complex partial status. Seizure 1994;3:79—80.

108. Ferrie CD, Robinson RO, Panayiotopoulos CP. Psychotic and severe behavioural reactions with vigabatrin-a review. Acta Neurol Scand 1996;93—108.

109. Wong ICK. Retrospective study of vigabatrin and psychiatric behavioural disturbances. Epilepsy Res 1995;21:227—30.

110. Levinson DFL, Mumford JP. Vigabatrin and psychosis. Epilepsia 1995;36 Suppl 4:32.

111. Canova-Martinez A, Ordovas-Baines JP, Beltran-Marques M, Escriva-Aparisi A, Delgado-Cordon F. Vigabatrin-associated reversible acute psychosis in a child. Ann Pharmacother 1995; 29:1115—7.

112. Rentmeester TW, Hulsman JARJ. Survey of 5 years experience with vigabatrin in an epilepsy center. Epilepsia 1995;36 Suppl 4:31.

113. Hommel L, Ruffieux P, Masouye I, Jallon P, Saurat JH. Acute bullous skin eruption after treatment with Sabril. Epilepsia 1995;36 Suppl 3:109.

114. Foletti GB, Delisle MC, Bachmann C. Reduction of plasma alanine aminotransferase during vigabatrin treatment. Epilepsia 1995;36:804—9.

115. Vallat C, Rivier F, Bellet H, Magnan de Bornier B, Mion H, Echenne B. Treatment with vigabatrin may mimic alpha-aminoadipic aciduria. Epilepsia 1996;37:803—5.

116. Bartoli A, Gatti G, Barzaghi N, Cipolla G, Veliz G, Mumford JP, Perucca E. Vigabatrin does not affect in vivo parameters of enzyme induction in humans. Epilepsia 1995;36 Suppl 3:162.

A.H. Ghodse and R.E. Edwards

8 Opioid analgesics and narcotic antagonists

OPIOID ANALGESICS *(SED-13, 160; SEDA-17, 78; SEDA-18, 80; SEDA-19, 82)*

Many publications on opioids during the past year, although of interest with regard to their analgesic effects, do not illustrate any new adverse effects, and this review therefore focuses on the adverse effects encountered with newer drugs, novel routes of administration, and new uses of the currently available opioids.

GENERAL

Use has been made of what is usually considered an adverse effect of opioids, namely a *reduction in ventilatory drive*, to relieve the sensation of dyspnea in patients with chronic obstructive pulmonary disease (1[R]). In addition to the reduction in central respiratory drive, morphine may also relieve the individual's perception of dyspnea. There is, of course, a significant risk of *carbon dioxide retention*, leading to coma and death, although this may be an acceptable outcome when other forms of treatment have failed.

In a study of opioid usage and the incidence of adverse effects after urological, gynecological, orthopedic, and general surgical operations, 180 chronic opioid users were matched with controls who did not have pain or use opioids (2[Cr]). The opioid users had higher pain scores, and used more opioid medication. They had fewer adverse effects than the control group, with a significantly lower incidence of *nausea and vomiting* and *pruritus*. This is not surprising, since tolerance develops to adverse effects as well as to analgesia.

FULL OPIOID AGONISTS

Alfentanil *(SED-13, 173; SEDA-17, 79; SEDA-18, 84; SEDA-19, 82)*

The plasma concentration profile of a bolus dose of epidural alfentanil followed by an infusion has been studied in women in labor (3[cr]). The effects of this method of pain relief on the fetal heart tracing were also described. Two groups of women (12 in each group) received either 500 µg of alfentanil in 10 ml of 0.125% bupivacaine or fentanyl 50 µg in 10 ml of 0.125% bupivacaine as a bolus dose. This was followed by a continuous infusion of 6−12 ml/h of alfentanil 20 µg/ml or fentanyl 2 µg/ml in 0.125% bupivacaine to maintain a sensory block to the tenth thoracic dermatome. There was no difference between the two groups in fetal heart rate variability and decelerations. In one patient in the alfentanil group there were variable decelerations after epidural placement, and there was also a fall in baseline heart rate and an increase in variability in one woman in the fentanyl group. There were no other changes in the fetal heart tracing within 1 h of epidural placement in the two groups. Steady-state plasma concentrations of alfentanil were reached quickly by this technique and were well below those associated with respiratory depression. The mean duration of infusion in this study was short (3.7 h), but in theory the infusion could continue much longer without the risk of higher plasma opioid concentrations.

Side Effects of Drugs, Annual 20
J.K. Aronson, ed.

Fentanyl *(SED-13, 174; SEDA-17, 80; SEDA-18, 80; SEDA-19, 82)*

Pain after thoracotomy is a therapeutic challenge, as the ideal method of pain relief should enable the patient to take deep breaths and cough without causing respiratory depression. Fentanyl or saline were randomly administered via a microspinal catheter to 30 patients scheduled for thoracotomy; a third group acted as a control (4^{Cr}). All the patients received patient-controlled morphine. The patients with a spinal catheter received either 1-ml boluses of 50 µg/ml fentanyl or normal saline at 10-min intervals to a maximum of three doses. The quality and duration of analgesia in the fentanyl group was excellent. Furthermore, the reduction in pulmonary function postoperatively was less in this group. Post-spinal headaches occurred in 25% of patients and responded to simple analgesia and fluids. Pruritus occurred in three patients who received intrathecal fentanyl and one who received saline. There were no clinically significant cases of respiratory depression.

℞ *Buccal and transdermal administration of fentanyl*

Buccal administration Fentanyl is a synthetic opioid with a potency 100 times that of morphine. It has a high tissue solubility and is heat resistant; it can therefore be administered by incorporation into a candy matrix to make a 'lollipop' for absorption via the buccal mucosa. First-pass metabolism is therefore avoided. Oral transmucosal fentanyl citrate 15—20 µg/kg or placebo was given to 48 children before lumbar puncture or bone-marrow aspiration (5^{CR}). A larger study had initially been planned, as it had been designed at a time when premedication for painful procedures was not routine. During the study, however, intravenous sedation became accepted practice and it was no longer ethical to include a placebo group. Not surprisingly, the pain ratings with placebo were significantly higher than with fentanyl. The adverse effects of fentanyl, in order of frequency, were pruritus (65%), nausea and vomiting (31%), nausea alone (12%), and a low oxygen saturation (7%). There were significant differences between the two groups in the incidences of pruritus and of nausea and vomiting. Two children in the fentanyl group had oxygen saturations of less than 95% (94 and 93%). No child required intervention for respiratory depression.

Two doses of oral transmucosal fentanyl citrate have been compared in 30 children aged 2—8 years undergoing laceration repair in a pediatric emergency department; fentanyl was given 30 min before the procedure (6^{cr}). There was no significant difference between the two groups in pain and sedation scores, and the physician's assessment of the child's sedation and pain score was excellent in 83%. Respiratory rate fell significantly in both groups after fentanyl, although only one child in the low-dose group had persistent oxygen saturations below 95% and required extra oxygen. Of those who received high-dose fentanyl, 47% vomited compared with 20% in the low-dose group; although this difference was not statistically significant, this may have been a Type 2 error, because the sample size was small. Three of the seven children in the high-dose group who vomited did so repeatedly. Pruritus was a common adverse effect in both groups (67 and 60%), although only two children had significant generalized pruritus.

Oral transmucosal fentanyl citrate has also been evaluated for use in adults undergoing painful procedures. Two doses (400 or 800 µg) were evaluated in 30 patients undergoing dermatological procedures as out-patients (7^{c}). Sedation and anxiety scores were comparable: 63% of patients in the low-dose group and 71% in the high-dose group became more sedated, and about half the patients in each group became less apprehensive. Nausea, vomiting, dizziness, and pruritus were the most common adverse effects. Four patients in the low-dose group and eight patients in the high-dose group were prompted to breathe when their oxygen saturations fell below 90%. Two patients required additional oxygen to maintain a saturation above 90%, which is still very low. It was not documented how many patients had a saturation below 95%.

Transdermal administration Another relatively novel route of administration of fentanyl is the transdermal route. Fentanyl is highly lipid soluble with a low molecular weight, which makes it suitable for transdermal use. In the fentanyl transdermal therapeutic system *fentanyl base is incorporated in 25% ethanol to increase its solubility. Fentanyl is released at a rate of 25 μg/h/cm^2 and the dose is therefore increased by increasing the surface area of the system.*

Guidelines for the use of transdermal fentanyl in patients with cancer have been published (8[r]) and it is proposed that this route offers an alternative non-invasive method of pain relief to oral therapy, which is of particular value in patients who are unable to swallow or who have nausea and vomiting. In a multicenter study, 39 patients with cancer pain were stabilized on morphine for at least 3 days, then converted to an equianalgesic dose of transdermal fentanyl (9[c]). The fentanyl patch was changed every 3 days. The median duration of fentanyl use was 84 days (range 5—365) and the median final dose was 100 μg/h (range 25—600 μg/h). One patient developed an exacerbation of a generalized dermatophytic reaction and one patient required naloxone for respiratory depression, although this was attributed to the patient's illness rather than to the fentanyl. No other untoward reactions were attributed to the fentanyl patch.

In 38 patients with malignant disease transdermal fentanyl was used in a dosage chosen in accordance with their previous morphine dosage (10[Cr]). There was no significant difference between the two drugs in the incidence of nausea, vomiting, diarrhea, or pruritus, but fentanyl was associated with significantly less constipation.

Transdermal fentanyl has been further evaluated in a study for pain relief in 50 patients with cancers (11[C]). The optimal dose for each patient was chosen by using intravenous patient-controlled fentanyl for 24 h and then calculating the dosage of transdermal fentanyl from the total dose used during this period. The mean duration of usage was 65 days (range 2—534). No serious adverse effects were observed. A respiratory rate of less than 8/min was documented in three sleeping patients. There was markedly less constipation, nausea, and vomiting during fentanyl treatment. Other symptoms were also reported, such as sweating, dizziness, fatigue, and pruritus, although these were not changed from the pre-study period. Nine patients experienced mild skin changes, but no treatment was required.

Another fentanyl transdermal therapeutic system (Janssen Duragesic TTS), which delivers 100 μg/h has been evaluated after upper abdominal surgery in 22 patients (12[c]). The system was applied 1 h before surgery and additional morphine was given on the patient's request in the recovery room (2.5 mg intravenously every 10 min) and on the ward (5 mg intramuscularly 2-hourly). The quality of analgesia was better with transdermal fentanyl than with intermittent dosing of morphine. However, three patients given fentanyl had respiratory rates of 7—9/min. Patients in both groups had saturations of about 93%, although the time spent with oxygen saturations of less than 90% was greater in the fentanyl group. The fentanyl group also had increased transcutaneous carbon dioxide concentrations. The study was terminated when a previously healthy woman became very sedated with a respiratory rate of 8—9/min, a P_aCO_2 of 7.4—7.6, and a P_aO_2 as low as 5.8 kPa. The use of the Janssen Duragesic TTS system has now been restricted by the FDA to patients with chronic cancer pain.

A newer fentanyl transdermal therapeutic system with a faster onset and shorter duration of action has been evaluated for postoperative analgesia in 144 women scheduled for gynecological laparotomy (13[Cr]). They were randomized to receive either 70—80 or 90—100 μg/kg/h in a double-blind placebo-controlled manner. Patient-controlled morphine was also available. The quality of analgesia in the higher-dose fentanyl group was significantly better than placebo at 8, 12, 16, 20, and 24 h postoperatively, and the quality of analgesia in the lower-dose group was significantly better than placebo at 16 and 24 h. There was a higher incidence of respiratory depression, pruritus, and erythema with fentanyl than placebo. Respiratory depression, defined as a respiratory rate of less than 8/min or SPO_2 less than 90%, was significantly more frequent in the higher-dose fentanyl group. The authors concluded that the patch shows promise for the relief of postoperative pain, but that the dosages used in this study were excessive.

Another fentanyl transdermal therapeutic system (Cygnus) has been evaluated for postoperative analgesia in 15 men undergoing a range of surgical procedures (14[cr]). The Cygnus system does not incorporate a rate-con-

trolling membrane. The 60-cm² patch was applied 24 h after the induction of anesthesia. Three patients had clinically significant fentanyl toxicity requiring removal of the patch. Two of these had respiratory depression, one requiring naloxone for 2 h; the third complained of dizziness. There was great variability in the rate of fentanyl absorption, with very variable plasma concentrations. This transdermal therapeutic system therefore does not afford greater safety than other systems for postoperative use.

An unusual reaction to transdermal fentanyl has been reported (15ᶜ). A 14-year-old boy with metastatic adenocarcinoma was treated with transdermal fentanyl in a starting dose of 25 μg/h, increased to 100 μg/h over 2 months. On the day after the dosage was increased from 75 to 100 μg/h he became agitated, and this progressed over 1 week to extreme agitation and hyperactivity. He was sedated with midazolam and pentobarbital and the fentanyl patch was removed. His symptoms resolved 24 h later. All other causes for his acute delirium were excluded. However, he did have mild hepatic and renal impairment, and it was postulated that this may have allowed accumulation of norfentanyl, the chief metabolite of fentanyl. On the other hand, it is uncertain whether norfentanyl has any effects on the central nervous system.

Oral transmucosal fentanyl citrate therefore seems to be suitable for producing analgesia and sedation in both adults and children undergoing short painful outpatient procedures. Transdermal fentanyl, on the other hand, provides excellent analgesia in patients with chronic pain due to malignancy, but is not suitable for postoperative analgesia, owing to the high incidence of adverse effects.

Methadone *(SED-13, 176; SEDA-17, 81; SEDA-18, 81; SEDA-19, 83)*

Four patients with methadone *withdrawal psychosis* have been described (16ᶜ). One patient had schizophrenia but had been asymptomatic on methadone treatment, one patient had had a previous psychotic episode 21 years previously, and two patients had no history of psychosis. The authors discussed the cause of this opioid withdrawal psychosis.

Morphine *(SED-13, 176; SEDA-17, 82; SEDA-18, 81; SEDA-19, 83)*

There has been a study of the use of epidural morphine in 146 consecutive patients with cancer, selected for epidural opioid when other routes of administration had failed to provide adequate pain relief with acceptable adverse effects (17ᶜᴿ). Epidural morphine was continued in 121 patients after the initial 10-day trial period. In 19 of these the opioid was changed to buprenorphine or methadone because of *nausea* (six), *hallucinations* (six), *sedation* (three), *rash* (two), *pruritus* (one), and an unspecified reason (one). The catheters were tunnelled subcutaneously, and infection along the catheter canal occurred in only two patients. Intolerable adverse effects were responsible for withdrawal from epidural morphine therapy; three patients were confused and one had severe nausea. No patients had respiratory depression.

Major abdominal surgery is associated with postoperative ileus and delayed recovery of gastrointestinal function. It has been suggested that epidural analgesia may accelerate the recovery of function. A prospective randomized study of different methods of analgesia after abdominal surgery has shown that patients who received epidural morphine with bupivacaine or epidural bupivacaine alone recovered gastrointestinal function significantly more quickly and fulfilled discharge criteria 1.5 days earlier than patients who received either intravenous or epidural morphine alone (18ᶜᴿ). Not surprisingly, there was a higher incidence of *pruritus* in the epidural morphine group. There was a lower incidence of adverse effects in the combined morphine/bupivacaine epidural group.

In a spot survey of the incidence of *constipation* in 32 orthopedic patients receiving postoperative opioid analgesia, 63% suffered from postoperative constipation (19ᶜ). Of the 78% of patients who received morphine, 76% were constipated. Of the 25 patients who received morphine seven were given it epidurally. Only 31% took a laxative to relieve the constipation.

In a prospective study of 500 children aged 6 months to 16 years receiving either 0.03 or 0.04 mg/kg of morphine caudally there were no cases of respiratory depression (20ᶜ). Analgesia was provided for 6—24 h, as assessed by the time to requiring additional analgesia. In all, 23% of patients had *nausea and vomiting*, 7% had *pruritus*, and 3% required *bladder catheterization*.

Two novel routes for the administration of morphine or bupivacaine have been studied for the provision of analgesia after laparoscopic cholecystectomy (21[CR]). The patients received either intraperitoneal morphine (1 mg in 20 ml of saline) or bupivacaine (20 ml 0.25%), interpleural morphine (1.5 mg in 30 ml of saline) or bupivacaine (30 ml 0.25%) with equivalent volumes of intravenous saline, or an equivalent volume of intraperitoneal and interpleural saline with 1.0 or 1.5 mg of morphine intravenously, respectively. Only interpleural bupivacaine produced satisfactory analgesia after the operation. There were no adverse effects, such as nausea, pruritus, or urinary retention, attributable to the drugs.

Morphine-6-glucuronide is an active metabolite of morphine; it is synthesized in the liver and excreted by the kidneys. Adverse effects associated with morphine may be due to morphine-6-glucuronide. A study has been carried out in 109 patients with cancer receiving either oral or parenteral morphine, in order to elucidate whether cognitive impairment or myoclonus, two adverse effects of morphine, were due to an increase in the morphine-6-glucuronide/morphine ratio or related to the concentration of morphine-6-glucuronide (22[Cr]). The mean doses of morphine were 486 mg for the oral group and 931 mg for the parenteral group. Neither adverse effect was significantly associated with the ratio of morphine-6-glucuronide:morphine. High concentrations of morphine-6-glucuronide (over 2000 ng/ml) were associated with *respiratory depression* and *obtundation* mainly when metabolic dysfunction due to organ failure was present. Patients who received oral morphine were three times more likely to have *myoclonus*, but the morphine-6-glucuronide:morphine ratio was not an independent predictor of myoclonus.

Oxycodone *(SED-13, 177; SEDA-19, 85)*

Rectal and intravenous oxycodone have been compared in a crossover study of 12 patients with cancer pain (23[CR]). The mean intravenous dose was 0.11 mg/kg and the rectal dose was 30 mg. Lower intravenous doses were given to patients with hepatic impairment. Adverse effects occurred within 4 h of intravenous drug administration and 8 h of rectal administration. There was no significant difference between the two routes in the total number of adverse effects, or in the mean verbal rating score for each adverse effect. The commonest adverse effect in both groups was *drowsiness*, followed by *light-headedness*. *Sweating* and *hot flushes* were reported with both routes, as were *pruritus* and *vomiting*. *Nausea* was commoner after the rectal route.

Pethidine (meperidine) *(SED-13, 178; SEDA-17, 83; SEDA-18, 178; SEDA-19, 85)*

Pethidine 75 mg plus promethazine 25 mg, or dihydroergotamine 0.5 mg plus metoclopramide 10 mg have been compared in a randomized study in 27 patients with acute migraine or a combination of migraine and tension headache (24[C]). Although there were no statistically significant differences in the relief of pain at 1 h or in the percentage of patients using pain medications at 24 h, there was a statistically significantly higher incidence of adverse effects in the pethidine/promethazine group. The adverse effects reported for the dihydroergotamine and pethidine groups respectively were nausea (1.3 vs. 1.9%), *dizziness* (1.0 vs. 2.3%), *lethargy* (1.6 vs. 2.9%), and *postural hypotension* (7.7 vs. 61.5%).

As pethidine is structurally similar to local anesthetics, a study has been carried out in 30 men scheduled for transurethral resection of the prostate or bladder tumours to determine whether the addition of adrenaline to intrathecal pethidine prolongs its action (25[cr]). The men were randomly allocated to receive 0.05 mg/kg of pethidine intrathecally with or without 0.2 ml of 1 in 10 000 adrenaline. The incidence of adverse effects were similar: *respiratory depression* (one in each group), *pruritus* (50%), *nausea* (21 vs. 19%), and *vomiting* (7.1 vs. 6.3%). Adrenaline did not prolong the duration of sensory blockade, although there was a significantly higher incidence of full motor blockade in the group that did not receive adrenaline.

Sufentanil *(SED-13, 178; SEDA-17, 84; SEDA-18, 83; SEDA-19, 85)*

A woman in labor was given two doses of intrathecal sufentanil 4 h apart; 20 min after the second injection she was unresponsive to verbal commands and had a *respiratory arrest* (26[c]). She responded immediately to 0.4 mg of naloxone. The most likely cause of the arrest was a high plasma concentration of sufentanil, because of its long duration of action of 7 h. However cephalad migration of the drug cannot be ruled out.

The incidence of *apneic episodes* has been documented after laparotomy in 30 patients (27[Cr]). The patients were randomly allocated to receive either morphine 10 mg intramuscularly on demand, or sufentanil 50 µg epidurally followed by a bolus of 10 µg either self-administered or nurse-administered on request. The mean doses in a 24-h period were 52 (range 30—80) mg for morphine, 275 (130—450) µg for self-administered sufentanil, and 144 (70—200) µg for nurse-administered sufentanil. Pain scores were similar in the three groups. There were no significant differences in the number or duration of apneic episodes across the three groups. Five patients in each group required additional oxygen for arterial oxygen saturations of less than 85%. Most of the episodes were obstructive. There was a significant difference in the pattern of episodes of apnea with respect to time across the groups: the incidence in the morphine group rose to a maximum at 2 h after the dose, while the peak incidence in the sufentanil group occurred a few minutes after administration, with a marked decrease at 30 min.

Tramadol *(SED-13, 178; SEDA-17, 84; SEDA-18, 83)*

The high incidence of *nausea* (30—35%) when tramadol is used for postoperative pain has recently been highlighted (28[R]). Other adverse effects are *vomiting*, *dry mouth*, *sweating*, *headache*, and *sedation*, although the sedative effect is less than that of morphine. *Hypertension* has also been reported.

Tramadol 50 or 100 mg has been compared with paracetamol 1000 mg plus codeine 60 mg for analgesia after orthopedic surgery (29[CR]).

Paracetamol plus codeine was superior, with fewer adverse effects. More than 50% of the patients who took tramadol had adverse effects. *Nausea and vomiting* were significantly more frequent with tramadol and *dizziness* was significantly more frequent with tramadol 100 mg than placebo.

The use of opioids in the treatment of neuropathic pain is recommended by some if analgesia is inadequate with antidepressants and neuroleptic drugs. However, their use is controversial. In addition to its opioid effect, tramadol inhibits noradrenaline reuptake and stimulates serotonin release; it therefore has similar effects to antidepressants. Tramadol has been compared with a combination of clomipramine plus levomepromazine in 35 patients with postherpetic neuralgia (30[Cr]). The patients were randomized to receive either tramadol in an initial dosage of 200 mg/day, increasing to a maximum of 600 mg/day, or clomipramine 50 mg/day, increasing to 100 mg/day if required. Levomepromazine was added if clomipramine did not relieve pain adequately. The incidence of adverse effects was 77% in the tramadol group and 83% in the clomipramine group. Treatment was terminated early because of *nausea*, *vomiting*, *tiredness*, or *dizziness* in 41% of patients in the tramadol group and 39% in the clomipramine group. The authors suggested that the incidence of adverse effects may have been influenced by the fact that most of the patients were over 65 years of age. In both groups of patients who completed the study, period pain improved from 'moderate to severe', to 'slight'.

The analgesic effects of intermittent boluses of tramadol or morphine after abdominal surgery have been compared in a multicenter study of 523 patients (31[Cr]). After surgery the patients received either intravenous tramadol 100 mg or morphine 5 mg, with repeated doses of 50 and 5 mg, respectively, during the first 90 min, up to three times on demand. During the next 24 h they were allowed further doses of tramadol intravenously or morphine intramuscularly, on demand, up to a maximum of 400 or 60 mg, respectively. The main measure of analgesic efficacy was the responder rate (no or slight pain) within the first 90 min. Tramadol caused more adverse effects (43 vs. 34%), although the difference was not statistically significant. The commonest adverse effects were *nausea* (32 and 22%), *vomiting* (4.9 and 3.8%), *urinary retention* (3.0 and 2.7%), and *sweating* (3.8 and 0.4%). There were two cases of severe vomiting with tramadol and one case of respiratory depression with morphine, leading to withdrawal from the study. Responder rates were 73% with tramadol and 81% with morphine. Overall, 98 (37%) of the 263 patients in the tramadol group did not receive adequate analgesia, as 165 of the 191 responders judged their overall pain relief to have been good or very good.

A spot survey of oral tramadol in the treatment of back pain found it to be an effective analgesic in dosages of 100—900 mg/day; adverse events occurred in 42% of patients (32[c]). The commonest adverse effect was nausea (24%) and the incidence of *constipation* was low (8%). Other reported adverse events were *headache* (18%), *eye symptoms* (unspecified) (14%), *confusion* (10%), *rash* (4%), *asthma* (2%), *micturition difficulties* (2%), and *sweating* (2%).

PARTIAL OPIOID AGONISTS

Buprenorphine *(SED-13, 180; SEDA-17, 87; SEDA-18, 86; SEDA-19, 89)*

When 120 consecutive patients were randomized to receive either 0.4 mg of buprenorphine or placebo as premedication before arthroscopy, the incidence of nausea was significantly higher with buprenorphine (13/40 vs. 3/42) (33[Cr]). This increased the median time to discharge from 150 min in the placebo group to 180 min in the buprenorphine group. There was also significantly more *respiratory depression* with buprenorphine, although this was not clinically significant and did not require intervention.

Buprenorphine has been used to treat depression in 10 subjects who had been unresponsive to at least two classes of antidepressants (34[CR]). Buprenorphine 0.15 mg was given either sublingually or intranasally in the morning and the dose was titrated to response to a maximum of 1.8 mg/day. Three patients discontinued the drug after one or two doses

because of *nausea, malaise,* or *dysphoria.* A further three discontinued treatment after 4 weeks, one each because of sedation, persistent nausea, and a personal crisis. Six of the seven subjects who completed at least 4 weeks treatment had clinical improvement, although in two patients the response was not sustained and one of these developed severe withdrawal symptoms on discontinuing buprenorphine.

Butorphanol *(SED-13, 181; SEDA-17, 87; SEDA-19, 89)*

The most common adverse effects of transnasal butorphanol have been outlined in two articles (35[R]), (36[R]), the latter an extensive review. Adverse events are frequent but are reported as mild to moderate. Butorphanol increases cardiac index and left ventricular end diastolic pressure and therefore *increases cardiac workload. Respiratory depression* does occur but has a ceiling effect that is reached with a dose of 2 mg. The most commonly reported adverse effects are *somnolence, dizziness,* and *nausea and/or vomiting.* Drowsiness and dizziness are dose related and may be minimized by administering two 1-mg boluses with a 60-min interval. Nasal adverse effects are related to duration of use; *nasal congestion and irritation, rhinitis,* and *epistaxis* have been reported with long-term administration.

Butorphanol (2 mg in 50 ml over 24 h) has been given by continuous infusion with or without 0.5% mepivacaine into the axillary sheath after upper extremity surgery and has been compared with mepivacaine alone (50 ml 0.5% over 24 h) (37[Cr]). The quality of analgesia was superior with the local anesthetic/opioid combination at 3 h, but there was no significant difference in analgesia provided by the combination compared with butorphanol alone at or after 6 h. The incidence of *nausea* was higher with butorphanol compared with mepivacaine, but there was no significant difference in the incidence of *nausea* in the two groups who received the same dose of butorphanol. The authors postulated that this may have been because better analgesia in those who received both local anesthetic and opioid caused fewer postoperative nociceptive impulses.

Equianalgesic doses of butorphanol and

morphine have been administered to 156 children aged 1.5–13 years who underwent day-care inguinal herniorrhaphy or orchidopexy (38[Cr]). Morphine 150 μg/kg or butorphanol 30 μg/kg was administered after induction of anesthesia, and the subjects were followed up for 4 h postoperatively. The quality of analgesia was significantly better with butorphanol at 10 min after surgery. No patient required additional oxygen for longer than 10 min postoperatively. The patients who received morphine had twice the incidence of *vomiting* as those who received butorphanol (28 vs. 14%); prolonged vomiting in two patients in the morphine group necessitated unscheduled hospital admission. Despite less pain and vomiting in the butorphanol group, there was no significant difference in the duration of stay in the recovery room or day-care unit, possibly because of the sedative effect of butorphanol. A flaw in the study, admitted by the authors, was the brief follow-up period of only 4 h.

Transnasal butorphanol has been compared with placebo in the treatment of migraine in 157 patients (39[C]). There was a significant reduction in the severity of the headache with butorphanol compared with placebo. Adverse effects were common, although confounded by the presence of migraine. The commonest adverse effects compared with placebo were *dizziness* (58 vs. 4%), *nausea and/or vomiting* (38 vs. 18%), and *drowsiness* (29 vs. 0%).

Transnasal butorphanol 1 mg with or without subcutaneous sumatriptan 6 mg has been investigated in the treatment of migraine in a crossover study with a 2-week washout period in 24 subjects (40[CR]). There was no pharmacokinetic interaction between the two drugs and no difference in the adverse effect profile of butorphanol when given with or without sumatriptan. There were 35 adverse experiences after butorphanol and sumatriptan and 29 after butorphanol alone. The most commonly reported adverse effects were *headache, dizziness, nausea,* and *vomiting*.

In a prospective, randomized, double-blind study of 71 patients undergoing cesarean section epidural butorphanol 1, 2 or 3 mg did not significantly reduce the adverse effects of epidural morphine 3 mg (41[CR]). The incidence of *sedation* with butorphanol plus morphine was significantly higher than with morphine alone at 8 h. However, in children aged 2–17 years undergoing spinal, abdominal, or thoracic procedures, butorphanol 40 μg/kg added to epidural morphine 80 μg/kg reduced the frequency of *nausea and vomiting* (20 vs. 0%) and *pruritus* (30 vs. 0%) (42[CR]). The children who received butorphanol and morphine as opposed to morphine alone required oxygen less frequently to maintain oxygen saturations above 90% (20 vs. 0%). Sedation was greater with butorphanol, although all the children were easily aroused. However, in another study of 60 children there was no overall reduction in the incidence of adverse effects (43[CR]). The patients, aged 6 weeks to 7 years, received epidural morphine 60 μg/kg with either epidural butorphanol 30 μg/kg or intravenous butorphanol 30 μg/kg. There was a significant reduction in the incidence of *pruritus* with epidural butorphanol and sedation was most marked in this group. However, there were too few patients without nasogastric tubes or urinary catheters to evaluate vomiting and urinary retention reliably, and the age of the patients precluded reporting of the subjective complaint of nausea.

Nalbuphine *(SED-13, 182; SEDA-17, 87)*

A prospective, randomized, double-blind comparison of patient-controlled morphine and nalbuphine has been performed in 24 patients after cholecystectomy and umbilical herniorrhaphy and in 24 patients after hysterectomy (44[Cr]). Loading doses of the drugs (3 mg) were given, followed by self-administered boluses (1 mg), with a lock-out time of 5 min for the first 30 min then 10 min. Analgesia was comparable in all groups. There was no clinical significant difference in respiratory frequency between the two drugs: there were no other measures of respiratory depression. There was also no significant difference in the incidence of nausea and vomiting.

OPIOID ANTAGONISTS

Naltrexone *(SED-13, 180; SEDA-18, 87)*

Animal studies have suggested that the neurotoxic adverse effects of interferon-α may be mediated by an action at opioid receptors.

Naltrexone, an opioid antagonist has been given to nine patients with hematological malignancies who had adverse effects from interferon-α; seven patients had moderate or complete relief (45^{cr}). Two patients had *headache* and *anxiety/visual hallucinations*, respectively, which resolved when naltrexone was withdrawn. In two patients the dose of naltrexone had to be increased above 100 mg/day for symptom relief and the major adverse effects were gastrointestinal, including *epigastric pain* and *constipation*.

In a short review of the use of naltrexone for the treatment of alcohol dependence, it has been reported that 5—10% of patients in clinical trials discontinued treatment because of adverse effects (46^{r}). *Nausea* is common and the other adverse effects of naltrexone include *dizziness*, *headache*, and *weight loss*.

REFERENCES

1. Nicotra MB, Carter R. The use of opiates in chronic obstructive pulmonary disease. Clin Pulm Med 1995;2:143—51.
2. Rapp SE, Ready LB, Nessly M. Acute pain management in patients with prior opioid consumption: a case-controlled retrospective review. Pain 1995;61:195—201.
3. Wilhite AO, Moore CH, Blass NH, Christmas JT. Plasma concentration profile of epidural alfentanil. Bolus followed by continuous infusion technique in the parturient: effect of epidural alfentanil and fentanyl on fetal heart rate. Reg Anesth 1994;19:164—8.
4. Sudarshan G, Browne BL, Matthews JNS, Conacher ID. Intrathecal fentanyl for post-thoracotomy pain. Br J Anaesth 1995;75:19—22.
5. Schechter NL, Weisman SJ, Rosenblum M, Bernstein B, Conard PL. The use of oral transmucosal rentanyl citrate for painful procedures in children. Pediatrics 1995;95:335—9.
6. Schutzman SA, Burg J, Liebelt E, Strafford M, Schechter N, Wisk M, Fleisher G. Oral transmucosal fentanyl citrate for premedication of children undergoing laceration repair. Ann Emerg Med 1994;24:6.
7. Gerwels J, Bezzant J, Le Maire L, Pauley L, Streisand J. Oral transmucosal fentanyl citrate premedication in patients undergoing outpatient dermatologic procedures. J Dermatol Surg Oncol 1994;20:823—6.
8. Payne R, Chandler S, Einhaus M. Guidlines for the clinical use of transdermal fentanyl. Anticancer Drugs 1995;6 Suppl 3:50—3.
9. Simmonds MA. Transdermal fentanyl: clinical development in the United States. Anticancer Drugs 1995;6 Suppl 3:35—8.
10. Zenz M, Donner B. Transdermal fentanyl: a new step on the therapeutic ladder. Anticancer Drugs 1995;6 Suppl 3:39—43.
11. Zech DFJ, Lehmann KA. Transdermal fentanyl in combination with initial intravenous dose titration by patient-controlled analgesia. Anticancer Drugs 1995;6 Suppl 3:44—9.
12. Bulow HH, Linnemann M, Berg H, Lang-Jensen T, Lacour S, Jonsson T. Respiratory changes during treatment of postoperative pain with high dose transdermal fentanyl. Acta Anaesthesiol Scand 1995;39:835—9.
13. Miguel R, Kreitzer JM, Reinhart D, Sebel PS, Bowie J, Freedman G, Eisenkraft JB. Postoperative pain control with a new transdermal fentanyl delivery system. Anesthesiology 1995;83:470—7.
14. Fiset P, Cohane C, Browne S, Brand SC, Shafer SL. Biopharmaceutics of a new transdermal fentanyl device. Anesthesiology 1995;83:59—69.
15. Kuzma PJ, Kline MD, Stamatos JM, Auth DA. Acute toxic delirium: an uncommon reaction to transdermal fentanyl. Anesthesiology 1995;83:869—71.
16. Levihnson I, Galynker II, Rosenthal RN. Methadone withdrawal psychosis. J Clin Psychiatry 1995;56:73—6.
17. Samuelsson H, Malmberg F, Eriksson M, Hedner T. Outcomes of epidural morphine treatment in cancer pain: nine years of clinical experience. J Pain Symptom Manage 1995;10:105—12.
18. Liu SS, Carpenter RL, Mackey DL, Thirlby RC, Rupp SM, Shine TSY, Feinglass NG, Metzger PP, Fulmer JT, Smith SL. Effects of perioperative analgesic technique on rate of recovery after colon surgery. Anesthesiology 1995;83:757—65.
19. Richards S. Constipation following orthopaedic surgery in patients receiving opiates—a 'spot' survey. Br J Med Econ 1995;9:55—8.
20. Mayhew JF, Brodsky RC, Blakey D, Petersen W. Low-dose caudal morphine for postoperative analgesia in infants and children: a report of 500 cases. J Clin Anesth 1995;7:640—2.
21. Schulte-Steinberg H, Weninger E, Jokisch D, Hogstetter B, Misera A, Lange V, Stein C. Intraperitoneal versus interpleural morphine or bupivacaine for pain after laparascopic cholecystectomy. Anesthesiology 1995;82:634—40.
22. Tiseo PJ, Thaler HT, Lapin J, Inturrisi CE, Portenowy RK, Foley KM. Morphine-6-glucuronide concentrations and opioid-related side effects: a survey in cancer patients. Pain 1995;61:47—54.
23. Leow KP, Cramond T, Smith MT. Pharmacokinetics and pharmacodynamics of oxycodone when given intravenously and rectally to adult

patients with cancer pain. Anesth Analg 1995; 80:296—302.

24. Scherl ER, Wilson JF. Comparison of dihydroergotamine with metoclopramide versus meperidine with promethazine in the treatment of acute migraine. Headache 1995;35:256—9.

25. Bostrom MA, Pakiz AM, Melnyk DL, Benke G, Cohen S. Spinal anesthesia with meperidine: will epinephrine prolong its duration? J Am Assoc Nurse Anesth 1995;62:267—72.

26. Baker MN, Sarna MC. Respiratory arrest after second dose on intrathecal sufentanil. Anesthesiology 1995;83:231—2.

27. Slade JM, Read MS, Klepper ID, Rosen M. Extradural sufentanil by patient-controlled analgesia or nurse-administered compared with optimal morphine in a high dependency unit: effects on oxygenation and pain relief after abdominal surgery. Br J Anaesth 1995;73:634—8.

28. Eggers KA, Power I. Tramadol. Br J Anaesth 1995;74:247—9.

29. Stubhaug A, Grimstad J, Breivik H. Lack of analgesic effect of 50 and 100 mg oral tramadol after orthopaedic surgery: a randomized, double-blind, placebo and standard active drug comparison. Pain 1995;62:111—18.

30. Gobel H, Stadler T. Treatment of pain due to postherpetic neuralgia with tramadol: results of an open, parallel pilot study vs clomipramine with or without levomepromazine. Clin Drug Invest 1995;10:208—14.

31. Vickers MD, Paravicini D. Comparison of tramadol with morphine for post-operative pain following abdominal surgery. Eur J Anaesthesiol 1995;12:265—71.

32. Price PM, Budd K. Tramadol in the treatment of spinal pain: a short report based on the results of a survey of 50 patients. Br J Med Econ 1995;9:17—20.

33. Juhlin-Dannfelt M, Adamsen S, Olvon E, Beskow A, Brodln B. Premedication with sublingual buprenorphine for out-patient arthroscopy: reduced need for postoperative pethidine but higher incidence of nausea. Acta Anaesthesiol Scand 1995;39:633—6.

34. Bodkin JA, Zornberg GL, Lukas SE, Cole JO. Buprenorphine treatment of refractory depression. J Clin Psychopharmacol 1995;15:49—57.

35. Anonymous. Transnasal butorphanol offers noninvasive route for opioid administration. Drugs Ther Perspect 1995;6:4—7.

36. Gillis JC, Benfield P, Goa KL. Transnasal butorphanol: a review of its pharmacodynamic and pharmacokinetic properties, and therapeutic potential in acute pain management. Drug Eval 1995;50:157—75.

37. Wajina Z, Shitara T, Nakjimay, Kim C, Kobayashi N, Kadotani H, Adachi H, Ishiawa G, Kaneko K, Inoue T, Ogawa R. Comparison of continuous brachial plexus infusion of butorphanol, mepivacaine and mepivacaine-butorphanol mixtures for postoperative analgesia. Br J Anaesth 1995;75:548—51.

38. Splinter WM, O'Brian HV, Komacar L. Butorphanol: an opioid for day-care paediatric surgery. Can J Anaesth 1995;42:483—6.

39. Hoffert MJ, Couch JR, Diamond S, Elkind AH, Godstein J, Koglerman NJ, Saper JR, Solomon S. Transnasal butorphanol in the treatment of acute migraine. Headache 1995;35:65—9.

40. Srinivas NR, Shyu WC, Upmalis D, Lee JS, Barbhaiya RH. Lack of pharmacokinetic interaction between butorphanol tartrate nasal spray and sumatriptan succinate. J Clin Pharmacol 1995; 35:432—7.

41. Gambling DR, Howell P, Huber C, Kozak S. Epidural butorphanol does not reduce side effects from epidural morthine after cesarean birth. Anesth Analg 1995;78:1099—104.

42. Lawhorn CD, Brown RE. Epidural morphine with butorphanol in pediatric patients. J Clin Anesth 1994;6:91—4.

43. Bailey AG, Valley RD, Freid EB, Calhoun P. Epidural morphine combined with epidural or intravenous butorphanol for postoperative analgesia in pediatric patients. Anesth Analg 1994;79:340—4.

44. Niv D, Wolmand I, Alon E, Weinbroum A, Rudick V, Varassi G, Geller E. Morphine versus nalbuphine for postoperative pain relief using the patient-controlled analgesia method. Eur J Pain 1995;16:1—2.

45. Valentine AD, Meyers CA, Talpaz M. Treatment of neurotoxic side effects of interferon-α with naltrexone. Cancer Invest 1995;13:561—6.

46. Anonymous. Naltrexone for alcohol dependence. Med Lett 1995;37:64—6.

A. Del Favero

9 Anti-inflammatory and antipyretic analgesics and drugs used in gout

NON-STEROIDAL ANTI-INFLAMMATORY DRUGS (NSAIDs)

℞ *NSAIDs and gastrointestinal damage*

Issues related to gastrointestinal damage by NSAIDs remain topical. I have previously reviewed the most important problems (SEDA-1, 102; SEDA-18, 99; SEDA-19, 93), but an update of some of them is worth while.

Are erosions an important prognostic factor for gastroduodenal ulceration? *Endoscopic studies in patients taking short- or long-term NSAIDs have clearly shown that erosions are the commonest abnormalities related to exposure to NSAIDs, and the number of erosions is included in endoscopic scales aimed at scoring gastroduodenal damage* $(1^C)-(3^C)$*. It is therefore important to ascertain whether the presence or absence of erosions, as well their number, can be considered as risk factors for the development of ulcers in patients taking NSAIDs. In fact, progression from erosion to ulceration is by no means inevitable and can be interrupted by mucosal adaptation and repair* (4^C)*. Several studies have documented that erosions are often transient* $(1^C)-(6^C)$ *and this leads to the impression that they are comparatively trivial lesions. Although this is probably true in subjects exposed to short courses of NSAIDs, the significance of erosions in long-term users is not clear. Three recent*

long-term endoscopic studies have provided some useful information on this topic and deserve attention.

The first is a prevention study of NSAID-induced ulcers, in which 253 patients took misoprostol or sucralfate prophylaxis (7^C)*. The presence of endoscopically documented gastric mucosal erosions (39% of patients) at the time of baseline endoscopic evaluation was associated with an increased risk of subsequent development of a gastric ulcer at endoscopic examination repeated after 3 months. The overall odds ratio (the chance of an ulcer with erosions divided by the chance of an ulcer without erosions) was 2.75. Data on duodenal ulcers were not evaluable because of their low number.*

The second study (8^C) *was a placebo-controlled trial of two dosages of famotidine for the prevention of gastric and duodenal lesions caused by 24 weeks of treatment with NSAIDs. The presence of duodenal erosions (or hemorrhagic lesions) at the initial endoscopic examination was predictive of both duodenal and gastric ulceration. In fact, in the famotidine group of 193 patients, ulcers developed in 23% of the patients who had duodenal lesions at base-line endoscopy and in 11% of those who did not (hazard ratio 2.9; 95% CI 1.2—6.9). The same trend was found in placebo-treated patients. There was also a trend towards an increased risk of ulceration among patients with Helicobacter pylori infection (hazard ratio 1.7; 95% CI 0.8—3.5).*

The third study was an observational study on a group of 50 long-term users of NSAIDs who underwent endoscopy at 0, 4, 12, and 24 weeks while continuing to take NSAIDs (9^C)*. The incidence of gastric and duodenal ulcers was assessed in relation to the presence of erosions at base-line endoscopy, as was the pre-*

Side Effects of Drugs, Annual 20
J.K. Aronson, ed.

sence or absence of *H. pylori*. Ulcers developed in 39% of patients with pre-existing erosions, compared with 22% without erosions, but ulcer development was not influenced by the initial number of erosions per subject, indicating that the presence or absence of erosions is a better predictor of the risk of ulceration than the numbers of erosions. However, in six of 15 ulcers (40%) in the study, no erosions were identified before ulcer development. *H. pylori* infection was found in 30 patients, and they had significantly more lesions, ulcers, and ulcers complicating previous erosions than non-infected patients. Duodenal erosions in patients infected with *H. pylori* were more likely to predict ulceration than their gastric counterparts. In fact, of six patients with duodenal erosions, five were positive for *H. pylori* and all of them developed ulceration (two gastric, three duodenal) at subsequent endoscopic examinations.

In summary, these studies suggest that ulcers are more likely to develop in NSAID users with erosions, despite the fact that such lesions may be transient or recurrent. Furthermore, as ulceration is more likely to occur in patients with duodenal erosions infected by *H. pylori*, these results could have practical implications, since they should allow us to identify patients who are at greater risk of ulceration, in whom a prophylactic approach aimed at protecting the gastroduodenal mucosa and eradicating *H. pylori* might prove useful. However, they should be interpreted with caution, as in the first two studies patients were taking anti-ulcer prophylaxis, which could have modified the natural history of NSAID-induced peptic ulceration and in the third study the number of patients was small. When the results of these studies are considered together it remains unclear which definition of injury correlates best with subsequent ulcer complication.

Moreover, even if in two studies *H. pylori* infection increased the risk of ulceration, other contrasting data continue to be published (7^C), $(10^C)-(14^C)$. More data on this important issue from large prospective studies are needed to draw any firm conclusions. In the meantime, in individual patients the endoscopic finding of erosions is a minor risk factor for ulceration in the long term. In fact, in a high percentage of patients with ulcers no erosions were identified before ulcer development. Erosions result from a dynamic variable process of mucosal adaptation; consequently, a snapshot view of this process by endoscopy is probably inadequate for ascertaining the risk of further ulceration. Finally, endoscopy is an invasive procedure, not without risks in some patients, for example those with rheumatoid arthritis. The identification of the other well-known risk factors (age, history of peptic ulcer or gastrointestinal bleeding, and concomitant cardiac disease) (SEDA-19, 92) remain the best guidance for identifying patients at high risk of gastroduodenal damage.

The role of histamine H_2 receptor antagonists in the prevention of gastric and duodenal ulcers caused by NSAIDs   *I have previously reviewed the problems related to the prevention of gastric and duodenal ulcer, as well as of serious gastrointestinal complications (bleeding and perforation) caused by NSAIDs (SEDA-18, 99; SEDA-19, 92). There is evidence, albeit controversial, that H_2 receptor antagonists, in particular ranitidine and famotidine, can reduce the frequency of duodenal ulcer, but not of gastric ulcer (the most common type of NSAID-induced ulcer) in users of NSAIDs $(15^C)-(17^C)$. Furthermore, there are no data on their ability to prevent the clinically important complications of gastrointestinal bleeding and perforation. On the other hand, misoprostol, a synthetic analog of prostaglandin E_1, not only protects against NSAID-induced gastric and duodenal ulcers, but also against their severe complications (18^C). The very few adequate trials in which these drugs have been directly compared have shown greater efficacy for misoprostol in preventing damage (16^C), (19^C). However, new contrasting data have recently been published. In a placebo-controlled trial, treatment with high-dose famotidine (40 mg tds) significantly reduced the cumulative incidence of both gastric and duodenal ulcers in patients taking long-term NSAIDs (8^C). These results are in direct contrast with those of another large trial with famotidine (17^C) and experience with other H_2 receptor antagonists (16^{CR}). Not only that, but in general practice H_2 receptor antagonists are often prescribed for NSAID users either as symptomatic treatment for dyspeptic symptoms or as prophylaxis for gastroduodenal ulceration. A recent large prospective observational cohort study on 1921 patients followed for 2.5 years in the US showed that antacids and H_2*

receptor antagonists were used in combination with NSAIDs by more than 30% of patients (20[C]). Patients taking these antiulcer drugs did not have a lower risk of significant gastrointestinal events. Indeed, asymptomatic patients who started to take antacids and H_2 receptor antagonists prophylactically had a higher risk of a serious gastrointestinal complication than those who did not (odds ratio 2.69; 95% CI 1.36—5.81). The association between the use of these medications and a higher gastrointestinal complication rate persisted after adjustment for patient characteristics that may be independently associated with both the use of these drugs and the incidence of gastrointestinal complications (adjusted odds ratio: 2.14; 95% CI 1.06—4.32). The increased risk of complications could have been due to the fact that these medications suppress gastrointestinal symptoms and so encourage the use of higher doses of NSAIDs for longer periods, ultimately resulting in more severe gastrointestinal complications.

What are the practical implications of these data? Although the famotidine study has been criticized (21[C]), when used in high dosages famotidine probably prevents gastric ulceration in patients taking NSAIDs. The extension of protection to the stomach could have been due to the greater acid suppression achieved by high dosages, a finding that accounts for similar results obtained with omeprazole, a potent inhibitor of acid secretion (22[C]). Should we then modify our approach to prophylaxis of gastrointestinal complications in NSAID users? Probably not. In fact, there is no evidence that either H_2 receptor antagonists or omeprazole prevent severe gastrointestinal complications, the primary therapeutic endpoint of any form of prophylaxis. To prevent gastric ulcers would require the prescription of very high dosages of famotidine or the use of omeprazole, but their long-term safety is still unknown. Not only that, but a word of caution seems wise with respect to the uncritical prescription of H_2 receptor antagonists and antacids for asymptomatic patients for prophylaxis, since they are potentially dangerous (20[C]). Misoprostol therefore remains the first choice drug for preventing gastrointestinal damage by NSAIDs. However, even then prophylaxis should be restricted to high-risk patients (SEDA-19, 92).

NSAID-induced colonic strictures *Several case reports have documented an association between strictures of the small bowel and the long-term use of NSAIDs (SEDA-15, 92; SEDA-16, 110). This problem has been termed 'diaphragm disease' (23[C]), and since its first description and characterization it has also been reported in the ascending colon, albeit rarely (24[C])—(29[C]), (30[CR]). These colonic lesions are identical to those reported in the small bowel and are found only in patients who have taken NSAIDs for more than a year. The disease is characterized by multiple, thin (2—4 mm), diaphragm-like strictures, which produce luminal occlusion that varies from 3 mm to a width approximating the normal bowel diameter. Most of the mucosa between these strictures is normal, but occasionally ulcers and inflammatory changes are noted (26[C]), (28[C])—(30[C]). The colonic involvement is most marked in the vicinity of the ileocecal valve and tends to reduce in severity towards the hepatic flexure. An association between colonic and small bowel involvement has been described (29[C]).*

The pathogenesis of strictures in the lower gastrointestinal tract is unknown. However, some features suggest topical damage by NSAIDs: patients with strictures are long-term users of modified-release NSAIDs, which are likely to be delivered unabsorbed to the intestine (30[C]); sometimes colonic strictures and ulcerations contain tablet fragments (28[C]); and lesions are concentrated in the ascending colon, which acts as a fecal reservoir, facilitating prolonged contact between unabsorbed tablets and the intestinal mucosa.

The usual presentation is with iron-deficiency anemia or chronic diarrhea and not intestinal obstruction or abdominal pain. The correct diagnosis has been greatly facilitated by colonoscopy, as X-rays can miss the diagnosis and underestimate the number of strictures (28[C]).

Discontinuation of NSAIDs is imperative and generally leads to clinical improvement. Sometimes segmental resection of the bowel or dilatation with a balloon dilator have been found necessary.

NSAIDs and renal damage

Membranous nephropathy   NSAID-induced nephrotic syndrome is usually associated with minimal-change glomerulopathy, with or without interstitial nephritis, membranous nephropathy being rare (SEDA-11, 85). In consequence, our knowledge of NSAID-induced membranous nephropathy is derived from a few case reports (SEDA-6, 96; SEDA-12, 84, 86, 88; SEDA-15, 100, 102; $(31^C)-(38^C)$).*

A recently published retrospective chart review in two large teaching hospitals in the US has provided more data on the frequency and clinical characteristics of membranous nephropathy associated with NSAIDs (39^C). Of 125 patients diagnosed during the last 20 years as having stage I or early stage II membranous nephropathy by renal biopsy, 13 met the strict criteria for NSAID-associated membranous nephropathy.

The patients with membranous nephropathy were aged 55 (range 36—68) years, with equal sex distribution. The following NSAIDs had been used: fenoprofen (four patients), ibuprofen (three), tolmetin (three), and diclofenac, nabumetone, and naproxen (one each). The median duration of treatment before the onset of symptoms was 43 weeks (range 4 weeks to 3 years). Symptoms occurred without prodromal illness and more than 90% of patients presented with nephrotic syndrome with a mean proteinuria of 10 g/day. No patients had signs or symptoms such as rash or fever or, except for one patient, acute renal failure. Mild peripheral blood eosinophilia was found in only five patients. Renal biopsy showed tubulointerstitial nephritis in three patients only. Prompt withdrawal of the NSAID caused a quick fall in proteinuria to less than 1 g/day, which occurred on average by 25 (range 9—64) weeks. None of these patients had any evidence of renal insufficiency or significant proteinuria after follow-up periods ranging from 5 months to 13 years.

The pathogenesis of membranous nephropathy is unknown, but given the characteristic deposition of IgG and C3 the reaction seems to be immune mediated. Whether the NSAID itself acts as an antigen or facilitates the immune response in some way is not clear.

Nephrotic syndrome due to membranous nephropathy should be recognized as an idiosyncratic, albeit rare, reaction to many NSAIDs.

Combination analgesics and renal failure   Although phenacetin is no longer marketed world wide, interest in analgesic nephropathy continues in relation to the abuse of fixed combinations of analgesics that include paracetamol with aspirin and/or caffeine, which have replaced the earlier phenacetin-containing combinations and which are widely advertised directly to the public (40^R). In Italy, for example, 15 different medications containing fixed combinations of caffeine plus various analgesics (paracetamol, aspirin, or propyphenazone) are marketed as over-the-counter drugs. The claim that these new compound analgesics are harmless is not convincing (SEDA-15, 89; SEDA-16, 104). In Germany, up to 10% of about 42 000 dialysis patients have suffered from kidney failure due to analgesic nephropathy, despite the fact that phenacetin was banned many years ago, and recently German nephrologists have demanded the withdrawal of these medications from the market, following the example of their American colleagues in the National Kidney Foundation, who have suggested that these medications should not be sold over the counter or advertised to the public and should be labelled with a warning about the risk of kidney failure if they are used regularly in the long term (41^c).*

Interactions with NSAIDs

Methotrexate   Low-dose methotrexate is one of the most effective treatments for rheumatoid arthritis and is widely used. NSAIDs are commonly prescribed in association with methotrexate, and interactions are possible, as both are secreted by the organic acid secretory pathway in the kidney and both bind to a high degree to plasma albumin. Severe toxicity has been attributed to the concomitant use of high dosages (42^C), intermediate dosages (43^C), and low dosages $(44^C)-(47^C)$ of methotrexate with various NSAIDs. The mechanisms of interaction are unclear. Although the possible pharmacokinetic interactions have been studied for some NSAIDs, in most studies few patients have been enrolled, not all significant kinetic measurements have been made, and the results have been conflicting $(48^C)-(55^C)$.

In a recent well-conducted study on the pharmacokinetics of total and unbound methotrexate, with or without piroxicam, in patients with rheumatoid arthritis there was no significant pharmacokinetic interaction between a single low dose of methotrexate (10 mg intramuscularly) and piroxicam (20 mg orally at steady state) (56^C).

While waiting for similar studies to be performed in patients taking the most widely used NSAIDs, should we follow the suggestion that simultaneous dosing of methotrexate and NSAIDs must be avoided (SED-13, 204)? It seems wise to do so, since methotrexate toxicity can be severe and there are alternative medications for the control of pain and inflammation during short-term interruption of NSAID therapy.

Calcium channel antagonists NSAIDs can alter the effects of many antihypertensive drugs (SEDA-19, 92; (57^R)). A recent randomized, placebo-controlled, short-term (3 weeks) study (58^C) has confirmed earlier observations $(59^C)-(62^C)$ that there was no significant change in blood pressure in patients taking calcium channel antagonists (verapamil or nifedipine) with NSAIDs such as diclofenac, ibuprofen, indomethacin, naproxen, piroxicam, and sulindac.

Chronopharmacology of NSAIDs

The clinical impressions of some rheumatologists that evening administration of NSAIDs is better tolerated (63^C) has some support from experimental studies on time-dependent changes in the clinical pharmacokinetics and tolerability of NSAIDs. There is evidence that the kinetics of some NSAIDs (indomethacin, ketoprofen, flurbiprofen, tenoxicam) is not constant during the day (64^{CR}). In agreement with animal studies, the data show that NSAID absorption is probably better in the morning. At the same time, patients who take indomethacin at 08:00 h have more adverse effects (33%) than those who take it at 12:00 h (approximately 20%) or at 20:00 h (about 7%). About 75% of the undesirable effects were represented by vertigo, headache, and anxiety. Similar data have

been documented in patients taking ketoprofen for 3 weeks. The number of patients suffering from gastrointestinal adverse effects was twice as high in those who took ketoprofen in the morning.

Similar results have been found in an endoscopic study in patients taking acetylsalicylic acid. Oral administration at 10:00 h caused gastric mucosal lesions twice as large as those that occurred after the 22:00 h dosing. However, the results of these studies must be interpreted with caution: they are small studies, often not blinded, of short duration, and possibly confounded by other factors (for example, sleeping can reduce the awareness of pain or other symptoms). It is difficult to explain also why the within-day changes in pharmacokinetics do not depend on the pharmaceutical formulation of the NSAID, as they are found after the administration of regular formulations or modified-release formulations and even after constant infusion of NSAIDs.

INDIVIDUAL DRUGS AND CLASSES

ACETYLSALICYLIC ACID AND RELATED COMPOUNDS *(SED-13, 170; SEDA-17, 94; SEDA-18, 90; SEDA-19, 97)*

Aspirin idiosyncrasy in systemic mast cell disease Long-term therapy with aspirin has been recommended to prevent recurrent attacks of flushing and severe hypotension in systemic mast cell disease. However, although this approach may be successful, some of these patients suffer from an idiosyncratic reaction, even to small doses of aspirin or other NSAIDs, associated with profound hypotension $(65^C)-(68^C)$. The mechanism of this hypotension is unknown, but it may result from the combined effects of several mediators (histamine, prostaglandin D2, and calcitonin gene-related peptide) (69^C). Only a few reports have described successful aspirin desensitization in these patients (68^C), (69^C). Attempts at desensitization cause acute severe hypotension, flushing, tachycardia, shortness of breath, and headache. However, when aspirin was continued it was tolerated and hypotensive attacks were prevented.

Lysine acetylsalicylate

Lysine acetylsalicylate is usually given intravenously to control acute pain. However, it has also been given intrathecally as a single dose (10 mg/kg) to a few patients with intractable cancer pain ([70C]), ([71C]). The adverse effects were important even if short-lived: severe pain, weakness or paralysis of the legs, a diffuse, burning, itching sensation, nervousness, and depression. The benefit:risk ratio of this approach to relieving cancer pain seems unacceptable.

ARYLALKANOIC ACID DERIVATIVES AND RELATED COMPOUNDS *(SED-13, 227; SEDA-17, 109; SEDA-18, 103; SEDA-19, 98)*

Aceclofenac *(SEDA-18, 103)*

Gastrointestinal Intestinal *microbleeding* in 20 healthy volunteers taking short-term aceclofenac and diclofenac tended to be slightly less with aceclofenac ([72C]). However, as experience with aceclofenac accumulates, it appears that its adverse effects profile is similar to that of other NSAIDs. In particular, symptoms of gastrointestinal intolerance are the most common reason for interrupting treatment; the rate of withdrawal is 3—15% ([73c])—([75c]).

Skin and appendages Palpable purpura of the lower and upper limbs developed in a 52-year-old man after 5 days of therapy with aceclofenac. Skin biopsy showed *leukocytoclastic vasculitis*. Microscopic hematuria was also present ([76C]), making this reaction similar to one previously described (SEDA-18, 103). Aceclofenac was stopped and the rash disappeared over 10 days with corticosteroid treatment.

Aceclofenac cream seems to be well tolerated. *Erythema*, *itching*, and a *burning sensation* occur in under 3% of patients ([77C]).

Bufexamac *(SEDA-18, 103)*

Long-term topical use of bufexamac in children was well tolerated with few mild local adverse effects ([78c]).

Diclofenac *(SED-13, 232; SEDA-17, 109; SEDA-18, 103; SEDA-19, 98)*

Liver damage due to diclofenac   ℞

A relatively large number of cases of hepatic injury attributed to diclofenac have been reported (SED-13, 232) or have been collected through spontaneous adverse reactions reporting systems in various countries (SEDA-12, 85; ([79C])). A recent retrospective study has illustrated the clinical features, the characteristics of the biochemical pattern of injury, and the histological changes in 434 reports of diclofenac-associated hepatic injury submitted to the voluntary reporting system of the FDA between November 1989 and June 1991 ([80Cr]).

After validation of the data, 254 cases were eliminated for various reasons (duplication, reporting unrelated to the drug, foreign source) and 180 cases were left for analysis. Of these, 79% were women, 71% were aged 60 years or older, and 77% were taking diclofenac for osteoarthritis. Two-thirds of the cases were detected by symptoms and the remainder by increased activities of liver transaminases noted incidentally (15%) or during monitoring (18%). The illness developed more than 5 weeks after starting diclofenac in more than 75% of the patients and the duration of therapy before the detection of liver injury was under 6 months in 85% of cases. The most frequent manifestation in symptomatic patients (120 patients) was jaundice (40 patients), and this was the only complaint in 14 of them (17%). Other symptoms in the majority of patients were anorexia, nausea, and vomiting, with or without fever. Much less frequent complaints included abdominal pain, pruritus, and malaise. Hallmarks of hypersensitivity (fever, rash, and eosinophilia) were very uncommon. Liver injury was classified on the basis of the biochemical data (serum bilirubin concentration and aspartate transaminase, alanine transaminase, and alkaline phosphatase activities): hepatocellular (54%), cholestatic (8%), mixed (12%), or indeterminate (26%) ([81C]). Specimens of hepatic tissue were available from 21 cases. All but six had hepatocellular injury, nine had acute hepatocellular injury, and six had changes of chronic hepatitis. The factors that affected susceptibility to liver damage by diclo-

fenac were sex and type of disease. In fact, although these factors may be confounded by the overlap of age, sex, and disease in arthritic patients, the relative risk of liver damage for women and patients with osteoarthritis was significantly greater than for men and patients with rheumatoid arthritis. There is no good explanation for this finding. The mechanism of diclofenac-induced liver injury is unknown, but since the incidence is very low an idiosyncratic mechanism rather then intrinsic toxicity of the drug seems likely. Furthermore, in view of the rarity of hallmarks of hypersensitivity, the delayed development of injury (more than 1 month after starting the drug in 76% of cases), and the delayed response to rechallenge in all but one of the 19 patients who responded to readministration, a metabolic effect rather than immunological idiosyncrasy seems more likely in most cases.

The results of this and other reports (SEDA-12, 85; (79ᶜ)), which have outlined the prominence of cases of hepatic injury attributed to diclofenac, seem at odds with the results of another study (82ᶜ), which recorded hardly any cases attributable to diclofenac. A possible explanation may be the different characteristics of the population studied or, more likely, the duration of use of the drug. In fact, in a review of safety experience with diclofenac in phase III studies in the US in more than 2400 patients, the incidence of hepatitis was 0.26% in long-term studies, while not a single case of hepatitis was documented in short-term studies (SEDA-12, 85).

Despite its potential hepatotoxicity, diclofenac has a good safety profile and is used world wide. However, it seems wise to suggest that prescribers advise patients to report new symptoms promptly, particularly anorexia, nausea, vomiting, and malaise. The usefulness of monitoring serum enzymes is unknown, but it might be prudent to do so during the first 6 months of treatment.

Hematological *Autoimmune hemolytic anemia* is an uncommon adverse reaction to diclofenac (SED-13, 232; SEDA-5, 103; SEDA-16, 109). A new case of severe autoimmune hemolytic anemia with acute renal failure has been described in a 64-year-old woman (83ᶜ).

Gastrointestinal A prospective 12-week endoscopic study has documented better gastrointestinal tolerability of diclofenac than naproxen (84ᶜ). The endoscopy grade of *gastric injury* increased over the baseline value in 65% of naproxen-treated patients versus 29% of patients treated with diclofenac, and gastroduodenal ulcers developed in 40% of patients in the naproxen group and in 13% in the diclofenac group. In contrast, there were *increases in serum transaminases* (to three times the upper end of the reference ranges) in about 10% of patients taking diclofenac and in none of those taking naproxen.

Dispersible diclofenac is a new formulation that forms a fine microcrystalline drinkable suspension when it is added to water. Absorption is almost immediate and significantly more rapid than with the usual formulation. Experience is still limited, but not unexpectedly the most frequent adverse effects are gastrointestinal (*nausea, abdominal pain, dyspepsia, diarrhea*) (85ᶜ).

Urinary system Oliguric functional *renal failure* after the use of diclofenac in patients with burns has been described (86ᶜ). Hypovolemia and septic complications of burns may predispose patients to functional renal failure if they are treated with NSAIDs. There is no convincing evidence that burns can be a predisposing factor per se.

Special senses Diclofenac eye-drops seem to be well tolerated by most patients. The few adverse effects have been local *hyperemia* and *burning* (87ᶜ).

Etodolac *(SED-13, 238; SEDA-18, 104; SEDA-19, 98)*

Liver Etodolac so far has a favorable safety profile. In particular, hepatotoxicity, in the form of a reversible rise in transaminases or bilirubin, occurs rarely (SED-13, 238). A case of fatal *acute liver failure* has now been reported in a 67-year-old woman (88ᶜ). She had taken etodolac for 4 months and developed nausea, vomiting, anorexia, weakness, and confusion. She was jaundiced but afebrile and without any hallmarks of hypersensitivity. Biochemical measurements were consistent with hepatocellular injury. Her condition rapidly deteriorated and she died 13 days later. At autopsy the main findings were diffuse micronodular areas of necrosis microscopically characterized by submassive bridging necrosis and early fibrosis.

Flurbiprofen *(SED-13, 230; SEDA-17, 109; SEDA-18, 104)*

Intramuscular flurbiprofen is effective and well tolerated in the treatment of ureteric colic. Local adverse effects include *pain* (30% of patients), *itching* (7.5%), a *burning sensation* (6%) and *edema-erythema-induration* (less than 3%); their intensity was judged slight (89[c]).

Ibuprofen *(SED-13, 228; SEDA-17, 110; SEDA-18, 104; SEDA-19, 98)*

A regimen of high-dosage ibuprofen (16—32 mg/kg) for 4 years significantly slowed the progression of lung disease in 41 patients with cystic fibrosis (mean age 15, range 5—39 years). Only two adverse effects (*conjunctivitis* and *epistaxis*) were related to ibuprofen (90[c]). However, this study was too small to detect even a common drug-related complication and the negative data should therefore be interpreted with caution. Careful monitoring of these patients remains mandatory.

Ibuprofen lysine is more rapidly absorbed than ibuprofen free acid. Clinical experience is still too limited to evaluate the comparative tolerability of the two formulations (91[c]).

Ketoprofen *(SED-13, 229; SEDA-17, 110; SEDA-18, 104)*

Different regulatory authorities sometimes take opposite decisions on the same matter, as in the case of the classification of ketoprofen as an over-the-counter drug. Non-prescription strengths of this NSAID have been approved for over-the-counter sales in the US by the FDA (92), whereas in Italy the Health Ministry has transferred two ketoprofen-containing products from non-prescription to prescription status (93). The reasons for this difference are not clear.

Ketorolac *(SED-13, 240; SEDA-17, 112; SEDA-18, 104; SEDA-19, 99)*

Hematological Further controlled studies have shown that perioperative administration of ketorolac puts the patient at greater risk of *bleeding* (94[c])—(97[c]). Although in many cases the blood loss was not serious, the increased risk was often not compensated by better control of pain (94[c]), (97[c]) with respect to other analgesics (diamorphine, paracetamol).

Nabumetone *(SED-13, 239)*

A total of 6148 patients with osteoarthritis or rheumatoid arthritis treated with nabumetone in long-term clinical trials had a 3-month cumulative incidence of clinically detected *perforations*, *ulcers*, and *bleeding* of 0.1% and a 6-month incidence of 0.2% (98[Cr]).

Naproxen *(SED-13, 231; SEDA-17, 112; SEDA-18, 105; SEDA-19, 99)*

The safety profile of naproxen sodium for over-the-counter use has been evaluated in 48 randomized, double-blind, comparative studies in 4138 patients with conditions appropriate to and conditions common to the use of non-prescription analgesics (99[c]). Comparator drugs were placebo, ibuprofen, or paracetamol. The incidence rates of adverse events were similar. There were no serious adverse reactions. Similar data have been reported in a post-marketing surveillance study in Australia (99[c]). If properly advised on the appropriate and prudent use of naproxen, patients can use the over-the-counter formulation without serious risks.

Pancreas Another case of *acute pancreatitis* has been described in a young woman who had taken naproxen for dysmenorrhea (100[c]). Her abdominal pain disappeared and her amylase activity reverted to normal soon after withdrawal. Acute pancreatitis is very rare in patients taking naproxen (SEDA-18, 105).

Oxaprozin *(SED-13, 238)*

Liver In phase II and III studies of oxaprozin *rises in serum transaminases* occurred in 10—20% of patients. *Anicteric hepatitis* has also been described (SEDA-11, 94). A similar incidence (9%) of asymptomatic liver enzyme rises has been reported in a comparative 6-week study of oxaprozin in 110 patients with osteoarthritis (101[c]). In about half of these the increase in transaminases was three times greater than the upper limit of the reference range. There were mild asymptomatic *increases in creatine phosphokinase* (to less than three times the upper limit of the reference range) in three of 109 patients.

Tiaprofenic acid *(SED-13, 235; SEDA-18, 106)*

The adverse effects profile of tiaprofenic acid have been reviewed, with particular attention to *chronic non-bacterial cystitis* (102[R]).

INDOMETHACIN AND RELATED COMPOUNDS *(SED-13, 221; SEDA-18, 101; SEDA-17, 108)*

Proglumetacin *(SED-13, 227)*

There are very few data on the efficacy and tolerability of proglumetacin. In a report of an uncontrolled, open-label, multicenter, 1-week study in 711 out-patients with cervical or low back pain treated with proglumetacin the most frequent adverse effects were *gastro-intestinal* (in about 10% of patients). Other adverse effects, which occurred in a minority of patients, included *fatigue, dizziness, allergic manifestations* (unspecified), and *headache* (103[c]). Worthy of note is the fact that central nervous system adverse effects seem to be less frequent with proglumetacin than with indomethacin.

Sulindac *(SED-13, 225; SEDA-18, 103)*

Low-dose rectal sulindac maintenance therapy achieved complete adenoma remission without relapse in 87% of 15 colectomized patients with familial adenomatous polyposis (104[c]). Two patients had histologically proven mild *gastritis* which responded to antacids.

OXICAM DERIVATIVES *(SED-13, 244; SEDA-17, 113; SEDA-18, 107; SEDA-19, 99)*

Cinnoxicam *(SED-13, 246)*

Cinnoxicam cream can cause *itchy erythema, edema, vesicles*, and *exudation* (105[c]), (106[c]). There was no cross-allergy on patch testing with other NSAIDs (fenoprofen, flurbiprofen, ibuprofen, ibuproxam, ketoprofen, naproxen, and piroxicam).

Lornoxicam *(SED-13, 247)*

Very little is known about the adverse effects of lornoxicam. In a dose-ranging placebo-controlled study *dizziness* and *gastrointestinal symptoms* were the most frequent adverse effects (107[c]).

Meloxicam *(SEDA 19, 93)*

Meloxicam has recently been marketed in some countries (for example, France, Italy) and promoted as an NSAID with a novel pharmacodynamic effect and an improved safety profile over current NSAIDs (108[R]). The basis for these claims is that in a number of experimental models meloxicam inhibits inducible COX-2 preferentially over the constitutional COX-1 isoform of cyclo-oxygenase (COX) (SEDA-19, 93; (109)). Meloxicam has a long elimination half-life (20 h), is highly protein bound, and is metabolized to inactive compounds, which are excreted in both urine and feces. Neither hepatic insufficiency nor moderate renal dysfunction appears to have any effects on its pharmacokinetics, and it has been said that dosage adjustments in the elderly may not be required (109), (110). However, in one study plasma concentrations of meloxicam were 26% higher in patients aged over 65 years than in younger patients (111[c]). Despite the theoretical advantage in terms of tolerability offered by a drug that selectively inhibits COX-2 relative to COX-1, the safety profile of any new NSAID must be judged on the basis of reliable clinical data in a large number of patients. Meloxicam is not an exception, and clinical experience is still limited (111[c])−(115[c]), (116[cr]).

Gastrointestinal   Gastrointestinal adverse effects were the most frequently reported (in about 15−20% of patients) but their incidence was lower with meloxicam than with all comparators (piroxicam, naproxen, diclofenac) in double-blind long-term studies (112[c])−(115[c]).

Gastrointestinal averse events were more frequent with a dosage of 15 than 7.5 mg/day. Gastrointestinal adverse events were judged severe in 1.7% and led to withdrawal in about 4% of patients. Symptoms included *abdominal pain*, *dyspepsia*, *eructation*, *nausea*, and *vomiting*. *Upper gastrointestinal perforation*, *ulceration*, and *bleeding* occurred rarely with meloxicam, and their incidence was dose related and lower than with the comparators. However, the total number of these severe complications was too small to allow the confident conclusion that meloxicam is less toxic than other NSAIDs.

The results of a double-blind endoscopic *microbleeding* comparison of meloxicam (7.5 mg/day for 4 weeks) and piroxicam (20 mg) in 51 healthy volunteers have supported the better gastrointestinal tolerability of meloxicam. Both fecal blood loss and endoscopy scores were higher in piroxicam-treated patients, and during the 4-week study six piroxicam volunteers versus one treated with meloxicam withdrew because of severe gastrointestinal toxicity (117[c]). However, it must be remembered that this type of study has many limitations and may only be useful for generating hypotheses that must be confirmed by appropriate epidemiological data.

One case of *colitis* was judged to have been probably related to treatment with meloxicam (113[c]).

Meloxicam suppositories can cause *abdominal pain* and *rectal bleeding* in a few patients (118[c]).

Other adverse effects   Central nervous system adverse events were found in about 7% patients and included *dizziness* and *headache*. *Rash*, *pruritus*, and other skin problems occurred in about 6.5% patients. In 16 (0.4%) patients there was *deterioration in renal*

function, reversible on withdrawal. One case of mild *leukopenia* and *neutropenia* was attributed to meloxicam (119[c]).

Intramuscular administration of meloxicam into the gluteal muscles has been studied and local tolerability was classified as good (120[c]). Slight local *pain*, *swelling*, and *reddened skin* were recorded in under 10% of patients. Slight *increases in serum CPK activity* can occur.

Systemic symptoms related to intramuscular administration of meloxicam, including *headache*, *dizziness*, *gastrointestinal disorders*, and *skin rashes*, have been reported by a very few patients (119[c]), (120[c]).

Piroxicam *(SED-13, 244; SEDA-17, 114; SEDA-18, 107; SEDA-19, 99)*

A new fast-dissolving dosage form of piroxicam has been evaluated in a number of trials (121[c]), (122[cr]), (123[cr]), with the claim that it is associated with better compliance in patients who have difficulties in swallowing tablets or capsules, or whenever a liquid formulation is not available, as the formulation can be taken under the tongue. Its systemic availability is the same as for other oral formulations of piroxicam. Local (oral) adverse effects are infrequent and include *stomatitis*, *mucosal erythema*, and *dysesthesia*, which in some cases has necessitated drug withdrawal.

Tenoxicam *(SED-13, 246; SEDA-17, 114; SEDA-18, 107; SEDA-19, 99)*

Urinary system   The renal adverse effects of tenoxicam have been comprehensively reviewed (124[R]). Data from phase III studies and from a large number of patients in phase IV clinical trials showed a very low prevalence of renal effects (a total of 0.07%). The most common events were *dysuria* and *renal pain*. Although tenoxicam has been used in some studies at younger adult recommended dosages in elderly patients and in patients with mild to moderate degrees of pre-existing renal impairment without renal adverse effects, awareness of potential nephrotoxicity of all NSAIDs is pertinent to tenoxicam.

ANILINE DERIVATIVES *(SED-13, 199; SEDA-18, 94; SEDA-17, 98)*

Paracetamol (acetaminophen)

Potentiation of paracetamol hepatotoxicity by alcohol and fasting Paracetamol in dosages over 10 g/day can cause severe liver toxicity. Alcohol abuse can predispose to paracetamol hepatotoxicity, even when the amounts ingested are less than 10 g/day (125[C])—(132[C]), and there have been anecdotal reports of severe hepatotoxicity in chronic ethanol abusers after ingestion of a therapeutic dose of paracetamol (4 g/day) (133[Cr]). The reason for enhanced paracetamol hepatotoxicity with chronic alcohol use may be that ethanol induces cytochrome CYP2E1 expression, resulting in production of *N*-acetyl-*p*-benzoquinone-imine, the reactive compound responsible for toxicity in many organs, including the liver, at a rate too fast for detoxification, because of reduced availability of glutathione, due to alcohol-related liver damage. Recent alcohol use may have the same effect on cytochrome induction, but acute alcohol intoxication may protect against hepatotoxicity by inhibiting hepatic enzymes (134[C]), (135[C]). However, alcohol (or other agents known to induce liver microsomal enzymes) is not used by all patients who develop paracetamol-related liver toxicity (SEDA-12, 76), and two of the largest published series of patients with paracetamol hepatotoxicity (136[C]), (137[C]) did not show any significant association between alcohol use and increased susceptibility to paracetamol hepatotoxicity.

A recent retrospective study on 21 cases of paracetamol hepatotoxicity (138[CR]), not due to intentional overdosage, has shown that fasting was significantly more common than recent alcohol use among patients who developed hepatotoxicity after a dosage of 4—10 g/day of paracetamol. The importance of fasting in potentiating the toxic effects of paracetamol has been also demonstrated in animal models (139), (140). Among the 21 patients, none of those who had used alcohol developed hepatotoxicity while taking the recommended dose of paracetamol (under 4 g/day). However, all the patients who developed toxicity while taking more than 10 g/day of paracetamol were alcohol users. It is worth noting that alcoholics are more likely to exceed the recommended dosage of paracetamol and consequently may be at higher risk of hepatotoxicity than non-alcoholics (132[C]), (141[C]).

Should paracetamol therefore be forbidden in alcoholic patients? Probably not, for at least three reasons. First, paracetamol hepatotoxicity almost never occurs when chronic alcoholics take paracetamol in the recommended dosage of 4 g/day (138[C]), (142[C])—(145[C]). Secondly, induction of CYP2E1 by alcohol ingestion may not be the primary factor in predisposing patients to hepatotoxicity, as other factors (drugs, illness resulting in prolonged fasting, genetic factors such as reduced glucuronidation capacity) may increase the susceptibility to paracetamol hepatotoxicity. Thirdly, to switch alcoholic patients from paracetamol to other analgesics, such as NSAIDs, does not seem wise, since NSAIDs are associated with severe gastrointestinal complications (bleeding, perforation), which are not common but which certainly occur with a significantly greater incidence than paracetamol-induced hepatotoxicity (146[C]), and more often still in alcoholics (147[C]).

In conclusion, paracetamol is a safe analgesic and antipyretic, even in alcoholics and after fasting. However all patients, especially alcoholics, should be warned to use it in the lowest effective dose, never to exceed the recommended dosage of 4 g/day, and to use it only for as long as is strictly necessary. As paracetamol is an over-the-counter drug, the public should be warned about this.

MISCELLANEOUS DRUGS

Tenidap *(SEDA-19, 100)*

Further studies have documented the potential toxicity of this compound (148[C]), (149[C]). Recently, Pfizer have abandoned tenidap for use in rheumatoid arthritis, following the issue of a non-approval letter from the FDA, issued because of unresolved questions about safety (150[C]). The decision related only to the 120-mg dose. The FDA's arthritis drugs advisory committee also voted against approving tenidap for osteoarthritis.

While there is as yet no clear evidence that tenidap is more effective than current agents in the treatment of rheumatoid arthritis, its safety profile is open to question. Gastrointestinal toxicity can be severe, and 2—3% of patients suffer from *ulceration*, *perforation*, or *bleeding*. *Proteinuria*, albeit mild, non-progressive, and with no evidence of deterioration of renal function, occurs in the majority of patients. *Increases in serum transaminases* can occur, and severe abnormalities of liver function tests have been reported (SEDA-19, 100; (148[C]), (149[C])).

REFERENCES

1. Caruso I, Bianchi Porro G. Gastroscopic evaluation of anti-inflammatory agents. Br Med J 1980;280:75—8.

2. Lanza FL. A review of gastric ulcer and gastroduodenal injury in normal volunteers receiving aspirin and other non-steroidal anti-inflammatory drugs. Scand J Gastroenterol 1989;24 Suppl 163:24—31.

3. Lanza F, Graham DY, Davis RE, Dack MF. Endoscopic comparison of cimetidine and sucralfate for prevention of naproxen-induced acute gastroduodenal injury: effect of scoring method. Dig Dis Sci 1990;35:1494—9.

4. Graham DY, Smith JL, Spjut HJ, Torres E. Gastric adaptation: studies in humans during continuous aspirin administration. Gastroenterology 1988;95:327—33.

5. Laine L, Weinstein WM. Subepithelial haemorrahages and erosions of the human stomach. Dig Dis Sci 1988;33:490—503.

6. Bardhan KD, Bjarnason I, Scott DL, Griffin WM, Fenn GC, Shield MJ. The prevention and healing of NSAID damage by misoprostol. Br J Rheumatol 1993;32:990—5.

7. Agrawal NM, Roth S, Graham DY, White RH, Germain B, Brown JA, Stromatt SC. Misoprostol compared with sucralfate in the prevention of nonsteroidal anti-inflammatory drug-induced gastric ulcer. Ann Intern Med 1991;115:195—200.

8. Taha AS, Hudson N, Hawkey CJ, Swannel AJ, Trye PN, Cottrell JM, Mann SG, Simon TJ, Sturrock RD, Russell RI. Famotidine for the prevention of gastric and duodenal ulcers caused by nonsteroidal antiinflammatory drugs. New Engl J Med 1996;334:1435—9.

9. Taha AS, Sturrock RD, Russell RI. Mucosal erosions in longterm non-steroidal anti-inflammatory drug users: predisposition to ulceration and relation to *Helicobacter pylori*. Gut 1995;36:334—6.

10. Taha AS, Russell RI. *Helicobacter pylori* and non-steroidal anti-inflammatory drugs: uncomfortable partners in peptic ulcer disease. Gut 1993;34:580—3.

11. Lanza FL, Evans DG, Graham DY. Effect of *Helicobacter pylori* infection on the severity of gastroduodenal mucosal injury after the acute administration of naproxen and aspirin to normal volunteers. Am J Gastroenterol 1991;86:735—7.

12. Taha AS, Angerson W, Nakshabendi I, Beekman H, Morran C, Sturrock RD. Gastric and duodenal mucosal blood flow in patients receiving non-steroidal anti-inflammatory drugs-influence of age, smoking, ulceration and *Helicobacter pylori*. Aliment Pharmacol Ther 1993;7:41—5.

13. Taha AS, Dahill S, Nakshabendi I, Lee FD, Sturrock RD, Russell RI. Duodenal histology, ulceration, and *Helicobacter pylori* in the presence or absence of non-steroidal anti-inflammatory drugs. Gut 1993;34:1162—6.

14. Mizokami Y, Kazutami T, Fukuda Y, Yamamoto I, Shimoyama T. Non-steroidal anti-inflammatory drugs associated with gastroduodenal injury and *Helicobacter pylori*. Eur J Gastroenterol Hepatol 1994;6 Suppl:S109—12.

15. Agrawal NM. Epidemiology and prevention of non-steroidal antiinflammatory drug effects in gastrointestinal tract. Br J Rheumatol 1995;34 Suppl 1:5—10.

16. Koch M, Capurso L, Dezi A, Ferrario F, Scarpignato C. Prevention of NSAID-induced gastroduodenal mucosal injury: meta-analysis of clinical trials with misoprostol and H_2-receptor antagonists. Dig Dis 1995;13 Suppl 1:62—74.

17. Simon TJ, Berger ML, Hoover ME, Stauffer LA, Berline RG. A dose ranging study of famotidine in prevention of gastroduodenal lesions associated with non-steroidal anti-inflammatory drugs (NSAIDs): results of a US multicenter trial. Am J Gastroenterol 1994;89:1644.

18. Silverstein FE, Graham DY, Senior JR, Davies HW, Struthers BJ, Bittman RM, Geis GS. Misoprostol reduces serious gastrointestinal complications in patients with rheumatoid arthritis receiving nonsteroidal anti-inflammatory drugs: a randomized, double-blind, placebo-controlled trial. Ann Intern Med 1995;123:241—9.

19. Raskin JB, White JB, Jaszewski R, Korsten MA, Schubert TT, Fort JG. Misoprostol and ranitidine in the prevention of NSAID-induced ulcers: a prospective, double-blind, multicenter study. Am J Gastroenterol 1996;91:223—7.

20. Singh G, Ramey DR, Morfeld D, Shi H, Hatoum HT, Fries JF. Gastrointestinal tract complications of nonsteroidal anti-inflammatory drug treatment in rheumatoid arthritis. Arch Intern Med 1996;156:1530—6.

21. Graham DY. Famotidine to prevent peptic ulcer caused by NSAIDs. New Engl J Med 1996;335:1322.

22. Cullen D, Bardhan KD, Eisner M, Kogut DG, Peacock RA, Thomson JM, Hawkey CJ. Primary gastroduodenal prophylaxis with omeprazole for NSAID users. Gastroenterology 1996;110 Suppl A:86.

23. Bjarnason I, Price AB, Zanelli G, Smethurst P, Burke M, Gumpel JM, Levi AJ. Clinicopatho-

logical feature of non-steroidal anti-inflammatory drug-induced small intestinal stricture. Gastroenterology 1988;94:1070—4.

24. Fellows IW, Clarke JMF, Roberts PF. Nonsteroidal anti-inflammatory drug-induced jejunal and colonic diaphragm disease: a report of two cases. Gut 1992;33:1424—6.

25. Sheers R, Williams WR. NSAID gut damage. Lancet 1989;ii:1154.

26. Hubert T, Ruchti C, Halter F. Nonsteroidal antiinflammatory drug-induced colonic stricture. Gastroenterology 1991;100:119—22.

27. Monahan D, Starnes E, Parker A. Colonic stricture in a patient on long-term non-steroidal anti-inflammatory drugs. Gastrointest Endosc 1992;38:385—8.

28. Whitcomb D, Martin S, Trellis DR, Evans BA, Becich MJ. Diaphragm-like stricture and ulcer of the colon during diclofenac treatment. Arch Intern Med 1992;152:2341—3.

29. Halter F, Weber B, Huber T, Eigenmann F, Frey MP, Ruchti C. Diaphragm disease of the ascending colon. Association with sustained-release diclofenac. J Clin Gastroenterol 1993; 16:74—80.

30. Gargot D, Chaussade S, d'Alteroche L, Desbazeille F, Grandjouan S, Louvel A, Douvin J, Causse X, Festin D, Chapuis Y, Legoux JL. Nonsteroidal anti-inflammatory drug-induced colonic strictures: two cases and literature review. Am J Gastroenterol 1995;90:2035—8.

31. Cahen R, Trolliet P, Francois B, Chazot C. Fenoprofen-induced membranous glomerulonephritis. Nephrol Dial Transplant 1988; 3:705—6.

32. Tettersall J, Greenwood R, Farrington K. Membranous nephropathy associated with diclofenac. Postgrad Med J 1992;68:392—3.

33. Miatello VR, Carbajal BF, Gotlieb D, Sadler TN. Sindrome nefrotico consecutivo a la ingestion de fenilbutazone. Prensa Med Argent 1959; 46:2551—8.

34. Schillinger F, Montagnac R, Milcent T. Membranous glomerulonephritis after diclofenac treatment. Kidney Int 1987;32:428—9.

35. Garrouste O, Bauwens M, Touchard G, Pourrat O, Patte D. Glomérulite extra-membraneuse et néphrite interstitielle aiguë après prise de diclofénac. Ann Med Interne (Paris) 1990;141:627—8.

36. Champion de Crispigny PJ, Becker GJ, Ihle BU, Walter NM, Wright CA, Kincaid-Smith P. Renal failure and nephrotic syndrome associated with sulindac. Clin Nephrol 1988;30:52—5.

37. Hurault de Ligny B, Faure G, Béné MC, Kessler M, Huriet C. Glomerulonephrite extra-membraneuse au course du traitement d'une polyarthrite rhumatoide par diclofénac. Nephrologie 1984;5:135—6.

38. Hay NM, Bailey RR, Lynn KL, Robson RA. Membranous nephropathy: a 19 year prospective study in 51 patients. NZ Med J 1992;105:489—91.

39. Radford MG Jr, Keith EH, Grande JP, Larson TS, Wagoner RD, Donadio JV, McCarthy JT. Reversibile membranous nephropathy asso-

ciated with the use of nonsteroidal anti-inflammatory drugs. J Am Med Assoc 1996;276:466—9.

40. Appel RG, Bleyer AJ, McCabe JC. Case report: analgesic nephropathy: a soda and a powder. Am J Med Sci 1995;310:161—6.

41. Tuffs A. German nephrologists demand pain-killer ban. Lancet 1996;348:952.

42. Thyss A, Milano G, Kubar J, Namer M, Schneider M. Clinical and pharmacokinetic evidence of a life-threatening interaction between methotrexate and ketoprofen. Lancet 1986; i:256—8.

43. Ellison NM, Servi RJ. Acute renal failure and death following sequential intermediate-dose methotrexate and 5-FU: a possible effect due to concomitant indomethacin administration. Cancer Treat Rep 1985;69:342—3.

44. Gabrielli A, Leoni P, Danieli G. Methotrexate and NSAIDs. Br Med J 1987;294:776.

45. Taillan B, Chichmanian RM, Fuzibet JG, Vinti H, Pesce A, Dujardin P. Pancytopénie au cours d'une polyarthrite rhumatoide traitée par des faibles doses de méthotrexate. Rev Rhum Mal Ostéoartic 1989;56:717.

46. Kraus A, Alarcon-Segovia D. Low-dose MTX and NSAID induced 'mild' renal insufficiency and severe neutropenia. J Rheumatol 1991;18:1274.

47. Singh RR, Malaviya AN, Pandey JN, Guleria JS. Fatal interaction between methotrexate and naproxen. Lancet 1986;i:1390.

48. Ahern M, Booth J, Loxton A, McCarthy P, Meffin P, Kevat S. Methotrexate kinetics in rheumatoid arthritis: is there an interaction with non-steroidal antiinflammatory drugs? J Rheumatol 1988;15:1356—60.

49. Skeith KJ, Russell AS, Jamali F, Coates J, Friedman H. Lack of significant interaction between low dose methotrexate and ibuprofen or flurbiprofen in patients with arthritis. J Rheumatol 1990;17:1008—10.

50. Furst DE, Herman R, Koehnke R, Ericksen N, Hash L, Riggs CE, Porras A, Veng-Pedersen P. Effects of aspirin and sulindac on methotrexate clearance. J Pharm Sci 1990;79:782—6.

51. Stewart CF, Fleming RA, Germain BF, Arkin CR, Evans WE. Coadministration of naproxen and low-dose methotrexate in patients with rheumatoid arthritis. Clin Pharmacol Ther 1990; 47:540—6.

52. Stewart CF, Fleming RA, Germain BF, Seleznick MJ, Evans WE. Aspirin alters methotrexate disposition in rheumatoid arthritis patients. Arthritis Rheum 1991;34:1514—20.

53. Tracy TS, Krohn K, Jones DR, Bradley JD, Hall SD, Brater DC. The effects of salicylate, ibuprofen and naproxen on the disposition of methotrexate in rheumatoid arthritis. Eur J Clin Pharmacol 1992;42:21—5.

54. Wallace CA, Smith AL, Sherry DD. Pilot investigation of naproxen/methotrexate interaction in patients with juvenile rheumatoid arthritis. J Rheumatol 1993;20;1764—8.

55. Anaya JM, Fabre D, Bressolle F, Bologna C, Alric R, Cocciglio M, Dropsy R, Sany J. Effects

of etodolac on methotrexate pharmacokinetics in rheumatoid arthritis patients. J Rheumatol 1994;21:203−8.

56. Combe B, Edno L, Lafforgue P, Bologna C, Bernard JC, Acquaviva P, Sany J, Bressolle F. Total and free methotrexate pharmacokinetics, with and without piroxicam, in rheumatoid arthritis patients. Br J Rheumatol 1995;34:421−8.

57. Menè P, Pugliese F, Patrono C. The effects of nonsteroidal anti-inflammatory drugs on human hypertensive vascular disease. Semin Nephrol 1995;15:244−52.

58. Houston MC, Weir, Gray J, Ginsberg D, Szeto C, Kaihlenen PM, Sugimoto D, Runde M, Lefkowitz M. The effects of nonsteroidal anti-inflammatory drugs on blood pressures of patients with hypertension controlled by verapamil. Arch Intern Med 1995, 155:1049−54.

59. Baez MA, Alvarez CR, Weidler DG. Effects of non-steroidal anti-inflammatory drugs, piroxicam or sulindac, on the anti-hypertensive actions of propranolol and verapamil. J Hypertens 1987;2:560−6.

60. Salvetti A, Magagna A, Abdel-Haq B, Lenzi M, Giovannetti R. Nifedipine interactions in hypertensive patients. Cardiovasc Drugs Ther 1990;4 Suppl 5:963−8.

61. Houston MC. Nonsteroidal anti-inflammatory drugs and antihypertensives. Am J Med 1991;90 Suppl 5A:42−7.

62. Takeuchi K, Abe K, Yasujima M, Sato M, Tanno M, Sato K, Yoshinaga K. No adverse effect of nonsteroidal anti-inflammatory drugs, sulindac and diclofenac sodium, on blood pressure control with a calcium antagonist nifedipine in elderly hypertensive patients. Tohoku J Exp Med 1991;165:201−8.

63. Huskisson EC, Chronopharmacology of antirheumatic drugs with special reference to indomethacin. In: Inflammatory arthropathies, Huskisson EC, Velò GP, editors. Amsterdam. Excerpta Medica, 1976:99−105.

64. Labrecque G, Bureau JP, Reinberg AE. Biological rhythms in the inflammatory response and in the effects of non-steroidal anti-inflammatory drugs. Pharmacol Ther 1995;66:285−300.

65. Roberts LJ, Fields JP, Oates JA. Mastocytosis without urticaria pigmentosa: a frequently unrecognized causa of recurrent syncope. Trans Assoc Am Phys 1982;95:36−41.

66. Hamrin B. Relase of histamine in urticaria pigmentosa. Lancet 1957;i:867−8.

67. Sutter MC, Beaulieu G, Birt AR. Histamine liberation by codeine and polymixin B in urticaria pigmentosa. Arch Dermatol 1962;86:217−21.

68. Crawhall JC, Wilkinson RD. Systemic mastocytosis: management of an unusual case with histamine (H_1 and H_2) antagonists and cyclooxygenase inhibition. Clin Invest Med 1987;10:1−4.

69. Butterfield JH, Kao PA, Klee GG, Yocum MW. Aspirin idiosyncrasy in systemic mast cell disease: a new look at mediator release during aspirin desentization. Mayo Clin Proc 1995;70:481−7.

70. Pellerin M, Hardy F, Abergel A, Boule D, Palacci JH, Babinet P, Wingtin LN, Glowinski J, Amiot JF, Mechali D, et al. Douleur chronique rebelle des cancereux. Interêt de l' injection intraradichidienne d'acetylsalycilate de lysine. Soixante observations. Presse Méd 1987;30:1465−8.

71. Mercadante S. Effects of intrathecal lysine acetylsalicylate in intractable cancer pain. Pain Digest 1995;5:181−5.

72. Wassif W, Bjarnason I. A comparison of the effects of aceclofenac and diclofenac on gastrointestinal blood loss. Br J Clin Res 1992;23:109−14.

73. Pasero G, Marcolongo R, Serni U, Parnham MJ, Ferrer F. A multi centre, double blind comparative study of the efficacy and safety of aceclofenac and diclofenac in the treatment of rheumatoid arthritis. Curr Med Res Opin 1995;13:305−15.

74. Martin-Mola E, Gijon-Banos J, Ansoleaga JJ. Aceclofenac in comparison to ketoprofen in the treatment of rheumatoid arthritis. Rheumatol Int 1995;15:111−16.

75. Ward DE, Veys EM, Bowdler JM, Roma J. Comparison of aceclofenac with diclofenac in the treatment of osteoarthritis. Clin Rheumatol 1995;14:656- 62.

76. Núñez M, Miralles ES, Harto A, Ledo A. Hypersensitivity vasculitis associated with aceclofenac. J Dermatol Treat 1995;I:54.

77. Tessari L, Ceciliani L, Belluati A, Letizia G, Martorana U, Pagliara L, Pognani A, Thovez G, Siclari A, Torri G, Solimeno L, Montull E. Aceclofenac cream versus piroxicam cream in the treatment of patients with minor traumas and phlogistic affection of soft tissues: a double blind study. Curr Ther Res 1995;56:702−12.

78. Riedl-Seifert RJ. Neurodermatitis in infants: a study of bufexamac. Tw Dermatol 1995;25:16−18.

79. Katz LM, Love PY. NSAIDs and the liver. In: Famaey JP, Paulus HE, editors. Therapeutic applications of NSAIDs: subpopulation and new formulation. New York: Marcel Dekker, 1992: 247−63.

80. Banks AT, Zimmerman HJ, Ishak KG, Harter JG. Diclofenac associated hepatotoxicity: analysis of 180 cases reported to the Food and Drug Administration as adverse reaction. Hepatology 1995;22:820−7.

81. Zimmerman HJ. Hepatotoxicity. Adverse effects of drugs and other chemicals on the liver. New York: Appleton Century Crofts, 1978:353.

82. Jick H, Derby LE, Garcia Rodriguez LA, Jick SS, Dean AD. Liver disease associated with diclofenac, naproxen and piroxicam. Pharmacotherapy 1992;12:207−12.

83. Lopez A, Linares M, Sánchez H, Blanquer A. Autoimmune hemolytic anemia induced by diclofenac. Ann Pharmacother 1995;29:787.

84. Roth SH, Bennett RE, Caldron PH, Mitchell CS, Swenson CM. Endoscopic evaluation of the long effects of diclofenac sodium and naproxen in elderly patients with arthritis. Clin Drug Invest 1995;9:171−9.

85. Marchini M, Tozzi L, Bakshi R, Pisati R, Fedele L. Comparative efficacy of diclofenac dispersible 50 mg and ibuprofen 400 mg in patients with primary dysmenorrhea. Int J Clin Pharmacol Ther 1995;33:491—7.

86. Jonsson CE, Ericsson F. Impairment of renal function after treatment of a burn patient with diclofenac, a non steroidal antiinflammatory drug. Burns 1995;21:471—3.

87. Sichart U. Voltaren ophtha sine Augentropfen nach fremdkorperverletzung bzw. Verblitzung Spektrum-Augenheilkd 1995;9:265—9.

88. Mabee CL, Mabee SW, Baker PB, Kirkpatrick RB, Levine EJ. Fulminant hepatic failure associetd with etodolac use. Am J Gastroenterol 1995;90:659—61.

89. Mora-Durban MJ, Extramiana-Cameno J, Arrizabalaga-Moreno M, Paniagua-Andres P, Camp-Herrero J, Milla-Santos J, del Nogal-Saez F, Gimeno-Albo F, Moreno-Carretero E, Dominguez-Granados R. Flubiprofeno vs dipirona asociada a hioscina: eficacia analgèsica en el còlico nefrìtico. Arch Esp Urol 1995;48:867—73.

90. Konstan MW, Byard PJ, Hoppel CL, Davis PB. Effects of high-dose ibuprofen in patients with cystic fibrosis. New Engl J Med 1995; 332:848—54.

91. Mehlisch DR, Jasper RD, Brown P, Korn SH, McCarroll K, Murakami AA. Comparative study of ibuprofen lysine and acetaminophen in patients with postoperative dental pain. Clin Ther 1995;17:852—60.

92. Anonymous. US ketoprofen switch approved. SCRIP 1995;2069:21.

93. Anonymous. Ketoprofen switched to Rx in Italy. SCRIP 1995;1993:21.

94. Rogers JEG, Fleming BG, Macintosh KC, Johnston B, Morgan-Hughes JO. Effect of timing of ketorolac administration on patient-controlled opioid use. Br J Anaesth 1995;75:15—18.

95. Fragen RJ, Stulberg D, Wixson R, Glisson S, Librojo E. Effect of ketorolac tromethamine on bleeding and on requirements for analgesia after total knee arthroplasty. J Bone Jt Surg 1995;77:998—1002.

96. Gallagher JE, Blauth J, Fornadley JA. Perioperative ketorolac tromethamine and postoperative hemorrhage in cases of tonsillectomy and adenoidectomy. Laryngoscope 1995;105:606—9.

97. Rusy LM, Houck CS, Sullivan LJ, Ohlms LA, Jones DT, McGill TJ, Berde CB. A double-blind evaluation of ketorolac tromethamine versus acetaminophen in pediatric tonsillectomy: analgesia and bleeding. Anesth Analg 1995;80:226—9.

98. Lipani JA, Poland M. Clinical update of the relative safety of nabumetone in long-term clinical trials. Inflammopharmacology 1995;3:351—61.

99. De Armond B, Francisco CA, Lin JS, Huang FY, Halladay S, Bartizek RD, Skare KL. Safety profile of over-the-counter naproxen sodium. Clin Ther 1995;17:4.

100. Castiella A, Lopez P, Bujanda L, Arenas JI. Possible association of acute pancreatitis with naproxen. J Clin Gastroenterol 1995;21:258.

101. Weaver A, Rubin B, Caldwell J, McMahon FG, Lee D, Makarowski W, Offenberg H, Sack M, Sikes D, Trapp R, Rush S, Kuss M, Ganju J, Bocanegra TS. Comparison of the efficacy and safety of oxaprozin and nabumetone in the treatment of patients with osteoarthritis of the knee. Clin Ther 1995;17:735—45.

102. Plosker GL, Wagstaff AJ. Tiaprofenic acid. A reappraisal of its pharmacological properties and use in the management of rheumatic diseases. Drugs 1995;50:1050—75.

103. Ginsberg F, Lefebvre D. A large, open-label study of proglumetacin in the treatment of patients with cervical and low-back pain. Curr Ther Res Clin Exp 1995;56:1237—46.

104. Winde G, Schmid KW, Schlegel W, Fischer R, Osswald H, Bünte H. Complete reversion and prevention of rectal adenomas in colectomized patients with familial adenomatous polyposis by rectal low-dose sulindac maintenance treatment. Dis Colon Rectum 1995;38:813—30.

105. Pigatto PD, Mozzanica N, Bigardi AS, Legori A, Valsecchi R, Cusano F, Tosti A, Guarrera M, Balato N, Sertoli A. Topical NSAID allergic contact dermatitis: Italian experience. Contact Dermatitis 1993;29:39—41.

106. Valsecchi R, Pansera B, Di Landro A, Cainelli T. Contact allergy to cinnoxicam. Contact Dermatitis 1995;32:63.

107. Nørholt SE, Sindet-Pedersen S, Bugge C, Branebjerg PE, Ersbøll BK, Bastian HL. A randomized, double-blind, placebo controlled, dose-response study of the analgesic effect of lornoxicam after surgical removal of mandibular third molars. J Clin Pharmacol 1995;35:606—14.

108. Noble S, Balfour JA. Meloxicam. Drugs 1996;51:424—30.

109. Engelhardt G. Pharmacology of meloxicam, a new non-steroidal anti-inflammatory drug with an improved safety profile through preferential inhibition of COX-2. Br J Rheumatol 1996;35 Suppl 1:4—12.

110. Bevis PJ, Bird HA, Lapham G. An open study to assess the safety and tolerability of meloxicam 15 mg in subjects with rheumatic disease and mild renal impairment. Br J Rheumatol 1996;35 Suppl 1:56—60.

111. Huskisson EC, Ghozlan R, Kurthen R, Degner FL, Bluhmki E. A long-term study to evaluate the safety and efficacy of meloxicam therapy in patients with rheumatoid arthritis. Br J Rheumatol 1996;35 Suppl 1:29—34.

112. Wojtulewski JA, Schattenkirchner, Barcelo P, Le Loët X, Bevis PJR, Bluhmki E, Distel M. A six-month double-blind trial to compare the efficacy and safety of meloxicam 7.5 mg daily and naproxen 750 mg daily in patients with rheumatoid arthritis. Br J Rheumatol 1996;35 Suppl 1:22—8.

113. Reginster JY, Distel M, Bluhmki E. A double-blind, three-week study to compare the efficacy and safety of meloxicam 7.5 mg and meloxicam 15 mg in patients with rheumatoid arthritis. Br J Rheumatol 1996;35 Suppl 1:17—21.

114. Lindén B, Distel M, Bluhmki E. A double-blind study to compare the efficacy and safety of meloxicam 15 mg with piroxicam 20 mg in patients with osteoarthritis of the hip. Br J Rheumatol 1996;35 Suppl 1:35−8.

115. Hosie J, Distel M, Bluhmki E. Meloxicam in osteoarthritis: a 6-month, double-blind comparison with diclofenac sodium. Br J Rheumatol 1996;35 Suppl 1:39−43.

116. Distel M, Mueller C, Bluhmki E, Fries J. Safety of meloxicam: a global analysis of clinical trials. Br J Rheumatol 1996;35 Suppl 1:68−77.

117. Patoia L, Santucci L, Furno P, Dionisi MS, Dell'Orso S, Romagnoli M, Sattarini A, Marini MG. A 4-week, double-blind, parallel-group study to compare the gastrointestinal effects of meloxicam 7.5 mg meloxicam 15 mg, piroxicam 20 mg and placebo by means of faecal blood loss, endoscopy and symptom evaluation in healthy volunteers. Br J Rheumatol 1996;35 Suppl 1:61−7.

118. Carrabba M, Paresce E, Angelini M, Galanti A, Marini MG, Cigarini P. A comparison of the local tolerability, safety and efficacy of meloxicam and piroxicam suppositories in patients with osteoarthritis: a single-blind, randomized, multicentre study. Curr Med Res Opin 1995;13:343−55.

119. Auvinet B, Ziller R, Appelboom T, Vélicitat P. Comparison of the onset and intensity of action of intramuscolar meloxicam and oral meloxicam in patients with acute sciatica. Clin Ther 1995;17:1078−90.

120. Ghozlan PR, Bernhardt M, Velicita P, Bluhmki E. Tolerability of multiple administration of intramuscular meloxicam: a comparison with intramuscular piroxicam in patients with rheumatoid arthritis or osteoarthritis. Br J Rheumatol 1996;35 Suppl 1:51−5.

121. Auvinet B, Crielaard JM, Manteuffel GE, Müller P, on behalf of the Multicenter Piroxicam FDDE European Study Group. A double-blind comparison of piroxicam fast dissolving dosage form and diclofenac enteric-coated tablets in the treatment of patients with acute musculoskeletal disorders. Curr Ther Res Clin Exp 1995;56:1142−53.

122. Porzio F. Sublingual piroxicam FDDF in the management of pain associated with rheumatic and nonrheumatic conditions: the Italian experience. Eur J Rheumatol Inflamm 1995;15:11−17.

123. Silva H. Worldwide clinical experience with piroxicam FDDF. Eur J Rheumatol Inflamm 1995;15:3−10.

124. Heintz RC. Tenoxicam and renal function. Drug Saf 1995;12:110−19.

125. Emby DJ, Fraser BN. Hepatotoxicity of paracetamol enhanced by ingestion of alcohol: report of two cases. S Afr Med J 1977;51:208−9.

126. Barker JJ, de Carle D, Anuras S. Chronic excessive acetaminophen use and liver damage. Ann Intern Med 1977;87:299−301.

127. Goldfinger R, Ahmed KS, Pitchumoni CS, Wesely SA. Concomitant alcohol and drug abuse enhancing acetaminophen toxicity: report of a case. Am J Gastroenterol 1978;70:385−8.

128. McClain CJ, Kromhout JP, Peterson FJ, Hoitzman JL. Potentiation of acetaminophen hepatotoxicity by alcohol. J Am Med Assoc 1980;244:251−3.

129. Licht H, Seeff LB, Zimmerman HJ. Apparent potentiation of acetaminophen hepatotoxicity by alcohol. Ann Intern Med 1980;92:511.

130. Johnson MW, Freidman PA, Mithc WE. Alcoholism, nonprescription drugs, and hepatotoxicity the risk from unknown acetaminophen ingestion. Am J Gastroenterol 1981;76:530−3.

131. Leist MH, Gluskin LE, Payne JA. Enhanced toxicity of acetaminophen in alcoholics: report of three cases. J Clin Gastroenterol 1985;7:55−9.

132. Seeff LB, Cuccherini BA, Zimmerman HJ, Alcer E, Benjamin SB. Acetaminophen hepatotoxicity in alcoholics: a therapeutic misadventure. Ann Intern Med 1986;104:399−404.

133. Zimmerman HJ, Maddrey WC. Acetaminophen (paracetamol) hepatotoxicity with regular intake of alcohol: analysis of instances of therapeutic misadventure. Hepatology 1995;22:767−9.

134. Kartsonis A, Reddy KR, Schiff ER. Alcohol, acetaminophen, and hepatic necrosis. Ann Intern Med 1986;105:138−9.

135. Sato C, Lieber CS. Mechanism of the preventive effect of ethanol on acetaminophen-induced hepatotoxicity. J Pharmacol Exp Ther 1981;218:811−15.

136. Rumack BH, Peterson RC, Koch GG, Amara IA. Acetaminophen overdose: 662 cases with evaluation of oral acetylcysteine treatment. Arch Intern Med 1981;141:380−5.

137. Read RB, Tredger JM, Williams R. Analysis of factor responsible for continuing mortality after paracetamol overdose. Hum Toxicol 1986;5:201−6.

138. Whitcomb DC, Block GD. Association of acetaminophen hepatotoxicity with fasting and ethanol use. J Am Med Assoc 1994, 271:1845−50.

139. Price V, Miller M, Jollow D. Mechanisms of fasting-induced potentiation of acetaminophen hepatotoxicity in the rat. Biochem Pharmacol 1987;36:427−33.

140. Price V, Jollow D. Effect of glucose and gluconeogenic substrates on fasting-induced suppression of acetaminophen glucuronidation in the rat. Biochem Pharmacol 1989;38:289−97.

141. Seeff L, Zimmerman H. Acetaminophen hepatotoxicity in alcoholics. Ann Intern Med 1986;105:624−5.

142. Benson G. Acetaminophen in chronic liver disease. Clin Pharmacol Ther 1983;33:95−101.

143. Hall AH, Kulig KW, Rumack BH. Acetaminophen hepatotoxicity. J Am Med Assoc 1986;256:1893−4.

144. Hall AH, Kulig KW, Rumack BH. Acetaminophen hepatotoxicity in alcoholics. Ann Intern Med 1986;105:624.

145. Hall AH, Kulig KW, Rumack BH. Acetaminophen and alcoholics. Dig Dis Sci 1987;32:558.

146. Strom BL. Adverse reaction to over the counter analgesics taken for therapeutic purposes. J Am Med Assoc 1994;272:1866−7.

147. Henry D, Dobson A, Turner C. Variability in the risk of major gastrointestinal complications from nonaspirin anti-inflammatory drugs. Gastroenterology 1993;105:1078—88.

148. Balckburn WD, Prupas HM, Silverfield JC, Poiley JE, Caldwell JR, Collins RL, Miller MJ, Sikes DH, Kaplan H, Fleischmann R, et al. Tenidap in rheumatoid arthritis. A 24-week double-blind comparison with hydroxychloroquine-plus-piroxicam, and piroxicam alone. Arthritis Rheum 1995;38:1447—56.

149. Wylie G, Appelboom T, Bolten W, Breedveld FC, Feely J, Leeming MRG, Le Loët X, Manthorpe R, Marcolongo R, Smolen J. A comparative study of tenidap, a cytokine-modulating anti-rheumatic drug, and diclofenac in rhematoid arthritis: a 24-week analysis of a 1-year clinical trial. Br J Rheumatol 1995;34:554—63.

150. Anonymous. Pfizer drops tenidap for RA. SCRIP 1996;2169:24.

10 General anesthetics and therapeutic gases

GENERAL TOPICS

Anesthesia in special circumstances *Children* Reviews have recently appeared on sedation and analgesia for children in intensive care units (1[R]) and on the use of new pharmacological agents in pediatric anesthesia (2[R]).

The use of total intravenous anesthesia with ketamine, etomidate, or propofol for short diagnostic or therapeutic procedures has been studied in 971 children with cancers (3[C]). There were 279 anesthesia-related adverse events, mostly vomiting, hypoxemia, tachycardia, agitation, or myoclonus. Ketamine was associated with vomiting (15%), agitation (15%), and tachycardia (20%). Etomidate was associated with vomiting (10%) and agitation (1.2%). Hypoxemia was rare, except in those given propofol (16%). Propofol caused vomiting in only 0.5% and agitation in 1.2% of cases.

Intramuscular sedation with ketamine, midazolam, and glycopyrrolate has been studied in 37 children aged 1–7 years during emergency procedures for facial injuries (4[C]). A single injection was given, followed by another dose of ketamine alone if necessary. Anesthesia occurred within 6 min in 73% of the children who received one injection. The most common adverse effects were random movements (14%), a transient rash (11%), and hypersalivation (11%). Other events included muscle hypertonicity and vomiting, either during recovery or later at home. There were no cases of delirium or hallucinations, which can occur with ketamine in adults.

Spinal and general anesthesia have been compared in 18 infants who had been born prematurely and who subsequently required inguinal herniorrhaphy (5[C]). The infants who were given general anesthesia had lower postoperative minimum hemoglobin oxygen saturations and minimum heart rates. There was no difference in the incidence of postoperative central apnea. The authors suggested that until it has been determined whether or not close monitoring is necessary after spinal anesthesia, all children should be carefully monitored after surgery, regardless of the anesthetic technique used, to look for postoperative hypoxemia.

Sedation for endoscopic procedures Intravenous midazolam and lidocaine spray have been compared with their respective placebos for sedation in patients undergoing gastroscopy (6[C]). Tolerance was greater in those given both active compounds compared with either alone, or with double placebo. There were no major adverse effects.

Various techniques have been used for sedation during colonoscopy, including diazepam with and without pethidine, midazolam with and without pethidine, and pethidine alone (7[R]). Although colonoscopy can be successfully achieved without sedation, sedation is associated with a higher percentage of completed examinations. Because of adverse cardiorespiratory effects some prefer not to use an opiate in addition to a sedative.

Propofol in combination with fentanyl or ketamine has been used to produce anesthesia in 60 patients undergoing urological endoscopy (8[C]). The main adverse effect was apnea lasting for more than 60 s in 14 of the 30 patients who received fentanyl and propofol.

Day-case surgery The use of newer anesthetics in day-case surgery has been reviewed (9[R]). The authors considered that propofol, although expensive, had made a significant improvement in this area. The newer inhalational anesthetics, such as isoflurane and sevoflurane, were promising and required further study. Midazolam was thought to produce more profound sedation, anxiolysis, and amnesia than propofol, but was associated with more prolonged recovery; nevertheless, they did not feel that flumazenil should be used to facilitate earlier discharge after sedation.

Critically ill patients Sedation in critically ill patients with neurological problems (10^R) and inhalational anesthesia in the intensive care unit (11^R) have been reviewed. Specific neurological problems that were considered were:

- the Guillain-Barré syndrome, in which the need for pain relief with opiates has to be balanced against the problem of potential respiratory depression and in which drugs that affect the blood pressure may be contraindicated;
- delirium tremens, in which cross-tolerance of anesthetic agents (for example, the benzodiazepines) with alcohol may be a problem;
- head injury, with the risks of hypotension;
- respiratory depression.

According to Kong (11^R) of all the inhalational agents available only isoflurane can be recommended, although it is not ideal and can in particular cause rising concentrations of plasma fluoride and nephrotoxicity during long-term sedation.

Coronary artery bypass grafting Propofol has been compared with enflurane, fentanyl, and thiopentone for its effects on hemodynamic stability and recovery after anesthesia for elective coronary artery bypass grafting (12^C). In 90 patients there was less intraoperative *hypertension* in the patients given propofol, but the incidence of *hypotension* was not different across the groups. However, vasopressor drugs were required during the period before bypass in those given fentanyl and propofol, and during bypass this was also the case for the patients treated with fentanyl alone. Those given propofol were extubated sooner. The authors concluded that the shorter-acting drugs (propofol and enflurane) helped earlier recovery without compromising hemodynamics during anesthesia.

Microvascular surgery The use of anesthesia in microvascular surgery has been reviewed (13^R). The main problems are the prolonged duration of such operations, the degree of

tissue trauma, and the extensive losses of blood and fluid. Nitrous oxide is often used in such operations, although it may have adverse effects on the bone-marrow during long procedures through vitamin B_{12} deficiency. Isoflurane is an alternative and was considered by the authors to be the volatile anesthetic of choice in these patients.

Cardiovascular A case of *Raynaud's syndrome* has been reported during general anesthesia (14^c).

A 14-year-old boy who had been given general anesthesia including propofol, nitrous oxide, and isoflurane developed Raynaud's syndrome. Within a few seconds of induction his hands and feet became pale, cold, and cyanosed; 15 min later they became red and vasodilated. The peripheral pulses were palpable throughout and areas to which EMLA cream had been applied were not affected. The peripheral vasodilatation persisted for several hours after the anesthetic, which lasted 30 min. The same occurred during two further general anesthetics. Investigations for primary Raynaud's disease were negative.

It was not clear whether this was a reaction to one of the drugs given (on each occasion fentanyl and either isoflurane or enflurane were used) or to some general effect of anesthesia, but this effect does not seem to have been reported before.

Respiratory The use of anesthetics in patients with *asthma* has been reviewed (15^R). Patients with asthma can be classified into one of three groups.

- Patients with a remote history, who have not had symptoms for several years, and are taking no drugs; in these patients normal spirometry is enough to warrant surgery.
- Patients without active wheezing but a history of recurrent attacks of bronchospasm requiring prophylactic drugs; spirometry should be comparable to the results of previous tests, and if results are within 80% of the predicted values or show no differences from previous values, anesthesia may be performed without alteration in the usual bronchodilatory drug regimen.
- Patients who are actively wheezing, or who have pulmonary function tests below

80% of predicted, or have deteriorated significantly; here anesthesia should be delayed or postponed in order to allow for optimization of drug treatment, although in an emergency that may not be possible.

Because some anesthetics (e.g. thiopentone) can cause bronchospasm through release of histamine, ketamine and propofol have become more popular for these patients.

Anesthetic technique in patients with asthma has been reviewed (16[R]). For induction of anesthesia benzodiazepines and propofol are safe, as are intravenous barbiturates, although thiobarbiturates should be avoided, since they can cause histamine release, leading to bronchospasm. In a randomized controlled trial of 59 asymptomatic asthmatics and 96 non-asthmatic patients of ASA status 1 and 2, propofol caused less wheezing in the asthmatic and non-asthmatic patients than thiobarbiturates did (17[C]).

Ketamine relaxes airway smooth muscle and may therefore be a useful induction agent in children with asthma.

If endotracheal intubation is required, lidocaine $1-2$ mg/kg intravenously before intubation has been recommended, although the use of a laryngeal mask airway may be more appropriate.

There is no appreciable difference in the effects of the various volatile anesthetics on bronchial airways. No type of anesthesia is associated with a lower rate of postoperative complications in these patients. Where possible regional anesthesia should be used.

Nervous system   The neurological and psychiatric adverse effects of anesthetics have been reviewed, including *intraoperative awareness* (an adverse effect of inadequate anesthesia), *postoperative delirium*, *psychotomimesis*, and *long-term postoperative cognitive/psychomotor impairment* (18[R]).

Parkinsonian symptoms have been reported in an apparently healthy 54-year-old man while he was emerging from anesthesia for an open cholecystectomy (19[C]). He developed sustained rigid extension of his limbs, and when he was able to move did so slowly and was unable to speak; 18 months later he developed definite Parkinson's disease. Although there have been reports of muscle rigidity postoperatively in patients with established Parkinson's disease, this seems to have been the first report in an individual who had not yet developed florid symptoms. The authors proposed that this was due to the effect of the inhalational anesthetics, perhaps in association with already reduced dopamine transport; dopamine receptor antagonists were not used in this case.

Previously undiagnosed meningiomas announced themselves in two women, aged 48 and 65 years, who became unrousable within 48 h after general anesthesia for non-neurosurgical operations (20[C]). This was attributed to *cerebral edema* in the tumors, in one case possibly exacerbated by hyponatremia and in one case by the use of glyceryl trinitrate, which has been reported to increase intracranial pressure.

Liver   The hepatotoxicity of inhaled anesthetics, particularly halothane, enflurane, and isoflurane, has been reviewed (21[R]), (22[R]) (see below under each drug). With all three drugs, antibodies to trifluoroacetylated liver microsomal proteins have been demonstrated, suggesting a common mechanism.

Musculoskeletal   Mutations in the ryanodine receptor have been sought in 101 patients who were positive for susceptibility to *malignant hyperthermia* and 137 patients who had negative tests (23[C]). Two specific mutations (C1840T and C487T) occurred in a total of 3% of those with positive caffeine contracture tests and in none of those who were negative. However, in two cases with C1840T mutations the responses to triggering anesthetics were very weak or non-existent, suggesting that this mutation is not particularly important in malignant hyperthermia.

Immunological and hypersensitivity reactions   *Histaminoid reactions* in general anesthesia have been reviewed (24[R]). The incidence of severe allergic reactions in anesthesia has been variably estimated as being as high as one in 350 or as low as one in 20 000 anesthetics. In one study mortality was $3-9\%$. Four mechanisms have been proposed.

(1) Type I hypersensitivity involving IgE. For example, 50% of thiopentone reactions have been associated with increases in serum IgE.

(2) Classical complement activation involving IgG or IgM. Thiopentone has been reported to cause alterations in complement in 30% of reactions. Reactions to Althesin and propanidid were probably due to the solvent in which they were formulated, polyethoxylated castor oil, via activation of complement.

(3) Alternative complement activation without antibody involvement.

(4) Direct pharmacological effects. For example, thiobarbiturates can release histamine, as can both depolarizing and nondepolarizing muscle relaxants. In contrast, propofol and etomidate are thought not to cause histamine release.

Most reactions involve *cardiovascular collapse*, which occurs in 90% of cases, and is the only presenting feature in about 10%. *Dysrhythmias* are common, supraventricular tachycardia occurring in over 80%, and cardiac arrest occurs in 11%. *Bronchospasm* occurs in 50% of patients and is the only presenting feature in 3%. *Generalized erythema or flushing* is very common, but typical *pruritic wheals* are uncommon. Occasionally there may be *conjunctival swelling and inflammation, eyelid edema, and lacrimation*. Other effects include *nausea, vomiting, abdominal pain*, and *blood loss from the gut*. Rarely *disseminated intravascular coagulation* may occur.

Risk factors The effects of *porphyrias* on anesthetic medication have been reviewed (25[R]). Drugs that are unsafe or probably unsafe in the acute hepatic porphyrias include barbiturates, etomidate, some benzodiazepines (chlordiazepoxide, flunitrazepam, nitrazepam), and enflurane. The safety of diazepam, ketamine, isoflurane, and halothane is uncertain. Midazolam, propofol, and nitrous oxide are safe.

Interactions Single agents are often insufficient in anesthesia, because different problems require separate treatments, because individual drugs may cause adverse effects, the severity of which may be reduced by the use of combinations, or because repeated administration of a single agent may lead to cumulative effects. Drug interactions in anesthesia have again been reviewed, both systematically (26[R]) and as uncritical listings (27[R]), (28[R]).

Many of the interactions are beneficial, the concurrent use of two or more different agents improving the quality of anesthesia. Several reviews of this have recently appeared (29[R])–(31[R]).

Disadvantages of combinations include unpredictability of synergistic actions or toxicity, mutual alterations in pharmacokinetics, increased likelihood of errors in drug administration, and difficulties in planning drug therapy when adverse effects occur and are not attributable to a particular drug. The combination of midazolam with propofol in the induction of anesthesia has been discussed in particular detail (31[R]).

In a different approach the effect of epidural eptazocine, as an adjunct to total intravenous anesthesia with ketamine, diazepam, droperidol, and vecuronium, has been studied in 115 patients (32[C]). In 46 of those who were given the intravenous anesthesia alone, the blood pressure, heart rate, and blood glucose concentration were all significantly higher than in those given eptazocine. Those given intravenous anesthesia alone required more vasodilators, nitrous oxide, and postoperative analgesia.

ANESTHETIC VAPORS *(SED-13, 265; SEDA-17, 122; SEDA-18, 114; SEDA-19, 104)*

Halogenated anesthetics, fluoride, and renal damage ℞

Renal damage, which was relatively common with methoxyflurane but is less so with the newer halogenated anesthetics, has been reviewed (22[R]). It has been attributed to the nephrotoxic effects of fluoride, which is a metabolic by-product. The risk of nephrotoxicity varies with different halogenated anesthetics, mostly because they are metabolized to different extents. For example, in a study of 120 children given sevoflurane or halothane, the mean peak plasma fluoride concentration after sevoflurane was 15 µmol/l compared with 2 µmol/l with halothane (33[C]). Halothane has not been reported to cause nephrotoxicity (22[R]).

However, even when plasma fluoride concentrations are comparable, nephrotoxicity varies from anesthetic to anesthetic. For example, there were only mild changes in concentrating ability and in the secretion of N-acetyl-β-glucosaminidase in association with plasma fluoride concentrations over 50 µmol/l in patients who had been given sevoflurane (34[C]). Similarly, no cases of nephrotoxicity were reported in patients in whom prolonged exposure to isoflurane had produced plasma fluoride concentrations over 50 µmol/l (35[C]). In contrast, renal impairment has been associated with plasma fluoride concentrations over 50 µmol/l after the administration of methoxyflurane (36[r]).

It has been suggested that this difference may be due to differential metabolism of the drugs in the kidney. This is because drugs like sevoflurane and enflurane are primarily metabolized by CYP2E1, while methoxyflurane is metabolized by more than one cytochrome P450 isoform. Thus, defluorination by several isoforms might occur in the kidney, contributing to the greater degree of renal impairment associated with methoxyflurane. The renal metabolism of methoxyflurane has been studied in cadaver kidneys (37[C])r. The defluorination of methoxyflurane by the renal microsomes was considerably higher for methoxyflurane than it was for sevoflurane. The defluorination of both anesthetics was inhibited by diethyldithiocarbamate, an inhibitor of CYP2E1. Inhibitors of CYP2A6 and CYP3A inhibited the metabolism of methoxyflurane to a greater extent than that of sevoflurane, supporting the hypothesis.

Drugs that induce the activity of CYP2E1 (such as isoniazid and ethanol) may increase the plasma concentration of fluoride. However, in one study of patients treated with isoniazid who were anesthetized with sevoflurane there were no cases of nephrotoxicity, despite plasma fluoride concentrations in excess of 100 µmol/l (38[C]). In contrast, disulfiram, an inhibitor of CYP2E1, reduced the formation of fluoride from sevoflurane in 22 patients undergoing anesthesia (39[C]) and also reduced the formation of fluoride from enflurane (40[C]);

however, it is not clear that this is likely to be clinically important.

Although patients with normal renal function are probably not at risk during normal anesthesia with sevoflurane, there is concern that those with pre-existing renal impairment may be at risk. However, in a group of 21 patients with pre-existing renal impairment who were given sevoflurane during an average period of 151 min there was no deterioration in renal function; peak serum concentrations of inorganic fluoride were only 25 µmol/l (41[C]). By comparison, in 20 patients given enflurane, the peak serum concentration was 13 µmol/l and the highest concentration 52 µmol/l.

In 40 patients with a mean age of 61 years the peak concentration of fluoride in the serum correlated with the duration of exposure to the anesthetic (42[C]). In 23 patients who had anesthesia with sevoflurane for at least 5 h, average 102 min) eight patients had peak fluoride concentrations over 50 µmol/l (mean 58), and 14 had concentrations below 50 µmol/l (mean 37) (34[C]). There was a weak but significant inverse correlation between peak fluoride concentration and maximal urinary osmolality after an injection of vasopressin at the end of anesthesia. In addition, there was a dose-related increase in the urinary excretion of N-acetyl-β-glucosaminidase. Although the effect on urine osmolality tended to be lower in those with a high peak fluoride concentration, the difference across the groups was not quite statistically significant. Urine osmolality response in the patients who had a low fluoride concentration after sevoflurane was the same as in 11 patients who were given isoflurane anesthesia and had peak fluoride concentration of 6 µmol/l. These results suggest that even with relatively prolonged exposure to sevoflurane, abnormalities of renal function in patients with normal pre-existing function are small and likely to be clinically unimportant. Whether more prolonged anesthesia in individuals with pre-existing renal impairment is of importance remains to be determined.

It should be noted that it is not clear that renal damage in patients who are exposed to sevoflurane is necessarily due to the fluoride; a fluorinated metabolite of sevoflurane (so-called compound CA), which is nephrotoxic in rats, may contribute.

Interactions   Interactions with the halogenated anesthetics have been reviewed (43[R]). Virtually all of the pharmacodynamic interactions are with other drugs that are used in general or local anesthesia. There have been very few pharmacokinetic studies in man, but animal studies suggest that some halogenated inhalational anesthetics (enflurane and desflurane) may displace drugs such as diazepam from plasma proteins, increasing their clearance rate, while halothane may inhibit drug elimination by a direct effect on the liver. Isoflurane and sevoflurane had neither of these effects. The halogenated anesthetics may also reduce the biliary elimination of glucuronidated metabolites of compounds such as paracetamol.

Desflurane *(SED-13, 272; SEDA-17, 122; SEDA-18, 114; SEDA-19, 105)*

Desflurane is identical in structure to isoflurane, except that it is halogenated completely with fluorine instead of fluorine and chlorine. Its advantages are that it has a lower blood gas partition coefficient than nitrous oxide and the lowest of any of the halogenated anesthetics, that it is resistant to in vivo degradation, that recovery is fast, and that it appears not to have hepatotoxic or nephrotoxic effects. Because of its low solubility it can be used in low-flow systems. Its main adverse effects are those on the upper respiratory tract detailed below. However, in high concentrations it can also cause transient activation of the sympathetic nervous system, predisposing to *hypertension* and *dysrhythmias*.

Desflurane is exceptionally pungent and often causes *coughing*, *spluttering*, *salivation*, and *laryngospasm*. In one study five of the first six patients who were given desflurane developed laryngospasm, breath-holding, coughing, and increased secretions; in four patients oxygen saturation fell to 92% or lower; in four patients there was significant *tachycardia* and *hypotension*, with *bradydysrhythmias* in three (44[c]). One patient developed *hiccups* and *bronchospasm*. Nebulized lidocaine did not alter these reactions.

Enflurane *(SED-13, 268; SEDA-17, 122; SEDA-18, 115; SEDA-19, 106)*

Nervous system   A case of *motor neurone disease* has been attributed to enflurane (45[c]).

A 71-year-old woman who habitually drank more than 70 g of alcohol a day was anesthetized with enflurane and propofol. On the first postoperative day after transurethral resection of a papillary bladder carcinoma she developed bilateral arm weakness, and over the next 3 years progressive weakness in the shoulders, arms, legs, and laryngeal and pharyngeal muscles. Her reflexes were reduced and there were no pyramidal signs. Co-ordination and sensation were normal.

The authors proposed that enflurane-induced release of glutamate may have caused changes in the spinal cord motor neurones and they did not think that the condition was either paraneoplastic or due to encephalomyelitis. It is not clear what role alcohol abuse had in this case.

Liver   Liver damage due to enflurane has been reviewed (21[R]), (22[R]). The incidence of hepatotoxicity with enflurane (about one in 800 000 exposures) is less than with halothane, but it has been associated with antibodies to trifluoroacetylated liver microsomal proteins, suggesting a common mechanism.

Postoperative hepatic necrosis has been attributed to enflurane (46[c]).

A 66-year-old woman underwent anesthesia with enflurane and nitrous oxide after induction with fentanyl and midazolam. On the third postoperative day she became drowsy and then unrousable, hypertensive, and hypothermic. She had profound lactic acidosis and hypoglycemia and her serum AsT activity was greatly increased. There were only slight increases in her serum alkaline phosphatase and γ-glutamyl transferase, and serology for cytomegalovirus and hepatitis A, B, and C viruses were all negative. She died on the fifth day. At autopsy there was massive widespread centrilobular necrosis and necrosis of Zone 2 of the acini in some areas. There was minimal infiltration in the portal tracts.

The histological features reported here were characteristic of the necrosis that the halogenated anesthetics have been reported to cause. The reactive acylated metabolite that is thought to be associated with liver damage due to the halogenated anesthetics is produced by the action of CYP2E1. In this case the presence of diabetes mellitus was proposed to have increased the defluorination of enflurane through induction of CYP2E1, which may also have enhanced the potential for hepatotoxicity.

Halothane *(SED-13, 269; SEDA-17, 122; SEDA-18, 116; SEDA-19, 107)*

Cardiovascular   Halothane has a *negative inotropic effect* and can cause cardiac arrest when used in excess. This is generally preceded by bradycardia, and it has been thought that the cardiotoxic effects of halothane might be mitigated in patients in whom atropine has been used. However, there has been a recent report of three infants in whom electromechanical dissociation occurred after exposure to halothane despite pretreatment with atropine (47[c]).

Respiratory   There was a *reduced acute ventilatory response to isocapnic hypoxia* after exposure to subhypnotic concentrations of halothane in 12 healthy adults; the effect was concentration-dependent (48[c]). The clinical relevance of this effect is not clear, but the authors pointed out that arousal, likely to be mediated, at least in part, by a peripheral chemoreflex response to hypoxia, is an important defence to airway obstruction, and that the ventilatory response, if intact, might help to alleviate postoperative hypoxemia due to factors other than airway obstruction.

Liver   Halothane-induced liver damage has been reviewed (21[R]), (22[R]) as have the pathogenesis and treatment of halothane-induced hepatitis (49[R]), (50[R]).

Halothane can cause two types of liver damage. Mild liver damage is common (occurring in up to 30% of cases) and causes small transient rises in the activities of serum transaminases. In contrast, severe toxicity, which is rare, can result in massive hepatic necrosis. It is this latter form of damage that is known as 'halothane hepatitis'. The damage is thought to be caused by oxidative metabolites of halothane that contain trifluoroacetyl groups, which react with liver microsomes, stimulating the production of antibodies. The risk of hepatitis is increased with repeated exposure to halothane and there is also a genetic component; women and older patients are also at greater risk, and other factors include obesity and enzyme induction.

In the past the diagnosis of halothane hepatitis has been made on the basis of the history and exclusion of other causes. However, the availability of tests for antibodies is improving diagnostic ability. In one study of sera from 15 patients with halothane hepatitis autoantibodies to human hepatic polypeptides were detected in ten (51[c]). In contrast, autoantibodies were not detected in the sera of 16 healthy blood donors, but were detected in three of six samples from patients who had been exposed to halothane but who had not developed hepatitis. In contrast to cases of hepatitis due to other drugs, in which autoantibodies were found to single major human hepatic polypeptide antigens, in the halothane-associated cases there was a marked degree of individual variation in both the intensity of the response and the number and nature of the microsomal proteins involved. The role of these multiple autoantibodies in the pathogenesis of the hepatitis is not clear.

A similar form of hepatitis has been more rarely reported following exposure to two other halogenated anesthetics, enflurane and isoflurane. In a study in guinea-pigs, the administration of enflurane and isoflurane resulted in the formation of fluoride-containing moieties, which were covalently bound to liver proteins (52). However, the proportion of bound fluoride groups was much less with enflurane and isoflurane than with halothane. The relative frequency of cases of hepatitis from drug to drug (halothane greater than enflurane, much greater than isoflurane) was comparable with the degree of formation of neoantigens.

Because halothane is administered in a formulation that has been stabilized with 0.01% thymol as an antioxidant, it has been proposed that the thymol may contribute to the hepatitis induced by halothane (53[r]). This is because thymol is immunogenic and binds to globulins. This is an untested hypothesis.

Musculoskeletal   A case of *rigidity* following exposure to halothane has been described in a 4-year-old boy with Smith-Lemli-Opitz syndrome (54[c]). Succinylcholine was not used and the serum creatine kinase activity did not rise during the episode. There was no fever. Other features of malignant hyperthermia were also absent. Muscle biopsy was not performed and so a susceptibility to malignant hyperthermia could not be ruled out.

Risk factors *Children* Halothane caused a greater degree of respiratory depression in 15 infants aged 2—6 months than in 15 children aged 1—5 years (55[C]). The authors attributed this to a reduction in ventilatory drive in the infants, the cause of which was not clear. However, paradoxical movement of the chest wall during anesthesia may have contributed.

Isoflurane *(SED-13, 271; SEDA-17, 123; SEDA-18, 117; SEDA-19, 108)*

Cardiovascular There was evidence of *myocardial ischemia* during emergence from anesthesia with isoflurane for carotid endarterectomy in six of 13 patients, mean age 65 years (56[C]). In addition, 10 of the 13 patients were hypertensive during extubation and required vasodilator therapy. All these events were short-lived.

Liver Liver damage due to isoflurane has been reviewed (21[R]), (22[R]). Although hepatitis is rare after exposure to isoflurane, a few cases have been reported (SEDA-18, 117), and there has been a further report in a 47-year-old man who had had a previous history of halothane-associated hepatitis (57[c]). Antitrifluoroacetyl antibodies were detected in the serum at the time of maximum changes in the activities of serum AlT and AsT. There was an eosinophilia, which peaked at 9%. These findings are consistent with an immune mechanism for this adverse effect. They suggest that previous sensitization to halothane may predispose patients to hepatitis on exposure to other halogenated anesthetics.

Sevoflurane *(SED-13, 273; SEDA-17, 124; SEDA-18, 119; SEDA-19, 110)*

Sevoflurane has been the subject of several general reviews (58[R]), (59[r]), (60[r]), (61[R]), (62[r]), as well as reviews of its use in specific circumstances, such as out-patient anesthesia (63[R]) and in children (64[R]). Its advantages are that it has a low blood gas partition coefficient, although not as low as desflurane or nitrous oxide, that it is not pungent and therefore (in contrast to desflurane) can be used both for induction and maintenance anesthesia and can also be used in children, and that it tends not to cause cardiac dysrhythmias.

Cardiovascular The cardiovascular effects of sevoflurane have been reviewed (65[R]). In contrast to isoflurane and desflurane, sevoflurane tends not to increase the heart rate. However, it has a similar effect on regional blood flow to other halogenated anesthetics, although it is perhaps slightly less of a coronary vasodilator than isoflurane. It *reduces myocardial contractility* and does not potentiate adrenaline-induced cardiac dysrhythmias. It also *reduces baroreflex function*, and in that respect is similar to other halogenated anesthetics. Coronary artery disease is not a risk factor for the use of these agents.

Some of these cardiovascular effects of sevoflurane have been confirmed in a study of 21 healthy volunteers aged 19—34 years who did not undergo surgery (66[C]).

Respiratory The ventilatory effects of sevoflurane have been reviewed (67[R]). It causes less airway irritation than other inhaled anesthetics and is effective in reversing bronchospasm.

Nervous system Sevoflurane alone has been compared with sevoflurane plus nitrous oxide and halothane plus nitrous oxide in 120 children aged 1—12 years (33[C]). The incidence of adverse effects was similar in all three groups, except for the occurrence of *excitement* during induction, which occurred in 35% of the children given sevoflurane alone, compared with 5% in each of the other groups. During maintenance 12.5% of the children given sevoflurane alone showed some degree of movement at the time of skin incision, compared with none in the other two groups. Other adverse effects were equally distributed through the groups, including *coughing during induction* (10—18%), *postoperative nausea* (13—18%), and *postoperative vomiting* (45—65%). In contrast, in a study of 40 adults anesthetized with sevoflurane, the addition of nitrous oxide made no difference to the incidence of adverse effects; however, there were no cases of excitement during induction (63[C]).

Liver In 150 patients given sevoflurane anesthesia, abnormal *increases in serum AsT and AlT activities* occurred in only two patients (68[C]).

Musculoskeletal Sevoflurane has been reported to cause *malignant hyperthermia* in a 20-year-old woman without a family history (69[c]). The diagnosis was confirmed by positive in vitro caffeine and halothane contracture tests.

Carpal spasm has been reported in a 63-year-old woman who was anesthetized with sevoflurane and who had a normal plasma calcium concentration (70[c]). The authors' hypothesis was that this occurred because fluoride ions had combined with calcium, effectively reducing the serum calcium concentration. This was consistent with the persistence of the carpal spasm for 56 h, fluoride having a half-life of up to 9 h.

Interaction The addition of *nitrous oxide* to sevoflurane for single-breath induction in 19 volunteers compared with 21 controls altered neither the number of complications nor the speed of induction (71[C]).

GASES

Nitrous oxide *(SED-13, 274; SEDA-17, 124; SEDA-18, 118; SEDA-19, 109)*

Nitrous oxide has been used during single-lung ventilation for elective thoracic surgery, in order to prevent the oxygen toxicity that occurs during the administration of 100% oxygen and inhaled anesthetics. However, this can result in hypoxemia. In order to circumvent this, continuous positive airway pressure has been used in 20 patients aged 33—73 years (72[C]). During anesthesia the mean P_aO_2 was 100—143 mmHg. However, the technique was not compared in a controlled fashion with the usual technique. None of these patients had obstructive lung disease.

Nervous system Long-term exposure to ni-

trous oxide *inactivates vitamin B$_{12}$*, leading to bone-marrow suppression and adverse effects on the nervous system, including myelopathy, peripheral neuropathy, and encephalopathy. These well-known effects have again been observed in an 18-year-old man who was exposed daily to nitrous oxide over a period of 7 months (73[c]). He developed a peripheral neuropathy indistinguishable from subacute combined degeneration of the cord and also had megaloblastic changes in the bone-marrow and a peripheral neutropenia. His serum B$_{12}$ concentration was well below the reference range. Pernicious anemia was ruled out and the nitrous oxide was implicated. If long-term nitrous oxide exposure is contemplated, it has been suggested that prophylaxis with cobalamin, folinic acid, or methionine should be given (74[r]). A similar case occurred in a 31-year-old woman who received nitrous oxide by inhalation for only 135 min (75[c]). She gradually developed a myelopathy over the next several months in association with a macrocytic anemia and a serum B$_{12}$ concentration below the reference range. These effects improved with vitamin B$_{12}$ administration.

Special senses *Rupture of the tympanic membrane* has been attributed to nitrous oxide in a 28-year-old woman with a history of tonsillectomy and a recent respiratory tract infection who underwent dilatation and curettage under diagnostic laparoscopy (76[c]). When nitrous oxide enters body spaces it alters the pressure within them. The middle ear normally contains nitrogen, whose blood gas partition coefficient is 0.014. Nitrous oxide, gas coefficient 0.47, can enter the space 34 times more rapidly than nitrogen can leave it. The ruptured eardrum in this case was attributed to an increase in pressure with impaired drainage via the Eustachian tube. The authors therefore suggested that care should be taken when using nitrous oxide in patients who are known to have diseases that can reduce patency of the Eustachian tube.

Interaction The effect of *nitrous oxide* on the dosage of propofol and recovery after total intravenous anesthesia has been studied in 42 patients aged 18—62 years undergoing inguinal herniotomy (77[C]). Nitrous oxide did not alter the propofol dosage requirements but prolonged early recovery.

INTRAVENOUS AGENTS

BARBITURATES *(SED-13, 275; SEDA-17, 128; SEDA-18, 129; SEDA-19, 119)*

Methohexital

The efficacy and adverse effects of methohexital 30 mg/kg given rectally have been studied in 648 children (78[C]). *Defecation* (10%) and *hiccups* (13%) were common, as has previously been noted. There were no cases of seizures or apnea.

In another study of the use of methohexital in 20 elderly patients undergoing cataract extraction, *respiratory depression* occurred in 30%, compared with 5% of 20 patients who were given midazolam/ketamine (79[C]). Movements during anesthesia were observed in 45% of the patients given methohexital, compared with 10% in the other group.

BENZODIAZEPINES

Midazolam *(SED-13, 277; SEDA-17, 125; SEDA-18, 120; SEDA-19, 112)*

Proposed criteria for the use of continuous midazolam infusion in adults have been published by the American Society of Health-System Pharmacists (80[R]).

Cardiovascular In 40 patients undergoing coronary artery bypass grafting, midazolam (0.1 mg/kg) *reduced left ventricular contractility* without changing cardiac index, perhaps because after-load was also reduced (81[C]). These effects were not exaggerated in patients who had a reduced ejection fraction before surgery.

Nervous system *Anterograde amnesia* is a well-known effect of benzodiazepines, and is a welcome feature when they are used for anesthesia. It is common with midazolam. For example, in one study of 15 patients, mean age 61 years, who were given 2—5 ml of midazolam intramuscularly 15 min before the start of anesthesia, 14 had no memory of the events immediately before anesthesia (82[C]).

Hematological In a 40-month-old boy a withdrawal syndrome with neurological symptoms (see below) was accompanied by a *thrombocytosis*, which peaked at $1230 \times 10^9/l$ (83[c]). Recovery from the withdrawal syndrome was accompanied by a normalization of the platelet count. The relevance of this change in platelet count was not clear.

Miscellaneous *Inhibition of normal thermoregulatory control* has been reported in eight healthy women, mean age 24 years, who were given midazolam to a target plasma concentration of 0.3 μg/ml (84[C]). The sweating threshold fell by 0.3°C, the shivering threshold by 0.6°C, and the core temperature that triggered vasoconstriction by 0.8°C; the sweating-to-vasoconstriction range increased from 0.2 to 0.7°C. This last value should be compared with the much larger changes produced by the volatile anesthetics, propofol, and opioids (3—5°C).

Risk factors *Age* In a study of 20 patients aged 19—47 and 20 aged 53—75 years, the older patients performed less well after sedation with midazolam for gastroscopy on a battery of neuropsychological tests of verbal ability and face recognition (85[C]). The effect was dose related. However, the effects were limited to a few of the tests used, and overall the results did not support increased susceptibility of older subjects to the amnesic effects of midazolam.

In contrast, there was an inverse relation between age and Glasgow Coma Scale scores during the administration of midazolam to 17 patients, mean age 52 years, undergoing mechanical ventilation (86[C]). This was not explained by differences in infusion rate. Data were collected on the use of other CNS depressant drugs during withdrawal of midazolam in 10 patients; eight of them required additional doses of other drugs, suggestive of withdrawal effects of midazolam. Six out of six patients in whom midazolam was abruptly discontinued required additional therapy, compared with two out of four in whom withdrawal had been gradual.

Sex In 30 healthy volunteers given midazolam (0.1—0.2 mg/kg) there were differences in sedation and breathing patterns between the men and women, the men being more sensitive to the drug (87[C]). The measurements were made by monitoring the movements of the rib cage and abdominal wall, the arterial partial pressure of oxygen, and the incidence of snoring. The authors attributed these differences to greater upper airway obstruction in the men.

Renal failure The conjugates of the main metabolite of midazolam, α-hydroxymidazolam, accumulate in renal failure. In five patients with severe renal failure (creatinine clearance 7 ml/min or less), in whom prolonged sedation after midazolam was immediately reversed by flumazenil, there were high serum concentrations of glucuronidated α-hydroxymidazolam, even at times when the concentrations of the unconjugated metabolite and midazolam itself were low (88[C]). Glucuronidated α-hydroxymidazolam is about one-tenth as potent as midazolam and unconjugated α-hydroxymidazolam, and accumulation of the conjugated metabolite in renal failure may be important.

Withdrawal effects Neurological symptoms have been observed after the withdrawal of midazolam (83[c]), (89[c]).

A 40-month-old boy was sedated with midazolam (0.5 µg/kg/min, increasing to 2 µg/kg/min because of tolerance) and fentanyl (1 µg/kg/h). After about 9 days the infusion was stopped and he subsequently became agitated and complained of temporary blindness. Later he became unresponsive and had non-purposeful movements and global aphasia. All neurological investigations were negative and he slowly recovered without specific therapy over the next several weeks.

A 36-year-old woman who required mechanical ventilation after an overdose of amitriptyline was given an infusion of midazolam (at first 15 mg/h and then after 5 days 20 mg/h). When the infusion was tailed off and withdrawn after 30 days she became agitated and unresponsive to verbal stimulation, with deviation of upward gaze and left-sided myoclonic movements. Midazolam was reintroduced, but when it was accidentally discontinued 10 h later she developed anxiety and tremor. At all times there was evidence of seizure activity in the electroencephalogram. The midazolam was replaced with clonazepam, after the withdrawal of which she recovered.

Interaction The addition of *clonidine* (5

µg/kg) to intravenous midazolam has been studied in eight healthy volunteers (90[C]). The dose of midazolam required to produce sedation was significantly reduced by clonidine from 0.078 to 0.043 mg/kg. Blood pressure, heart rate, respiration, and pulse oximetry were not altered. All the subjects suffered from amnesia after the procedure. The recovery time from midazolam was shortened by clonidine. The authors suggested that this effect might have been brought about by enhanced release of GABA by the α_2-adrenoceptor agonist.

Etomidate *(SED-13, 276; SEDA-17, 126; SEDA-18, 123; SEDA-19, 114)*

Etomidate is administered intravenously in propylene glycol as vehicle. A case of propylene glycol toxicity has been reported in a 9-year-old boy who was given intravenous etomidate for cerebral protection during angiography and embolization and resection of an arteriovenous malformation (91[c]). The first adverse effect was *hemoglobinuria* due to *acute hemolysis*; subsequently he developed a progressive *metabolic acidosis* and *hyperosmolality*, with a peak serum osmolality of 347 mOsm/kg. This was accounted for by the serum glycol concentration of 2.3 g/l, accounting for 30 mOsm/kg.

Ketamine *(SED-13, 277; SEDA-17, 126; SEDA-18, 124; SEDA-19, 114)*

The pharmacology and clinical uses of ketamine in anesthetic and subanesthetic doses have been reviewed (92[R]), (93[R]).

In one series of 32 patients given ketamine (50—100 mg) for a variety of procedures in patients suffering from burns, adverse effects were common (94[C]). One 50-year-old man without a history of hypertension developed transient *hypertension*. Excessive *salivation* occurred in two patients, *vomiting* in two, *hallucinations* in six (all of whom were women), and *nightmares* in two, in one case accompanied by *anxiety*.

Interactions In 40 patients who underwent elective superficial surgery with ketamine as anesthetic, *dexmedetomidine* (2.5 µg/kg) or *midazolam* (0.07 mg/kg) were given intramuscularly 45 min before anesthesia (95[C]). Although they had equal sedative and anxiolytic effects, dexmedetomidine was associated with significantly less preoperative cycle motor impairment and less anterograde amnesia than midazolam. Dexmedetomidine also reduced the need for intraoperative ketamine and was more effective than midazolam in reducing ketamine-induced adverse nervous system effects. It was also more effective than midazolam in attenuating the hemodynamic responses to intubation and the cardiostimulatory effect of ketamine. However it increased the incidence of intraoperative and postoperative bradycardia. The authors attributed these effects to the α_2-adrenoceptor agonist action of dexmedetomidine, comparable to that of clonidine.

In 28 patients who were anesthetized with intravenous ketamine, half were given a mixture of *physostigmine* with glycopyrronium and half saline 0.9% (96[C]). Although the mean duration of anesthesia and the total doses of all anesthetics used were the same in the two groups, those who were given physostigmine recovered significantly more quickly after anesthesia (16 vs. 34 min). The authors were unable to say whether physostigmine had reversed the ketamine component. Ketamine may have at least in part a central anticholinergic action, which would be reversed by physostigmine. However, physostigmine has also been shown to reverse the actions of benzodiazepines non-specifically (97[C]), and that might have contributed.

Propofol *(SED-13, 278; SEDA-17, 126; SEDA-18, 125; SEDA-19, 115)*

The pharmacology, clinical pharmacology, uses, and adverse effects of propofol have again been reviewed (98[R]), (99[R]).

Cardiovascular   Four deaths due to *cardiovascular collapse* during induction have been reported in patients aged 78—92 years given propofol 1.1—1.8 mg/kg (100[c]). The patients were of ASA classes 3 or 4. The total number of patients anesthetized with propofol during the years in which the deaths occurred (1990 and 1991) was not stated, and so an incidence figure cannot be calculated.

In another case a 9-year-old boy was given 50 mg of propofol followed by a continuous infusion of propofol, shortly after which his heart rate fell from 100/min to 55/min and *complete heart block* developed (101[c]). Three hours later he developed asystole and died. The myocardium showed some lymphocytic infiltration but no evidence of myocarditis or damage to the conducting system. The suggestion that this event, of which five similar cases have previously been reported (102[c]), was related to the administration of propofol has been challenged (103).

The use of propofol in rapid-sequence induction is sometimes associated with *hypotension*. In a study of 12 patients, ephedrine 70 mg/kg was given intravenously just before induction of anesthesia; 12 other patients were not given pretreatment and 12 patients were volume loaded with Ringer's lactate (12 ml/kg) over the 10—15 min before the administration of propofol (104[C]). In the control group the mean systolic blood pressure just after induction was 115 mmHg, increasing after intubation to 113 mmHg and falling 10 min later to 82 mmHg. In those given ephedrine the blood pressure reached a peak of 165 mmHg after intubation, and 10 min later fell to 108 mmHg. Ringer's lactate did not significantly increase the blood pressure during induction or after intubation, and although the blood pressure was slightly increased during the next few minutes, by 10 min it had reached the post-induction baseline. The heart rate fell slightly in the controls and with volume loading, but with ephedrine the post-intubation heart rate was significantly increased; by 10 min after intubation the heart rates were the same in all groups. The authors concluded that pre-induction volume loading with Ringer's lactate was preferable to ephedrine in providing hemodynamic stability during the administration of propofol.

Propofol with or without nitrous oxide has been used in 20 patients each, and compared with isoflurane plus nitrous oxide in another 20 (105[C]). The drugs were given in the interval between induction and skin incision. In those given propofol alone significantly more ephedrine was used to treat hypotension, while in those given propofol and nitrous oxide glycopyrrolate was given to significantly more patients to treat bradycardia. The results were the same whether or not the patients with cardiac disease were excluded from the analysis.

Respiratory   There was a *reduction in the acute ventilatory response to isocapnic hypoxia* by subhypnotic concentrations of propofol in 12 healthy adults; the effect was concentration-dependent (48[C]) (see above under halothane).

Pulmonary fat embolism following the use of propofol has been attributed to the milky emulsion in which the propofol was dissolved (106[c]).

A 66-year-old man with a history of chronic cor pulmonale became progressively breathless and developed ankle edema. When he required controlled mechanical ventilation propofol was used as an anesthetic, and a loading dose of 1 mg/kg was followed by a continuous infusion at a rate of 1 mg/kg/h, with supplementary bolus doses of 0.5 mg/kg before painful procedures and mobilization. The total amount of propofol given over 14 days was 27 g. Three weeks after admission he died from multi-organ failure. At post-mortem there was evidence of acute lung injury and obliteration of the capillaries and arteries by lipid-filled vacuoles. There was no evidence of amiodarone toxicity.

Nervous system   The most common adverse effect of propofol is *pain on injection*. It is particularly the case when propofol is injected into veins on the back of the hand, compared with the forearm or antecubital fossa. The incidence is 25—74% of cases and in one recent series of 18 patients, mean age 46 years, to whom propofol was given into a vein in the back of the hand over 30 s, pain was reported in 10 cases (107[C]).

The pain can be reduced by the use of a local anesthetic such as lidocaine, which should be given about half a minute before the propofol or mixed with the propofol immediately before administration. In a study of 183 patients aged 15—65 years who were given propofol into a vein on the back of the hand, lidocaine was added to the solution before injection in concentrations of 0.05, 0.10, 0.15, and 0.20% and compared with saline in the same concentrations (108[C]). Severe pain in those given lidocaine occurred in 11—30% compared with 35—67% in those given saline, and overall the incidence of pain was reduced significantly by lidocaine. However,

there was no benefit in using lidocaine in a concentration above 0.05%.

Among other methods that have been reported to reduce propofol-associated pain (opioids, metoclopramide, topical glyceryl trinitrate or EMLA), co-induction with thiopentone has also been reported to be effective. In 90 women aged 15—34 years given propofol into a vein in the back of the hand, co-induction with thiopentone reduced the severity of the pain but not its frequency (109[C]). However, lidocaine reduced both the severity (to a greater extent than thiopentone) and the frequency.

Lidocaine and prilocaine in 70 patients aged 19—65 years, given either separately or together, reduced the amount of pain produced by propofol (110[C]). In contrast, ketorolac given intramuscularly 45—60 min before propofol had no effect, suggesting that propofol-induced pain is not mediated by prostaglandins.

Propofol has occasionally been reported to cause *myoclonus* after induction of anesthesia, and another case has been reported in association with *meningism* (111[c]).

A 15-year-old boy who had been given propofol 175 mg developed generalized myoclonic jerking 5 min later. The contractions involved the muscles of the limbs and trunk and were worsened by attempts to rouse him. He had marked disconjugate gaze and pupillary dilatation. He regained consciousness 35 min later, but continued to suffer myoclonus. At that time he complained of severe occipital headache, and had marked neck stiffness. A CT scan of the brain and a lumbar puncture were normal, and the CSF did not yield any micro-organisms. The myoclonus and meningism gradually resolved over the next few days without any specific therapy.

The authors had no doubt that the myoclonus was associated with the propofol, but were unable to explain the accompanying meningism.

Liver   Propofol is not frankly hepatotoxic, but a subclinical *rise in the serum activity of glutathione transferase α* has been demonstrated in 10 healthy women who were given either propofol or its lipid vehicle (112[C]). The mechanism of this effect is not known.

Special senses   Increased intraocular pressure before eye surgery may lead to complications, and anesthetics should preferably not increase the intraocular pressure. In 20 patients, mean age 69 years, intravenous propofol 1 mg/kg caused a small fall in intraocular pressure for at least 7 min after induction (113[C]). This confirms the effects of higher doses in previous studies. The mechanism is thought to be relaxation of the extraocular muscles through central nervous system depression.

Of 100 patients who received intravenous propofol, 58 experienced a *sensation of taste* within the circulation time (114[C]). Of these, 16 disliked the taste, three liked it, and the rest were indifferent. Tasters were significantly younger than non-tasters and were more likely to be women. The nature of the taste differed from individual to individual.

Miscellaneous   Of 239 patients sedated with propofol before face-lift surgery (rhytidectomy or other procedures), 10 developed expanding *hematomas* compared with three out of 147 of those who were sedated with diazepam, meperidine, and methohexital (115[C]). However, although this was a two-fold difference, analysis of the data by chi-squared test shows that it was not significant.

Propofol (16 ml, total dose not stated) was inadvertently infused into an artery in a 52-year-old hypertensive man who was anesthetized for ventilation after tonic-clonic convulsions (116[C]). Although the infusion was continued for 6 h there was no apparent effect of this infusion.

Steroid anesthetics *(SED-13, 276; SEDA-16, 125)*

The steroid anesthetic mixture Althesin (alphadolone—alphaxalone) was withdrawn a few years ago because of adverse reactions to its vehicle, Cremophor EL (polyethoxylated castor oil). However, there has been renewed interest recently in steroid anesthetics, and their history, pharmacology, clinical pharmacology, and uses have been reviewed (117[R]). The first water-soluble steroid for anesthesia was minaxolone, which had a slower onset of action than Althesin and a more prolonged recovery time. However, it was withdrawn in 1981 because of toxicological findings in rats. More recently, eltanolone, a pregnanolone derivative, has been developed for formulation as an emulsion in Intralipid. Recovery time after eltanolone is probably slower than after Althesin. There have been few studies of the actions of these drugs in man. Newer agents are under development.

REFERENCES

1. Tobias JD. Sedation and analgesia for children in the pediatric intensive care unit. J Intensive Care Med 1995;10:294—314.
2. De Soto H. New pharmacologic agents and their use in pediatric anesthesia. Am J Anesthesiol 1995;22:305—11.
3. McDowall RH, Scher CS, Barst SM. Total intravenous anesthesia for children undergoing brief diagnostic or therapeutic procedures. J Clin Anesth 1995;7:273—80.
4. Pruitt JW, Goldwasser MS, Sabol SR, Prstojevich SJ, Campbell RL. Intramuscular ketamine, midazolam, and glycopyrrolate for pediatric sedation in the emergency department. J Oral Maxillofac Surg 1995;53:13—18.
5. Krane EJ, Haberkern CM, Jacobson LE. Postoperative apnea, bradycardia, and oxygen desaturation in formerly premature infants: prospective comparison of spinal and general anesthesia. Anesth Analg 1995;80:7—13.
6. Froehlich F, Schwizer W, Thorens J, Kohler M, Gonvers JJ, Fried M. Conscious sedation for gastroscopy: patient tolerance and cardiorespiratory parameters. Gastroenterology 1995;108:697—704.
7. Phillips MS. Drugs and sedation for colonoscopy. Prim Care Clin Off Pract 1995;22:433—43.
8. Fabbri LP, Batacchi S, Linden M, Bucciardini L, Fontanari P, Venneri F, Marsili M. Anaesthesia for urological endoscopic procedures in adult outpatients. Eur J Anaesthesiol 1995;12:319—24.
9. Smith I, White PF. New anaesthetics, analgesics and muscle relaxants for ambulatory surgery. Curr Opin Anaesthesiol 1995;8:298—303.
10. Mirski MA, Muffelman B, Ulatowski JA, Hanley DF. Sedation for the critically ill neurologic patient. Crit Care Med 1995;23:2038—53.
11. Kong KL. Inhalational anesthetics in the intensive care unit. Crit Care Clin 1995;11:887—902.
12. Mora CT, Dudek C, Torjman MC, White PF. The effects of anesthetic technique on the hemodynamic response and recovery profile in coron-

ary revascularization patients. Anesth Analg 1995;81:900—10.

13. Sigurdsson GH, Thomson D. Anaesthesia and microvascular surgery: clinical practice and research. Eur J Anaesthesiol 1995;12:101—22.

14. Bedforth NM, Lockey DJ. Raynaud's syndrome following intravenous induction of anaesthesia. Anaesthesia 1995;50:248—9.

15. Lee-Chiong TL Jr, McCloskey G. Preoperative and perioperative management of the asthmatic patient. Clin Pulm Med 1995;2:195—200.

16. Kremer M. What's new with reactive airways and anesthesia? CRNA Clin Forum Nurse Anesth 1995;6:118—24.

17. Pizov R, Brown RH, Weiss YS, Baranov D, Hennes H, Baker S, Hirshman CA. Wheezing during induction of general anesthesia in patients with and without asthma: a randomized, blinded trial. Anesthesiology 1995;82:1111—16.

18. Klafta JM, Zacny JP, Young CJ. Neurological and psychiatric adverse effects of anaesthetics. Epidemiology and treatment. Drug Saf 1995; 13:281—95.

19. Muravchick S, Smith DS. Parkinsonian symptoms during emergence from general anesthesia. Anesthesiology 1995;82:305—7.

20. Razis PA, Robinson DL, Alberry R. Clinical presentation of 'silent' meningiomas after general anaesthesia. Br J Anaesth 1995;74:335—7.

21. Holt C, Csete M, Martin P. Hepatotoxicity of anesthetics and other central nervous system drugs. Gastroenterol Clin North Am 1995; 24:853—74.

22. Kenna JG, Jones RM. The organ toxicity of inhaled anesthetics. Anesth Analg 1995;81:S51-S66.

23. Fletcher JE, Tripolitis L, Hubert M, Vita GM, Levitt RC, Rosenberg H. Genotype and phenotype relationships for mutations in the ryanodine receptor in patients referred for diagnosis of malignant hyperthermia. Br J Anaesth 1995;75:307 10.

24. McKinnon RP, Wildsmith JAW. Histaminoid reactions in anaesthesia. Br J Anaesth 1995; 74:217—28.

25. Jensen NF, Fiddler DS, Striepe V. Anesthetic considerations in porphyrias. Anesth Analg 1995; 80:591—9.

26. Hindle AT, Columb MO, Shah MV. Drug interactions and anaesthesia. Curr Anaesth Crit Care 1995;6:103—12.

27. McAuliffe MS, Hartshorn EA. Anesthetic drug interactions. CRNA Clin Forum Nurse Anesth 1995;6:103—7.

28. McAuliffe MS, Hartshorn EA. Anesthetic drug interactions. CRNA Clin Forum Nurse Anesth 1995;6:139—42.

29. Stoltzfus DP. Advantages and disadvantages of combining sedative agents. Crit Care Clin 1995;11:903—12.

30. Whitwam JG. Co-induction of anaesthesia: day-case surgery. Eur J Anaesthesiol 1995;12 Suppl:25—34.

31. Amrein R, Hetzel W, Allen SR. Co-induction of anaesthesia: the rationale. Eur J Anaesthesiol 1995;12 Suppl:5—11.

32. Aida S, Tomiyama T, Shimoji K. Total intravenous anesthesia combined with epidural eptazocine. J Anesth 1995;9:311—17.

33. Sarner JB, Levine M, Davis PJ, Lerman J, Cook DR, Motoyama EK. Clinical characteristics of sevoflurane in children: a comparison with halothane. Anesthesiology 1995;82:38—46.

34. Higuchi H, Sumikura H, Sumita S, Arimura S, Takamatsu F, Kanno M, Satoh T. Renal function in patients with high serum fluoride concentrations after prolonged sevoflurane anesthesia. Anesthesiology 1995;83:449—58.

35. Murray JM, Trinick TR. Plasma fluoride concentrations during and after prolonged anesthesia: a comparison of halothane and isoflurane. Anesth Analg 1992;74:236—40.

36. Mazze RI, Jamison R. Renal effects of sevoflurane. Anesthesiology 1995;83:443—5.

37. Kharasch ED, Hankins DC, Thummel KE. Human kidney methoxyflurane and sevoflurane metabolism: intrarenal fluoride production as a possible mechanism of methoxyflurane nephrotoxicity. Anesthesiology 1995;82:689—99.

38. Mazze RI, Woodruff RE, Heerdt ME. Isoniazid-induced enflurane defluorination in humans. Anesthesiology 1982;57:5—8.

39. Kharasch ED, Armstrong AS, Gunn K, Artru A, Cox K, Karol MD. Clinical sevoflurane metabolism and disposition: II. The role of cytochrome P450 2E1 in fluoride and hexafluoroisopropanol formation. Anesthesiology 1995;82:1379—88.

40. Kharasch ED, Thummel KE, Mautz D, Bosse S. Clinical enflurane metabolism by cytochrome P450 2E1. Clin Pharmacol Ther 1994;55:434—40.

41. Conzen PF, Nuscheler M, Melotte A, Verhaegen M, Leupolt T, Van Aken H, Peter K. Renal function and serum fluoride concentrations in patients with stable renal insufficiency after anesthesia with sevoflurane or enflurane. Anesth Analg 1995;81:569—75.

42. Blanco E, Vidal MI, Blanco J, Fagundo S, Campana O, Alvarez J. Comparison of maintenance and recovery characteristics of sevoflurane-nitrous oxide and enflurane-nitrous oxide anaesthesia. Eur J Anaesthesiol 1995;12:517—23.

43. Dale O. Drug interactions in anaesthesia: focus on desflurane and sevoflurane. Baillière's Clin Anaesthesiol 1995;9:105—17.

44. Bunting HE, Kelly MC, Milligan KR. Effect of nebulized lignocaine on airway irritation and haemodynamic changes during induction of anaesthesia with desflurane. Br J Anaesth 1995;75:631—3.

45. Schnorf H, Landis Th. Motor neuron disease after enflurane/propofol anaesthesia in patient with alcohol abuse. Lancet 1995;346:850—1.

46. Schneider M. Fatal hepatic necrosis following cardiac surgery and enflurane anaesthesia. Anaesth Intensive Care 1995;23:225—7.

47. Audenaert SM. Atropine, halothane, and pul-

seless electrical activity. Anesth Analg 1995; 80:634−5.

48. Nagyova B, Dorrington KL, Gill EW, Robbins PA. Comparison of the effects of sub-hypnotic concentrations of propofol and halothane on the acute ventilatory response to hypoxia. Br J Anaesth 1995;75:713−18.

49. Kenna JG, Neuberger JM. Immunopathogenesis and treatment of halothane hepatitis. Clin Immunother 1995;3:108−24.

50. Farnsworth ST, Johnson JO. Halothane hepatitis: updating an old nemesis. Am J Anesthesiol 1995;22:139−44.

51. Kitteringham NR, Kenna JG, Park BK. Detection of autoantibodies directed against human hepatic endoplasmic reticulum in sera from patients with halothane-associated hepatitis. Br J Clin Pharmacol 1995;40:379−86.

52. Clarke JB, Thomas C, Chen M, Hastings KL, Gandolfi AJ. Halogenated anesthetics form liver adducts and antigens that cross-react with halothane-induced antibodies. Int Arch Allergy Immunol 1995;108:24−32.

53. Hutter CDD. Hypothesis: halothane hepatitis—has thymol been overlooked? Anaesthesia 1995;50:1098.

54. Petersen WC, Crouch ER Jr. Anesthesia-induced rigidity, unrelated to succinylcholine, associated with Smith-Lemli-Opitz syndrome and malignant hyperthermia. Anesth Analg 1995;80:606−8.

55. Brown KA, Reich O, Bates JHT. Ventilatory depression by halothane in infants and children. Can J Anaesth 1995;42:588−96.

56. Mutch WAC, White IWC, Donen N, Thomson IR, Rosenbloom M, Cheang M, West M. Haemodynamic instability and myocardial ischaemia during carotid endarterectomy: a comparison of propofol and isoflurane. Can J Anaesth 1995;42:577−87.

57. Gunaratnam NT, Benson J, Gandolfi AJ, Chen M. Suspected isoflurane hepatitis in an obese patient with a history of halothane hepatitis. Anesthesiology 1995;83:1361−4.

58. Young CJ, Apfelbaum JL. Inhalational anesthetics: desflurane and sevoflurane. J Clin Anesth 1995;7:564−77.

59. Jones R. The new inhalational agents: desflurane and sevoflurane. What is the clinical role of 3rd generation fluorinated anaesthetics and how do they compare with 2nd generation agents? Acta Anaesthesiol Scand 1995;39 Suppl:130−1.

60. Korttila K. Desflurane and sevoflurane in adult day surgery. Acta Anaesthesiol Scand 1995;39 Suppl:128−9.

61. Brown Br Jr, Frink EJ Jr. Sevoflurane: an update. Baillière's Clin Anaesthesiol 1995;9:1−14.

62. Anonymous. Sevoflurane for general anesthesia. Med Lett Drugs Ther 1995;37:96−7.

63. Smith I, Nathanson MH, White PF. The role of sevoflurane in outpatient anesthesia. Anesth Analg 1995;81:S67−72.

64. Lerman J. Sevoflurane in pediatric anesthesia. Anesth Analg 1995;81:S4-S10.

65. Ebert TJ, Harkin CP, Muzi M. Cardiovascular responses to sevoflurane: a review. Anesth Analg 1995;81:S11−22.

66. Malan TP Jr, DiNardo JA, Isner RJ, Frink EJ Jr, Goldberg M, Fenster PE, Brown EA, Depa R, Hammond LC, Mata H. Cardiovascular effects of sevoflurane compared with those of isoflurane in volunteers. Anesthesiology 1995;83:918−28.

67. Green WB Jr. The ventilatory effects of sevoflurane. Anesth Analg 1995;81:S23−6.

68. Tsujimoto S, Kato H, Minamoto Y, Miki H, Kitamura R. Comparison of postoperative liver dysfunction following halothane and sevoflurane anesthesia in women undergoing mastectomy for cancer. J Anesth 1995;9:129−34.

69. Ducart A, Adnet P, Renaud B, Riou B, Krivosic-Horber R. Malignant hyperthermia during sevoflurane administration. Anesth Analg 1995; 80:609−11.

70. Watanabe S, Ashiura H, Inomata S, Taguchi M, Shibata K. Carpal spasm observed during and after sevoflurane anesthesia. J Anesth 1995; 9:75−7.

71. Yurino M, Kimura H. Comparison of induction time and characteristics between sevoflurane and sevoflurane/nitrous oxide. Acta Anaesthesiol Scand 1995;39:356−8.

72. Taneyama C, Fujita T, Kohno N, Otagiri T, Goto H. Continuous positive airway pressure oxygenation during one-lung ventilation with 50% nitrous oxide and isoflurane in oxygen. J Anesth 1995;9:285−8.

73. King M, Coulter C, Boyle RS, Michael Whitby R. Neurotoxicity from overuse nitrous oxide. Med J Aust 1995;163:50−1.

74. Seppelt IM. Neurotoxicity from overuse of nitrous oxide. Med J Aust 1995;163:280.

75. McMorrow AM, Adams RJ, Rubenstein MN. Combined system disease after nitrous oxide anesthesia: a case report. Neurology 1995;45:1224−5.

76. Ohryn M. Tympanic membrane rupture following general anesthesia with nitrous oxide. J Am Assoc Nurse Anesth 1995;63:42−4.

77. Lindekaer AL, Skielboe M, Guldager H, Jensen EW. The influence of nitrous oxide on propofol dosage and recovery after total intravenous anaesthesia for day-case surgery. Anaesthesia 1995;50:397−9.

78. Audenaert SM, Montgomery CL, Thompson DE, Sutherland J. A prospective study of rectal methohexital: efficacy and side effects in 648 cases. Anesth Analg 1995;81:957−61.

79. Rosenberg MK, Raymond C, Bridge PD. Comparison of midazolam/ketamine with methohexital for sedation during peribulbar block. Anesth Analg 1995;81:173−4.

80. Woodward C. Criteria for use of continuous midazolam infusion in adult inpatients. Am J Health Syst Pharm 1995;52:754−5.

81. Messina AG, Paranicas M, Yao FS, Illner P, Roman MJ, Saba PS, Devereux RB. The effect of midazolam on left ventricular pump performance

and contractility in anesthetized patients with coronary artery disease: effect of preoperative ejection fraction. Anesth Analg 1995;81:793—9.

82. Nishiyama T. The post-operative analgesic action of midazolam following epidural administration. Eur J Anaesthesiol 1995;12:369—74.

83. Ducharme MP, Munzenberger P. Severe withdrawal syndrome possibly associated with cessation of a midazolam and fentanyl infusion. Pharmacotherapy 1995;15:665—8.

84. Kurz A, Sessler DI, Annadata R, Dechert M, Christensen R, Bjorksten AR. Midazolam minimally impairs thermoregulatory control. Anesth Analg 1995;81:393—8.

85. Kirkby KC, Hennessy MJ, Montgomery IM, Daniels BA. Amnesia following gastroscopy with midazolam: a comparison in two age groups. J Psychopharmacol 1995;9:32—7.

86. Macak IA, Bayliff CD, Block GD. Surveillance of midazolam infusions in ICU. Can J Hosp Pharm 1995;48:218—23.

87. Masuda A, Haji A, Wakasugi M, Shibuya N, Shakunaga K, Ito Y. Differences in midazolam-induced breathing patterns in healthy volunteers. Acta Anaesthesiol Scand 1995;39:785—90.

88. Bauer TM, Ritz R, Haberthur C, Ha HR, Hunkeler W, Sleight AJ, Scollo-Lavizzari G, Haefeli WE. Prolonged sedation due to accumulation of conjugated metabolites of midazolam. Lancet 1995;346:145—7.

89. Hantson Ph, Clemessy JL, Baud FJ. Withdrawal syndrome following midazolam infusion. Intensive Care Med 1995;21:190—1.

90. Murai T, Kyoda N, Misaki T, Takada K, Sawada S, Machida T. Effects of clonidine on intravenous sedation with midazolam. Anesth Prog 1995;42:135—8.

91. Van de Wiele B, Rubinstein E, Peacock W, Martin N. Propylene glycol toxicity caused by prolonged infusion of etomidate. J Neurosurg Anesthesiol 1995;7:259—62.

92. Idvall J. Ketamine—a review of clinical applications. Anaesth Pharmacol Rev 1995;3:82—9.

93. Eide PK, Stubhaug A, Oye I. The NMDA-antagonist ketamine for prevention and treatment of acute and chronic post-operative pain. Baillière's Clin Anaesthesiol 1995;9:539—54.

94. Ashraf Ganatra M, Bhatti BT, Durrani KM. Ketamine in burn wound management. Specialist 1995;11:327—33.

95. Levanen J, Makela ML, Scheinin H. Dexmedetomidine premedication attenuates ketamine-induced cardiostimulatory effects and postanesthetic delirium. Anesthesiology 1995;82:1117—25.

96. Hamilton-Davies C, Bailie R, Restall J. Physostigmine in recovery from anaesthesia. Anaesthesia 1995;50:456—8.

97. Wiklund L. Reversal of sedation and respiratory depression after anaesthesia by the combined use of physostigmine and naloxone in neurosurgical patients. Acta Anaesthesiol Scand 1986;30:374—7.

98. Bryson HM, Fulton BR, Faulds D. Propofol: an update of its use in anaesthesia and conscious sedation. Drugs 1995;50:513—59.

99. Fulton B, Sorkin EM. Propofol. An overview of its pharmacology and a review of its clinical efficacy in intensive care sedation. Drugs 1995;50:636—57.

100. Warden JC, Pickford DR. Fatal cardiovascular collapse following propofol induction in high-risk patients and dilemmas in the selection of a short-acting induction agent. Anaesth Intensive Care 1995;23:485—7.

101. Bray RJ. Fatal myocardial failure associated with a propofol infusion in a child. Anaesthesia 1995;50:94.

102. Parke TJ, Stevens JE, Rice ASC, Greenaway CL, Bray RJ, Smith PJ, Waldmann CS, Verghese C. Metabolic acidosis and fatal myocardial failure after propofol infusions in children: five case reports. Br Med J 1992;305:613—16.

103. Hawkins WJ, Cohen T. Fatal myocardial failure associated with a propofol infusion in a child. Anaesthesia 1995;50:564.

104. El-Beheiry H, Kim J, Milne B, Seegobin R. Prophylaxis against the systemic hypotension induced by propofol during rapid-sequence intubation. Can J Anaesth 1995;42:875—8.

105. Jensen AG, Granfeldt H, Kalman SH, Nystrom PO, Eintrei C. A comparison of propofol and isoflurane anaesthesia: the need for ephedrine and glycopyrrolate. Eur J Anaesthesiol 1995;12:291—9.

106. El-Ebiary M, Torres A, Ramirez J, Xaubet A, Rodriguez Roisin R. Lipid deposition during the long-term infusion of propofol. Crit Care Med 1995;23:1928—30.

107. Sear JW, Jewkes C, Wanigasekera V. Hemodynamic effects during induction, laryngoscopy, and intubation with eltanolone (5β-pregnanolone) or propofol. A study in ASA I and II patients. J Clin Anesth 1995;7:126—31.

108. Tham CS, Khoo ST. Modulating effects of lignocaine on propofol. Anaesth Intensive Care 1995;23:154—7.

109. Haugen RD, Vaghadia H, Waters T, Merrick PM. Thiopentone pretreatment for propofol injection pain in ambulatory patients. Can J Anaesth 1995;42:1108—12.

110. Eriksson M. Prilocaine reduces injection pain caused by propofol. Acta Anaesthesiol Scand 1995;39:210—13.

111. Hughes NJ, Lyons JB. Prolonged myoclonus and meningism following propofol. Can J Anaesth 1995;42:744—6.

112. Tiainen P, Lindgren L, Rosenberg PH. Disturbance of hepatocellular integrity associated with propofol anaesthesia in surgical patients. Acta Anaesthesiol Scand 1995;39:840—4.

113. Neel S, Deitch R Jr, Moorthy SS, Dierdorf S, Yee R. Changes in intraocular pressure during low dose intravenous sedation with propofol before cataract surgery. Br J Ophthalmol 1995;79:1093—7.

114. Low SW. The taste of propofol. Anaesth Intensive Care 1995;23:753—4.

115. Kamer FM, Kushnick SD. The effect of propofol on hematoma formation in rhytidectomy. Arch Otolaryngol Head Neck Surg 1995;121:658—61.

116. Vohra SB. Inadvertent intra-arterial infusion of propofol. Br J Intensive Care 1995;5:306—7.

117. Sear JW. Steroidal anaesthetic agents. Anaesth Pharmacol Rev 1995;3:57—66.

Stephan A. Schug and David Sidebotham

11 Local anesthetics

℞ *Drug combinations in epidural or spinal local anesthesia*

The effects of combinations of local anesthetics with opioids and/or clonidine for epidural and spinal anesthesia have been described in further publications, mirroring a trend noted in previous editions of SEDA.

Anesthetic/opioid combinations (SEDA-18, 141) In 54 patients who underwent bowel surgery, analgesia was provided with epidural morphine, epidural bupivacaine, a combination of both, or intravenous patient-controlled analgesia (1[C]). Quality of pain relief, return of gut function, and discharge fitness were all greatest in the bupivacaine and morphine/bupivacaine combination groups. The incidence of orthostatic hypotension was greatest in the bupivacaine group (57%) and the incidence of pruritus greatest in the morphine group (58%). The rates of nausea and hypotension (systolic pressure below 90 mmHg) were similar between the groups.

A combination of either morphine 0.1 or 0.2 mg/ml plus bupivacaine 0.75% was infused at 0.8 ml/h epidurally in 60 patients after thoracotomy (2[C]). Quality of analgesia during exercise was better with the higher dose of morphine. The combined incidence of pruritus, nausea, and somnolence was low (below 20%) and not statistically different between groups. Interestingly, the incidence of nausea was significantly higher in the low-dose morphine group. Both groups had a significant rise in P_aCO_2 postoperatively compared with preoperative values.

*A combination of morphine 2 mg with bupivacaine 10 mg, administered as required via a surgeon-placed epidural catheter, has been assessed for analgesic efficacy following scoliosis surgery (3[C]). All 22 patients had ade-*quate pain relief. Reported adverse effects (nausea, vomiting, and pruritus) each occurred in under 20% of patients.

A combination of morphine 4 mg plus bupivacaine 20 mg epidurally, for postoperative analgesia, was given to patients after cesarean section under either epidural or general anesthesia (with an epidural cannula in situ but unused during the operation in the latter group) (4[C]). This analgesic combination was most effective after epidural anesthesia, but the incidence of pruritus was also highest in this group. The authors commented that the finding of a higher incidence of pruritus with epidural morphine after epidural anesthesia (as opposed to general anesthesia) has been reported previously.

Patient controlled epidural analgesia with bupivacaine 0.17% plus sufentanil 1 µg/ml has been assessed in 537 patients after major surgery (5[C]). The most frequent adverse effects were pruritus (21%), vomiting (14%), nausea (13%), and urinary retention after removal of catheter (8%). Five patients had an increased P_aCO_2 (indicating respiratory depression), requiring discontinuation of the epidural; four were older than 70 years. Disorientation, dizziness, and hallucinations each occurred in under 5% of patients. The authors concluded that the technique is safe and effective, although they suggested that sufentanil should be avoided in elderly people. They did not mention hypotension.

Bupivacaine and sufentanil have also been combined during intrathecal analgesia in labor (6[C]). A combination of bupivacaine 2.5 mg plus sufentanil 10 µg provided prolonged analgesia with no increase in clinically relevant adverse effects compared with either agent alone.

The effect of epidural lidocaine 200 mg, morphine 2 mg, or a combination of the two on ventilatory response has been assessed in 24 women preoperatively (7[C]). There were no changes in tidal volume at rest. The ventilatory response to progressive hypercapnia was re-

Side Effects of Drugs, Annual 20
J.K. Aronson, ed.

duced by morphine, increased by lidocaine, and unchanged by the combination. The authors concluded that the combination of epidural morphine with lidocaine does not increase the risk of respiratory depression associated with morphine.

The use of epidural bupivacaine 0.125% in combination with either fentanyl or sufentanil has been compared for analgesia in labor (8[C]). The quality of pain relief and the incidence of adverse effects were similar between groups, suggesting that either opioid is an appropriate choice. The overall incidence of pruritus was high (50%).

For continuous epidural analgesia after orthopedic surgery, fentanyl or meperidine, both in combination with bupivacaine 0.125%, have been compared (9[C]). Analgesia was better with bupivacaine/fentanyl, while adverse effects (urinary retention, 20 vs. 0%, and nausea and vomiting, 15 vs. 0%) were more common in the bupivacaine/meperidine group.

In a comparison in postoperative general surgical patients of equianalgesic doses of epidural fentanyl, bupivacaine, or a combination of the two, both the magnitude and frequency of hypotension were greatest in the bupivacaine only group (10[C]). Other adverse effects, such as pruritus and nausea, were similar across the groups.

These findings strongly suggest that the combination of a local anesthetic and an opioid provides enhanced analgesia, but similar or reduced adverse effects compared with either agent administered alone. This is in contrast to reports mentioned in previous Annuals, which suggested that the combination of agents may be associated with an increased risk of adverse effects for only an inconsistent benefit (SEDA-18, 141). It is becoming more and more obvious that a continuous infusion of a local anesthetic and a lipid-soluble opioid, such as fentanyl or sufentanil, both in low concentrations, is a good way of providing epidural analgesia with a minimum of adverse effects.

Anesthetic/opioid/clonidine combinations (SEDA-18, 142) There have been two recent studies on the addition of clonidine to epidural analgesia with bupivacaine plus an opioid.

After cesarean section 60 women received bupivacaine 25 mg with morphine 2 mg with or without the addition of clonidine (75 or 150 µg) (11[C]). Analgesia was greatly prolonged (more than a two-fold increase) and adverse effects were similar in both clonidine groups, although there was a tendency for increased pruritus and drowsiness in the clonidine-treated patients.

Fentanyl and/or clonidine was added to bupivacaine for 48 women in labor (12[C]). The duration of bupivacaine analgesia was prolonged by the addition of either agent, although the effect was greatest when a combination of all three agents was used. Sedation was also greatest when all three drugs were used (all the patients were drowsy or asleep at 90—180 min) and two patients had hypotension. Similarly, when clonidine was added to bupivacaine spinal anesthesia, not only was the duration of anesthesia prolonged, but the degree of hypotension and sedation increased (13[C]).

These findings of prolonged analgesia at the cost of increased sedation and hypotension are similar to those of previous reports, suggesting that combinations that include clonidine are of only limited benefit and should be used with care.

Anesthetic/corticosteroid combinations The use of epidural corticosteroids plus local anesthetics in the management of back pain has been the subject of a recent review (14[r]). The authors noted that catastrophic neurological complications, such as epidural hematoma, are extremely rare, while minor complications, such as dural puncture, vasovagal episodes, and steroid-induced adverse effects, are not uncommon. No mention was made of the current controversy surrounding possible arachnoiditis induced by this technique; this suggests again that this risk is negligible.

The efficacy of lidocaine 200 mg plus methylprednisolone 80 mg epidurally (via caudal injection), has been investigated in 85 patients with lumbosciatic pain (15[C]). The technique was highly successful: 63% of patients with symptoms of less than 3 months duration had a good or excellent result at 1 year follow-up; adverse effects were minimal: two patients experienced hypotension and three had transient paresthesia during insertion.

Anesthetic/butyrophenone combinations The addition of droperidol to an epidural mixture *of bupivacaine plus fentanyl significantly reduced the incidence of nausea and vomiting in 184 patients with epidural catheters for postlaminectomy syndrome (16[C]).*

Nervous system   The incidence of local anesthetic-induced systemic toxicity has been assessed in 25—697 patients undergoing brachial plexus, epidural, or caudal anesthesia; there were 26 seizures (17[C]). The incidence of *seizures* was significantly higher with caudal than with brachial than with epidural administration (6.9 vs. 2.0 vs. 0.1 per 1000 procedures). Within the types of brachial plexus anesthesia, seizures occurred more often with the supraclavicular and interscalene approaches than with the axillary approach (7.9 and 7.6 per 1000 vs. 1.2 per 1000 procedures). In most of the patients who had seizures (15/26) bupivacaine had been used. The combination of bupivacaine with 2-chloroprocaine resulted in an even higher rate of seizures, thereby contradicting data from previous animal experiments. Importantly, no adverse events in the cardiovascular, pulmonary, or nervous systems were linked to any of the seizures.

Immunological and hypersensitivity reactions *(SED-13, 286; SEDA-18, 135)* Long-term evaluation of 19 patients with a previous history of adverse reactions to local anesthetics has shown that no patient experienced a second reaction after re-exposure (18[C]). The authors concluded that many so-called allergic reactions to local anesthetics are in fact misdiagnoses, confirming previous experience.

Stability of solutions of local anesthetics   The stability and pH at which precipitation of alkalinized solutions of lidocaine and bupivacaine occurs has been reported (19[cr]). The authors showed that the likelihood of precipitation depends on the initial pH (which in turn depends on the particular drug, its concentration, and any additives, for example epinephrine), the amount of bicarbonate added, and the freshness of the solution. They showed that microprecipitation may not be seen by the user, particularly if the solution is drawn into a plastic syringe. Finally, they described the potential complications of using precipi-

tated solutions of local anesthetics, including vascular embolization, granuloma formation, and skin hyperpigmentation. They concluded that alkalinized solutions should be used shortly after preparation and provided a nomogram showing the amount of bicarbonate required to cause precipitation in various solutions of lidocaine and bupivacaine.

Addition of epinephrine to solutions of local anesthetics   Epinephrine is commonly added to local anesthetic solutions in an attempt to reduce the risk of systemic toxicity and prolong their clinical effect. The local and systemic effects of various concentrations of epinephrine added to 1% lidocaine has been studied in 23 patients (20[c]). There were no differences in cutaneous blood flow or systemic hemodynamics using epinephrine concentrations varying from 1:50 000 to 1:400 000. Given that effective vasoconstriction was produced by the weakest concentration of epinephrine (compared with the plain solution), it seems a logical choice for infiltration anesthesia, particularly when large doses of local anesthetic are used.

EFFECTS RELATED TO DIFFERENT MODES OF USE

Brachial plexus anesthesia *(SED-13, 287; SEDA-17, 139; SEDA-18, 142; SEDA-19, 127)*

Forty patients undergoing shoulder surgery under interscalene block received bupivacaine 200 mg with or without morphine 5 mg (21[C]). The quality of analgesia was similar in both groups. There were two cases of *Horner's syndrome* and three of temporary *phrenic nerve blockade* (one requiring supplemental oxygen). Half of those who received morphine had *nausea* postoperatively, compared with 25% in the plain morphine group. Three patients in the morphine-free group complained of *pruritus*.

A combination of mepivacaine plus butorphanol infused into the axillary sheath has been compared with either agent alone after upper limb surgery (22[C]). The quality of analgesia was greatest in the combination group.

The use of butorphanol alone resulted in the worst analgesia and the highest incidence of *nausea*.

Caudal anesthesia

The safety of caudal anesthesia in 165 children with bupivacaine 4 mg/kg plus fentanyl 1 µg/kg has been assessed (23[C]). Four patients experienced vomiting and two required postoperative ventilation; in both cases this was felt to be related to their underlying pathology rather than to the regional technique. The authors concluded that the technique is safe and effective. However, it is important to point out that the dose of bupivacaine used was higher than the manufacturers recommend (2 mg/kg) and higher than most pediatric anesthetists would routinely use (2.5—3 mg/kg). The authors did not report on the occurrence of bradycardia, hypotension, or postoperative irritability, all of which could be expected to occur at high doses of bupivacaine.

The duration of pain relief with caudal bupivacaine 2.5 mg/kg, combined with either epinephrine 5 µg/ml, clonidine 2 µg/kg, or ketamine 0.5 mg/kg, has been compared in 60 boys undergoing orchidopexy (24[C]). The duration of analgesia was greatly prolonged in the ketamine group and moderately so in the clonidine group. Adverse effects, such as *delayed awakening*, *increased sedation scores*, *urinary retention*, and *leg weakness* were uncommon and similar between the groups.

Caudal bupivacaine 1.8 mg/kg plus buprenorphine 7.2 µg/kg has been compared with bupivacaine alone for postoperative analgesia in 30 adults after hip and knee arthroplasty (25[C]). The duration of analgesia was longest in the combination group. The incidence of *vomiting* was highest in the bupivacaine-only group (10/15 vs. 6/15). One patient in the combination group suffered *bradypnea* (respiratory rate 6/min) but had normal blood gases. The increased incidence of nausea and vomiting in the opioid-free group in this study (or the low-dose opioid group in a previously mentioned study (2[C])) could have reflected the increased pain experienced by those patients.

Dental anesthesia *(SEDA-13, 288; SEDA-17, 140; SEDA-19, 127)*

In a 21-year retrospective study of reports of the use of local anesthetics in dentistry, 143 reports of *paresthesia* (mainly in the tongue and lips), not associated with the surgery performed, were identified; the predicted incidence was one in 785 000 (26[C]). The paresthesia was painful in 22% of cases. In all cases anesthesia involved the mandibular arch; prilocaine and articaine resulted in a greater frequency of paresthesia than other agents. The authors suggested that this finding implies an increased potential for mild neurotoxicity of some local anesthetic formulations.

In a similar case review, 12 patients with *altered sensation* in the distribution of the inferior alveolar or lingual nerves after local anesthesia for restorative dental treatment were identified (27[C]). This implies that the incidence of this complication is probably underestimated.

Epidural and spinal anesthesia
(SED-13, 290; SEDA-17, 136, 138; SEDA-18, 143; SEDA-19, 127)

Epidural

Epidural bupivacaine and ropivacaine have been compared in three studies.

Ropivacaine 150 mg and bupivacaine 150 mg were compared in 60 women undergoing cesarean section (28[C]). Maternal *hypotension* was common (over 90% of patients had a fall in blood pressure to below 90 mmHg or by more than 30% of baseline), but equal in both groups and easily treated with ephedrine. The onset and duration of motor block were shorter in the ropivacaine group. Pharmacokinetic differences were slight and not of clinical importance; peak blood concentrations were well below the toxic range.

In a comparison of bolus doses of ropivacaine 50 mg or bupivacaine 50 mg followed by 25 mg top-ups for analgesia during labor, there were no clinically important differences between the two drugs (29[C]). In particular, the degree of motor block was similar between the two groups.

A radiologically confirmed case of unintentional subdural block during attempted epidural catheter insertion has been described in a middle-aged man. After injection of local anesthetic an intense, prolonged, and extensive block to the of level C2 rapidly developed and the resulting paralysis made intubation and ventilation necessary (30[c]).

An unexplained case of severe and *persistent back pain* and posterior thigh *muscle spasm* 10 min after the epidural injection of 296 mg of mepivacaine (20 ml of a 1.48% alkalinized solution with epinephrine) has been reported in a 75-year-old man (31[c]). Epidural hematoma and unintentional injection of an irritant were excluded; initially the symptoms required general anesthesia, but they resolved completely within 1 h.

Unexplained prolonged *unilateral leg paresis* accompanied by *neurogenic pain* occurred in a man who was receiving an epidural infusion on the fourth postoperative day (32[c]). The authors went to considerable lengths to explain the findings, but were unable to clarify the cause.

Accidental subdural injection occurred while epidural injection was being attempted in a woman, resulting in patchy unilateral block of greater magnitude than expected (33[c]). The necessity for early recognition of this complication, especially in a day-stay setting, was emphasized to avoid serious complications.

Cardiovascular Bupivacaine thoracic epidural anesthesia has been examined in 30 patients undergoing coronary artery bypass grafting and found not to alter coronary hemodynamics or myocardial metabolism (34[c]). However the issue of using an epidural in patients who are about to undergo total heparinization remains unresolved. To minimize the risk of an epidural hematoma the authors positioned the epidural catheter at least 16 h before heparinization. Japanese authors, however, have described a case of coronary artery spasm after lumbar epidural anesthesia, with chest discomfort and ST segment elevation on the cardiogram, probably caused by sympathetic denervation of the heart (35[c]).

Spinal

Discussion on the potential neurotoxicity of hyperbaric 5% lidocaine for spinal anesthesia continues, and another case report of *leg pain* after spinal anesthesia with lidocaine has been published (36[c]). In a randomized comparison of 5% lidocaine in 7.5% dextrose (hyperbaric) with 5% lidocaine in 2.7% dextrose (isobaric) plus 0.5% bupivacaine in 8.25% dextrose (hyperbaric) for spinal anesthesia, transient *radicular irritation* was observed only in the two lidocaine groups, but not in the bupivacaine group (37[C]). These findings contradict the assumption that neurotoxicity is a result of the high osmolarity of the commonly used hyperbaric lidocaine formulation, but concur with recent literature in which the neurotoxic potential of high concentrations of lidocaine itself has been described. This impression has been confirmed in a letter to the editor of the British Journal of Anaesthesia (38[r]) and by a further study, in which hyperbaric lidocaine 5% was compared with hyperbaric bupivacaine 0.5% for spinal anesthesia in 270 patients (39[C]). A blinded observer identified transient neurological symptoms in 37% of the lidocaine group, but in only one patient of the bupivacaine group.

Nevertheless, others have reported a case of neurogenic pain in the back and legs after uncomplicated bupivacaine and morphine spinal anesthesia, with complete resolution of symptoms during 3 months of amitriptyline therapy (40[c]). This suggests other potential mechanisms of neurotoxicity after spinal anesthesia.

The effectiveness of 1—2.5-ml boluses of 0.25% bupivacaine administered via a 28-gauge continuous spinal catheter has been assessed in 100 patients after hip and knee surgery (41[C]). Analgesia was satisfactory in the majority of patients, although technical problems (usually difficulty in aspirating through the catheter) occurred in 12 patients. *Backache* occurred in 12 patients, and most experienced marked *leg weakness*. The authors noted that serious neurological problems (for example, cauda equina syndrome) after continuous spinal anesthesia with microcatheters has led to the withdrawal of these products from the US market. They argued, however, that such problems have not been reported with the use of low concentrations of isobaric local anesthetics, such as in their study. This issue aside, the value of this technique is severely limited by the marked motor blockade it produces.

Two techniques for the prevention of hypotension in 30 elderly patients receiving bupivacaine spinal anesthesia have been compared (42[C]). A bolus of ephedrine 0.2 mg/kg followed by a colloid infusion (Haemaccel 8 ml/kg) was superior to ephedrine bolus and infusion (0.5 mg/kg/h).

Intra-articular anesthesia *(SED-13, 288)*

The analgesic properties of intra-articular morphine 1 mg, bupivacaine 50 mg, or a combination of the two have been evaluated in 40 patients after knee arthroscopy (43[C]). The combination group had satisfactory analgesia throughout the study period, significantly better than that produced with either agent alone. No adverse effects were reported.

An injection of intra-articular lidocaine 200 mg has been compared with systemic meperidine/diazepam for the reduction of acute secondary shoulder dislocations (44[C]). Both techniques were successful in the majority of patients. No local or systemic complications were reported in the lidocaine group. In contrast, 3/26 patients in the meperidine/diazepam group suffered *respiratory depression*. The authors concluded that intra-articular lidocaine is safe and effective.

Interpleural and paravertebral analgesia *(SED-13, 288, 289; SEDA-17, 139)*

After thoracotomy, 53 patients received postoperative analgesia with either interpleural or paravertebral bupivacaine, 150 mg intraoperatively, followed by an infusion of 0.5 mg/kg/h for 2 days (45[C]). Pain scores and the use of rescue analgesia were similar in both groups, but postoperative spirometry, respiratory morbidity, and hospital stay were all improved in the paravertebral group. Five patients in the interpleural group became *confused* postoperatively; the authors sug-

gested that this may have been due to bupivacaine toxicity, which is quite possible with this unusually high infusion rate.

The effect of epinephrine (1:200 000) on the pharmacokinetics of lidocaine administered into the interpleural space in 10 patients with pancreatic cancer has been studied (46[C]). Lidocaine uptake into and elimination from plasma and CSF were delayed in the epinephrine group. These findings were used to develop a model in which plasma and CSF concentrations on a multiple lidocaine dose regimen (200 mg 8-hourly) could be predicted. The results showed that the addition of epinephrine would result in the accumulation of lidocaine in the CSF, with a subsequent risk of toxicity.

These two studies carry important messages: first that local anesthetics administered via the interpleural route produce relatively high serum drug concentrations, with an attendant risk of toxicity, and secondly (and rather surprisingly) that the addition of epinephrine may actually increase this risk.

Ocular anesthesia *(SED-13, 1420; SEDA-17, 139, 542; SEDA-18, 144; SEDA-19, 129)*

Diplopia after cataract surgery under local anesthesia was diagnosed in four patients without pre-existing strabismus (47[C]). While injury to the vertical rectus muscle is commonly assumed to be the cause of this complication, careful investigations in these patients showed contracture (three patients) and paresis (one patient) of the inferior oblique muscle to be the cause. Contracture could result from local anesthetic myotoxicity and paresis from mechanical trauma.

Retrobulbar block with bupivacaine plus lidocaine in a 78-year-old woman, with previous surgical removal of the bone of the orbital roof, resulted in *cardiopulmonary arrest* requiring resuscitation and ventilation for 18 h with no sequelae (48[C]). The authors proposed several mechanisms for the transgression of local anesthetics into the CNS and recommended caution with this technique in patients with orbital roof defects.

A combined topical and subconjunctival

technique using 4% lidocaine plus 0.75% bupivacaine for cataract extraction has been described in a series of 73 patients (49[C]). The majority reported no pain during the operation and no patient required peribulbar or retrobulbar supplementation. Postoperatively, 21 patients complained of *pain*, five of *headache*, and one of *vomiting*. The author commented that despite a lack of akinesia the technique seems safe and effective.

The warming of topical anesthetic eye drops (amethocaine 1%, oxybuprocaine 0.4%, or lidocaine 4%) from room temperature to 42°C did not reduce the discomfort experienced in 60 patients (50[C]).

Nasal anesthesia

The use of intranasal lidocaine 4% to relieve migraine (51[c]) or cluster headache (52[c]) has been reported; migraine attacks were aborted in about half of 23 patients. Adverse effects were minor: a *bitter taste* was reported by all patients and 30% experienced minor *nasal burning* and *oropharyngeal numbness*. For cluster headache, half of 30 patients gained some benefit, five did not like the taste, and two each felt *dizzy* and mildly *anxious*.

Regional anesthesia

A *tension pneumothorax* has been described as a rare and unusual complication of breast infiltration with lidocaine plus epinephrine before breast augmentation (53[c]). The iatrogenic pneumothorax resulted in hemodynamic instability and was successfully treated by drainage.

Topical anesthesia *(SEDA-17, 140; SEDA-18, 145; SEDA-19, 131)*

Topical anesthesia of the airway is commonly used to facilitate endoscopy. A comparative study in nine patients has shown that 100 mg of 5% lidocaine liquid and 100 mg of 2% lidocaine paste both resulted in a similar significant increase in airway flow resistance

lasting for over 10 min (54[C]). As the two patients with the worst responses had inspiratory laryngeal collapse during endoscopy, the authors assumed that laryngeal dysfunction had been involved; this might have explained poor respiratory tolerance in some patients during this diagnostic procedure.

EMLA cream (lidocaine 2.5% plus prilocaine 2.5%) has been regarded by some authors as being contraindicated in neonates, because of the potential development of significant *methemoglobinemia*. In a French study, 116 neonates in an intensive care unit were pretreated with EMLA cream before skin puncture (55[C]). Methemoglobin concentrations measured 18—24 h and 2—3 days after application of EMLA never exceeded 5% and were not related to gestational age or the duration of application. The authors concluded that EMLA cream is safe in neonates, including preterm babies, when applied in a small amount once a day.

Minor adverse effects (*itch and burning*) of EMLA cream (SEDA-19, 131) continue to be reported (56[C]).

Recently 4% amethocaine gel has been introduced as a topical anesthetic. Compared with placebo, amethocaine was effective in reducing the pain of venous cannulation (57[C]). Two out of 21 patients receiving amethocaine reported *itch* and one had *erythema*.

Compared with EMLA cream, 4% amethocaine gel was more effective in reducing the pain of venous cannulation in children (58[C]). Thirty-seven percent of those receiving amethocaine had localized *erythema*, compared with 4% in the EMLA group. The authors note that erythema, as a consequence of vasodilatation, may actually be an advantage of amethocaine over EMLA in allowing easier cannula placement. The concern that the topical placement of an ester local anesthetic, such as amethocaine, may result in dermatitis was not realised.

Wound anesthesia *(SEDA-19, 131)*

Intermittent instillation of 20 ml of 0.25% bupivacaine has been compared with placebo as an adjuvant to patient-controlled analgesia with morphine in the management of pain after cesarean section (59[C]). Pain scores, morphine consumption, nausea, and sedation were all less in the bupivacaine-treated patients.

INDIVIDUAL COMPOUNDS

Bupivacaine and etidocaine *(SED-13, 293; SEDA-17, 141; SEDA-18, 145; SEDA-19, 131)*

Toxic reactions to bupivacaine and etidocaine have recently been reviewed from a dental perspective (60[R]). The authors noted the increased risk of life-threatening cardiac events with either agent compared with lidocaine. For bupivacaine they recommended a safe upper dose of 1.25 mg/kg in dental practice. This is in contrast to the international data sheet for bupivacaine, which suggests an upper dose limit of 2 mg/kg and makes no distinction for dental infiltration.

Cocaine *(SED-13, 294; SEDA-17, 142; SEDA-19, 132)*

One possible factor that contributes to cocaine toxicity during anesthetic use is the wide variation in the rate and amount of cocaine absorbed systemically. The kinetics of cocaine have been measured in 12 patients of ASA grade 1 undergoing major intranasal surgery with topical anesthesia with cocaine HCl (33% solution) (61[C]). The mean dose of cocaine was 5.85 mg/kg. The mean (SD) C_{max} was 859 (503) ng/ml at a t_{max} of 47 (17) min. The mean elimination half-life was 87 (19) min. The total clearance and the volume of distribution were respectively 4521 (1858) ml/min and 568 (273) l. There was no clinical evidence of toxicity. This variability in pharmacokinetics may be related to the type and concentration of vasoconstrictor used with cocaine, reducing its systemic absorption, and explaining the differences in the kinetics of cocaine in these patients compared with cocaine addicts (62[C]).

Cardiovascular Although cocaine, along with other vasoconstrictors, has attractive features as a topical anesthetic, it can occasionally produce catastrophic adverse effects, such as myocardial infarction, stroke, and death, well-documented toxic effects of illicit use of cocaine.

Cardiac dysrhythmias have been described in three patients who were given cocaine and epinephrine for nasal surgery (63[Cr]). Two children went into ventricular fibrillation and were successfully resuscitated; an adult developed tachycardia, extra beats, cardiographic ST segment depression, and hypertension. The authors suggested that these events were compounded by the combined use of cocaine and epinephrine and advised against it. However, this suggestion was subsequently disputed in correspondence, and it was suggested that excessive doses had been used in the reported cases (64)−(67). The latter opinion has been supported by the results of another study, in which tachycardia was identified as the only adverse effect of the use of 200 mg of cocaine with 1 mg of epinephrine in 178 patients undergoing sinus surgery (68[C]). In various previous reports of the toxic cardiovascular effects of cocaine used as a topical anesthetic (69[c])−(72[c]), cocaine was used in concentrations of 1−25% in a volume of 4 ml.

In another case, myocardial infarction was attributed to cocaine (73[cr]).

A 23-year-old woman without a history of coronary artery disease had an acute non-Q-wave myocardial infarction and stunned myocardium after receiving topical phenylephrine and cocaine anesthesia for elective nasal septoplasty. Before surgery her nose was prepared with 4% cocaine HCl solution. Surgery was successful and uneventful. For further decongestion and control of bleeding phenylephrine packing (0.25% solution) was applied before extubation; 15 min later she had an acute increase in blood pressure and heart rate, and subsequently a cardiac arrest with ventricular tachycardia and ventricular fibrillation. She was treated with dopamine, dobutamine, and lidocaine; her hemodynamic status improved during the next 48 h and she recovered. Subsequent cardiac catheterization showed normal coronary arteries.

Lidocaine *(SEDA-17, 142; SEDA-18, 146; SEDA-19, 132)*

The alkalinization of local anesthetic solutions has been shown in some studies to provide faster-onset, prolonged anesthesia, and reduced pain of injection. Lidocaine 2%, alkalinized with 1 mmol of sodium bicarbonate per 10 ml of lidocaine, prepared either fresh or 1 h before use, has been compared with a non-alkalinized solution in 15 women undergoing cesarean section (74[C]). There were no differences in the onset or quality of anesthesia or the incidence of adverse effects between the three groups. The pH of the older alkalinized solution was higher than that of the fresh solution and thus potentially closer to the precipitation threshold (see above).

Prilocaine *(SED-13, 294; SEDA-18, 146)*

Prilocaine is widely used in a commercial formulation containing methylparaben as a preservative. In a comparison of 0.5% prilocaine, with and without methylparaben, for intravenous regional anesthesia, there was an increased incidence of *erythematous skin reactions* in the methylparaben group (4 vs. 17%) (75[C]). These reactions were always restricted to the exposed arm and lasted under 1 h. Patients never had positive intradermal tests, suggesting a non-IgE-mediated anaphylactoid reaction to the preservative.

Methemoglobinemia is a dose-related adverse effect of prilocaine and results in erroneous measurement of oxygen saturation by pulse oximetry. The magnitude of the error has been suggested as a way of determining methemoglobin concentration. The value of this technique has been assessed in 171 patients receiving prilocaine axillary plexus blockade for hand surgery (76[C]). For each of the three oximeter models tested there was a relation between the methemoglobin concentration and the magnitude of the error in measuring oxygen saturation, but the authors

were unable to demonstrate a consistent correlation across models. this was most likely because different manufacturers use different algorithms. The authors cautioned against the use of pulse oximetry to determine methemoglobin concentrations, since a distinction between methemoglobinemia and hypoxia is not possible without recourse to blood gas analysis.

Methemoglobinemia (peak methemoglobin concentration 17%) has been described in a full-term neonate after the use of prilocaine for circumcision (77[C]). The baby developed tachypnea and cyanosis unresponsive to oxygen; the arterial oxygen saturation was 80%. The situation improved without treatment or sequelae.

A similar case has been reported in a 15-year-old boy after dental treatment with prilocaine plus bupivacaine anesthesia (78[c]). The patient presented 4 h later with an oxygen saturation of 75% and a methemoglobin concentration of 15%, which resolved spontaneously. The incident was thought to be more the consequence of a relative overdose of prilocaine (8.6 mg/kg) in a patient with a borderline low hemoglobin concentration, rather than linked to the patient's previous renal transplant.

Ropivacaine *(SED-13, 295; SEDA-18, 147)*

High concentrations of ropivacaine can lead to an increased incidence of *hypotension*. In 126 patients undergoing hip replacement surgery, 70% of those receiving 0.75% ropivacaine and 100% of those receiving 1.0% ropivacaine suffered hypotension; about 50% also experienced bradycardia (79[C]). Great caution should therefore be exercised when using concentrations of ropivacaine over 0.5%.

REFERENCES

1. Liu SS, Carpenter RL, Mackey DC, Thirlby RC, Rupp SM, Shine TSJ, Feinglass NG, Metzger PP, Fulmer JT, Smith SL. Effects of perioperative technique on rate of recovery after colon surgery. Anesthesiology 1995;83:757—65.

2. Geurts AM, Jessen HJG, Megens JHAM, Hasenbos MAWM, Gielen MJM. Continuous high thoracic epidural administration of morphine with bupivacaine after thoracotomy. Reg Anesth 1995;20:27—32.

3. Adu-Gyamfi Y. Epidural morphine plus bupivacaine for relief of post-operative pain following Harrington rod insertion for correction of idiopathic scoliosis. J Int Med Res 1995;23:211—17.

4. Asantila R, Eklund P, Latvala H, Rosenberg PH. Epidural analgesia with 4 mg of morphine

after caesarean section: modulating effect of epidural block compared to general anaesthesia. Int J Obst Anesth 1995;4:89—92.

5. Deroover I, Wiebalck A, Van Aken H. Efficiency and safety of patients controlled epidural analgesia with a mixture of bupivacaine 0.17% and sufentanil 1 μg/ml. Acta Anaesthesiol Belg 1995;46:102.

6. Cambell DC, Camann WR, Datta S. The addition of bupivacaine to intrathecal sufentanil for labor analgesia. Anesth Analg 1995;81:305—9.

7. Saito Y, Sakura S, Kaneko M, Kosaka Y. Interaction of extradural morphine and lignocaine on ventilatory response. Br J Anaesth 1995; 75:394—8.

8. Kudialis SJ, Wirth RK. Comparison of sufentanil verses fentanyl with 0.125% bupivacaine for continuous labor epidural anesthesia. CRNA 1995;16:26—30.

9. Uckunkaya N, Yilmazlar A, Sahin S. Epidural continuous infusion of fentanyl-bupivacaine and meperidine, bupivacaine for postoperative pain control. Turk J Med Sci 1995;23:121—4.

10. Torda TA, Hann P, Mills G, De Leon G, Penman D. Comparison of extradural fentanyl, bupivacaine and two fentanyl-bupivacaine mixtures for pain after abdominal surgery. Br J Anaesth 1995;74:35—40.

11. Capogna G, Danilo C, Zangrillo A, Costantino P, Foresta S. Addition of clonidine to epidural morphine enhances postoperative analgesia after cesarean delivery. Reg Anesth 1995;20:57—61.

12. Celleno D, Capogna G, Costantino P, Zangrillo A. Comparison of fentanyl with clonidine as adjuvants for epidural analgesia with 0.125% bupivacaine in the first stage of labor. Int J Obstet Anesth 1995;4:26—9.

13. Liu S, Chiu AA, Neal JM, Carpenter RL, Bainton BG, Gerancher JC. Oral clonidine prolongs lidocaine spinal anesthesia in human volunteers. Anesthesiology 1995;82:1353—9.

14. Woodward JL, Weinstein SM. Epidural injections for the diagnosis and management of axial and radicular pain syndromes. Phys Med Rehabil Clin North Am 1995;6:691—713.

15. Mam MK. Results of epidural injection of local anaesthetic and corticosteroid in patients with lumbosciatic pain. J Indian Med Assoc 1995;93:17—18.

16. Aldrete JA. Reduction of nausea and vomiting from epidural opioids by adding droperidol to the infusate in home-bound patients. J Pain Symptom Manage 1995;10:544—7.

17. Brown DL, Ransom DM, Hall JA, Leicht CH, Schroeder DR, Offord KP. Regional anesthesia and local anesthetic-induced systemic toxicity: seizure frequency and accompanying cardiovascular changes. Anesth Analg 1995;81:321—8.

18. Wasserfallen JB. Long-term evaluation of usefulness of skin and incremental challange tests in patients with history of adverse reactions to local anesthetics. Allergy 1995;50:162—5.

19. Hinshaw KD, Fiscella R, Sugar J. Preparation of pH-adjusted local anesthetics. Ophthalmic Surg 1995;26:194—9.

20. O'Malley TP, Postma GN, Holten M, Girod DA. Effect of local epinephrine on cutaneous bloodflow in the human neck. Laryngoscope 1995;105:140—3.

21. Flory N, Van Gessel E, Donald F, Hoffmeyer P, Gamulin Z. Does the addition of morphine to brachial plexis block improve analgesia after shoulder surgery? Br J Anaesth 1995;75:23—6.

22. Wajima Z, Shitara T, Nakajima Y, Kobayashi N, Kadotani H, Adachi H, Ishikawa G, Kaneko K, Inoue T, Ogawa R. Comparison of continuous brachial plexus infusion of butorphanol, mepivacaine and mepivacaine-butorphanol mixtures for postoperative analgesia. Br J Anaesth 1995; 75:548—51.

23. Melman E, Berrocal M. Analgesia preventiva: evaluación bupivacaina-fentanyl epidural caudal para analgesia intra y postoperatoria en el paciente peditrico. Rev Mex Anestesiol 1995;18:51—6.

24. Cook B, Grubb DJ, Aldridge LA, Doyle E. Comparison of the effects of adrenaline, clonidine and ketamine on the duration of caudal analgesia produced by bupivacaine in children. Br J Anaesth 1995;75:698—701.

25. Gao F, Waters B, Seager J, Dowling C, Vickerst MD. Comparison of bupivacaine plus buprenorphine with bupivacaine alone by caudal blockade for post-operative pain relief after hip and knee arthroscopy. Eur J Anaesthesiol 1995;12:471—6.

26. Haas DA, Lennon D. A 21 year retrospective study of reports of paresthesia following local anesthetic administration. J Can Dent Assoc 1995; 61:319—20, 323—6, 329—30.

27. Pogrel MA, Bryan J, Regezi J. Nerve damage associated with inferior alveolar nerve blocks. J Am Dent Assoc 1995;126:1150—5.

28. Datta S, Camann W, Bader A, Vander Burgh L. Clinical effects and maternal and fetal plasma concentrations of epidural ropivacaine versus bupivacaine for cesarean sections. Anesthesiology 1995;82:1346—52.

29. McCrae AF, Jozwiak H, McClure JH. Comparison of ropivacaine in extradural analgesia for the relief of pain in labour. Br J Anaesth 1995;74:261—5.

30. Chauhan S, Gaur A, Tripathi M, Kaushik S. Unintentional combined epidural and subdural block. Case report. Reg Anesth 1995;20:249—51.

31. Beers RA, Thomas PS, Martin RJ, Gorji R. Severe lumbar back pain following epidural injection of local anesthetic for epidural anesthesia. Case report and literature review. Reg Anesth 1995;20:69—74.

32. Lyons B, Phelan D, McCarroll M, Stack J, Murphy S, O'Moore BT, Gorey TF. Prolonged unilateral lower limb paresis following abdominal surgery with epidural and general anaesthesia. Anaesth Intens Care 1995;23:507—9.

33. Lehmann LJ, Pallares VS. Subdural injection of a local anesthetic with steroids: complicaion of

epidural anesthesia. South Med J 1995;88:467—9.

34. Stenseth R, Berg EM, Bjella L, Christensen O, Levang OW, Gisvold SE. Effects of thoracic epidural analgesia on coronary hemodynamics and myocardial metabolism in coronary artery bypass surgery. J Cardiothorac Vasc Anesth 1995;9:503—9.

35. Hoka S, Izumi K, Matsukado T, Matsuda K, Takahashi S. Coronary artery spasm induced after lumbar epidural anaesthesia. Eur J Anaesthesiol 1995;12:609—12.

36. Cozanitis DA. Leg pains after spinal anaesthesia. Can J Anaesth 1995;42:657.

37. Hampl KF, Schneider MC, Thorin D, Ummenhofer W, Drewe J. Hyperosmolarity does not contribute to transient radicular irritation after spinal anesthesia with hyperbaric 5% lidocaine. Reg Anesth 1995;20:363—8.

38. Strichartz GR, Lambert DH. Neurotoxicity of 5% lignocaine. Br J Anaesth 1995;75:376.

39. Hampl KF, Schneider MC, Ummenhofer W, Drewe J. Transient neurologic symptoms after spinal anesthesia. Anesth Analg 1995;81:1148—53.

40. Ong B, Baker C. Temporary back and leg pain after bupivacaine and morphine spinal anaesthesia. Can J Anaesth 1995;42:805—7.

41. Standl T, Eckert S, Schulte am Esch J. Microcatheter continuous spinal anaesthesia in the postoperative period: a prospective study of its effectiveness and complications. Eur J Anaesthesiol 1995;12:273—9.

42. Critchley LAH, Stuart JC, Conway F, Short TC. Hypotension during subarachnoid anaesthesia: haemodynamic effects of ephedrine. Br J Anaesth 1995;74:373—8.

43. Chan ST. Intra-articular morphine and bupivacaine for pain relief after therapeutic arthroscopic knee surgery. Singapore Med J 1995;36:35—7.

44. Suder PA, Mikkelsen JB, Hougaard K, Jensen PE. Reduction of traumatic secondary shoulder dislocations with lidocaine. Arch Orthop Trauma Surg 1995;114:233—6.

45. Richardson J, Sabanathan S, Mearns AJ, Shah RD, Goulden C. A prospective, randomized comparison of interpleural and paravertebral analgesia in thoracic surgery. Br J Anaesth 1995;75:405—8.

46. Calvo B, Pedraz JL, Gascon AR, Hernandez RM, Garcia-Ortega E, Muriel CM, Dominguez-Gil A. The influence of adrenaline on the pharmacokinetics of interpleurally administered lidocaine in patients with pancreatic neoplasia. J Clin Pharmacol 1995;35:436—1.

47. Hunter DG, Lam GC, Guyton DL. Inferior oblique muscle injury from local anesthesia for cataract. Ophthalmology 1995;102:501—9.

48. Weidenthal DT, King J. Cardiopulmonary arrest after retrobulbar anesthesia in a patient with an orbital roof defect. Am J Ophthalmol 1995;120:535—6.

49. Anderson CJ. Combined topical and subconjunctival anesthesia in cataract surgery. Ophthalmic Surg 1995;26:205—8.

50. Callear AB. The effect of temperature on the discomfort of caused by topical local anaesthesia. J Roy Soc Med 1995;88:709—11.

51. Kudrow L, Kudrow D, Sandweiss JH. Rapid and sustained relief of migraine attacks with intranasal lidocaine: preliminary findings. Headache 1995;35:79—82.

52. Robbins L. Intranasal lidocaine for cluster headache. Headache 1995;35:83—4.

53. Kaye AD, Eaton WM, Jahr JS, Nossaman BD, Youngberg JA. Local anesthesia infiltration as a cause of intraoperative tension pneumothorax in a young healthy woman undergoing breast augmentation with general anesthesia. J Clin Anesth 1995;7:422—4.

54. Beydon L, Lorino AM, Verra F, Labroue M, Catoire P, Lofaso F, Bonnet F. Topical upper airway anaesthesia with lidocaine increases airway resistance by impairing glottic function. Intens Care Med 1995;21:920—6.

55. Gourrier E, Karoubi P, el Henache A, Merbouche S, Mouchnino G, Dhabhi S, Leraillez J. Use of EMLA cream in premature and full-term infants. Study of efficacy and tolerance. Arch Pediatr 1995;2:1041—6.

56. Gupta AK, Sibbald RG. Application of a eutectic mixture of lidocaine/prilocaine cream to the moustache area prior to electrolysis provides effective analgesia. J Dermatol Treat 1995;6:89—94.

57. O'Connor B, Tomlinson AA. Evaluation of the efficacy and the safety of amethocaine gel applied topically before venous cannulation in adults. Br J Anaesth 1995;74:706—8.

58. Lawson LA, Smart NG. Evaluation of an amethocaine gel preparation for percutaneous analgesia before venous cannulation in children. Br J Anaesth 1995;75:282—5.

59. Mecklem DWJ, Humphrey MD, Hicks RW. Efficacy of bupivacaine delivered by wound catheter for post-caesarean section analgesia. Aust NZ J Obstet Gynaecol 1995;35:416—21.

60. Bacsik CJ, Swift JQ, Hargreaves KM. Toxic systemic reactions of bupivacaine and etidocaine. Oral Surg Oral Med Oral Pathol 1995;79:18—23.

61. Le Pelley E, Kossek JM, Bouquet S, Ferrier B, Fusciardi J. Anaesthesia de contact à la cocaine pour chirugie endonasalae. Cinetique et tolerance clinique d'une solution concentr*e. Ann Fr Anesth Reanim 1995;14:472—7.

62. Benowitz NL. Clinical pharmacology and toxicology of cocaine. Pharmacol Toxicol 1993;72:3—12.

63. Nicholson KEA, Rogers JEG. Cocaine and adrenaline paste: a fatal combination? Br Med J 1995;311:250—1.

64. Burton M, Marks R. Dangers of cocaine and adrenaline paste. Br Med J 1995;311:1089.

65. Williamson P, Slack R. Dangers of cocaine and adrenaline paste. Accurate measurement of dose and patience are important. Br Med J 1995;311:1089.

66. Farrell RWR. Dangers of cocaine and adrenaline paste. Combination is still widely used. Br Med J 1995;311:1089.

67. Ellis PDM, Wilkey BR. Dangers of cocaine and adrenaline paste. Other aspects of anaesthetic technique may have added to danger. Br Med J 1995;311:1089.

68. Kubo N, Nakamura A, Yamashita T. Efficacy and complications of topical cocaine anesthesia in functional endoscopic sinus surgery. Nippon Jibiinkoka Gakkai Kaiho 1995;98:1263—9.

69. Young D, Glauber JJ. Electrocardiographic changes resulting from acute cocaine intoxication. Am Heart J 1946;34:272—9.

70. Chiu YC, Brecht K, Dasgupta DS, Mhoon E. Myocardial infarction with topical cocaine anesthesia for nasal surgery 1986;112:988—90.

71. Littlewood SC, Tabb HD. Myocardial ischemia with epinephrine and cocaine during septoplasty. J La State Med Sci 1987;139:15—18.

72. Minor RL, Scott DB, Brown DD, Winniford MD. Cocaine-induced myocardial infarction in patients with normal coronary arteries. Ann Intern Med 1991;115:797—806.

73. Aschi M, Wiedmann HP, James KB. Cardiac complications from use of cocaine and phenylephrine in nasal septoplasty. Arch Otolaryngol Head Neck Surg 1995;121:681—4.

74. Gaggero G, Meyer O, Van Gessel E, Rifat K. Alkinization of lidocaine 2% does not influence the quality of epidural anaesthesia for elective caesarean section. Can J Anaesth 1995;42:1080—4.

75. Kajimoto Y, Rosenberg ME, Kytta J, Randell T, Tuominen M, Reunala T, Rosenberg PH. Anaphylactoid skin reactions after intravenous regional anaesthesia using 0.5% prilocaine with or without preservative-a double blind study. Acta Anaesthesiol Scand 1995;39:782—4.

76. Rudlof B, Lampert R, Brandt L. Untersuchungen zum Einsatz der Pulsoxymetrie bei prilocaininduzierter Methämoglobinämie. Anaesthesist 1995;44:887—91.

77. Tse S, Barrington K, Byrne P. Methemoglobinemia associated with prilocaine use in neonatal circumcision. Am J Perinatol 1995;12:331—2.

78. Hardwick FK, Beaudreau RW. Methemoglobinemia in a renal transplant patient: case report. Pediatr Dent 1995;17:460—3.

79. Wolff AP, Hasselström L, Kerkkamp HE, Gielen MJ. Extradural ropivacaine and bupivacaine in hip surgery. Br J Anaesth 1995;74:458—60.

M. Leuwer and O. Zuzan

12 Neuromuscular blocking agents and skeletal muscle relaxants

GENERAL TOPICS

℞ *Muscle relaxants in emergency medicine*

The use of neuromuscular blocking agents to aid airway management in emergency situations has been under discussion for some time. While the proponents of muscle relaxants in this area argue that neuromuscular blockade is essential for safe and atraumatic rapid-sequence intubation, the opponents emphasize the potential adverse effects. One particular concern is the risk of succinylcholine-induced hyperkalemia.

Indeed, there has been a case report of hyperkalemic cardiac arrest related to succinylcholine-aided emergency intubation (1[c]).

A 42-year-old woman went into profound shock because of severe hemorrhage some hours after a cesarean section. After she had collapsed and lost consciousness, succinylcholine was given to aid emergency endotracheal intubation. Shortly after she became pulseless, and cardiopulmonary resuscitation was initiated. Her serum potassium concentration was 8.2 mmol/l. Despite maximum efforts she could not be resuscitated and died 45 min later.

While pre-succinylcholine potassium concentrations were not available in this case, the authors assumed that this patient could have had pre-existing hyperkalemia, resulting from metabolic acidosis, exacerbated by succinylcholine-induced potassium release. This assumption received experimental support from an animal study, in which profound hyperkale-

mia occurred after succinylcholine injection to hemorrhagic acidotic rabbits (2).

In contrast to this, a recent study in 100 emergency patients with a variety of conditions such as trauma, neurological emergencies, drug overdose, cardiac and respiratory emergencies did not show any succinylcholine-associated hyperkalemic complications after rapid-sequence intubation (3[c]). The patients were closely observed for changes in serum potassium concentrations and disturbances of cardiac rhythm. The largest increase in serum potassium concentration was 1.1 mmol/l, and only two patients had post-succinylcholine potassium concentrations above 5 mmol/l (5.6 and 5.1 mmol/l). None of the patients had succinylcholine-associated asystole, ventricular tachycardia, or ventricular fibrillation. Based on this, the authors concluded that succinylcholine-induced hyperkalemia is an uncommon phenomenon in emergency patients. They cautiously admitted that the incidence of hyperkalemic complications might have been higher had they not excluded patients whose disease processes had lasted longer than 24 h.

There are, of course, certain clinical conditions in which hyperkalemic complications have been reported, such as burns, multiple trauma, and hemiplegia or paraplegia (SED-13, 306). In these cases, hyperkalemia occurred at least several days after the onset of the disease process. However, intubation in the emergency department or in prehospital emergency medicine is performed almost exclusively in patients with acute problems. Therefore, emergency patients do not necessarily have an increased risk of succinylcholine-induced hyperkalemia.

This is supported by further studies in a variety of emergencies, in which there were no

Side Effects of Drugs, Annual 20
J.K. Aronson, ed.

133

severe succinylcholine-induced complications. In a retrospective analysis of 213 succinylcholine-assisted emergency intubations, several complications (such as hypotension) were noted after endotracheal intubation, owing to the nature of the critical condition and the underlying disease (4[C]). One death occurred in a woman with chronic obstructive pulmonary disease and congestive heart failure who died of progressive respiratory failure shortly after emergency intubation. A detailed examination of this case led the authors to conclude that the fatal outcome had been caused by the severity of the disease and was unrelated to the use of a paralysing agent. Three patients had bradycardia and two had a short period of ventricular bigeminy. None of the patients experienced hyperkalemic complications. The authors concluded that rapid-sequence intubation aided by succinylcholine is a safe method of airway management in emergency patients, without serious adverse effects.

In a retrospective analysis of 654 prehospital intubations in children, succinylcholine was administered by paramedics to aid intubation in 47% of the cases (5[C]). There were no adverse effects.

Another risk possibly associated with the use of muscle relaxants in emergency patients is not really an adverse effect, but rather the result of the desired pharmacodynamic effect itself, namely generalized muscle paralysis. As the dosages of muscle relaxants commonly used to facilitate endotracheal intubation result in paralysis of all skeletal muscles, including the respiratory muscles, the return of spontaneous ventilation is precluded for some time. If the attempted intubation turns out to be unsuccessful, there is an urgent need to provide ventilation and oxygenation by means other than the endotracheal tube. Failure to do so will result in hypoxic brain damage or death. On the other hand, inadequate muscle relaxation itself can lead to difficult intubating conditions. The emergency care provider, therefore, has to choose one of two potentially dangerous methods of airway management. This raises the question of whether emergency tracheal intubation using a neuromuscular blocking agent can be considered to be a safe technique.

*Several publications have discussed this issue. In 219 muscle relaxant-aided emergency intubations there was no case of failed intu*bation (4[C]). In urgent intubations in trauma patients there were three esophageal intubations and one failed intubation requiring cricothyroidotomy among 198 cases of intubation with paralysis; multiple attempts were needed for endotracheal intubation in 14 cases (6[C]). In a further investigation on intubation in trauma patients, six cricothyroidotomies had to be performed, while 223 patients were successfully intubated; muscle relaxants were used in 175 patients, but there was no information in the paper whether the six cricothyroidotomies were performed on paralysed patients (7[C]). In 297 emergency intubations, 80% of which were performed using a muscle relaxant, translaryngeal intubation was accomplished in all cases; 8% of the intubations proved difficult, requiring more than two attempts (8[C]). In 95 succinylcholine-aided intubations performed by paramedics in the prehospital setting, there was successful endotracheal tube placement in 96% of the cases (9[C]). A comparison of emergency intubations with or without a sedative and a muscle relaxant showed a 100% success rate with drug-facilitated intubation (10[C]). Oral intubation was attempted in 54 patients. When drugs were used to facilitate intubation (n = 36), the success rate was 92% on the first attempt, and 100% on the second attempt. When drugs were not used (n = 18), 39% could not be intubated. Similarly, succinylcholine-facilitated orotracheal intubation in 52 overdose patients with Glasgow Coma Scale scores of 12 or less had a 100% success rate with no complications, compared with a 65% success rate and complications in 86% of the cases in which blind nasotracheal intubation was used (11[C]).*

In summary, there is a risk of failed or difficult intubation in paralysed emergency patients. However, this risk does not appear to be high enough to exclude emergency patients from the beneficial effects of a fast and atraumatic muscle relaxant-aided intubation. It should be stressed that every emergency care provider who performs endotracheal intubations, with or without the aid of a muscle relaxant, should be familiar with alternative techniques of maintaining ventilation and oxygenation, in case the intubation attempt is unsuccessful.

Until now, the anecdotal evidence of succinylcholine-induced hyperkalemia in patients with severe hemorrhagic shock has not been confirmed in clinical studies. Taking into ac count its pharmacodynamic properties and the lack of evidence of an increased risk of hyperkalemic complications, succinylcholine should be regarded as an appropriate drug for urgent intubation in emergency patients (12[R]). There are, of course, absolute contraindications for the use of succinylcholine, such as known hyperkalemia, allergy, susceptibility to malignant hyperthermia, and certain neuromuscular disorders. In patients with severe trauma, burns, or paraplegia, hemiplegia, or quadriplegia, succinylcholine should be avoided if the onset of the condition dates back more than 1 or 2 days, and also in patients who have been immobilized for more than a few days. Furthermore, care should be taken in using succinylcholine in cases of suspected hyperkalemia.

The management of rapid-sequence intubation in emergencies in children, including the adverse effects of muscle relaxants and measures for the failed intubation situation, has been recently reviewed (13[R]).

Muscle relaxants in intensive care

Extensive reports continue to feature in the current literature on the adverse effects of muscle relaxants in intensive care patients. Most of the papers have focused on the acute generalized *myopathy* that is associated with the use of non-depolarizing neuromuscular blocking agents.

Although it has been assumed by some that non-steroidal relaxants might be of advantage when compared with steroidal agents (SEDA-19, 141), a recent report has extended the list of manifestations of acute quadriplegic myopathy in intensive care patients after the use of benzylisoquinolone-relaxants (14[c]).

Two patients, a 74-year-old woman and a 73-year-old man were treated with doxacurium by infusion for 6 and 10 days, respectively. Both received concomitant glucocorticoid therapy, and both developed generalized flaccid paralysis, which became obvious after discontinuation of doxacurium. Electromyographic studies showed reduced evoked compound action potentials, with no evidence of residual neuromuscular blockade. Muscle biopsies showed a severe, non-inflammatory, focally necrotizing myopathy. One patient's neurological condition failed to improve over several weeks and supportive therapy was withdrawn at the request of her family. The other was discharged to a rehabilitation

hospital, having regained some of his baseline motor function over a period of 3 months.

These two cases clearly show the impact of muscle relaxant-associated myopathy. The economic consequences of these disturbances have been investigated (15[c]). Ten patients who developed prolonged neuromuscular weakness after continuous administration of non-depolarizing neuromuscular blockers were compared with 10 who did not develop motor weakness after paralysis. Apart from the medical and humanitarian aspects of prolonged ICU and hospital stay and prolonged ventilator dependency, patients with prolonged weakness after neuromuscular blockade caused increased health-care costs, an excess of \$66 000 per patient compared with patients without prolonged paralysis.

The importance of recognizing risk factors has been illustrated by report of a 60-year-old man who had prolonged paralysis after long-term vecuronium treatment, caused by accumulation of an active metabolite of vecuronium, owing to renal and hepatic failure (16[c]). This particular problem is known to be associated with vecuronium and pancuronium (17[c]), (18[c]); however, prolonged neuromuscular blockade is not excluded by the long-term use of atracurium (19[c]).

The pharmacodynamics and pharmacokinetics of *cis*-atracurium and atracurium have been compared in 12 intensive care patients (20[c]). There were no clinically important pharmacokinetic differences between the groups. Furthermore, the pharmacokinetics did not differ notably from the results of an earlier study in healthy adults (21[c]). However, before it can be concluded that both atracurium and *cis*-atracurium are safe drugs for long-term administration in ICU patients from a pharmacokinetic point of view, one should consider the comparatively short duration of infusion in this study (longest duration 48 h for *cis*-atracurium and 34 h for atracurium, respectively). Moreover, some cases of prolonged paralysis might have been detected had a greater number of patients been included. Plasma laudanosine concentrations tended to be higher in the atracurium group.

Probably any neuromuscular blocking agent can contribute to the development of critical illness myopathy. There were 20 cases of muscular weakness in 107 patients with severe asthma requiring mechanical ventilation, and significantly more cases in patients treated with neuromuscular blocking agents (29 vs. 0%) (22[C]). There were no clear differences between atracurium, vecuronium, and pancuronium, and the incidence of muscle weakness increased with the duration of neuromuscular blockade (6% in patients paralysed for less than 24 h, 38% in patients paralysed for 24—48 h, and 85% in patients paralysed for more than 2 days).

The question of which drug is the most appropriate for ICU patients has been discussed in two letters (23), (24), in the first of which the authors reiterated the hypothesis that the adverse sequelae of prolonged neuromuscular blockade are substantially reduced if neuromuscular function is carefully monitored in the critically ill patient, an assumption that has been supported by a recent study, in which routine train-of-four-monitoring was performed on 90 ICU patients (25[C]). The incidence of prolonged paralysis (over 12 h) was compared with the incidence in a historical cohort without neuromuscular monitoring. All patients who received either more than six doses of vecuronium or atracurium over a 24-h period or a continuous infusion of either drug were included. Before the implementation of neuromuscular monitoring there were five instances of neuromuscular weakness in 43 patients. With monitoring, no weakness was observed in 90 patients. The use of a retrospective comparison might give rise to criticism; however, this study represents some evidence of a potential beneficial effect of neuromuscular monitoring. For that reason, neuromuscular monitoring is strongly recommended once the use of a muscle relaxant is regarded as unavoidable in the intensive care patient.

While continuous muscle relaxation is achieved exclusively by the administration of non-depolarizing neuromuscular blocking agents, there are instances in which only short-term relaxation is required to facilitate airway management or other maneuvers in the ICU. Succinylcholine is mainly used for short-term relaxation. However, in patients who have been treated for more than a couple of days in the ICU, succinylcholine can result in life-threatening hyperkalemia (26[C]).

A 69-year-old woman was admitted to the ICU with a septic pericardial effusion and right thoracic empyema. Because of respiratory failure she received continuous mechanical ventilation and required a high concentration of inspired oxygen. Nineteen days after admission, she was given succinylcholine to facilitate an urgent change of tracheal tube. Shortly after the succinylcholine injection she developed a cardiac arrest and did not respond to standard resuscitation, atropine, and adrenaline. Her serum potassium concentration 7 min after succinylcholine was 8.3 mmol/l. She was given calcium chloride, and after an episode of ventricular tachycardia a synchronized shock resulted in stable sinus rhythm with a satisfactory blood pressure.

There have been previous reports of *hyperkalemia* causing complications in intensive care patients (27[c]), (28[c]). Immobilization results in changes in the post-junctional acetylcholine receptor, i.e. enlargement of the ACh-sensitive area, ACh receptor proliferation, and shifts in the dose-response curves to ACh and succinylcholine (29[R]). Because of these changes, a depolarizing agent can cause massive and long-lasting release of potassium from muscle cells. Succinylcholine should therefore be strictly avoided in patients who have been immobilized in the intensive care unit for more than a few days. It still has to be evaluated whether this is true for intensive care patients who have not been fully immobilized. In addition, there is evidence that succinylcholine-induced hyperkalemia after immobilization may be exacerbated by long-term treatment with non-depolarizing neuromuscular blocking agents (SEDA-19, 141).

Heterotopic ossification has been reported after the long-term administration of muscle relaxants to intensive care patients (SEDA-19, 142; (30[c])). A recent case illustrates the drastic consequences for the patient (31[c]).

A 21-year-old man developed adult respiratory distress syndrome after receiving a gunshot wound to the neck. Pancuronium was given continuously until extubation on the 50th postoperative day. After extubation, he complained of myalgia and arthralgia in many places. He had limited range of movement in his shoulders, elbows, hips, and knees, and radiography showed extensive periarticular heterotopic ossification in these joints. All active or passive joint movements caused severe pain. His serum alkaline phosphatase was increased at that time, as it had been for the previous 6 weeks. During the next 4 months his joint mobility decreased even more, accompanied by a continuously increased alkaline phosphatase. The periarticular ectopic bone continued to mature radiographically. Two years after the injury, the ectopic bone was removed surgically, supported by radiotherapy and indomethacin, which finally restored his movements, allowing him to be ambulatory and self-sufficient.

Heterotopic ossification is a known complication in a wide variety of conditions, the common factor among which appears to be prolonged immobility. Therefore, complete pharmacologically-induced immobilization might be a contributing element. Considering the severity of this potential adverse effect of long-term muscle relaxation, it should be regarded as one more reason for avoiding neuromuscular blocking drugs in intensive care patients over longer periods.

Interactions among muscle relaxants

Mivacurium is a non-depolarizing neuromuscular blocking agent with a comparatively short duration of action. However, a recent study has shown that it has a significantly prolonged duration of action when given after pancuronium (32[C]). The mean time to 95% EMG recovery after mivacurium 70 µg/kg was 97 min when preceded by an ED_{95}-dose of pancuronium compared with 20 min without previous pancuronium. One explanation for this observation may be that the first relaxant dominates the block for some time (SED-13, 311). Furthermore, pancuronium inhibits plasma cholinesterase activity (SED-13, 317) With this mechanism, the rate of metabolism of mivacurium could be reduced and its duration of action prolonged. While it might appear tempting to use a top-up dose of the assumed short-acting mivacurium when muscle relaxation is required towards the end of surgery, these results show that this is not an appropriate technique when a long-acting agent has been used before mivacurium. Similarly, prolonged duration of action has been reported when mivacurium was preceded by either atracurium or vecuronium in 45 patients randomly allocated to one of three equal groups: mivacurium, atracurium, or vecuronium, in each case followed by mivacurium (33[C]).

The effects of non-depolarizer pretreatment on the course of action of succinylcholine have been reported in 64 patients (34[C]). The mean

time to 90% twitch recovery was significantly shorter after pretreatment with atracurium or vecuronium (7.5 and 8.2 min) compared with a control group without pretreatment (11.8 min). In contrast, pancuronium resulted in a significantly prolonged time to 90% twitch recovery (13.5 min). The authors therefore concluded that the duration of action of succinylcholine can be influenced according to clinical needs by the choice of drug for non-depolarizer pretreatment.

DEPOLARIZING NEURO-MUSCULAR BLOCKING AGENTS *(SED-13, 301; SEDA-18, 150; SEDA-19, 136)*

Succinylcholine *(SED-13, 301; SEDA-18, 150; SEDA-19, 136)*

Musculoskeletal *Fasciculations and myalgia* Rocuronium pretreatment has been compared with vecuronium and placebo in the prevention of succinylcholine-induced myalgia in 150 patients (35[C]). The incidence of myalgia on the first postoperative day was significantly less after rocuronium (20%) than after vecuronium (42%) or placebo (70%). The potential benefit of non-depolarizer pretreatment in individual patients has also been illustrated by a case report (36[c]).

A 19-year-old woman received succinylcholine on several occasions for electroconvulsive therapy. Each succinylcholine administration without pretreatment was followed by severe and distressing muscle pain. Therefore, in the next sessions she was given vecuronium 1 mg 3 min before succinylcholine. In these cases, recovery from anesthesia was prompt and uneventful, with no muscle pain. When pretreatment was omitted on one occasion her myalgia recurred.

The choice of muscle relaxant for surgery of short duration with regard to succinylcholine-induced myalgia has been discussed in two letters (37), (38). In the first, the authors suggested that myalgia after succinylcholine is best avoided by using atracurium or mivacurium instead of succinylcholine. In the second, the authors emphasized that succinylcholine is still recognized as the only muscle relaxant available that allows intubation and subsequent rapid return of spontaneous ventilation. For reduction of myalgia, they suggested the pretreatment use of intravenous lidocaine.

Malignant hyperthermia   Succinylcholine is a potent trigger of malignant hyperthermia (SED-13, 305). Interestingly, chlorocresol, an additive in a commercial formulation of succinylcholine, may itself trigger release of calcium from the sarcoplasmic reticulum in individuals who are susceptible to malignant hyperthermia. In in vitro contracture tests on muscle biopsies from patients susceptible chlorocresol caused muscle contractures without the addition of caffeine and intensified caffeine-induced contractures (39). In the isolated rabbit sarcoplasmic reticulum, chlorocresol magnified caffeine-induced calcium release. The authors therefore concluded that the use of this formulation could increase the risk of activation of malignant hyperthermia in susceptible patients. Their article was accompanied by an editorial review of the molecular mechanisms involved in the pathogenesis of malignant hyperthermia (40[R]).

Risk factors   The use of succinylcholine in children has been discussed controversially (SEDA-19, 138). The issue is obviously of clinical relevance for many anesthesiologists, as reflected by further correspondence (41)—(43). Meanwhile, another undesired effect of succinylcholine in children has been reported (44[c]). Two children (30 and 20 kg, respectively) experienced *respiratory arrest* some hours after the end of surgery, when succinylcholine was flushed into the circulation from the dead space of the intravenous cannula. Both were resuscitated with bag-and-mask ventilation and made a full recovery. The authors measured a dead space of 0.24 ml in the cannula and the non-reflux valve, corresponding to 12 mg of succinylcholine given a 5% solution was used. Thus, when such unusually high concentrations of succinylcholine are used, succinylcholine might remain in the dead space in amounts sufficient to put children at risk. The practical consequence should be routine flushing of the intravenous line after the use of succinylcholine. Moreover, the use of 1% succinylcholine is strongly recommended, as it allows more precise dosing;

5% succinylcholine is impractical in both children and adults.

NON-DEPOLARIZING NEUROMUSCULAR BLOCKING AGENTS *(SED-13, 310; SEDA-17, 150; SEDA-18, 153; SEDA-19, 140)*

Interactions   *Anticonvulsants*   There is reduced sensitivity to non-depolarizing neuromuscular blocking agents in patients taking long-term anticonvulsants (SED-13, 319). The underlying mechanism is still speculative, but new information has recently become available. The pharmacokinetics and pharmacodynamics of a bolus dose of vecuronium have been compared in 10 epileptic patients taking chronic carbamazepine and in 10 non-epileptic patients in whom craniotomy was necessary for a variety of neurosurgical procedures (45[C]). The recovery times were significantly shorter in the carbamazepine group (the mean times to recovery of twitch height to 25% of baseline were 28 and 47 min, respectively). Total vecuronium clearance was 9 versus 3.8 ml/kg/min in the controls. The vecuronium concentrations at 50% block did not differ. Thus, the clinical experience of many anesthesiologists, that patients taking anticonvulsants need more maintenance doses of neuromuscular blocking agents, may be explained by altered pharmacokinetics rather than decreased sensitivity of the neuromuscular junction to non-depolarizing muscle relaxants, a mechanism that had been suggested on the basis of animal studies (46). However, no information was provided in the paper on intraoperative blood loss and volume replacement; the study was performed in patients undergoing major neurosurgery (craniotomy), and important blood loss, which cannot be excluded, could have a significant impact on pharmacokinetic calculations.

Magnesium sulfate   Magnesium has muscle-relaxing effects (SED-13, 315). On the background of increasing popularity of magnesium sulfate as an antiarrhythmic drug, its influence on neuromuscular transmission has been investigated in 20 patients receiving general anesthesia (47[C]). When given at recovery of train-of-four ratio to 0.7 after injection of vecuronium 0.1 mg/kg, magnesium sulfate 60 mg/kg resulted in a profound reduction in twitch height (mean minimum twitch height 24%) and a reduction in the number of detectable responses to train-of-four stimulation. In a second group of patients, the same effect was seen when magnesium sulfate was given 1 h after recovery of train-of-four ratio to 0.7 (mean minimum twitch height 34%). The authors concluded that magnesium sulfate can result in muscle weakness and associated complications when given postoperatively during recovery from neuromuscular blockade.

Risk factors *Smoking* The pharmacodynamics of vecuronium have been compared in 12 smokers and 12 non-smokers (48[C]). Both ED_{95} values and the dosage requirements for maintaining 90—98% block were significantly higher in smokers than in non-smokers (ED_{95}, 61 μg/kg vs. 97 μg/kg/min; dosage requirements for 90—98% block, 48 μg/kg vs. 72 μg/kg/min). While these results await confirmation, there could be practical consequences. If smokers really require larger doses for the induction and maintenance of neuromuscular blockade, one should consider modifying routine dosing of vecuronium in smokers, especially if profound block is necessary. Moreover, neuromuscular transmission should be monitored in these cases. Meanwhile, the underlying mechanism for altered sensitivity towards vecuronium can only be speculated on.

Mivacurium and plasma cholinesterase Mivacurium has a short duration of action because it is hydrolysed by plasma cholinesterase. Therefore, the effects of mivacurium are prolonged in patients with atypical plasma cholinesterase activity, an example of which has recently been reported (49[c]). Furthermore, it has been shown that the dose—response relation is significantly altered in patients who are homozygous for the atypical or the silent cholinesterase gene (50[C]). Using an incremental dosage technique, the mean estimated ED_{50} was 15 μg/kg in seven patients phenotypically homozygous for the atypical gene and 13 μg/kg in one patient homozygous for the silent gene, corresponding to one-quarter to one-fifth of the values determined in patients with normal plasma cholinesterase ac-

tivity. Based on their data, the authors concluded that mivacurium appears to be 4—5 times more potent in patients phenotypically homozygous for the atypical gene or the silent gene than in patients with normal plasma cholinesterase activity and phenotype. However, as patients with atypical plasma cholinesterase are rarely identified before anesthesia, the management of prolonged blockade after mivacurium is important, and some aspects of it have been discussed in an accompanying editorial (51[R]).

In addition to genetic causes of reduced plasma cholinesterase activity, a variety of drugs may reduce the activity of this enzyme (SED-13, 308; SEDA-19, 139). Bambuterol, a β-adrenoceptor agonist, inhibited plasma cholinesterase activity by 83% in 14 patients 2 h before induction of general anesthesia (52[c]). After mivacurium 0.2 mg/kg, the first response to train-of-four stimulation occurred after 15 min in a control group compared with 75 min in patients who took bambuterol. Mivacurium may, therefore, have a prolonged duration of action in patients taking bambuterol. The same phenomenon has been reported with succinylcholine (SED-13, 308; (53[C])).

Neuromuscular disease The pharmacodynamics of neuromuscular blocking agents may be significantly altered in neuromuscular disease, but there have been conflicting reports in mitochondrial myopathy. Perioperative management in one case has recently been reported (54[c]).

In addition to routine procedures, an intra-arterial cannula was inserted before the induction of anesthesia in a 16-year-old boy with mitochondrial myopathy. Electrodes for non-invasive cardiac pacing were attached, in preparation for atrioventricular conduction block, which has been reported to occur in such patients. A nerve stimulator and a force displacement transducer were used to monitor neuromuscular function. After induction of anesthesia with propofol, train-of-four fade was present without the administration of a neuromuscular blocking agent (train-of-four ratio 0.59), which did not improve after 10 mg of edrophonium. Ten minutes later, mivacurium 15 μg/kg was given, resulting in a 98% reduction of twitch height. Recovery to 95% twitch height took 38 min. There was no evidence of residual paralysis after removal of the endotracheal tube. Cardiac rhythm was stable and the external pacemaker was not required.

Based on the observation of near total twitch depression after a small dose of mivacurium, which would have been expected to be subparalysing, the authors assumed that this patient had a significantly increased sensitivity to mivacurium. However, as an anticholinesterase drug was given before the administration of mivacurium, the effect might have been partly due to reduced degradation of mivacurium as a result of cholinesterase inhibition.

In another case report, the authors described their experience with mivacurium in a 53-year-old woman with late onset myopathy, i.e. congenital myopathy manifesting in an adult (55[c]). Incremental doses of mivacurium up to a total of 12 mg (about three times the usual ED_{95}) resulted in 88% reduction of twitch height as measured by electromyography and were followed by prompt recovery of neuromuscular transmission (23 min to 100% recovery of twitch height). However, the authors correctly cautioned readers not to accept these observations as evidence of a lack of complications of neuromuscular blockade in patients with myopathies. Responses to muscle relaxants may vary considerably, and so neuromuscular monitoring is strongly recommended. When discussing the choice of muscle relaxant, mivacurium might offer the advantage of shorter duration of action compared with other non-depolarizing agents. This could be of benefit in cases of increased sensitivity to muscle relaxants. While the relation between myopathies and susceptibility to malignant hyperthermia has not been further clarified, succinylcholine is best avoided in these patients.

Liver disease The pharmacokinetics and pharmacodynamics of *cis*-atracurium have been compared in 14 patients with end-stage liver disease and 11 control patients with normal hepatic and renal function undergoing elective surgery (56[C]). There were significant differences in the volume of distribution and plasma clearance (195 ml/kg and 6.6 ml/kg/min in liver disease vs. 161 ml/kg and 5.5 ml/kg/min in controls). Probably as a result of low statistical power, differences in recovery times, measured by relaxometry, did not reach statistical significance, but there was a trend to longer duration and greater variability of recovery times in the patients with liver disease. Apparently *cis*-atracurium does not have a predictably prolonged duration of action in patients with severe liver disease. In individual patients, however, the duration of action may be prolonged. Monitoring of neuromuscular transmission is therefore strongly recommended.

SKELETAL MUSCLE RELAXANTS *(SED-13, 328; SEDA-17, 155; SEDA-18, 156; SEDA-19, 143)*

Baclofen *(SED-13, 328; SEDA-17, 155; SEDA-19, 143)*

Since the early 1980s intrathecal baclofen has been used to control spinal spasticity associated with CNS lesions. While some adverse effects have been reported, there were no major adverse effects with long-term administration in two recent follow-up studies in 18 patients (57[C]) and 17 patients (58[C]).

Apart from some specific drug-induced adverse effects, certain complications may be associated with the mode of drug delivery. Cases of bacterial or viral meningitis have occurred, and a recent case of *aseptic meningitis* has been interpreted by the authors as being chemically induced (59[c]).

Intrathecal baclofen was given to a 29-year-old man with C5 paraplegia, using an epidural catheter. On the first day, a test dose of 50 μg was given, followed by 75 μg on the second day. After the second dose, the patient reported some reduction in the severity and frequency of his spasms. Ten hours after the second injection, however, his blood pressure increased by 20% and he had a bradycardia of 40/min, accompanied by chills, headache, and chest tightness. The intrathecal catheter was removed. Some hours later, he had a temperature of 39°C and neck stiffness. Cerebrospinal fluid showed increased protein and reduced glucose concentrations compared with a second sample 2 weeks later. Prophylactic triple antibiotic therapy was given. He made a full recovery.

The episode was diagnosed as aseptic, possibly chemical meningitis secondary to intrathecal baclofen, but spinal fluid viral culture was not obtained, and so a viral origin cannot be ruled out. The authors, however, thought that a viral cause was unlikely, taking into account the rapid onset and the rapid improvement after withdrawal of baclofen. While the exact diagnosis remains unclear, the possibility of baclofen-associated chemical meningitis should be kept in mind.

Overdosage Overdose of intrathecal baclofen may have serious consequences. While the administration of the benzodiazepine receptor antagonist flumazenil might be expected to be effective in the treatment of overdose of baclofen, a GABA receptor agonist, a recent case report has suggested the contrary (60[c]).

A 43-year-old woman with paraplegia secondary to long-standing multiple sclerosis had been treated with intrathecal baclofen for 15 months. After repair of a disconnected intrathecal catheter, an intrathecal dose of 600 μg was given. Over the next few hours she experienced progressively impaired consciousness down to a Glasgow coma score of 7. Flumazenil 500 μg was given intravenously, but resulted in no neurological improvement. She remained unconscious for another 3 h, but awoke spontaneously and was discharged the next day.

With regard to the lack of effect of flumazenil in this case of baclofen overdose, the authors suggested that these drugs act on different central GABA receptors. They therefore suggested that a specific baclofen antagonist should be developed.

Cyclobenzaprine *(SED-13, 330)*

Cyclobenzaprine is a tricyclic skeletal muscle relaxant structurally related to amitriptyline. Thus, an overdose of cyclobenzaprine might be assumed to have similar deleterious and life-threatening consequences as an overdose of a tricyclic antidepressant. However, in a retrospective review of 402 reports of cyclobenzaprine exposure to five poison centers in the US, there were no life-threatening cardiovascular or neurological effects, such as malignant dysrhythmias or seizures (61[C]). In doses up to 1 g, *lethargy*, *sinus tachycardia*, *agitation*, and both *hypertension* and *hypotension* were commonly observed. In spite of the lack of evidence of lethal complications in cyclobenzaprine intoxication in this investigation, it should be stressed that appropriate therapy is required. In the reported cases, this

included gastrointestinal decontamination as well as fluid and catecholamine therapy and sedation; 150 patients were admitted to the intensive care unit and 13 received mechanical ventilation.

Botulinum toxin *(SED-13, 330; SEDA-17, 156; SEDA-19, 144)*

The problem of immunological resistance to the effects of botulinum toxin associated with repeated injections has been reviewed (62[R]).

Gastrointestinal *Dysphagia* occurred in two men in their twenties after injections of botulinum toxin into muscles of the neck and the face (63[c]). In both cases, dysphagia was severe enough to require a gastrostomy tube for feeding. It took several months for the disturbance to resolve fully. In patients treated for spasmodic dysphonia, botulinum toxin-induced dysphagia is not uncommon, but it occurs more often and is more severe in patients who have complained of dysphagia before botulinum toxin injection (64[C]).

Urinary system *Urinary incontinence* after botulinum A toxin injection has been reported in 6-year-old twins treated for mild spastic diplegia (65[c]). Urinary incontinence occurred 14 and 16 days after injection of botulinum toxin into both thigh adductor muscles and lasted 3 weeks. In one twin urinary incontinence was accompanied by fecal incontinence. The authors thought that the disturbances had been caused by local spread of the toxin, as previous injections into more distal parts of the limbs had not resulted in any adverse effects.

Musculoskeletal In the presence of neuromuscular disorders, such as myasthenia gravis or Lambert-Eaton syndrome, botulinum toxin-induced inhibition of acetylcholine release may cause *generalized weakness*. In addition to that, a case of general weakness after injection of botulinum toxin in a patient with amyotrophic lateral sclerosis has been described (66[c]).

A 56-year-old woman with amyotrophic lateral sclerosis received an injection of botulinum toxin type A into the adductor muscles of the leg in an attempt to treat involuntary leg crossing due to spasticity. Three days later she was unable to walk, owing to weakness in the proximal muscles of the lower limb. One week after the injection, raising the arm also became difficult. As a result, she was temporarily bedridden. Two months after the botulinum toxin treatment, her weakness had resolved.

This case illustrates that in patients with a reduced margin of safety with regard to neuromuscular transmission, botulinum toxin can result in increased morbidity or even mortality. Therefore, botulinum toxin should, if at all, be used with extreme caution in patients with generalized neuromuscular disorders.

REFERENCES

1. Schwartz D, Kelly B, Caldwell J, Carlisle A, Cohen N. Succinylcholine-induced hyperkalemic arrest in a patient with severe metabolic acidosis and exsanguinating hemorrhage. Anesth Analg 1992;75:291—3.
2. Antognini J, Gronert G. Succinylcholine causes profound hyperkalemia in hemorrhagic, acidotic rabbits. Anesth Analg 1993;77:585—8.
3. Zink BJ, Snyder HS, Raccio Robak N. Lack of a hyperkalemic response in emergency department patients receiving succinylcholine. Acad Emerg Med 1995;2:974—8.
4. Dufour DG, Larose DL, Clement SC. Rapid sequence intubation in the emergency department. J Emerg Med 1995;13:705—10.
5. Brownstein D, Shugerman R, Cummings P, Rivara F, Copass M. Prehospital endotracheal intubation of children by paramedics. Ann Emerg Med 1996;28:34—9.
6. Rotondo MF, McGonigal MD, Schwab CW, Kauder DR, Hanson CW. Urgent paralysis and intubation of trauma patients: is it safe? J Trauma 1993;34:242—6.
7. Norwood S, Myers MB, Butler TJ. The safety of emergency neuromuscular blockade and orotracheal intubation in the acutely injured trauma patient. J Am Coll Surg 1994;179:646—52.
8. Schwartz D, Matthay M, Cohen N. Death and other complications of emergency airway management in critically ill adults. Anesthesiology 1995;82:367—6.
9. Hedges JR, Dronen SC, Feero S, Hawkins S, Syverud SA, Shultz B. Succinylcholine-assisted intubations in prehospital care. Ann Emerg Med 1988;17:469—72.
10. Ligier B, Buchman TG, Breslow MJ, Deutschman CS. The role of anesthetic induction agents and neuromuscular blockade in the endotracheal intubation of trauma victims. Surg Gynecol Obstet 1991;173:477—81.
11. Dronen SC, Merigian KS, Hedges JR, Hoekstra JW, Borron SW. A comparison of blind nasotracheal and succinylcholine-assisted intubation in the poisoned patient. Ann Emerg Med 1987; 16:650—2.
12. Rubin MA, Sadovnikoff N. Neuromuscular blocking agents in the emergency department. J Emerg Med 1996;14:193—9.
13. Gerardi MJ, Sacchetti AD, Cantor RM, Santamaria JP, Gausche M, Lucid W, Foltin GL. Rapid-sequence intubation of the pediatric patient. Ann Emerg Med 1996;28:55—74.
14. Marik PE. Doxacurium-corticosteroid acute myopathy: another piece to the puzzle. Crit Care Med 1996;24:1266—7.
15. Rudis M, Guslits B, Peterson E, Hathaway S, Angus E, Beis S, Zarowitz B. Economic impact of prolonged motor weakness complicating neuromuscular blockade in the intensive care unit. Crit Care Med 1996;24:1749—56.
16. Sanders KA, Aucker R. Early recognition of risk factors for persistent effects of vecuronium. South Med J 1996;89:411—14.
17. Segredo V, Caldwell JE, Matthay MA, Sharma ML, Gruenke LD, Miller RD. Persistent paralysis in critically ill patients after long-term administration of vecuronium. New Engl J Med 1992;327:524—8.
18. Vandenbrom RH, Wierda JM. Pancuronium bromide in the intensive care unit: a case of overdose. Anesthesiology 1988;69:996—7.
19. Rubio ER, Seelig CB. Persistent paralysis after prolonged use of atracurium in the absence of corticosteroids. South Med J 1996;89:624—6.
20. Boyd AH, Eastwood NB, Parker CJ, Hunter JM. Comparison of the pharmacodynamics and pharmacokinetics of an infusion of cis-atracurium (51W89) or atracurium in critically ill patients undergoing mechanical ventilation in an intensive therapy unit. Br J Anaesth 1996;76:382—8.
21. Eastwood NB, Boyd AH, Parker CJ, Hunter JM. Pharmacokinetics of 1-R-cis 1'R-cis atracurium besylate (51W89) and plasma laudanosine concentrations in health and chronic renal failure. Br J Anaesth 1995;75:431—5.
22. Leatherman JW, Fluegel WL, David WS, Davies SF, Iber C. Muscle weakness in mechanically ventilated patients with severe asthma. Am J Respir Crit Care Med 1996;153:1686—90.
23. Khuenl Brady KS, Sparr HJ, Waibel U. Neuromuscular blocking agents in the intensive care unit: a two-edged sword. Crit Care Med 1996;24:717—19.
24. Sladen R. Author's reply. Crit Care Med 1996;24:718—19.
25. Frankel H, Jeng J, Tilly E, St Andre A,

Champion H. The impact of implementation of neuromuscular blockade monitoring standards in a surgical intensive care unit. Am Surg 1996; 62:503—6.

26. Dornan RI, Royston D. Suxamethonium-related hyperkalaemic cardiac arrest in intensive care. Anaesthesia 1995;50:1006.

27. Hemming A, Charlton S, Kelly P. Hyperkalaemia, cardiac arrest, suxamethonium and intensive care. Anaesthesia 1990;45:990—1.

28. Horton W, Fergusson N. Hyperkalaemia and cardiac arrest after the use of suxamethonium in intensive care. Anaesthesia 1988;43:890—1.

29. Martyn J, White D, Gronert G, Jaffe R, Ward J. Up-and-down regulation of skeletal muscle acetylcholine receptors. Anesthesiology 1992;76:822—43.

30. Clements NC Jr, Camilli AE. Heterotopic ossification complicating critical illness. Chest 1993;104:1526—8.

31. Ray TD, Lowe WD, Anderson LD, Muller AL, Brogdon BG. Periarticular heterotopic ossification following pharmacologically induced paralysis. Skeletal Radiol 1995;24:609—12.

32. Erkola O, Rautoma P, Meretoja OA. Mivacurium when preceded by pancuronium becomes a long-acting muscle relaxant. Anesthesiology 1996;84:562—5.

33. Rautoma P, Meretoja OA, Erkola O, Kalli I. The duration of action of mivacurium is prolonged if preceded by atracurium or vecuronium. Acta Anaesthesiol Scand 1995;39:912—15.

34. Ebeling BJ, Keienburg T, Hausmann D, Apfelstaedt C. Das Wirkungsprofil von Succinylcholin nach Präcurarisierung mit Atracurium, Vecuronium oder Pancuronium. Anästhesiol Intensivmed Notfallmed Schmerzther 1996;31:304—8.

35. Findlay GP, Spittal MJ. Rocuronium pretreatment reduces suxamethonium-induced myalgia: comparison with vecuronium. Br J Anaesth 1996;76:526—9.

36. Herriot PM, Cowain T, McLeod D. Use of vecuronium to prevent suxamethonium-induced myalgia after ECT. Br J Psychiatry 1996; 168:653—4.

37. van den Berg AA, Iqbal S. Post suxamethonium myalgia—will we never learn? Anaesth Intensive Care 1996;24:116—17.

38. Campbell R, Rodrigo M. Post suxamethonium myalgia—reply. Anaesth Intensive Care 1996; 24:117.

39. Tegazzin V, Scutari E, Treves S, Zorzato F. Chlorocresol, an additive to commercial succinylcholine, induces contracture of human malignant hyperthermia-susceptible muscles via activation of the ryanodine receptor Ca^{2+} channel. Anesthesiology 1996;84:1380—5.

40. Pessah I, Lynch C, Gronert G. Complex pharmacology of malignant hyperthermia. Anesthesiology 1996;84:1275—9.

41. Farrell PT. Suxamethonium in children. Br J Anaesth 1996;76:883—4.

42. Fiacchino F, Consonni F, Dulcamara A, Grandi L. Suxamethonium in children. Br J Anaesth 1996;76:883.

43. Hopkins P. Suxamethonium in children. Author's reply. Br J Anaesth 1996;76:884.

44. Davidson A, Brown TC. Respiratory arrest in two children following postoperative flushing of suxamethonium from the deadspace of intravenous cannulae. Anaesth Intensive Care 1996; 24:97—8.

45. Alloul K, Whalley DG, Shutway F, Ebrahim Z, Varin F. Pharmacokinetic origin of carbamazepine-induced resistance to vecuronium neuromuscular blockade in anesthetized patients. Anesthesiology 1996;84:330—9.

46. Kim CS, Arnold FJ, Itani MS, Martyn JA. Decreased sensitivity to metocurine during long-term phenytoin therapy may be attributable to protein binding and acetylcholine receptor changes. Anesthesiology 1992;77:500—6.

47. Fuchs Buder T, Tassonyi E. Magnesium sulphate enhances residual neuromuscular block induced by vecuronium. Br J Anaesth 1996; 76:565—6.

48. Teiria H, Rautoma P, Yli Hankala A. Effect of smoking on dose requirements for vecuronium. Br J Anaesth 1996;76:154—5.

49. Robertson WS, Shaikh J, Purdie DW. Mivacurium sensitivity in a patient heterozygous for the atypical and silent genes for plasma cholinesterase. Ann Clin Biochem 1995;32:431—3.

50. Ostergaard D, Jensen FS, Skovgaard LT, Viby Mogensen J. Dose-response relationship for mivacurium in patients with phenotypically abnormal plasma cholinesterase activity. Acta Anaesthesiol Scand 1995;39:1016—18.

51. Viby Mogensen J. Mivacurium block in patients with abnormal plasma cholinesterase. Acta Anaesthesiol Scand 1995;39:1001—2.

52. Ostergaard D, Kristensen RW, Bang U, Pedersen NA, Viby Mogensen J. Influence of bambuterol on the pharmacokinetics and pharmacodynamics of mivacurium. Anesthesiology 1995; 83:A899.

53. Bang U, Viby Mogensen J, Wiren JE, Skovgaard LT. The effect of bambuterol (carbamylated terbutaline) on plasma cholinesterase activity and suxamethonium-induced neuromuscular blockade in genotypically normal patients. Acta Anaesthesiol Scand 1990;34:596—9.

54. Naguib M, el Dawlatly AA, Ashour M, al Bunyan M. Sensitivity to mivacurium in a patient with mitochondrial myopathy. Anesthesiology 1996;84:1506—9.

55. Parmar M, Scott RP. Mivacurium chloride and late onset congenital myopathy. Br J Anaesth 1996;76:160—2.

56. De Wolf AM, Freeman JA, Scott VL, Tullock W, Smith DA, Kisor DF, Kerls S, Cook DR. Pharmacokinetics and pharmacodynamics of cisatracurium in patients with end-stage liver disease undergoing liver transplantation. Br J Anaesth 1996;76:624—8.

57. Azouvi P, Mane M, Thiebaut JB, Denys P, Remy Neris O, Bussel B. Intrathecal baclofen administration for control of severe spinal spasticity: functional improvement and long-term follow-up. Arch Phys Med Rehabil 1996;77:35—9.

58. Mertens P, Parise M, Garcia Larrea L, Benneton C, Millet MF, Sindou M. Long-term clinical, electrophysiological and urodynamic effects of chronic intrathecal baclofen infusion for treatment of spinal spasticity. Acta Neurochir Suppl Wien 1995;64:17—25.

59. Naveira FA, Speight KL, Rauck RL, Carpenter RL. Meningitis after injection of intrathecal baclofen. Anesth Analg 1996;82:1297—9.

60. Byrnes SM, Watson GW, Hardy PA. Flumazenil: an unreliable antagonist in baclofen overdose. Anaesthesia 1996;51:481—2.

61. Spiller HA, Winter ML, Mann KV, Borys DJ, Muir S, Krenzelok EP. Five-year multicenter retrospective review of cyclobenzaprine toxicity. J Emerg Med 1995;13:781—5.

62. Borodic G, Johnson E, Goodnough M, Schantz E. Botulinum toxin therapy, immunologic resistance, and problems with available materials. Neurology 1996;46:26—9.

63. Tuite PJ, Lang AE. Severe and prolonged dysphagia complicating botulinum toxin A injections for dystonia in Machado-Joseph disease. Neurology 1996;46:846.

64. Holzer SE, Ludlow CL. The swallowing side effects of botulinum toxin type A injection in spasmodic dysphonia. Laryngoscope 1996;106:86—92.

65. Boyd RN, Britton TC, Robinson RO, Borzyskowski M. Transient urinary incontinence after botulinum A toxin. Lancet 1996;348:481—2.

66. Mezaki T, Kaji R, Kohara N, Kimura J. Development of general weakness in a patient with amyotrophic lateral sclerosis after focal botulinum toxin injection. Neurology 1996;46:845—6.

Michael Schachter

13 Drugs affecting autonomic functions or the extrapyramidal system

DRUGS ACTING ON ADRENOCEPTORS *(SED-13, 348; SEDA-17, 161; SEDA-18, 158; SEDA-19, 147)*

The many drugs that may cause *hypertension* have been reviewed ([1][R]). The sympathomimetic drugs form one major class of possible culprits, including ephedrine and pseudoephedrine, phenylpropanolamine, and phenylephrine; other related drugs, such as oxymetazoline, are also mentioned.

DRUGS STIMULATING BOTH α- AND β-ADRENOCEPTORS

Isoprenaline (isoproterenol) *(SED-13, 353)*

A 34-year-old Japanese man, who was being investigated for two syncopal and several near-syncopal episodes suffered a severe *vasovagal episode* during an infusion of isoproterenol, even without upright tilting ([2][c]). The authors pointed out that in such susceptible patients, reduced venous return may not be a prerequisite for a vasovagal response.

DRUGS PREDOMINANTLY STIMULATING β₁-ADRENOCEPTORS

Dobutamine *(SED-13, 354; SEDA-17, 163; SEDA-18, 158)*

The problem of *hypotension* during dobutamine stress echocardiography has been discussed in two reports. A group from Duke University studied over 100 patients undergoing this procedure; 15 had a significant hypotensive response ([3][c]). The authors concluded that this was not due to dynamic intraventricular obstruction, as has been proposed, but they did find a significant positive association with baseline systolic blood pressure. In the other study, 12 of 59 patients developed significant hypotension during dobutamine stress echocardiography ([4][c]). The authors suggested that several hemodynamic mechanisms may be responsible, alone or in combination, including impaired systolic reserve, reduced left ventricular filling time, and reflex bradycardia.

DRUGS PREDOMINANTLY STIMULATING β₂-ADRENOCEPTORS

It is well established that inhalation of bronchodilators, such as salbutamol, can produce significant plasma concentrations. In an Australian study of the effect of nebulized salbutamol in 12 children, mean age 5 years, there was a significant *rise in plasma glucose concentrations* from about 6 to 9 mmol/l, approximately in parallel with plasma salbutamol concentrations (5^C). The authors did not regard this as clinically significant, except as an indirect means of assessing previous β-agonist exposure and dosage. However, one would expect responses to be too variable to make this realistic.

Apart from bronchodilatation, the other major clinical indication for the β_2-agonists is in attempting to arrest premature labor. In a review of a series of over 8700 women treated with low-dose subcutaneous terbutaline the authors concluded that the incidence of cardiopulmonary adverse effects is well below 1%, and that in nearly half of these, other concurrent therapies may have contributed (6^{CR}). *Pulmonary edema* was the most common adverse effect, occurring in 0.32% of the study population. Understandably, the authors concluded that this is a very safe procedure, especially when compared with intravenous administration of the β_2-agonists.

The potential hazards of long-term bronchodilator therapy in patients with chronic obstructive pulmonary disease (COPD) have been considered in two reviews (7^R), (8^R). In the first of these, which focuses largely if not exclusively on asthma, the view that continuous bronchodilator therapy is potentially harmful in asthmatics has been supported. The authors recommended that patients should be instructed to inform their physicians if they need to use a short-acting bronchoilator more than once a day. However, the author of the second review has come to a different conclusion, although not of course for a strictly comparable population of patients. He has noted that there is much less information concerning patients with COPD but has suggested that the β_2-agonists can be used safely and effectively in these patients. In contrast, he doubts the value of adding inhaled steroids in such patients if they are taking optimal doses of bronchodilators such as the β_2-agonists and ipratropium, a view that is contrary to most current expert opinion.

DRUGS ACTING ON DOPAMINE RECEPTORS
(SED-13, 355; SEDA-17, 166; SEDA-18, 159; SEDA-19, 148)

Levodopa

Abnormal sweating was described in Parkinsonian patients long before the introduction of levodopa. Subsequently, some observers have noted an increased incidence of severe whole-body sweating associated with response fluctuations, although there has been dispute as to whether these occurred mostly during on or off periods. Four patients with *drenching sweats* have been described (9^C). The authors concluded that this distressing symptom is definitely an off phenomenon. In all cases the sweating disappeared when levodopa was replaced with a dopamine receptor agonist. In two of the patients dopamine agonists caused hallucinations, leading to re-institution of levodopa and resumption of sweating.

Another relatively little studied aspect of the levodopa on-off phenomenon is *fluctuation in mood*. In an uncontrolled study of 15 patients with motor fluctuations, improvement in mood and reduction in anxiety somewhat preceded the motor response to a levodopa infusion (10^C). The authors suggested that on the one hand depressed mood and increased anxiety may enhance motor disability, while on the other hand the mood-elevating effect of the drugs may encourage excessive self-administration, as previously reported (11^c).

There has been long-standing controversy concerning the optimal time for starting levodopa in Parkinsonian patients. Of two recent contributors, one favors delay, especially in younger patients, in whom response fluctuations and dyskinesias may occur sooner and in a more severe form (12^R). However, the other has contended that there is no evidence that this is a problem and can see no valid reason for delaying treatment (13^R). This issue is still far from being resolved.

OTHER DRUGS INCREASING DOPAMINE ACTIVITY

Amantadine *(SED-13, 357; SEDA-17, 170; SEDA-18, 160)*

Livedo reticularis is a common adverse effect in Parkinsonian patients treated with amantadine, though it is rarely very troublesome. A syndrome characterized by *livedo reticularis* and *multiple ischemic strokes* has been described, and this has subsequently been associated with the presence of *antiphospholipid antibodies* (14[C]). Of 24 patients taking amantadine 100—200 mg/day for at least 3 months, 14 had some evidence of livedo reticularis and five of these had antiphospholipid antibodies (15[c]). However, seven patients without skin symptoms also had antiphospholipid antibodies. In fact, there is no evidence for any increase in the risk of thrombotic episodes in patients taking amantadine, whether or not they develop livedo, and the authors very reasonably concluded that the occurrence of this adverse effect should not necessarily lead to withdrawal of the drug.

THE ERGOT ALKALOIDS AND RELATED DRUGS *(SED-13, 366; SEDA-17, 170; SEDA-18, 160)*

Yet another case report has emphasized the dangers of excessive use of ergotamine (16[c]). In this instance a 53-year-old woman developed severe *ischemia in one foot*; fortunately, there was a good response to heparin and chemical sympathectomy.

AGENTS WITH ANTICHOLINERGIC EFFECTS
(SED-13, 369; SEDA-17, 173; SEDA-18, 160; SEDA-19, 148)

Terodiline, a drug with antimuscarinic and calcium antagonist properties, has been used for the treatment of urinary incontinence associated with detrusor muscle instability. However, it was withdrawn in the UK in 1991 because of reports of drug-related *prolongation of the electrocardiographic QT interval* and cardiac dysrhythmias, notably *torsade de pointes*. A retrospective analysis of data from 19 patients has shown that the effect on the QT interval is dose-related (17[C]). The authors commented that terodiline has structural similarities to prenylamine, an antianginal drug previously shown to have prodysrhythmic properties, so that such problems should not have been wholly unexpected.

Interactions   Seven patients taking benztropine and one of the *selective serotonin re-uptake inhibitors* all developed delirium (18[C]). However, this observation elicited a report of a series of 14 patients taking fluoxetine and benztropine in whom this adverse effect was entirely absent (19[c]). In a reply appended to this observation the authors of the first paper pointed out that their own patients had been significantly older and therefore more vulnerable to delirium. In any case, clinicians who administer such combinations need to exercise some caution, especially in elderly patients, until the extent and nature of this problem become clearer.

REFERENCES

1.   Clyburn EB, DiPette DJ. Hypertension induced by drugs and other substances. Semin Nephrol 1995;15:72—86.

2.   Shihara M, Harasawa Y, Ando S-I, Mohri M, Takeshita A. Isoproterenol infusion provokes vasovagal response without upright tilt in a patient exhibiting syncopal episodes. Heart Vessels 1995;10:279—82.

3.   Heinle SK, Tice FD, Kisslo J. Hypotension during dobutamine stress echocardiography: is it related to dynamic intraventricular obstruction? Am Heart J 1995;130:314—17.

4.   Tanimoto M, Pai RG, Jintapakorn W, Shah PM. Mechanisms of hypotension during dobutamine stress echocardiography in patients with coronary artery disease. Am J Cardiol 1995;76:26—30.

5.   Dawson KP, Penna AC, Manglick P. Acute asthma, salbutamol and hyperglycaemia. Acta Paediatr 1995;84:305—7.

6.   Perry KG, Morrison JC, Rust OA, Sullivan CA, Martin RW, Naef RW. Incidence of adverse cardiopulmonary effects with low-dose terbutaline infusion. Am J Obstet Gynecol 1995;173:1273–7.

7.   van Schayck CP, Cloosterman SGM, Hofland ID, ven Herwaarden CLA, van weel C. How detrimental is chronic use of bronchodilators in asthma and chronic obstructive pulmonary disease? Am J Respir Crit Care Med 1995;151:1317–19.

8.   Ziment I. The agonist controversy. Impact in COPD. Chest 1995;107 Suppl:198S–205S.

9.   Sage JI, Mark MH. Drenching sweats as an off phenomenon in Parkinson's disease: treatment and relation to plasma levodopa profile. Ann Neurol 1995;37:120–2.

10.   Maricle RA, Nutt JG, Carter JH. Mood and anxiety fluctuation in Parkinson's disease associated with levodopa infusion: preliminary findings. Mov Disord 1995;10:329–32.

11.   Soyka M, Huppert D. L-dopa abuse in a patient with former alcoholism. Br J Addict 1992;87:117–18.

12.   Quinn NP. A case against early levodopa treatment of Parkinson's disease. Clin Neuropharmacol 1995;18 Suppl 3:S43–9.

13.   Caraceni T. A case for early levodopa treatment of Parkinson's disease. Clin Neuropharmacol 1995;18 Suppl 3:S38–42.

14.   Levine SR, Langer SL, Albers JW, Welch KM. Sneddon's syndrome: an antiphospholipid antibody syndrome? Neurology 1988;38:798–800.

15.   Paulson GW, Brandt JT. Amantadine, livedo reticularis, and antiphospholipid antibodies. Clin Neuropharmacol 1995;18:4667.

16.   Paraskevopoulos JA, Teasdale DE, Cuschieri RJ. Severe reversible arterial spasm with ergotamine. Br J Clin Pract 1995;49:214.

17.   Thomas SHL, Higham PD, Hartigan-Go K, Kamali F, Wood P, Campbell RWF, Ford GA. Concentration dependent cardiotoxicity of terodiline in patients treated for urinary incontinence. Br Heart J 1995;74:53–6.

18.   Roth A, Akyol S, Nelson JC. Delirium associated with the combination of a neuroleptic, an SSRI, and benztropine. J Clin Psychiatry 1994;55:492–5.

19.   Rothschild AJ. Delirium: an SSRI-benztropine adverse effect? J Clin Psychiatry 1995;56:537.

Anton C. de Groot

14 Dermatological drugs, topical agents, and cosmetics

℞ Contact allergy to fragrances

Perfumes are so much a part of our culture that we take them for granted, but if they were suddenly taken from us, society would suffer immeasurably. We do pay a price for their use, and part of that concerns adverse dermatological and other medical reactions. Adverse reactions include allergic contact dermatitis, irritant dermatitis, photocontact dermatitis, immediate contact reactions (contact urticaria), and pigmented cosmetic dermatitis. Here I shall discuss only allergic contact dermatitis. Reactions to fragrances have been reviewed elsewhere (1[R]), (2[R]), (3[r]).

What are fragrances? *Fragrances may be of natural origin (balsams, essential oils, concretes/absolutes) or synthetic. Natural fragrances are of botanical origin, with few exceptions (animal products such as musk, ambergris, civet, and castoreum, which can also be produced synthetically nowadays). A natural fragrance contains several hundred different chemicals, a few major and many minor ones, which are responsible for the complexity of the odor.*

Balsams are viscous, colored, and aromatic plant products soluble in alcohol but not in water. They are obtained from the exudate of trees by incising the bark. Balsams with a characteristic odor can be obtained from trees that are rich in resins, for example, balsam of Peru, balsam of Tolu, storax, galbanum, myrrh, and benzoin.

Essential oils come from a limited number of animals and from many different plants, and they can be synthesized from two fossil fuels (coal and petroleum). Essential oils can

become gaseous at room temperature; because they volatilize so easily, they are also known as volatile oils. There are five classic methods of extracting essential oils from plants and flowers: distillation, extraction, enfleurage, maceration, and expression (4), (5). Examples of essential oils obtained by stem distillation of various plant raw materials, such as blossoms, leaves, and fruits of flowers, are oils of roses, laurel, and lavender; from the wood and roots of trees come cedarwood oil and sandalwood oil.

Concretes or absolutes are obtained by solvent extraction of plant materials (which for absolutes is alcohol), with evaporation of the solvent. Materials manufactured in this way are subject to less change during their preparation than those that are distilled.

Synthetic fragrances are well-defined chemical compounds with simple odors.

Until the nineteenth century, fragrances were manufactured from essential oils and alcohol extracts of plant origin. Nowadays, synthetic chemicals are far often more used for reasons of cost, purity, compatibility, and quality control; they may account for as much as 90% of the composition of a perfume. The history of fragrances has been well described (4), (5).

The blending of a perfume *(4), (6) Perfumery is the art of making people and products attractive to the nose. Specific fragrances must be designed for individual products, as compatibility is essential and the product ingredients may affect the odor. These products may also be designed for a particular price range, which often determines the ingredients available to the perfumer. Among thousands of chemical substances that have an odor, about 3000 (of which 300—400 are of natural origin) are used in the fragrance industry.*

A perfume is a creative composition of fragrance materials, of which it may contain from

Side Effects of Drugs, Annual 20
J.K. Aronson, ed.

a few to over 300. On opening a bottle, the most volatile components or the 'top note' will be smelled. After 5—20 min the 'heart' or the 'body' of the perfume is perceptible. With a good perfume this heart will last for 2—4 h. What is left is the 'dry out', which will gradually disappear. There are distinct perfume materials that have a favorable influence on the perfume profile, tempering the top note, refining and extending the heart, and strengthening the dry out. Such materials are called 'fixatives' and include balsam of Peru, balsam of Tolu, storax, benzoin, coumarin, and musk.

Perfumes contain about 12—20% of the perfume compound. They are expensive and actually too concentrated. The more diluted products (perfume lotion, perfume de toilette, eau de toilette, colognes) are therefore much more popular. There are no legally defined concentrations of the perfume compounds for these products, but in general colognes will contain 2—5%, perfume lotion and perfume de toilette 5—8%. Most fragrance products are alcoholic solutions (70—96% ethanol), but perfume creams (sachets) and aerosols are also popular. Approximate concentrations of fragrance materials in cosmetics are 0.5% and in masking fragrances 0.1% or less.

Contact with fragrances and fragranced products   *The use of fragrances is ubiquitous and not limited to cosmetic products primarily used for their scent, such as perfumes, eaux de cologne, eaux de toilette, deodorants, and after-shave lotions. Virtually all cosmetics and toiletries contain fragrance materials; even 'unscented' or 'fragrance-free' products may contain a 'masking' perfume. Flavors used in oral hygiene products, toothpastes, mouthwashes, and dental flosses, are fragrance chemicals. Scented household products include detergents, cleaners, softeners, deodorizing sprays, polishes, solvents, and waxes. In industry, cutting fluids, electroplating fluids, paints, rubber, plastics, insecticides, herbicides, and additives used in air-conditioning water may all be scented. Eugenol is widely used by dentists. Paper and paper products, including diapers, facial tissues, moist toilet paper, and sanitary napkins may cause a reaction. Fabrics and clothes may contain fragrance materials, especially after they have been laundered or treated*

with a fabric softener. Topical drugs often contain perfumes, and ventilating systems may spread fragrances.

The distinction between fragrances and spices is often indistinct. Many synthetic fragrances are used as spices and flavours. Natural fragrances, such as cinnamon, clove, vanilla, and cardamom, are added to foods, soft drinks, lozenges, chewing gum, candies, ice cream, and tobacco.

Thus, it can be stated that everyone is in daily contact with fragrance materials.

Modes of contact   *Contact with fragrances may be from direct application of a product to the skin or mucous membranes (toothpaste, mouth-fresheners, feminine hygiene sprays, perfumed eyedrops), by occasional contact with an allergen-contaminated product, such as towels and pillows, contact with products used by partners, friends, or co-workers ('consort' or 'connubial' contact dermatitis), airborne contact, and systemic exposure by inhalation and ingestion (fragrances, flavors, and spices in foods and drinks, cough syrup).*

Sites of contact with fragrances   *Any part of the body may be in contact with fragranced cosmetics:*

- *the scalp: shampoo, hair lacquer, hair gel;*
- *the face: skin-care products, after-shave, perfumed tissue handkerchiefs, airborne from perfumes on clothing;*
- *the eyelids: eye cosmetics;*
- *the lips: lipstick, tooth-paste;*
- *the neck: after-shave, perfume;*
- *the trunk: body lotion;*
- *the axillae: deodorants and antiperspirants;*
- *the arms and legs: body lotion;*
- *the perianal area: fragranced (moistened) toilet tissue;*
- *the vulvar area: feminine hygiene sprays, sanitary napkins, topical drugs;*
- *the hands: moisturizing creams, soap;*
- *the feet: scented antiperspirants.*

Epidemiology of adverse reactions to fragrances in cosmetics and toiletries   *Adverse reactions to fragrances and fragranced cosmetics are far from rare. In a questionnaire study in 90 student nurses, 29 (32%) gave a history of cutaneous fragrance intolerance (7). When patch* tested with the 'fragrance mix' (a composition of eight commonly used fragrances to identify subjects with fragrance allergy), 15/90 (18%) gave a positive reaction. Of these 15, 12 (80%) had a positive history of fragrance sensitivity. Of the nurses with a negative patch test reaction, only 21% considered themselves to be fragrance sensitive.

Of 1609 adult subjects who were interviewed, 196 (12%) reported reactions to various kinds of cosmetics and toiletries in the preceding 5 years (8); 69 of these (35% of the reactors and 4.3% of the total population) attributed their reactions to products primarily used for their smell (45 deodorants, 16 after-shaves, and 8 perfumes).

The Medical Product Agency introduced a cosmetic control system in Sweden in 1989. Between 1989 and 1994, 191 reports of cosmetic adverse effects were evaluated (9). The majority of adverse effects involved only the skin, and 90% were eczematous reactions. Of the cases of dermatitis, 70% were classified as allergic. Patch testing with cosmetic ingredients showed that fragrances were the leading cause (22/79 positive reactions). Considering the extensive use of balsams, fragrances, spices, and flavor additives to food, the frequency of contact allergy to these groups of materials is relatively low. In absolute numbers, however, fragrance allergy is common. The prevalence in patients with dermatitis seen by dermatologists is high; in most countries the fragrance mix is among the 'Top five' allergens, usually number two after nickel sulfate, and yields 6—11% of positive reactions.

Indeed, fragrances are common causes of allergic contact dermatitis. At least 35% of all allergic reactions to cosmetics are due to perfume ingredients (10). In studies of contact allergy to cosmetic products, perfumes account for 4—18% of all reactions, and deodorants/antiperspirants cause 5—17% of all cases of allergic contact dermatitis (11). This may actually be an underestimate of the real importance of fragrance sensitivity. People rarely consult a dermatologist with a rash caused by perfume, toilet water, cologne, or deodorant. When they do get a rash the culprit is usually obvious, and they simply stop using the fragrance on their skin.

Even in the general population, fragrance sensitivity is not rare. In Denmark, 567 un-

selected individuals aged 15—69 years were tested with the fragrance mix (TRUE-test system), and six (1.1%) had a positive reaction (12). The frequency in men (1.1%) was identical to that in women (1.0%). In men, shaving with a razor is said to increase the risk of becoming sensitized by fragrances by a factor of three, possibly by creating small cuts in the skin, facilitating penetration of perfumes derived from soaps, shaving foams, and after-shave lotions (13).

Clinical features   In spite of daily contact of virtually everybody with fragrances, and despite the high frequency of positive patch test reactions to the fragrance mix in patients routinely tested for suspected contact dermatitis, literature on the clinical features of perfume dermatitis is scant. In not a single study in which the fragrance mix has been routinely used have the clinical features of patients with positive reactions to the mix been described and compared with contact dermatitis in patients who have not been sensitized to fragrances.

It can be expected, however, that the neck, the skin behind the ear, and the axillae will often be affected, since those areas are commonly exposed to products with high concentrations of fragrances (perfumes, deodorants). Also, the sensitive skin of the face and the eyelids is particularly susceptible to developing allergic contact dermatitis to fragrances in skin-care products, decorative cosmetics, and cleansing preparations, and from airborne contact. Micro-trauma from shaving facilitates (photo)-contact allergy to after-shave fragrances (13). Indeed, among 167 patients with suspect fragrance allergy the face was most frequently affected (40%) (14).

Of 28 patients with fragrance sensitivity 12 were sensitized to perfumes or perfumed products, five to perfumes in topical drugs, and seven to both; in four the relevance was uncertain (15). One patient had pruritus on the eyelids without a rash from fragrance sprayed on her clothes. Several had allergic contact dermatitis on the face and chest. Most of these were erythematous. In some cases the eruption resembled nummular eczema, seborrheic dermatitis, sycosis barbae, or lupus erythematosus. More acute lesions with papules, vesicles, and oozing may sometimes occur. Lesions in the *skin folds may be mistaken for atopic dermatitis. Dermatitis due to perfumes or toilet water tends to be 'streaky'. Facial psoriasis may be induced or aggravated by allergic contact dermatitis from fragrances.*

Eczema of the hands is common in fragrance-sensitive patients. In 54 patients who were sensitive to the fragrance mix, the hands were most often affected (41%), followed by the face (25%), diffuse (17%), axillae (9%), and legs (4%) (16). In another study, the hands were also the most frequently affected in patients with suspected allergic cosmetic fragrance dermatitis (17). Indeed, patients with eczema of the hands have an odds ratio of 2.6 of being sensitized to the fragrance mix, compared with patients without dermatitis of the hands but dermatitis elsewhere (18). This may be explained by contact with fragranced cosmetics and toiletries (soap, shampoo, hand cream), perfumed topical drugs, perfumed household products, flavoring materials used in the kitchen, and vegetable foods. Fragrances are probably rarely the sole cause of hand eczema, including occupational cases. Usually, patients first have irritant dermatitis or atopic dermatitis, which is later complicated by contact allergy to products used for treatment (fragranced topical drugs) or prevention (hand creams and lotions) of dermatitis of the hands, or to other perfumed products in the household, hobby, or work environment. Atopic dermatitis located at other body sites (for example, perianal dermatitis and vulvar dermatitis) may also be complicated by fragrance allergy.

Diagnosis *Contact allergy to fragrances is diagnosed with patch tests. The European standard series, which is routinely used in all patients suspected of allergic contact dermatitis, contains three 'markers' or 'indicators' for fragrance sensitivity: the fragrance mix, balsam of Peru, and colophony (rosin). The fragrance mix contains eight commonly used fragrance materials: eugenol, isoeugenol, oak moss, geraniol, hydroxycitronellal, α-amylcinnamic aldehyde, cinnamic aldehyde, and cinnamic alcohol. It has been estimated that this mix detects 70–80% of all cases of fragrance allergy; the frequency of positive reactions varies between 6 and 11%. In most studies, the fragrance mix is number two in the 'Top five' of*

frequent allergens after nickel sulfate. Of the ingredients of the mix, oak moss (a natural fragrance often used in after-shave lotions), isoeugenol, and cinnamic alcohol cause reactions most often.

Although the fragrance mix is extremely valuable, it has some disadvantages. Of all fragrance-sensitive subjects 20–30% remain undetected. Furthermore, both false-positive and false-negative reactions are not rare. To solve these problems, many investigators have tried to improve the mix, thus far with very little result. With the possible exception of citral, dihydrocoumarin, and possibly some essential oils (ylang-ylang oil, narcissus oil, sandalwood oil), no suitable new candidates for the fragrance mix have been identified, and the ingredients of the mix have remained the same for over 15 years. In addition to the European Standard Series and possibly a series of individual fragrances (over 50 of which are commercially available), the patient's contact materials (work, home, hobby) should always be patch tested. Products with higher concentrations of fragrances (perfume, deodorant, aftershave, eau de toilette) often induce positive reactions. When a fragranced product is highly suspect, but patch tests remain negative, a ROAT (Repeated Open Application Test) can then be performed: the suspected product is applied to the antecubital fossa twice daily for 1–2 weeks. When the patient is allergic, a positive reaction with itching, erythema, and papules will be observed within several days to 2 weeks. This test cannot be used for detergent-containing products, such as soap, shampoo, and cleaning products.

A positive patch test reaction should be followed by evaluation of its relevance. Often, however, no clear relation to the clinical symptoms can be found, and many fragrance-sensitive patients can tolerate the use of fragranced products. Possible explanations for this are:

- *the 'positive' reaction to the mix and/or the product were actually false-positive;*
- *the products used either do not contain the fragrances to which the patient is allergic, or are present in concentrations too low to cause clinically visible reactions;*
- *as the perfume ages, the allergen may become inactivated.*

It is assumed that at least 55—65% of positive reactions to the mix are relevant to the patient's complaints.

Contact allergy to other fragrances *Many investigators have presented the results of routine testing of certain fragrances. The relevance of positive reactions has often remained uncertain. The frequency of such reactions depends on the population tested, the country, and the allergens investigated. Fragrances that regularly cause allergic reactions include benzyl salicylate, citral, coumarin, dihydrocoumarin, hydroabietyl alcohol, jasmine (absolute/synthetic), lilial, methyl salicylate, and ylang-ylang oil. A total of 95 (well-defined) fragrance materials and 70 essential oils have been described as contact allergens (1[R]).*

ORAL PHOTOCHEMOTHERAPY (PUVA) *(SED-13, 380; SEDA-17, 182; SEDA-18, 166; SEDA-19, 154)*

A very helpful review article on PUVA for psoriasis, including a large section on adverse reactions, has recently been published (19[R]).

PUVA and follicular mycosis fungoides It is well-known that plaques of mycosis fungoides react more intensively by an inflammatory response to PUVA treatment than normal skin.

A 22-year-old man had rather inconspicuous, discrete, hypopigmented lesions on both legs, which had developed during the preceding 2 years (20[Cr]). The lesions then generalized and transformed into erythematous infiltrated and scaly plaques. Alopecia and follicular keratoses finally occurred. Several biopsies, including immunopathology, confirmed the diagnosis of mycosis fungoides. Topical corticosteroids combined with oral photochemotherapy (PUVA) were started. PUVA therapy induced a strong flare-up with erythema, scaling, and burning. In addition, new lesions were unmasked, revealing a much more extensive skin involvement than had been suspected on clinical inspection before therapy. Nevertheless, PUVA was continued, and several weeks later the alopecia and erythematous infiltrates were markedly improved and almost disappeared.

The mechanisms responsible for this inflammatory reaction are unknown, but are likely to involve the release of inflammatory mediators by T cells infiltrating the upper dermis or epidermis after photochemotherapy.

Generalized exanthematous pustulosis *(SEDA-16, 151)* Acute generalized exanthematous pustulosis is usually caused by drugs, notably antibiotics.

A 22-year-old man was treated with hydroxychloroquine and PUVA for actinic pseudolymphoma. Two days after a PUVA session, pustular erythema developed on the trunk, limited to the UVA-exposed areas. Curiously, the eruption did not involve the areas on which a phototest had been performed 1 month before. The lesions resolved rapidly after withdrawal of hydroxychloroquine and PUVA.

Photo-induced acute generalized exanthematous pustulosis with a photo-distribution has not been reported previously. The authors ascribed the reaction to the combination of hydroxychloroquine with PUVA (21[Cr]).

Verruciform xanthoma developing during PUVA therapy Verruciform xanthoma is a rare lesion that occurs primarily on the oral mucosa, the vulva, scrotum, penis, and digits. Although its cause is unknown, it has been suggested that repeated epidermal and/or dermal damage gives rise to a reactive process that involves the formation of lipid-laden cells or xanthoma cells by leakage of lipoproteins from small blood vessels. A 63-year-old man with psoriasis vulgaris developed verruciform xanthoma on the scrotum during PUVA therapy. Although it is uncertain whether the lesion was caused by PUVA, the authors speculated that UV light may be one of the causative factors that triggers verruciform xanthoma, as such lesions have been observed in sun-exposed areas (22[Cr]).

RETINOIDS *(SED-13, 382; SEDA-17, 183; SEDA-18, 168; SEDA-19, 156)*

Musculoskeletal Toxicity has proven a significant problem with long-term administration of retinoids. Bone abnormalities that mimic seronegative spondyloarthropathy or diffuse idiopathic skeletal hyperostoses have often been described, as have rheumatological complications, such as arthritis, myopathy, and vasculitis (Table 1). Rheumatological complications of vitamin A and the retinoids have been well reviewed (23[R]).

Extensive *spinal hyperostoses* were observed in a 31-year-old man after long-term treatment with retinoids for pityriasis rubra pilaris (24[Cr]). The most prominent abnormality was a bridging exostosis between the left acetabulum and collum. X-ray examinations of the spine during retinoid treatment showed no abnormalities. The authors stressed that a normal spinal X-ray is no guarantee that a patient has no hyperostoses, and that it is important to ask the patient on a regular basis about skeletal pain or restriction of mobility.

Conversely, on the basis of animal experiments, the development of *osteopenia (osteoporosis)* might be anticipated, and has been reported (25). A cross-sectional study was designed to assess bone mineral density during long-term therapy with etretinate or isotretinoin in 24 patients using the standard techniques and single- and dual-photon absorptiometry (26[Cr]). They received 50 g or more of etretinate (15 patients) or isotretinoin (nine patients) for 2 years or more. Compared with age-, sex-, and weight-matched controls, the bone mineral density of the etretinate group was significantly reduced at four of the five measurement sites: the femoral neck (91%), Ward's triangle (88%), the trochanter (88%), and the radius (85%). In contrast, the bone mineral densities in the isotretinoin group did not differ from control values, except for an increase in the lumbar spine. The authors concluded that long-term treatment with etretinate causes osteoporosis. No such effect was observed for isotretinoin. However, the isotretinoin-treated patients were younger and were treated for a shorter period than the etretinate-treated patients. Therefore, the authors stated that it is uncertain whether longer periods of exposure to isotretinoin will lead to osteoporosis. Short-term treatment with (low-dose) isotretinoin 0.4 mg/kg/day for 6 months did not result in osteoporosis of the lumbar spine in 15 men with severe acne (27[Cr]). However, even etretinate did not cause osteoporosis at this particular site (26[Cr]), which may indicate that the lumbar spine is not the optimal anatomical location to look for retinoid-induced osteoporosis.

Acitretin

Liver   *Hepatitis* caused by acitretin and etretinate has been reported (28[Cr]) but is not common (SEDA-17, 183; (29[CR])). Single cases of acitretin-induced hepatic injury, including pseudoallergic hepatitis (after a single dose of 10 mg acitretin) (30[C]) and worsening of hepatitis A (31[C]) have been reported recently.

Teratogenicity *(SEDA-17, 185)* Retinoids are teratogens, and women should avoid pregnancy during treatment or for a period of 2 years after discontinuation of acitretin. However, in some women retinoids can still be demonstrated in fat over 2 years after discontinuation of etretinate and/or acitretin. A negative finding in the plasma does not rule out the possibility that retinoids are still pre-

Table 1.   *Rheumatological complications of retinoids (23[R])*

Bone abnormalities	*Other rheumatological manifestations*
SNSA-like abnormalities	*Arthropathies*
Hyperostoses (24[Cr])	Arthralgias
DISH	Arthritis (77[Cr]) (SEDA-18, 168)
Extraspinal calcifications	Gout
Costochondritis	
Enthesopathy (76[c])	*Muscle abnormalities*
	Myalgia
Other bone changes	Increased muscle rigidity
Periostal bone resorption	Myopathy
Osteoporosis (25[Cr]), (26[Cr])	
Slender long bones	*Vasculitis*
Premature epiphyseal plate closure	Erythema nodosum
	Wegener's granulomatosis
	Leukocytoclastic vasculitis

Abbrevations: DISH, diffuse idiopathic skeletal hyperostosis; SNSA, seronegative spondyloarthropathy.

sent in fatty tissues, thus representing a potential teratogenic hazard. In consequence, it may be prudent in women who used to take acitretin/etretinate to look for retinoids in plasma and/or fatty tissues. The latter can be demonstrated in specimens taken by means of a punch biopsy of the skin and subcutaneous fat of the buttocks (32[r]), (33).

Etretinate

The results of a 5-year prospective study of a cohort of 956 patients with psoriasis treated with etretinate, in which the frequency and nature of adverse events were assessed, have been published (28[Cr]). There was no evidence of increased risks of cardiovascular disease, cancer, diabetes, or inflammatory bowel disease in association with long-term etretinate. Although some patients reported that *joint problems* improved with etretinate, a greater number associated its use with joint problems. It was concluded that with proper patient selection and monitoring long-term etretinate therapy (up to 4 years) does not appear to be accompanied by a substantial increased risk of major adverse effects.

Isotretinoin

Respiratory Eosinophilic pleural effusion has been linked to isotretinoin treatment (SED-13, 383). *Eosinophilic pneumonia* developed in a 19-year-old man 2 months after he started to take isotretinoin for acne. His symptoms rapidly disappeared after withdrawal and administration of corticosteroids. The authors suggested that isotretinoin was the primary initiating factor in this case (34[Cr]).

Psychiatric There have been several reports suggesting that isotretinoin may cause *depression*, with features similar to hypervitaminosis A. The feeling in dermatological circles is that the association is a tenuous one (35[R]), even though suicides have been described in young people taking retinoids (36[C]). Three patients taking isotretinoin for acne consulted a psychiatrist for depression (37[c]). None had a family history or a previous history. They had depression of varying chronicity, with the particular features of anergy, headache, irritability, and agitation. All said that symptoms had begun during a period of treatment with isotretinoin. One woman had discontinued treatment 5 months before attending, but in the other two there was a marked recovery in terms of mood after stopping isotretinoin. Two patients had been actively suicidal, but these feelings disappeared with antidepressant drug treatment. The authors, both psychiatrists, felt that there may well be a specific syndrome that develops in some young people who are taking isotretinoin, and warned that the effect of this psychological change may be life-threatening.

Endocrine, metabolic It is well known that the number and size of *epidermal cysts* can be increased with isotretinoin treatment.

A 23-year-old woman developed an asymptomatic anterior cervical mass during treatment with isotretinoin (38[c]). This involuted shortly after withdrawal. Two years later, when her acne recurred, she started to take isotretinoin again. Two months later in the second treatment, she noted a recurrence of the mass. This was surgically removed and proved to be a thyroglossal cyst.

The authors, while admitting that the mechanism of action remains speculative, suggested that isotretinoin could have revealed the presence of this thyroglossal cyst.

Skin and appendages A 17-year-old man developed *pemphigus vulgaris*, with typical clinical, histopathological, and immunopathological features and circulating antibodies, during isotretinoin therapy. Isotretinoin was immediately withdrawn, and azathioprine and prednisolone were given. The skin lesions improved within 3 weeks, and there was complete recovery within 3 months. The improvement in antibody titres was also quick, and they became negative about 6 months after the disease had started. One year later, the patient had no signs of pemphigus and the antibody titre was negative. A causal association between isotretinoin and the development of pemphigus in this case is highly likely (39[C]).

Overdosage In humans, acute hypervitaminosis A has been primarily described in the Inuit after ingestion of polar-bear meat or seal liver, known to be very rich in vitamin A.

Table 2. *Allergic reactions to antifungal imidazoles* (41[R])

Phenylethyl imidazoles	Number of cases of allergy
Econazole	37
Enilconazole	1
Isoconazole	22
Ketoconazole	6
Miconazole	51
Oxiconazole	4
Sulconazole	13
Tioconazole	33

Phenylmethyl imidazoles	Number of cases of allergy
Bifonazole	1
Clotrimazole	13
Croconazole	12

Increased intracranial pressure, drowsiness, weakness, loss of appetite, dizziness, nausea, and *vomiting* have been observed in the hours after intoxication. Later, *dryness of the mucosa, skin desquamation, cheilitis,* and *loss of hair* occurred. Other adverse effects included *edema, bone pain,* and *hepatosplenomegaly.* Laboratory tests showed *increased alkaline phosphatase, aspartate and alanine transaminases, serum lipids, and calcium.*

There have been four reported cases of (intentional) intoxication with isotretinoin. The toxicity of isotretinoin overdosage appears to be low, and symptoms are restricted to headache and mucocutaneous adverse effects (40[Cr]).

CONTACT ALLERGY (SED-13, 385; SEDA-17, 185; SEDA-18, 169; SEDA-19, 158)

Imidazoles used as antimycotic agents The literature up to 1994 on contact sensitivity to imidazoles has been reviewed (41[R]). Since they were first introduced in 1969, imidazoles have become the most widely used of all antifungal drugs in human and veterinary medicine. There are two main groups: phenylethyl imidazoles and the structurally different phenylmethyl imidazoles. The numbers of cases of contact allergy found in the literature are specified for each imidazole in Table 2. Contact allergy is relatively infrequent in view of their widespread use. The most common allergens are miconazole, econazole, tioconazole,

and isoconazole, but they are also the ones most commonly used. Croconazole sensitivity seems to occur only in the Far East, the only place in which it is marketed. Cross-sensitivity may occur between miconazole, econazole, and isoconazole; between sulconazole, miconazole, and econazole; and also between isoconazole and tioconazole. The test concentration and vehicle should be either 1% alcohol or 1% methyl ethyl ketone. With regard to therapeutic alternatives, patients who need antimycotic therapy and who are sensitive to phenylethyl imidazoles (except ketoconazole) can be advised to use ketoconazole, clotrimazole, bifonazole, or non-imidazole antifungals such as the allylamines (naftifine, terbinafine).

Kojic acid in skin-care products Kojic acid (5-hydroxy-2-(hydroxymethyl)-4-pyrone) is a fungal metabolic product that has been used as a skin-depigmenting agent in skin-care products in Japan since 1988. Of 220 women suspected of having cosmetic-related contact dermatitis, eight had used at least one skin care product containing kojic acid (42[Cr]). Of these, five had positive patch test reactions to aqueous kojic acid 1% and 5%. Controls were negative. The five kojic acid-sensitive patients developed facial dermatitis 1–12 months after application of the products containing kojic acid. Kojic acid is considered to have a high sensitizing potential.

Toothpastes

Most people in industrialized countries use toothpaste daily. Toothpastes contain:

- abrasive agents, used for cleaning the teeth and for removing discoloration;
- cleansing agents, to form foam and clean the teeth;
- binding agents, which give toothpaste suitable viscosity;
- flavourings;
- humectants, which keep toothpaste soft and prevent it from drying out;
- preservatives, which prevent the growth of microbes both in the toothpaste and in the mouth;
- colorings, which improve the appearance of toothpaste;
- fluoride salts, which prevent the formation of caries;

Table 3. *Ingredients in toothpastes that have caused contact allergic reactions (43[R])*

Acetamide
Aluminium
Anethole
Anise oil
Azulene
Benzoates
Caraway seed oil
Carvone
Chloroacetamide
Cinnamic aldehyde
Cinnamon (cassia) oil
Dichlorophene
Eugenol
Flavors (undefined or mixtures)
Fluorides
Formaldehyde
Guaiazulene
Herbs (undefined)
Hexylresorcinol
Laurel oil
Menthol
Orris root
Peppermint oil
Phenyl salicylate
Propolis
Spearmint oil
Thymol

- antiseptics and antacids, which reduce the sensitivity of the teeth;
- other agents, such as herb extracts.

The most common adverse effects of toothpastes are local effects, i.e. irritation and allergic reactions. The oral mucosa is more resistant to irritation than the skin, so that chemical irritation by toothpastes is rare. However, tartar-controlled toothpastes have been incriminated as a cause of irritant reactions. Fluorides in toothpastes have been reported to cause *acne-like eruptions*, *ulcerative stomatitis*, and *discoloration of the teeth*. Although toothpastes may contain several agents that have caused immediate contact reactions (balsam of Peru, menthol, cinnamic aldehyde), clinical reactions of immediate-type hypersensitivity have rarely been reported. Contact allergy to ingredients of toothpastes may cause *stomatitis, cheilitis, gingivitis, perioral dermatitis, ulceration, glossitis,* and *dermatitis* on the hand in which the toothbrush is held. Ingredients in toothpastes that have caused contact hypersensitivity reactions are shown in Table 3. The most common allergens in toothpaste are flavors (e.g., cinnamic

aldehyde, cinnamon oil, peppermint) and preservatives (43[R]).

Other contact allergens

Each year 'new' allergens (i.e. chemicals that have not previously been known to cause contact allergy) are described. These allergens and updated information on chemicals already known to be sensitizers in topical drugs and cosmetics are presented in Table 4.

MISCELLANEOUS

Topical drugs for psoriasis

The October 1995 issue of *Dermatologic Clinics* is devoted to psoriasis therapy and includes reviews on the adverse reactions of topical corticosteroids (71[R]), tars and anthralins (72[R]), and vitamin D3 analogs (73[R]).

Calcipotriol

A 50-year-old man developed a severe *headache* lasting for 3—4 hours, 15—20 min after applying calcipotriol ointment for psoriasis. After several days, he again applied the calcipotriol, and once more complained of headache. Such a reaction is extremely rare (74[c]).

Povidone-iodine A 25-year-old woman was referred for an abortion (75[C]). The vulva, vagina, and cervix were cleansed with povidone-iodine solution, and a menstrual aspiration progressed uneventfully. However, 10—15 min later, she developed periorbital edema, generalised pruritus, and urticaria over her abdomen and arms. Facial cyanosis and acrocyanosis, dyspnea, sweating, and faintness followed. Three weeks later, prick tests were negative to latex and a 1:10 dilution of the same povidone-iodine solution that had been used, but at full strength it caused urticaria and generalised pruritus. The clinical findings and test results established that povidone-iodine had caused *anaphylaxis* in this patient. This reaction has not been reported before. Whether the specific allergen was the povidone-iodine iodophor itself, elemental iodine, or polyvinylpyrrolidone (povidone) remained uncertain.

Table 4. *Contact allergy to ingredients of topical drugs and cosmetics*

Ingredient	Use	Concentration and vehicle	No.	Comments	Ref
Acetarsone	Trichomonacide	1% and 5% petrolatum	1	Systemic contact dermatitis from mucosal absorption	(44[Cr])
Anthrarobin	In Arning's tincture	1% and 10% petrolatum	1	Cross-reaction (?) to tincture of benzoin; first report of contact allergy; no controls; report possibly unreliable	(45[Cr])
Carboxyvinyl polymer	Increases viscosity in cosmetics	0.2% aqueous	1	First report of contact allergy; controls were negative	(46[Cr])
Cinchocaine	Anesthetic	5% petrolatum	1	Systemic contact dermatitis from mucosal absorption	(47[Cr])
Cinnoxicam	NSAID*	not tested	1	Diagnosis of allergy made by exclusion; dubious report	(48[c])
Clindamycin phosphate	Antibiotic	1% aqueous	1	Very rare contact allergen	(49[Cr])
Clotrimazole	Antifungal†	1% petrolatum	1	Very rare allergen; no cross-reactions	(50[Cr])
Cloxyquin (5-chloro-8-hydroxy-quinoline)	Antimicrobial	5% petrolatum	1	First report of contact allergy, possibly from cross-sentization to clioquinol	(51[Cr])
Colistin	Antibiotic	10—20% petrolatum	1	Very rare allergen	(52[Cr])
Cyclopiroxolamine	Antifungal	1% alcohol 40%	1	Very rare allergen	(53[Cr])
Dexpanthenol	Wound treatment	5% petrolatum	7	2/273 routinely tested patients with eczema were positive	(54[CR])
Dipropylene glycol	Solvent	10% aqueous	1	Only one reaction in 503 consecutive patients with eczema; relevance not established; test concentration slightly irritant; (see also SEDA-18, 172)	(55[Cr])
Eosin (tetra-bromofluorescein)	Dyestuff; antibacterial	1% petrolatum	1	Reactions to eosin are usually caused by an impurity	(56[CR])
Fenticonazole	Antifungal†	5% petrolatum	1		(57[c])
Hydroxyethyl salicylate	Anti-inflammatory; analgesic	1% petrolatum	1	First report of contact allergy; no controls, but report reliable; no cross-reactions to other salicylates; oral provocation with acetyl salicylic acid negative	(58[Cr])

Table 4.   *(Continued)*

Ingredient	Use	Concentration and vehicle	No.	Comments	Ref
Methyl glucose dioleate	Excipient in drugs and cosmetics	5% petrolatum	1	First report of contact allergy; 20 controls were negative	(59[C])
Mupirocin	Antibiotic	1% and 10% petrolatum	1	First report of contact allergy; no controls, but report reliable	(60[C])
Myristyl picolonium chloride	Preservative	1% petrolatum	1	Very rare allergen	(61[r])
Naftifine	Antifungal	5% alcohol	1	Allylamine antifungal	(62[Cr])
Piketoprofen	NSAID*	1% and 5% petrolatum	1	First report of contact allergy; five controls were negative; no cross-reactions to other NSAIDs	(63[C])
Retinoic acid	Anti-acne	0.05% petrolatum and alcohol	1	Test concentration used is irritant; dubious report	(64[c])
Sertaconazole	Antifungal†	1% and 5% petrolatum	1	First report of contact allergy; 20 controls were negative; cross-reactions to miconazole and econazole	(65[C])
Tacalcitol	Antipsoriatic	0.0002% alcohol	1	First report of contact allergy; no controls, but report reliable; cross-reaction to calcitriol	(66[Cr])
Thymol	Antibacterial	1% petrolatum	1	Rare contact allergen	(67[Cr])
Tiopronin (N-(2-mercapto-propionyl) glycine)	Aerosol mucolytic 'solution'	6.66 mg/ml	1	First report of contact allergy; six controls were negative	(68[Cr])
Tolnaftate	Antifungal	0.1% and 1% petrolatum	1	Rare allergen	(69[Cr])
Usnic acid	Antibacterial	1% petrolatum	1	Lichen acid, also used in fragrances	(70[Cr])

*For a review of the adverse effects of NSAIDs see SEDA-18, (pp. 163—5).
†See also (41[R]).

REFERENCES

1. De Groot AC, Frosch PJ. Adverse reactions to fragrances: a clinical review. Contact Dermatitis 1997;36:57—86.

2. De Groot AC, Frosch PJ. Fragrances as a cause of contact dermatitis in cosmetics: clinical aspects and epidemiological data. In: Frosch PJ, Johansen JD, White IR, editors. Fragrances-Beneficial and Adverse Effects. Heidelberg: Springer-Verlag, 1997:in press.

3. De Groot AC. Contactallergie voor parfumgrondstoffen in cosmetica en toiletartikelen. Ned Tijdschr Geneeskd 1997;141:571—4.

4. Guin JD. History, manufacture, and cutaneous reactions to perfumes. In: Frost P, Horwitz SW, editors. Principles of Cosmetics for the Dermatologist. St. Louis: The CV Mosby Company, 1982:111—29.

5. Scheinman PL. Allergic contact dermatitis to fragrance: a review. Am J Contact Dermatitis 1996;7:65—76.

6. Fisher T. Perfumed products. In: Guin JD, editor. Practical Contact Dermatitis. New York: McGraw-Hill, 1995:355−71.

7. Guin JD, Berry VK. Perfume sensitivity in adult females. A study of contact sensitivity to a perfume mix in two groups of student nurses. J Am Acad Dermatol 1980;3:299−302.

8. De Groot AC, Nater JP, van der Lende R, Rijcken B. Adverse effects of cosmetics: a retrospective study in the general population. Int J Cosmetic Sci 1987;9:255−9.

9. Berne B, Boström Å, Grahnén AF, Tammela M. Adverse effects of cosmetics and toiletries reported to the Swedish Medical Product Agency 1989-1994. Contact Dermatitis 1996;34:359−62.

10. Dooms-Goossens A, Kerre S, Drieghe J, Bossuyt L, Degreef H. Cosmetic products and their allergens. Eur J Dermatol 1992;2:465−8.

11. De Groot AC, Weyland JW, Nater JP. Unwanted Effects of Cosmetics and Drugs used in Dermatology, 3rd edn. Elsevier: Amsterdam, 1994:442−51.

12. Nielsen NH, Menné T. Allergic contact sensitization in an unselected Danish population. Acta Dermatol Venereol 1992;72:456−60.

13. Edman B. The influence of shaving method on perfume allergy. Contact Dermatitis 1994; 31:291−2.

14. Larsen W, Nakayama H, Lindberg M, Fischer T, Elsner P, Burrows D, Jordan W, Shaw S, Wilkinson J, Marks J Jr, Sugawara M, Nethercott J. Fragrance contact dermatitis. A worldwide multicenter investigation (Part I). Am J Contact Dermatitis 1996;7:77−83.

15. Meynadier J-M, Meynadier J, Peyron J-L, Peyron L. Formes cliniques des manifestations cutanées d'allergie aux parfums. Ann Dermatol Venereol 1986;113:31−9.

16. Santucci B, Cristaudo A, Cannistraci C, Picardo M. Contact dermatitis to fragrances. Contact Dermatitis 1987;16:93−5.

17. Malten KE, van Ketel WG, Nater JP, Liem DH. Reactions in selected patients to 22 fragrance materials. Contact Dermatitis 1984;11:1−10.

18. Christophersen J, Menné T, Tanghøj P, Andersen KE, Brandrup F, Kaaber K, Osmundsen PE, Thestrup-Pedersen K, Veien NK. Clinical patch test data evaluated by multivariate analysis. Contact Dermatitis 1989;21:291−9.

19. González E. PUVA for psoriasis. Dermatol Clin 1995;13:851−66.

20. Germing H, Hölzle E, Schulte-Huermann P, Ruzicka Th. Follicular mycosis fungoides−augmentation by PUVA therapy. Acta Dermatol Venereol 1995;75:164−5.

21. Bonnetblanc JM, Combeau A, Dang PM. Hydroxychloroquine-PUVA induced acute generalized exanthematous pustulosis. Ann Dermatol Venereol 1995;122:604−5.

22. Yamamoto T, Katayama I, Nishioka K. Verruciform xanthoma in a psoriatic patient under PUVA therapy. Dermatology 1995;191:254−6.

23. Nesher G, Zuckner J. Rheumatologic complications of vitamin A and retinoids. Semin Arthritis Rheum 1995;24:291−6.

24. Van Dooren-Geebe RJ, van de Kerkhof PCM. Extensive extraspinal hyperostoses after long-term oral retinoid treatment in a patient with pityriasis rubra pilaris. J Am Acad Dermatol 1995;32:322−5.

25. Sewell KL. Iatrogenic osteoporosis. Arch Dermatol 1995;131:1321−2.

26. DiGiovanni JJ, Sollitto RB, Abangan DL, Steinberg SM, Reynolds JC. Osteoporosis is a toxic effect of long-term etretinate therapy. Arch Dermatol 1995;131:1263−7.

27. Kocijancic M. 13-cis-retinoic acid and bone density. Int J Dermatol 1995;34:733−4.

28. Stern RS, Fitzgerald E, Ellis CN, Lowe N, Goldfarb MT, Baughman RD. The safety of etretinate as long-term therapy for psoriasis: results of the etretinate folow-up study. J Am Acad Dermatol 1995;33:44−52.

29. Sanchez MR, Ross B, Rotterdam H, Salik J, Brodie R, Freedberg IM. Retinoids hepatitis. J Am Acad Dermatol 1993;28:853−8.

30. Blum A, Scherwitz C, Rassner G. Pseudoallergic hepatitis after a single intake of 10 mg acitretin (Neotigason®) for treatment of psoriasis pustulosa. Acta Dermatol Venereol 1995;75:332.

31. Krüge-Krasagakes S, Grabbe J, Czarnetzki BM. Possible aggravation of hepatitis A by acitretin. Acta Dermatol Venereol 1995;75:82−3.

32. Anonymous. Acitretin (Neotigason®): after two years still in the body? Geneesmiddelenbulletin 1995;29:41−2.

33. Sturkenboom MCJM, de Jong-van den Berg LTW, Cornel MC, Stricker BHCh, Wesseling H. Inability to detect plasma etretinate and acitretin is a poor predictor of the absence of these teratogens in tissue and after stopping acitretin treatment. Br J Clin Pharmacol 1994;38:229−35.

34. Oliviero G, Constans P, Caby I, De Rohan Chabot P, Lacherade JC. Pneumopathie induite par l'isotrétinoine. Rev Mal Respir 1995;12:631−3.

35. Saurat H. Side effects of systemic retinoids and their clinical management. J Am Acad Dermatol 1992;27:S23−8.

36. Bravard P, Krug M, Rzeznick JC. L'Isotrétinoin et depression, soyons vigilantes. Nouv Dermatol 1993;12:215.

37. Byrne A, Hnatko G. Depression associated with isotretinoin therapy. Can J Psych 1995; 40:567.

38. Lafontaine N, Tousignant J, Rozenfarb E, Bernier-Buzzanga J. Thyroglossal cyst and isotretinoin. Eur J Dermatol 1995;5:225−6.

39. Georgala S, Gourgiotou K. Isotretinoin-induced pemphigus. Acta Dermatol Venereol 1995; 75:413.

40. Aubin S, Lorette G, Muller C, Vaillant L. Massive isotretinoin intoxication. Clin Exp Dermatol 1995;20:348−50.

41. Dooms-Goossens A, Matura M, Drieghe J, Degreef H. Contact allergy to imidazoles used as antimycotic agents. Contact Dermatitis 1995; 33:73−7.

42. Nakagawa M, Kawai K, Kawai K. Contact

allergy to kojic acid in skin care products. Contact Dermatitis 1995;32:9—13.

43. Sainio E-L, Kanerva L. Contact allergens in toothpastes and a review of their hypersensitivity. Contact Dermatitis 1995;35:100—5.

44. Sasseville D, Carey WD, Singer MI. Generalized contact dermatitis from acetarsone. Contact Dermatitis 1995;33:431—2.

45. Keller-Melchior R, Bräuninger W. Allergic contact dermatitis from anthrarobin. Contact Dermatitis 1995;33:361.

46. Hisa T, Mochida K, Taniguchi S, Goti Y, Hamada T, Yoshioka M, Shigenaga Y, Takigawa M. Contact dermatitis from carboxyvinyl polymer. Contact Dermatitis 1995;33:271.

47. Marques C, Faria E, Machado A, Gonçalo S. Allergic contact dermatitis and systemic contact dermatitis from cinchocaine. Contact Dermatitis 1995;33:443.

48. Valsecchi R, Pansera B, Di Landro A, Cainelli T. Contact allergy to cinnoxicam. Contact Dermatitis 1995;32:63.

49. Vejlstrup E, Menné T. Contact dermatitis from clindamycin. Contact Dermatitis 1995;32:110.

50. Baes H. Contact dermatitis from clotrimazole. Contact Dermatitis 1995;32:187—8.

51. Wantke F, Götz M, Jarisch R. Contact dermatitis from cloxyquin. Contact Dermatitis 1995; 32:112—3.

52. Inoue A, Shoji A. Allergic contact dermatitis from colistin. Contact Dermatitis 1995;33:200.

53. Jager SU, Pönningshaus JM, Koch P. Allergic contact dermatitis from cyclopiroxolamine. Contact Dermatitis 1995;33:349—50.

54. Schmid-Grendelmeier P, Wyss M, Elsner P. Contact allergy to dexpanthenol. A report of seven cases and review of the literature. Dermatosen 1995;43:175—8.

55. Johansen JD, Jemec GBE, Rastogi SC. Contact sensitization to dipropylene glycol in an eczema population. Contact Dermatitis 1995; 33:211—2.

56. Koch P, Bahmer FA, Hausen BM. Allergic contact dermatitis from purified eosin. Contact Dermatitis 1995;32:92—5.

57. Guidetti MS, Vincenzi C, Guerra L, Tosti A. Contact dermatitis due to imidazole antimycotics. Contact Dermatitis 1995;33:282.

58. Reichert C, Gall H. Contact dermatitis from hydroxyethyl salicylate. Contact Dermatitis 1995; 33:275—6.

59. Foti C, Vena GA, Mazzarella F, Angelini G. Contact allergy due to methyl glucose dioleate. Contact Dermatitis 1995;32:303—4.

60. Eedy DJ. Mupirocin allergy in the setting of venous ulceration. Contact Dermatitis 1995; 32:240—1.

61. Goulden V, Goodfield MJD. Delayed hypersensitivity reaction to the preservative myristyl picolonium chloride. Contact Dermatitis 1995; 33:209—10.

62. Willa-Craps C, Wyss M, Elsner P. Allergic contact dermatitis from naftifine. Contact Dermatitis 1995;32:369—70.

63. Navarro LA, Jorro G, Morales C, Pelez A. Allergic contact dermatitis due to piketoprofen. Contact Dermatitis 1995;32:181.

64. Balato N, Partruno C, Lembo G, Cuccurullo FM, Ayala F. Allergic contact dermatitis from retinoic acid. Contact Dermatitis 1995;32:51.

65. Goday JJ, Yanguas I, Aguirre A, Ilardia R, Soloeta R. Allergic contact dermatitis from sertaconazole with cross-sensitivity to miconazole and econazole. Contact Dermatitis 1995;32:370—1.

66. Kimura K, Katayama I, Nishioka K. Allergic contact dermatitis from tacalcitol. Contact Dermatitis 1995;33:441—2.

67. Lorenzi S, Placucci F, Vincenzi C, Bardazzi F, Tosti A. Allergic contact dermatitis due to thymol. Contact Dermatitis 1995;33:439—40.

68. Romano A, Pietrantonio F, Di Fonso M, Venuti A, Fabrizi G. Contact allergy to tiopronin: a case report. Contact Dermatitis 1995;33:269.

69. González Pérez R, Aguirre A, Oleaga JM, Eizaguirre X, Díaz Pérez JL. Allergic contact dermatitis from tolnaftate. Contact Dermatitis 1995; 32:173.

70. Rafanella S, Bacchilega R, Stanganelli I, Rafanelli A. Contact dermatitis from usnic acid in vaginal ovules. Contact Dermatitis 1995; 33:271—2.

71. Katz HI. Topical corticosteroids. Dermatol Clin 1995;13:805—15.

72. Silverman A, Menter A, Hairston JL. Tars and anthralins. Dermatol Clin 1995;13:817—33.

73. Kragballe K. Vitamin D3 analogues. Dermatol Clin 1995;13:835—9.

74. Anonymous. Calcipotriol (Daivonex®) and headache. Geneesmiddelenbulletin 1995;29(9).

75. Waran KD, Munsick RA. Anaphylaxis from povidone-iodine. Lancet 1995;345:1506.

76. Hernández Rodríguez I, Allegue F. Achilles and suprapatellar tendinitis due to isotretinoin. J Rheumatol 1995;22:2009—10.

77. Bewley AP, Rankin ECC, Levell NJ, Robinson TWE. Isotretinoin causing aseptic arthropathy. Clin Exp Dermatol 1995;20:279.

15 Antihistamines

GENERAL

Second-generation histamine H₁-antagonists: cardiac effects

Both astemizole and terfenadine have been associated with serious cardiovascular adverse events, including *prolongation of the QT interval*. These effects have been seen both in overdose and with therapeutic doses, when their effects are enhanced by certain factors: hepatic impairment, combination with drugs that inhibit their metabolism via cytochrome P450, and combination with drugs that block potassium channels, cause torsade de pointes, or prolong the QT interval. Precautions required to avoid adverse cardiovascular effects with terfenadine and astemizole have been discussed before (SEDA-17, 196).

Tachycardia has been associated with loratidine overdose. Current evidence, however, suggests that loratidine may be associated with a lower risk of cardiac effects than astemizole and terfenadine. Adverse cardiovascular events have not been reported with cetirizine or acrivastine (SEDA-17, 196; (1[R]), (2[c])).

Astemizole *(SED-13, 417; SEDA-18, 183; SEDA-19, 170)*

Reports to the Committee on Safety of Medicines (UK) on suspected adverse cutaneous reactions to astemizole include cases of *photosensitivity* and *urticaria*. A previously unreported association of *Stevens-Johnson syndrome* following astemizole therapy is presented below (3[c]).

A 28-year-old man on a walking holiday in England took astemizole 10 mg/day for hay-fever (no details given on the number of doses taken). He had used terfenadine on previous occasions with no adverse effects. He was taking no other medications and had no significant past medical history. He developed fever, headache, and mouth ulceration, followed within 24 h by a generalized rash. He was admitted to hospital 5 days after the last dose of astemizole, with fever, widespread blistering skin lesions, and mucosal ulceration. Stevens-Johnson syndrome was diagnosed. Despite high-dosage systemic corticosteroids, adult respiratory distress syndrome developed, necessitating prolonged mechanical ventilation. He eventually made a full recovery, apart from minor corneal scarring. Antibody titers for *Mycoplasma pneumoniae*, *Herpes simplex*, and anti-streptolysin O were all negative.

It is often difficult to establish definitively the cause of Stevens-Johnson syndrome; the severity of the illness precludes rechallenge with the suspect drug, as in this case.

Azelastine *(SED-13, 417; SEDA-17, 199; SEDA-18, 184; SEDA-19, 171)*

Azelastine nasal spray (0.14 mg in each nostril bd) has been compared with ebastine tablets (10 mg as a single night-time dose) in a Phase IV, open, randomized, parallel-group study lasting 14 days in 65 patients with seasonal allergic rhinitis (4[c]). Five patients were lost to follow-up: two had been randomised to ebastine but without benefit; three others, one of whom was taking ebastine, withdrew for reasons not related to the medication. Eight adverse events were reported with azelastine. Four patients taking azelastine complained of *bitter taste*, two had *pharyngeal pruritus*, one reported *nasal pruritus*, and another had *facial paresthesia* lasting several minutes after the first dose. The investigators thought that these effects were probably related to the drug and they judged them to be mild. The adverse effects of ebastine in this study are described below.

Ebastine *(SEDA-17, 200)*

Ebastine is a potent, selective H₁ receptor antagonist which undergoes rapid and almost

Side Effects of Drugs, Annual 20
J.K. Aronson, ed.

complete first-pass metabolism to the acid metabolite carebastine. After oral administration in both adults and children, plasma concentrations of carebastine reach a peak after 3—6 h and its half-life is 10—16 h.

The magnitude and duration of the effect of a single dose of ebastine (1, 3, 10, or 30 mg) in suppressing the skin reaction to histamine has been assessed in a double-blind, placebo-controlled, parallel study in 40 patients (5[C]). Skin reactivity was tested before treatment and at several times during the next 24 h. Ebastine caused dose-dependent suppression of cutaneous reactions to histamine for 24 h after all doses. This effect peaked at 6—12 h and was more consistent with doses of 10—30 mg. There were no differences from placebo in either the incidence of adverse effects or in the QTc interval in serial electrocardiograms. The incidence of adverse effects was low and there was no dose-dependence. *Drowsiness* was reported in four patients who took ebastine.

In the study described above under 'Azelastine' (4[C]), there were eight adverse effects in the ebastine-treated group: three patients felt *sleepy*, two patients had *headache*, and one each had *increased appetite*, *weakness*, and *epigastric pain*. The investigators thought that these effects were probably related to the drug and they judged them to be mild, except for one patient who experienced moderately severe sedation several hours after treatment.

Levocabastine *(SED-13, 417; SEDA-17, 210; SEDA-18, 184; SEDA-19, 494)*

Levocabastine is a highly-potent selective H_1-receptor antagonist which has been developed for topical administration by the ocular and nasal routes. Its effects occur rapidly and are predominantly due to local antihistaminic actions at the site of application. Levocabastine has an adverse effects profile comparable to that of sodium cromoglycate. As might be expected from the route of administration, *local irritation* is the most frequent adverse event with levocabastine eye-drops and nasal spray. Intranasal application does not have an adverse effect on ciliary activity either in vitro or in vivo, while ocular administration has no significant or consistent adverse effects in animals or humans. In therapeutic dosages, levocabastine has no significant systemic activity, and has no apparent effects on cardiovascular, psychomotor, or cognitive functions. Since levocabastine undergoes little hepatic metabolism, and only low plasma concentrations of the drug are reached after topical administration, drug interactions are unlikely (6[R]).

Mizolastine *(SEDA-19, 175)*

The pharmacodynamic interaction of mizolastine with ethanol has been assessed in a randomized, double-blind, three-way crossover, placebo-controlled study in 18 healthy young men, who received mizolastine (10 mg od), cetirizine (10 mg od), or placebo for 7 days with a 1-week wash-out interval (7[C]). An oral dose of ethanol or ethanol placebo, given 2 h after dosing on days five or seven of each treatment period, was administered to achieve a peak breath alcohol concentration of 16 mmol/l (0.7 g/l), and maintained for 1 h by two further doses of ethanol. Driving ability and psychomotor performance were evaluated using actual and simulated driving tests, critical flicker fusion threshold, adaptive tracking, and divided attention tasks.

A single oral dose of ethanol, which produced a peak breath alcohol concentration of 16 mmol/l, had detrimental effects in all the psychomotor and driving performance tests. Neither mizolastine nor cetirizine significantly impaired driving ability or arousal (critical flicker fusion threshold) compared with placebo. However, both drugs significantly impaired performance in the divided attention tasks 6 h after the dose. Tracking speed was significantly reduced by mizolastine and more consistently by cetirizine. Neither mizolastine nor cetirizine potentiated the effects of ethanol or had any effect on blood alcohol concentration.

Terfenadine *(SED-13, 417; SEDA-17, 203; SEDA-18, 186; SEDA-19, 176)*

Nervous system There has been renewed interest in histamine H_1 receptor antagonists since the recent discovery of second-generation antihistamines that cause little sedation. Histamine H_1 receptor occupancy in human brain has been measured in 20 healthy young men by positron emission tomography using $[^{11}C]$doxepin (8[c]). Single oral doses of a classical and a non-sedative antihistamine (chlorpheniramine and terfenadine) were tested. Oral chlorpheniramine 2 mg occupied 77% of the available H_1 receptors in the frontal cortex and intravenous chlorpheniramine 5 mg occupied 98%; in contrast, oral terfenadine 60 mg occupied 17% of the available receptors. There was no correlation between H_1 receptor occupancy by terfenadine and the plasma concentration of its active acid metabolite. These studies have shown the possible usefulness of quantifying H_1 receptor occupancy in estimating unwanted adverse effects of antihistamines, such as sedation and drowsiness.

Interactions Several hepatic enzyme-inhibiting drugs (for example, ketoconazole and erythromycin) cause cardiotoxicity when combined with terfenadine. Similarly, fluoxetine (half-life 48−72 h) or its active metabolite norfluoxetine (half-life 116 h) can alter the metabolism of terfenadine and precipitate cardiac toxicity. *Prolongation of the QTc interval*, probably associated with the combination of terfenadine with fluoxetine, has been reported (9[c]).

A 39-year-old woman was admitted for 28 days for in-patient treatment of substance abuse. Her past medical history included genital herpes, headaches, hay-fever, and hemorrhoids. Her medications included acyclovir 5% ointment prn, beclomethasone 2 puffs bd, pseudoephedrine 60 mg bd, and ibuprofen 800 mg prn. Other medications begun in hospital included fluoxetine 40 mg/day (begun on day 0), terfenadine 60 mg bd (begun on day 0), and disulfiram 250 mg/day (begun on day 6). Routine electrocardiography on day 14 showed a prolonged QT_c interval of 550 ms. She was asymptomatic, in no acute distress, and had no prior history of heart disease. Throughout her stay several urine toxicology screens were negative. Her physician discontinued only her terfenadine and repeated the electrocardiogram on day 21, when the QT_c was normal. She reported no adverse effects and was discharged on day 28 taking the same medications as during her stay, apart from terfenadine. Calcium concentrations, liver function abnormalities, and other concomitant drugs were ruled out as possible causative factors.

The authors speculated that fluoxetine, or more probably norfluoxetine (a potent in vitro inhibitor of CYP3A4), inhibited the metabolism of terfenadine and resulted in the prolonged QTc. The two electrocardiograms performed before and after the withdrawal of terfenadine support this view.

REFERENCES

1. Anonymous. Second-generation H_1-antagonists first line in the treatment of urticaria. Drugs Ther Perspect 1995;5:5−8.
2. Türktas I, Oguz D, Olguntürk R, Demirsoy S, Tunaoglu FS. Cardiotoxic and hepatotoxic effects of acrivastin and cetirizin. Turk Kardiyol Dernegi Ars 1995;23:100−3.
3. Cunliffe NA, Barnes AJ, Dunbar EM. Stevens-Johnson syndrome following astemizole therapy. Postgrad Med J 1995;71:383.
4. Conde Hernandez DL, Palma Aqilar JL, Delgado Romero J. Investigation on the efficacy and tolerance of azelastine (HCl) nasal spray versus ebastine tablets in patients with seasonal allergic rhinitis. Immunopathology 1995;23:51−9.
5. Nelson HS, Bucher B, Buchmeier A, Oppenheimer J, Garcia J. Suppression of the skin reaction to histamine by ebastine. Ann Allergy Asthma Immunol 1955;74:442−7.
6. Howarth PH. A review of the tolerability and safety of levocabastine eye drops and nasal spray. Implications for patient management. Mediators Inflamm 1995;4:S26−30.
7. Patat A, Stubbs D, Dunmore C, Ulliac N, Sexton B, Zieleniuk I, Irving A, Jones W. Lack of interaction between two antihistamines, mizolastine and cetirizine, and ethanol in psychomotor and driving performance in healthy subjects. Eur J Clin Pharmacol 1995;48:143−50.
8. Yanai K, Ryu JH, Watanabe T, Iwata R, Ido T, Sawai Y, Ito K, Itoh M. Histamine H_1 receptor occupancy in human brains after single oral doses of histamine H_1 antagonists measured by positron emission tomography. Br J Pharmacol 1995;116:1649−55.
9. Marchiando RJ, Cook MD. Probable terfenadine-fluoxetine associated cardiac toxicity. Ann Pharmacother 1995;29:937−8.

Gunnar Boman

16 Drugs acting on the respiratory tract

R *Asthma medications and exacerbations of asthma* (SED-13, 427; SEDA-17, 164; SEDA-18, 159; SEDA-19, 178)

Much of the discussion on the safety of asthma treatment has focused on fatal and near-fatal asthma, e.g. the oft-quoted series of case—control studies from New Zealand and the pharmacoepidemiological studies from Saskatchewan (SED-13, 427). Non-fatal exacerbations of asthma are common events, causing considerable adverse effects on patients' quality of life and health-care costs. A nested case-control study has been performed in a cohort of 680 asthmatics identified in a Dutch drug-dispensing database (1^C). Within the cohort, the proportion of patients dispensed inhaled corticosteroids rose from 12 to 27% between 1986 and 1991. The proportion of asthmatics using inhaled bronchodilators without inhaled corticosteroids also fell over this period. The intermittent use of oral corticosteroids was taken as a proxy for exacerbation of asthma. Chronic users of oral corticosteroids were excluded. Cases in which exacerbation had occurred (n = 133) were pair-wise matched with controls. After adjustment for disease severity, the use of inhaled fenoterol (OR 10) and of oral xanthines (OR 2.9) was associated with an increased probability of exacerbation. There was no significant association (negative or positive) with the use of inhaled salbutamol, corticosteroids, cromoglycate, or ipratropium bromide.

This study illustrates the possible risks of using inhaled β$_2$-adrenoceptor agonists in asthma, which none the less remain the most important bronchodilators currently available,

and sales of which continue to increase in many parts of the world, especially after the introduction of long-acting agonists such as salmeterol and formoterol. The prolonged and intense professional debate and the widespread public concern about their potential risks seem not to have diminished their clinical use. Each year a large number of experimental, clinical, and epidemiological studies of their use in asthma and other obstructive lung diseases appear, which may reflect not only their clinical value but also their large economical value for the pharmaceutical industry. The rapidly increasing bulk of often conflicting evidence is impossible to survey for the practising physician and poses a risk for selection bias for the scientific reviewer.

Two extensive and balanced reviews of this topic by two eminent experts are relevant (2^R), (3^R). The first concluded that "β-agonists will continue to be the bronchodilators of choice for many years because they are effective in all patients and have few or no adverse effects when used in low doses. It will be difficult to find a bronchodilator that improves on the efficacy and safety of inhaled β$_2$-agonists. Although some concerns have been expressed about the long-term effects of inhaled β-agonists, the evidence suggests that when used as required for symptom control, short-acting inhaled β-agonists are safe" (2^R). Observe the restrictions "when used as required" and "short-acting". The conclusions of the second reviewer were that "β-adrenergic agonists remain the most important class of bronchodilators currently available. When used appropriately, they provide safe and effective relief of the symptoms of airflow obstruction" (3^R). Note here the restriction "when used appropriately". The reader is advised to consider these two reviews before reading more clearly debate articles that are either for (4^r), (5^r) or against (6^r), (7^r) the use of β$_2$-agonists in asthma.

Side Effects of Drugs, Annual 20
J.K. Aronson, ed.

Table 1.   *Possible dangers of β_2-adrenoceptor agonists in asthma (adapted from 8[R])*

Hypothesis	Mechanism	Comment
Non-responders	Tachyphylaxis	Occurs only with short-acting agents and ephedrine
	Subsensitization of β_2-receptors	Occurs in exacerbations, e.g. viral damage to receptors
	Down-regulation of β_2-receptors	May occur with excessive use of aerosol β_2-agonists; usually a minor effect
Paradoxical response	Irritation causing bronchoconstriction	Cold aerosol or adjuvants may result in this non-specific response
	Specific reaction to β_2-agonists	Not explained
	Rebound increase in airway tone	Rarely described
β_2-blockade	By metabolites of β_2-agonists	Not shown to occur
	By therapeutically inactive enantiomers in marketed drugs	Theoretical and unlikely
Hyper-responsiveness	Antigen penetration increases in bronchodilated airways	Theoretical and unlikely; could occur with any effective airway dilator
	Rebound effect	Laboratory finding; doubtful clinical significance
Cardiotoxicity	Dysrhythmias	Rare; could result from hypoxia, hypokalemia, and prolongation of the QT_c interval
	Myocardial ischemia	Rare; could occur with excessive isoprenaline
Inflammatory effect	Bronchodilatation allows inflammation to occur unchecked	Could be a factor in progressive asthma; an indication for corticosteroid therapy
	Inhibition of release of mast cell heparin (anti-inflammatory)	Hypothetical
Psychosomatic	Poor recognition of worsening symptoms	May make patient ignore dangerous obstructive symptoms
	Laughter, excess effort causing sudden bronchospasm	May provoke severe irreversible spasm, i.e. "locked lung"

A third careful review of the β-agonist controversy includes a useful summary of the theoretical dangers of β-agonists (see Table 1) (8[R]). This review focuses on the use of β_2-agonists in chronic obstructive pulmonary disease, in which, in contrast to asthma, the bronchodilating effects are less obvious. By definition the bronchoconstriction in chronic obstructive pulmonary disease is more or less irreversible. In comparison with asthma patients, patients with chronic obstructive pulmonary disease are usually older, have progressive and more serious lung disease, and tend to use other medications for concomitant diseases. The balance between the benefits and risks of β_2-agonists may therefore be different in chronic obstructive airway disease than in asthma. However, this third review concluded reassuringly that β-agonists in standard doses have a basic role in the management of chronic obstructive airway disease and can be given safely on a regular basis.

Chlorofluorocarbon-free propellants *(SED-13, 427)   In order to reduce the harmful effects of chlorofluorocarbons (CFCs) on the ozone layer, the Montreal Protocol, first drawn up in 1987 and subsequently revised several times, set world-wide goals for the reduction in the use of CFCs with the intention of ending all use by 1996. However, an exemption has been temporarily granted for CFCs in metered-dose inhalers. Two propellants, hydrofluoroalkane (HFA)-134a and -227, have been identified to replace CFCs in metered-dose inhalers through the joint efforts of several pharmaceutical companies. However, the new propellants have different properties than the old ones, and the reformulation of inhaled drugs and devices has been difficult. The acute safety of the propellant HFA-134a has been tested in 12 healthy subjects (9[C]). Cumulative doses from metered-dose inhalers with HFA only, HFA with salbutamol, or a conventional CFC were compared in a double-blind, randomized design.*

There was no statistically significant difference in the change from baseline of any parameter between the two propellant systems. Blood samples for HFA-134a were collected to measure systemic absorption and whole blood concentrations of 200—700 ng/ml were detected in all subjects at 2 min after the dose but fell substantially by 12 min.

In a small clinical study in 26 patients with stable asthma, salbutamol in HFA-134a (the Airomir system) has been compared with conventional salbutamol in CFC-11/12 (Ventolin) (10^C*). Single doses were compared double-blind. The bronchodilator effect was clinically comparable and there were no "clinically meaningful differences" in safety between the two delivery systems. Salbutamol, salmeterol, and fluticasone propionate have all been reformulated with HFA-134a and tested in a variety of single and chronic dosing studies (11*^{c}*). According to the author, the HFA-134a formulations provide equivalent efficacy with a similar safety profile to existing formulations at equivalent doses.*

In view of the unsolved controversies during the 1960s and 1970s about the possible role of CFC propellants in fatal asthma, it is hoped that the new CFC-free propellants will be properly assessed regarding safety before they are introduced on to the market on a large scale.

β₂-ADRENOCEPTOR AGONISTS

Orciprenaline (metaproterenol) *(SED-13, 353; SEDA-17, 163)*

Orciprenaline is a less-selective β₂-agonist than, for example, terbutaline and salbutamol, and is therefore used less often in the treatment of acute asthma (12^r). There was a high incidence of *tachycardia* in an open-label series of 50 adult patients with acute asthma given three rapid-sequence treatments with orciprenaline by nebulizer, each dose being 15 mg (13^C). There were increases in pulse rate of more than 30 beats/min in 21% of the patients, and one patient developed a transient supraventricular tachycardia at a rate of 200 beats/min. Serum potassium concentration was not monitored. The authors concluded that although orciprenaline is effective in reversing bronchospasm, its adverse effects when it is used in rapid sequence are of major concern.

Salbutamol (albuterol) *(SED-13, 427; SEDA-17, 164; SEDA-19, 178)*

Inhalation therapy may cause adverse effects that are related more to the procedure than to the drug itself. One recent example was an outbreak of nosocomial respiratory tract infections with *Burkholderia* (*Pseudomonas*) organisms associated with nebulized salbutamol therapy (14^C). Respiratory tract colonization or infection with *B. cepacia* occurred in 42 mechanically ventilated patients. Observation of intensive care unit and respiratory care personnel showed faulty infection control procedures. For example, the same multiple-dose bottle of salbutamol was used for many patients. Medication nebulizers and bottles of salbutamol in use harbored *B. cepacia*. Molecular fingerprints of patient isolates and environmental isolates of *B. cepacia* were identical. No further isolates of *B. cepacia* were identified after the institution of appropriate infection control procedures.

ANTICHOLINERGIC DRUGS

Ipratropium bromide *(SED-13, 426; SEDA-17, 174)*

Inhaled ipratropium bromide from a metered-dose inhaler, a breath-activated powder device, or a nebulizer has been used for several years in the treatment of asthma as an alternative to inhaled β₂-adrenoceptor agonists in patients who fail to respond adequately to these drugs. It has been suggested that ipratropium is more effective than β₂-agonists in patients with chronic obstructive pulmonary disease. The drug has been well tolerated in most studies and the risk of systemic anticholinergic effects seems to be small, even after the administration of high doses by nebulization for acute severe asthma (12^r). The efficacy and safety of frequent nebulized ipratropium bromide added to high-dose salbutamol have been assessed in 120 children with severe acute asthma in a randomized, double-blind, placebo-controlled trial (15^C). Three regimens were studied: three doses of nebulized ipratropium within 60 min (250 µg/dose); one dose of ipratropium; and no ipratropium. All the children were also treated with three doses of nebulized salbutamol within 60 min (0.15 mg/kg per dose). The addition of ipratropium to high-dose salbutamol increased the predicted FEV_1 significantly, and even more so in children with an initial FEV_1 that was less than 30% of the predicted value. There were no adverse effects attributable to ipratropium.

An aqueous solution of ipratropium bromide has been used as a nasal spray in patients with allergic and perennial non-allergic rhinitis, as well as in the common cold. In a double-blind trial of 233 patients with perennial non-allergic rhinitis, 42 µg of ipratropium tds for 8 weeks produced a 30% reduction in rhinorrhea, a significantly greater effect than the saline vehicle produced (16[C]). There were no serious drug-related adverse effects and no nasal rebound after withdrawal. *Epistaxis* was reported in 9.4% of patients taking ipratropium compared with 2.6% of those taking the vehicle. In a similar but open-label study 285 patients were treated with nasal ipratropium for 1 year (17[C]). Ipratropium nasal spray was well tolerated and was not associated with any serious or systemic adverse effects, although 10% of the patients withdrew because of perceived adverse events. The two most frequent nasal adverse events were *nasal dryness* (10%) and *epistaxis* (4%). Rhinoscopy showed no detrimental effects of long-term nasal ipratropium. The safety and efficacy of a stronger solution (0.06%) of ipratropium have been studied in 96 patients with perennial allergic rhinitis, using an open-label protocol for 1 year (18[C]). Nasal dryness and epistaxis were the most common local adverse events. There were two cases of potential systemic anticholinergic adverse events. A double-blind dose-response study of ipratropium nasal spray (42, 84, or 168 µg to each nostril tds) in the treatment of the common cold has been performed in 955 patients from six centers (19[C]). There was a dose-dependent reduction in the severity of the rhinorrhea, measured both objectively and subjectively, but also a dose-dependent increase in nasal and systemic adverse events, none of them serious.

Tiotropium bromide

A newly developed long-acting antimuscarinic agent, tiotropium bromide, has been investigated in 35 patients with stable chronic obstructive pulmonary disease in a randomized, double-blind, crossover design (20[C]). The patients inhaled single doses of 10—80 µg of the drug, formulated in powder capsules. Pulmonary function testing was performed at regular intervals for up to 32 h after inhalation of the test drug. Compared with placebo, tiotropium bromide produced significant improvements in lung function in a dose-dependent fashion. Peak improvement in FEV_1 occurred 1—4 h after the inhalation and the duration of action extended to 32 h after the 20, 40, and 80 µg doses. *Dyspnea*, probably as a result of insufficient bronchodilatation, was the event most frequently reported in all treatment groups, but most commonly with placebo. There was no evidence of systemic anticholinergic effects at any dose.

CROMOGLYCATE AND RELATED DRUGS

Nedocromil *(SED-13, 422; SEDA-19, 183)*

Studies that confirm the excellent safety of nedocromil inhalation therapy for asthma continue to appear. The efficacy and safety of nedocromil has been compared with placebo in an 8-week study in 112 adult asthmatics (21[C]). As in previous studies, the only significant adverse effect was an *unpleasant taste sensation*, which was reported by 21% of the patients. In a double-blind study, 212 patients with asthma took either 4 mg of nedocromil or 180 µg of salbutamol qds for 12 weeks (22[C]). *Headache* (5 vs. 2%) and *unpleasant taste sensation* (5 vs. 2%) were the most common adverse events and were not significantly different between the two treatment groups.

Viral respiratory infections often cause exacerbations of asthma in children. The protective effects of 0.5% nedocromil nebulizer solution tds in preventing asthma exacerbations have been investigated in 93 children (6—12 years), who took either nedocromil or placebo for 24 weeks during the viral season (23[C]). Nedocromil did not prevent infections or exacerbation of asthma symptoms. However, patients treated with nedocromil had faster resolution of asthma symptoms after infection. There were treatment-related events in 21% of the nedocromil-treated patients. *Unpleasant taste, upper respiratory infections,* and *headache* were most commonly reported but were considered of no clinical importance.

INHALED CORTICOSTEROIDS *(SED-13, 428; SEDA-17, 450; SEDA-18, 190; SEDA-19, 181)*

Treatment with inhaled corticosteroids was originally introduced to reduce the need for oral corticosteroids in patients with severe asthma. The steroid-sparing action of fluticasone propionate, a new inhaled corticosteroid has been demonstrated in 96 patients dependent on oral prednisone who were treated for 16 weeks with placebo or fluticasone propionate aerosol (750 or 1000 μg bd) (24[C]). In all, 69 and 88% of patients treated with the two respective doses of fluticasone, compared with 3% of the placebo-treated patients, used no prednisone by the end of the study. The reduced dosage of prednisone was reflected in the fact that fewer patients on fluticasone than on placebo had abnormal plasma cortisol concentrations at the last visit. On the other hand, the percentages of patients with potentially drug-related local adverse events (*oral candidiasis, hoarseness,* and *sore throat*) were 53 and 44% with fluticasone compared with 16% with placebo.

Almost all experts agree that in severe asthma, maintenance therapy with inhaled corticosteroids has a more favourable benefit:risk ratio than the systemic corticosteroids. An important problem is that inhaled corticosteroids are not available to many patients in poor countries, owing to cost.

Even in mild asthma, inhaled corticosteroids are now recommended as the appropriate treatment for patients who need inhalations of β_2-agonists more than once daily, according to several national and international guidelines. The scientific basis of this recommendation is the recognition that inflammation of the airways is already present, even in mild forms of the disease, from the start of the illness. As a result of this increased interest in early treatment with corticosteroids, many

reports of therapeutic trials are published each year, also reflecting the great commercial potential of this field of therapy. A timely and well-referenced review of all aspects, including the adverse effects, of inhaled corticosteroids has been published (25[R]). The local adverse effects of inhaled corticosteroids (*dysphonia, thrush, sore throat*) are usually dose-dependent and are fairly easy to handle. However, there are constant concerns about their systemic effects, especially since they are likely to be used for very long periods and also in children. As more and more sensitive biochemical tests of the systemic effects become available, such effects will be identified more often, although they may not all be clinically important. Another difficulty is in differentiating between the adverse effects of inhaled corticosteroids and those of the systemic corticosteroids that patients may take during exacerbations. The systemic effect of any inhaled corticosteroid will depend on several factors: the pharmacokinetics of the substance, the daily dose, possibly the number of daily administrations, the delivery system, and the individual patient's response to the drug.

Musculoskeletal While plasma and urine markers of bone metabolism have been analysed in many studies of short- to medium-term therapy with inhaled corticosteroids, very few have studied the really important end-point, fractures. Cross-sectional studies of bone density in patients treated with inhaled corticosteroids have shown conflicting results, and prospective, long-term studies in large cohorts of patients are still lacking. In another cross-sectional study, bone density and lumbar fractures were measured in 26 men and 43 women (41 postmenopausal, all of whom had taken estrogen supplements) (26[C]). These patients had been treated, on average, for 10 years with an inhaled corticosteroid and for 11 years with oral prednisone. The results suggested that the daily dose, but not the duration, of inhaled corticosteroid therapy may adversely affect bone density, and that estrogen therapy may offset this bone-depleting effect in postmenopausal women.

EXPECTORANTS AND MUCOLYTIC DRUGS

N-Acetylcysteine *(SED-13, 430; SEDA-17, 207)*

Traditionally used as a mucolytic agent, *N*-acetylcysteine also has important antioxidant and scavenger properties. When taken orally it is rapidly absorbed, deacetylated, and incorporated into intracellular and extracellular glutathione stores. *N*-Acetylcysteine is widely used as an antidote in acute paracetamol (acetaminophen) poisoning. On the basis of experimental animal studies it has also emerged as one of the most promising cancer chemopreventive agents. Interim results regarding safety are available from EUROSCAN, a large European preventive study in patients previously treated for lung or head and neck cancer (27[c]). A total of 2191 patients were divided into four treatment groups for 2 years: *N*-acetylcysteine 600 mg daily; *N*-acetylcysteine 600 mg + retinol 300 000 IU daily; retinol only; or no drugs. Adverse effects were reported by 14% of the patients who took *N*-acetylcysteine, compared with 23% of the patients who took retinol and 25% of patients who took the combination. *Dyspepsia* was the most common adverse effect related to *N*-acetylcysteine. Higher daily doses than 600 mg seemed to have been less well tolerated. In a dose-finding study in healthy volunteers given 600 mg of *N*-acetylcysteine bd or tds for 4 weeks, 25 and 61%, respectively, reported gastrointestinal adverse effects.

Mesna *(SED-13, 431)*

Mesna is used to prevent hemorrhagic cystitis from cyclophosphamide and ifosfamide, but it has also been claimed to be a mucolytic agent. In a double-blind study in 20 patients on mechanical ventilation, one endotracheal instillation of mesna was compared with saline (28[c]). Mesna caused important *increases in maximal airways resistance* and *impairment of oxygenation* and a slight *increase in P_aCO_2*. There was a major adverse effect in one patient, who had an episode of *increased bronchial secretions* 10 min after the instillation of mesna. The instillation of saline had no positive or negative effects.

Sinupret

In a multicenter post-marketing surveillance study of 3187 patients with acute bronchitis, 1805 (57%) were treated with two tablets tds of Sinupret (a combination of five herbal ingredients), while 17% received *N*-acetylcysteine (200 mg tds) and 18% ambroxol (60 mg bd) (29[c]). Adverse events were reported during monotherapy with Sinupret in 0.8%, with ambroxol in 1.0%, and with *N*-acetylcysteine in 4.3%. When concomitant drugs were used, this rank order was unchanged, but the incidence rates markedly increased (3.4, 6.5, and 8.2%, respectively). The most frequent adverse reactions were *gastrointestinal symptoms*. Although reassuring regarding safety, it should be pointed out that the efficacy of these products was not assessed at all.

DESENSITIZATION (SPECIFIC IMMUNOTHERAPY) *(SED-13, 424; SEDA-17, 206; SEDA-19, 183)*

Specific immunotherapy is commonly indicated for the management of life-threatening reactions from *Hymenoptera* stings. Many randomized controlled clinical trials have shown the beneficial effect and limited risk of allergen immunotherapy for allergic rhinoconjunctivitis due to airborne pollens and house-dust mite allergens. In a double-blind, placebo-controlled trial of 40 adult patients with summer hay fever, immunotherapy with a depot grass pollen extract (Alutard SQ) reduced symptoms and the need for medications, with an acceptable incidence of adverse effects. The original placebo group, as well as those given immunotherapy, were then given immunotherapy in an open fashion for a further 3 years (30[c]). Efficacy was maintained throughout. Of the initial 40 patients, 32 completed the third year of treatment. In a total of 2598 injections, there were five immediate *systemic reactions*, all during the induction phase, and all responded promptly to adrenaline. After the 1477 injections during the maintenance phase the only adverse events were six extensive local reactions.

Alum-precipitated allergenic extracts (Allpyral) used for immunotherapy has been associated with subcutaneous nodule formation at injection sites. A patient who had taken injections for almost 10 years without proper medical supervision developed extensive *subcutaneous inflammation and fibrosis* with overlying skin changes that appeared to be permanent (31^c). Local nasal immunotherapy represents a potentially safer route of administration than the traditional subcutaneous injections. Thirty patients with birch allergic rhinitis took part in a placebo-controlled trial of an allergen extract in powder form for 22 weeks (32^C). Clinical efficacy was suggested by a significant reduction in medication score. There were mild adverse reactions, limited to the upper respiratory tract, but no asthmatic or systemic reactions.

The precise role of specific immunotherapy in allergic asthma remains controversial. A careful meta-analysis of 20 randomized, placebo-controlled, double-blind trials of allergen immunotherapy (mite, pollen, animal dander, or mold) has been published (33^C). The combined odds of symptomatic improvement from immunotherapy with any allergen was 3.2 (95% CI 2.2—4.9). *Systemic reactions* occurred in a mean of 32% (95% CI 20—44%) of all patients who received active immunotherapy. The authors pointed out that the benefits of allergen immunotherapy could be overestimated because of unpublished negative studies, but concluded that allergen immunotherapy is a treatment option in highly selected patients with allergic asthma. This rather positive conclusion has been questioned in an editorial, in which it was argued that the meta-analysis had included trials that had not used the same type of allergen extract or the same drug regimen for the treatment of asthma (34^r). The studies with the most positive results were those published in the 1970s. This could suggest that they were less rigorous in the experimental design. Considering that 32% of patients had systemic reactions, it was argued that the use of immunotherapy in allergic asthma should not be encouraged until the results of a large, randomized, controlled trial using standardized allergen extracts confirmed its effectiveness and safety.

REFERENCES

1. Van Ganse E, van der Linden PD, Leufkens HGM, Herings RMC, Vincken W, Ernst P. Asthma medications and disease exacerbations: an epidemiological study as a method for asthma surveillance. Eur Respir J 1995;8:1856—60.

2. Barnes PJ. Beta-adrenergic receptors and their regulation. Am J Respir Crit Care Med 1995;152:838—60.

3. Harold SN. Beta-adrenergic bronchodilators. New Engl J Med 1995;333:499—506.

4. Wanner A. Is the routine use of inhaled beta-adrenergic agonists appropriate in asthma treatment? Yes. Am J Respir Crit Care Med 1995; 151:597—9.

5. Johnson M. Pharmacology of long-acting beta-agonists. Ann Allergy Asthma Immunol 1995; 75:177—9.

6. Sears MR. Is the routine use of inhaled beta-adrenergic agonists appropriate in asthma treatment? No. Am J Respir Crit Care Med 1995; 151:600—1.

7. Barrett TE, Strom BL. Inhaled beta-adrenergic receptor agonists in asthma: more harm than good? Am J Respir Crit Care Med 1995; 151:574—7.

8. Ziment I. The beta-agonist controversy. Impact in COPD. Chest 1995;107:198S—205S.

9. Donnell D, Harrison LI, Ward S, Klinger NM, Ekholm BP, Cooper KM, Porietis I, McEwen J. Acute safety of the CFC-free propellant HFA-134a from a pressurized metered dose inhaler. Eur J Clin Pharmacol 1995;48:473—7.

10. Dockhorn R, Vanden Burgt JA, Ekholm BP, Donnell D, Cullen MT. Clinical equivalence of a novel non-chlorofluorocarbon-containing salbutamol sulfate metered-dose inhaler and a conventional chlorofluorocarbon inhaler in patients with asthma. J Allergy Clin Immunol 1995;96:50—5.

11. Jenkins M. Clinical evaluation of CFC-free metered dose inhalers. J Aerosol Med 1995;8 Suppl:41—7.

12. Corbridge TC, Hall JB. The assessment and management of adults with status asthmaticus. Am J Respir Crit Care Med 1995;151:1296—316.

13. Jerrard DA, Olshaker J, Welebob E, Caraballo V, Hooper F. Efficacy and safety of a rapid-sequence metaproterenol protocol in the treatment of acute adult asthma. Am J Emerg Med 1995;13:392—5.

14. Hamill RJ, Houston ED, Georghio PR,

Wright CE, Koza MA, Cadle RM, Goepfert PA, Lewis DA et al. An outbreak of *Burkholderia* (formerly *Pseudomonas*) *cepacia* respiratory tract colonization and infection associated with nebulized albuterol therapy. Ann Intern Med 1995; 122:762−6.

15.   Schuh S, Johnson DW, Callahan S, Canny G, Levison H. Efficacy of frequent nebulized ipratropium bromide added to frequent high-dose albuterol therapy in severe childhood asthma. J Pediatr 1995;126:639−45.

16.   Bronsky E, Druce H, Findlay SR, Hampel FC, Kaiser H, Ratner P, Valentine MD, Wood CC. A clinical trial of ipratropium bromide nasal spray in patients with perennial nonallergic rhinitis. J Allergy Clin Immunol 1995;95:1117−22.

17.   Grossman J, Banov C, Boggs P, Bronsky EA, Dockhorn RJ, Druce H, Findlay SR, Georgitis JW et al. Use of ipratropium bromide nasal spray in chronic treatment of nonallergic perennial rhinitis, alone and in combination withother perennial rhinitis medications. J Allergy Clin Immunol 1995;95:1123−7.

18.   Kaiser HB, Findlay SR, Georgitis JW, Grossman J, Ratner PH, Tinkelman DG, Roszko P, Zegarelli E et al. Long-term treatment of perennial allergic rhinitis with ipratropium bromide nasal spray 0.06%. J Allergy Clin Immunol 1995;95:1128−32.

19.   Diamond L, Dockhorn RJ, Grossman J, Kisicki JC, Posner M, Zinny MA, Koker P, Korts D et al. A dose-response study of the efficacy and safety of ipratropium bromide nasal spray in the treatment of the common cold. J Allergy Clin Immunol 1995;95:1139−46.

20.   Maesen FPV, Smeets JJ, Sledsens TJH, Wald FDM, Cornelissen PJG. Tiotropium bromide, a new long-acting antimuscarinic bronchodilator: a pharmacodynamic study in patients with chronic obstructive pulmonary disease (COPD). Eur Respir J 1995;8:1506−13.

21.   Creticos P, Burk J, Smith L, Comp R, Norman P, Findlay S. The use of twice daily nedocromil sodium in the treatment of asthma. J Allergy Clin Immunol 1995;95:829−36.

22.   Wasserman SI, Furukawa CT, Henochowicz SI, Marcoux JP, Prenner BM, Findlay SR, Gross GN, Hudson LD et al. Asthma symptoms and airway hyperresponsiveness are lower during treatment with nedocromil sodium than during treatment with regular inhaled albuterol. J Allergy Clin Immunol 1995;95:541−7.

23.   König P, Eigen H, Ellis MH, Ellis E, Blake K, Geller D, Shapiro G, Welch M et al. The effect of nedocromil sodium on childhood asthma during the viral season. Am J Respir Crit Care Med 1995;152:1879−86.

24.   Noonan M, Chervinsky P, Busse WW, Weisberg SC, Pinnas J, De Boisblanc BP, Boltansky H, Pearlman D et al. Fluticasone propionate reduces oral prednisone use while it improves asthma control and quality of life. Am J Respir Crit Care Med 1995;152:1467−73.

25.   Barnes PJ. Inhaled glucocorticoids for asthma. New Engl J Med 1995;332:868−75.

26.   Toogood JH, Baskerville JC, Markov AE, Hodsman AB, Fraher LJ, Jennings B, Haddad RG, Drost D. Bone mineral density and the risk of fracture in patients receiving long-term inhaled steroid therapy for asthma. J Allergy Clin Immunol 1995;96:157−66.

27.   van Zandwijk N. *N*-Acetylcysteine (NAC) and glutathione (GSH): antioxidant and chemopreventive properties, with special reference to lung cancer. J Cell Biochem 1995;Suppl 22:24−32.

28.   Fernandez R, Solé J, Blanch L, Artigas A. The effect of short-term instillation of a mucolytic agent (mesna) on airway resistance in mechanically ventilated patients. Chest 1995;107:1101−6.

29.   Ernst E, Sieder C, März R. Adverse drug reactions to herbal and synthetic expectorants. Int J Risk Saf Med 1995;7:219−25.

30.   Walker SM, Varney VA, Gaga M, Jacobson MR, Durham SR. Grass pollen immunotherapy: efficacy and safety during a 4-year follow-up study. Allergy 1995;50:405−13.

31.   Orfan NA, Dykewicz MS, Barnowsky L. Extensive subcutaneous fibrosis in a patient treated with alum precipitated allergenic extract. Ann Allergy Asthma Immunol 1995;75:453−6.

32.   Andri L, Senna G, Andri G, Dama A, Givanni S, Betteli C, Dimitri G, Falagiani P et al. Local nasal immunotherapy for birch allergic rhinitis with extract in powder form. Clin Exp Allergy 1995;25:1092−9.

33.   Abramson MJ, Puy RM, Weiner JM. Is allergen immunotherapy effective in asthma? A meta-analysis of randomized controlled trials. Am J Respir Crit Care Med 1995;151:969−74.

34.   Donner CF, Braghiroli A. Allergen immunotherapy in asthma. Eur Respir Top 1995;1:111.

J.K. Aronson

17 Positive inotropic drugs and drugs used in dysrhythmias

CARDIAC GLYCOSIDES *(SED-13, 438; SEDA-17, 215; SEDA-18, 196; SEDA-19, 188)*

Previous retrospective analyses of non-randomized studies of the effects of digitalis during long-term treatment in patients with heart failure and sinus rhythm suggested that there may be a small increase in mortality (SEDA-10, 142; SEDA-11, 153; SEDA-15, 165; SEDA-16, 173). However, there has now been a large multicenter, randomized, prospective, double-blind, controlled trial of digoxin versus placebo in 6800 patients, showing that there is no such increase in mortality (1[C]). The dosages to which the patients in this study were randomized produced plasma digoxin concentrations at the lower end of the usual target range (0.8 ng/ml) and that may have militated against any positive or negative effect of digoxin. Although there was a trend to a reduction in the number of deaths attributed to heart failure, there was a non-significant increase in sudden cardiovascular death attributed to dysrhythmias, and the two cancelled each other out. There was a significant reduction in the rate of hospitalization in the patients taking digoxin, but the effect was very small and led to a reduction in the number of hospital admissions of around nine per 1000. In view of the availability of other effective agents in the treatment of heart failure, digoxin probably has no place in the majority of patients with heart failure in sinus rhythm, although it may occasionally be useful for symptomatic relief when other therapy has not been completely effective. It may also be that digoxin is valuable in patients who cannot tolerate an ACE inhibitor, since there are no large prospective studies of mortality in patients taking digoxin and not taking an ACE inhibitor.

Recent studies have confirmed that even in patients who are not taking ACE inhibitors digoxin may none the less have a beneficial effect on cardiac and neurohumoral effects. In one study of 64 patients with heart failure of NYHA classes II and III, digoxin 0.25 mg/day for 6 months improved exercise tolerance and reduced plasma renin activity (2[C]), the latter effect having been shown before (3[c]). Digoxin also reduced the plasma noradrenaline concentration significantly. In another study of 22 patients with heart failure and sinus rhythm, NYHA classes II or III, digoxin significantly increased ejection fraction dose-dependently but did not have any effects on serum noradrenaline concentration or plasma renin activity; however, there was an increase in serum aldosterone concentration (4[C]). The chief difference between these two studies was that ACE inhibitors were not used in the first, but were in the second. Since over 90% of patients with heart failure are taking ACE inhibitors nowadays, it is not clear to what extent the results of the first study are relevant in most patients.

Special senses *Color vision abnormalities* are a well-known adverse effect of digitalis (SEDA-10, 143; SEDA-15, 166; SEDA-8, 197). In a further study healthy volunteers took one of four dosages of digitoxin between 0.03 and 0.1 mg/day for 2 weeks each (5[C]). Only with the highest dosage was there impairment of color vision, as tested by electroretinography. In view of the fact that color vision abnormalities with digoxin are concentration related (6[C]) this result is not surprising; furthermore, since digitoxin is more water-soluble than digoxin, it may penetrate the retina less well.

That digitalis can produce visual distur-

Side Effects of Drugs, Annual 20
J.K. Aronson, ed.

bances even in association with serum concentrations in the usual therapeutic range has been confirmed in a further report of six patients aged 66—85 years, five of whom had *photopsia* and one *reduced visual acuity* (7[c]). Four of five patients who were studied had prolonged cone b-wave times on the electroretinogram, consistent with an effect of digoxin.

Interactions   Drug interactions of clinical significance with cardiac glycosides have again been reviewed (8[R]).

In an interaction study in 12 healthy men *ziluton* had no important effects on the pharmacokinetics of digoxin (9[C]).

Treatment of digitalis toxicity   The use of Fab fragments of digoxin-specific antibodies in the treatment of digitalis toxicity has again been reviewed (10[R]), (11[R]).

In an 85-year-old woman with digitalis-associated delirium during treatment for congestive heart failure antidigoxin antibody reversed the delirium within 3 h of treatment (12[c]).

OTHER INOTROPIC DRUGS *(SED-13, 447; SEDA-17, 217; SEDA-18, 198; SEDA-19, 189)*

Thrombocytopenia has been reported in up to 1% of patients taking long-term milrinone (SEDA-16, 175). In a study of 27 patients undergoing cardiac surgery requiring cardiopulmonary bypass, the platelet count fell significantly from about 230×10^9/l to around 100×10^9/l at 2 and 24 h after bypass, accompanied by a significant increase in bleeding time; however, the acute administration of milrinone intravenously had no extra effect (13[C]).

DRUGS USED IN DYSRHYTHMIAS

The adverse effects of antidysrhythmic drugs have been prospectively studied in 300 patients. There were adverse effects in 41 (13.6%), serious in nine cases, including five *dysrhythmias*, one case of *pulmonary fibrosis*, one of *peripheral neuropathy*, and two of *acute heart failure* (14[c]). Adverse effects led to withdrawal of treatment in 26 cases (7.6%). Of the drugs used (amiodarone, cibenzoline,

disopyramide, flecainide, hydroquinidine, mexiletine, propafenone, quinidine, and sotalol), the drugs that were most commonly associated with adverse effects were disopyramide (46%) and propafenone (42%). Sotalol was less commonly associated with adverse effects (2%) than the other drugs (flecainide 20%, amiodarone 16%, cibenzoline 5%, hydroquinidine 4%). Adverse effects were more common when two drugs were used (39%) than one drug (13%).

The commonest form of dysrhythmia in response to antidysrhythmic drugs is *torsade de pointes*, the mechanisms of which have been reviewed (15[R]). An attempt has been made to differentiate between the prolongation of the QT_c interval produced by antidysrhythmic drugs in cases in which it does or does not lead to torsade de pointes (16[C]). The TU wave of the electrocardiogram was studied in 18 patients without a history of torsade de pointes or syncope (control group) and eight patients with torsade de pointes induced by class Ia drugs. The QT_c interval was prolonged in both groups, but to a greater extent in those who had had torsade de pointes. Furthermore the amplitude of the U wave in those patients also increased significantly. The authors suggested that the increased amplitude of the U wave may help to differentiate those patients who are more likely to develop torsade de pointes when the QT_c interval is prolonged. In those in the control group taking quinidine there was a positive correlation between the change in the QT_c interval and the serum quinidine concentration. However, there was no correlation with the change in amplitude of the U wave.

Adenosine *(SED-13, 450; SEDA-17, 219; SEDA-18, 200; SEDA-19, 190)*

The adverse effects of adenosine continue to be reported in large studies of its use as an antidysrhythmic drug (17[C]), in the diagnosis of coronary artery disease and myocardial ischemia (18[C]), and in the study of myocardial function after acute myocardial infarction (19[C]). As before (SEDA-16, 176; SEDA-18, 200), the common adverse effects are *headache, weakness, flushing, dyspnea and bronchospasm, chest or epigastric pain or discomfort, sore throat, paresthesia, light-headedness,* and *nausea*. Cardiac effects include *ventricular extra beats*, *atrioventricular block*, and *asystole*; occasionally *ST segment depression* may occur in the electrocardiogram. *Atrial fibrillation* and symptomatic *hypotension* occur occasionally (19[C]). The adverse effects of adenosine triphosphate are similar to those of adenosine (20[C]). In six patients with cerebrovascular disease adenosine increased cerebral blood flow without causing major adverse effects (21[C]).

Cardiovascular Serious cardiac dysrhythmias, including ventricular fibrillation, have occasionally been reported with adenosine (SEDA-18, 200). Another case of *ventricular fibrillation* has been reported in an 8-day-old infant with Wolff-Parkinson-White syndrome (22[c]). Digoxin was also used in this case, and the authors suggested that the adverse effect may have been due to an interaction of adenosine with digoxin; however, it is not clear what the mechanism of such an interaction might be.

In 20 patients who had coronary artery surgery, adenosine in dosages of 30—120 mg/kg/min caused dose-dependent increases in heart rate, cardiac output, and stroke volume, and reductions in arterial pressure and systemic and pulmonary vascular resistances (23[C]). There was a small but statistically significant depression of the mean ST segment during adenosine infusion and two patients developed clear ST segment changes consistent with new *ischemia*. However, there were no concomitant changes in regional or global wall motion.

Exercise has been found to reduce the non-cardiac effects and the incidence of major dysrhythmias in 407 patients who were randomized to adenosine by infusion for 6 min, adenosine with submaximal exercise, or adenosine with symptom-limited exercise (24[C]). Of the non-cardiac effects, faintness, flushing, headache, nausea, and anxiety were all significantly reduced by exercise. Atrioventricular block was reduced from 4.7 to 0.4%, and sinus bradycardia/arrest was similarly less common (4.7 vs. 0.4%). Shortening the duration of adenosine infusion from 6 to 4 min can also produce small reductions in the adverse effects profile (25[C]). In 1351 patients adverse effects occurred in about 90% no matter what the rate of infusion. Non-cardiac effects were not altered, but there was significantly less chest discomfort and ischemic ST segment changes in those given adenosine for only 4 min.

Amiodarone *(SED-13, 452; SEDA-17, 220; SEDA-18, 200; SEDA-19, 192)*

The pharmacology, clinical pharmacology, uses, and adverse effects and interactions of amiodarone have again been reviewed (26[R]), (27[R]).

Although the results of CAST showed that some class I antidysrhythmic drugs increased mortality in patients with asymptomatic ventricular dysrhythmias after myocardial infarction, some studies have shown that amiodarone, whose actions are predominantly of class III, may *reduce* mortality in such circumstances (28[R]). This was also the case in a study of 127 patients with poor left ventricular function and asymptomatic ventricular dysrhythmias who were randomized to amiodarone or placebo (29[C]). In contrast, in a study of 674 patients with congestive heart failure and asymptomatic ventricular dysrhythmias there was no significant difference in overall mortality in those given amiodarone compared with placebo (30[C]). This was despite the fact that amiodarone significantly suppressed ventricular dysrhythmias and increased the left ventricular ejection fraction by 42% after 2 years. The reasons for the discrepancy between the results of this study and those of others are not clear, but quite a high dosage of amiodarone was used, and there was a relatively high withdrawal rate due to adverse effects; it may therefore be that adverse effects of amiodarone counterbalanced any beneficial effect on mortality.

The adverse effects of high-dosage amiodarone have been reported in a study of 33 patients with refractory breast cancer who were treated with an infusion of doxorubicin or vinblastine with oral amiodarone to inhibit the P-glycoprotein, in the hope of reducing resistance to the cancer chemotherapy (31[C]). Amiodarone was given in a loading dose of 1000 mg/day for 2 weeks followed by 600—800 mg/day. Gastrointestinal adverse effects occurred in 21 of the 33 patients (*anorexia, nausea, vomiting,* or *diarrhea*). Cardiac complications were also quite common: eight patients developed *first-degree atrioventricular block* and there was one case of *junctional rhythm* and one of *second-degree atrioventricular block*. Amiodarone was discontinued in three patients with *ocular keratopathy*. *Hepatotoxicity* was suspected in one patient, but there were also extensive metastases. There were neurological symptoms (*weakness, paresthesia, dysesthesia*, or *muscle cramps in the leg*) in three patients. In those cases there was a trend towards higher plasma concentrations of total amiodarone plus desethylamiodarone, but there were no correlations of plasma concentrations with the presence of other adverse effects.

Cardiovascular With the licensing of amiodarone in an intravenous formulation in the US, further studies and reviews on the use of intravenous amiodarone have appeared (32^C), (33^R)−(36^R). As has often been noted before (SEDA-10, 147; SEDA-17, 220), *hypotension* is the commonest adverse effect of intravenous amiodarone; in one series it occurred in 13% (35^R). *Thrombophlebitis* (SEDA-13, 140) can be avoided by infusing the drug into a large vessel in a solution of low concentration. *Bradycardia* and *atrioventricular block* occur in about 5% of cases.

Respiratory Another case of *bronchiolitis obliterans organizing pneumonia* attributed to amiodarone has been reported (37^c).

A 61-year-old woman who had been taking amiodarone 200 mg/day on 5 days of the week (cumulative total dose 370 mg) developed an unproductive cough, left-sided pleuritic chest pain, a fever of 30°C, weakness, and anorexia. There were bilateral basal pulmonary infiltrates, and pulmonary function tests showed reduced diffusion. The amiodarone was withdrawn and she made a good recovery with prednisone (1 mg/kg/day). Two months later the pulmonary infiltrates had disappeared, and the lung function tests were normal.

Skin and appendages *Increased sensitivity of the skin to light* in patients taking amiodarone can be prevented by the use of topical zinc oxide or titanium oxide (SEDA-9, 166; SEDA-11, 156). There has recently been a report that narrow-band UVB phototherapy ameliorated the effects of amiodarone-induced photosensitivity in a 56-year-old man (38^c). After phototherapy (cumulative dose 6129 mJ/cm^2) he was able to increase his daily tolerance of direct sunlight from under 3 min to about 3−4 h.

Risk factors The risk factors for the non-cardiovascular adverse effects of amiodarone have been studied in 44 patients who took it for an average of 100 weeks for supraventricular dysrhythmias (39^C). The patients who developed adverse effects in the skin (9%) were more likely to be under 60 than over, and those who developed hepatic adverse effects (7%) had significantly reduced left ventricular function. In no case was there any relation between adverse effects and duration of therapy, cumulative dose, or serum concentration of amiodarone or amiodarone plus desethylamiodarone.

Second-generation effects In a survey of the patients treated by all adult and pediatric cardiologists in Canada, 12 pregnant women were identified as having taken amiodarone either for the entire duration of pregnancy (seven cases) or for 15−32 weeks (five cases) (40^C). Most of the women were taking 200−400 mg/day but one took 800 mg/day for 10 days followed by 600 mg/day for 5 days a week. Of six cases in which there was exposure in the first trimester one child had *congenital nystagmus* with *synchronous head titubation*. There was one case each of transient neonatal *hypothyroidism* and *hyperthyroidism*. One child who was exposed to amiodarone from 20 weeks of gestation onwards had developed *mental delay, hypotonia, hypertelorism*, and *micrognathia*. The authors considered that the possible link between amiodarone and neurotoxicity in one child was speculative. However, they thought that the occurrence of thyroid disease was likely to be associated with amiodarone. Anecdotal report of thyroid abnormalities in fetuses exposed to amiodarone during pregnancy have previously been reported (SEDA-13, 141; SEDA-14, 149).

Cibenzoline *(SED-13, 457; SEDA-15, 173; SEDA-17, 222; SEDA-18, 203)*

In 123 outpatients who were treated with oral cibenzoline for 3 months to prevent recurrence of supraventricular dysrhythmias, adverse effects occurred in 41% of cases and required withdrawal in 8% (41[C]). The most frequently reported adverse effects affected the gastrointestinal system (*nausea, vomiting, diarrhea*, and *abdominal pain*) and the nervous system (*vertigo, faintness*, and *nervousness*). Others included *muscular pain, hypoglycemia* (which has previously been reported quite commonly, SEDA-13, 142; SEDA, 18, 204), *pruritus, headache, hypertension, nightmares and insomnia, constipation*, and *foul-smelling sweat*.

Cardiovascular In 37 patients treated with intravenous cibenzoline for acute supraventricular tachydysrhythmias, there was a significant *increase in ventricular rate* in eight patients from 148 to 196 beats per minute on average (42[C]). This was poorly tolerated in two patients, requiring treatment with intravenous amiodarone in one case and cardioversion in the other. There was asymptomatic *prolongation of the QRS complex* in three cases, and in the group as a whole a significant *reduction in systolic blood pressure* from 130 to 121 mmHg. Success or failure in converting the rhythm to sinus rhythm was not associated with plasma cibenzoline concentration. There have previously been anecdotal reports of dysrhythmias in patients given cibenzoline (SEDA-17, 222; SEDA-18, 203).

Disopyramide *(SED-13, 457; SEDA-17, 222; SEDA-18, 204; SEDA-19, 194)*

The major metabolite of disopyramide, mono-*N*-dealkylated disopyramide has pharmacological activity and might contribute to the therapeutic or adverse effects of disopyramide. In a study of 79 patients with ventricular or supraventricular dysrhythmias, those in whom it was effective had a significantly higher average minimum serum concentration of disopyramide at steady state (2.14 vs. 1.74 mg/ml), although there was a large degree of overlap between the groups (43[C]). However, when the dosage of disopyramide was in-

creased in 14 patients in whom it had been ineffective (serum concentration 1.40 mg/l) it was effective in eight with a serum concentration of 1.72 mg/l, but ineffective in another three with a mean serum concentration of 2.56 mg/l. Adverse effects were mainly attributable to anticholinergic actions of disopyramide, namely *dry mouth* and *dysuria*; these occurred in 14 patients. There was no difference in the steady-state serum concentration of disopyramide in those with and without adverse effects, nor in the serum of the active metabolites.

Encainide *(SED-13, 458; SEDA-17, 222)*

Attempts continue to be made to elucidate the mechanisms of the *increased mortality* in patients given encainide and flecainide for asymptomatic ventricular dysrhythmias after myocardial infarction in the Cardiac Arrhythmia Suppression Trial (CAST). In one such study the time to the first event (dysrhythmia, ischemia, or heart failure) was analysed (44[R]). Although encainide and flecainide appeared to convert an ischemic event to death in more cases and more quickly than moricizine, an excess of deaths with flecainide and encainide occurred as often after heart failure as after an ischemic event. The authors were unable to identify any specific mechanism to explain the adverse effects in CAST. In another analysis the total numbers of non-fatal ischemic events and sudden deaths were the same in the placebo and treatment groups, but the deaths occurred more commonly in those who took active treatment (45[R]). The authors suggested that in some way encainide or flecainide may have interacted with active ischemia, converting non-fatal to fatal events. The authors proposed that this was not due to a prodysrhythmic action, despite the fact that they thought that the mechanism of death was a ventricular dysrhythmia. Because they thought that the effect was due to an interaction between ischemia and the drug they were reluctant to classify it with the traditional categories of prodysrhythmia.

Flecainide *(SED-13, 459; SEDA-17, 223; SEDA-18, 204; SEDA-19, 195)*

The mechanism of the increased mortality in CAST due to encainide and flecainide is discussed above under encainide.

In contrast to the increased risk of death in patients with ventricular dysrhythmias, flecainide may be safer in patients with supraventricular dysrhythmias (SEDA-16, 180; SEDA-17, 223). In an open, randomized comparison of flecainide and propafenone in 335 patients with paroxysmal atrial fibrillation or supraventricular tachycardia and no history of heart disease, 12 of 169 patients who were treated with flecainide 100—200 mg/day reported 16 adverse cardiac effects (46[C]). There were four cases of *bundle branch block*, three of *dysrhythmias*, two of *ankle edema*, and one each of *hypotension* and *left ventricular failure*. In five cases the effects were serious enough to merit withdrawal. Poor left ventricular function was not a risk factor in this study. Other less serious adverse effects that were reported were *headache* and *dizziness*.

Procainamide *(SED-13, 463; SEDA-17, 226; SEDA-18, 206; SEDA-19, 196)*

Cardiovascular   There has been a further report of two cases of *torsade de pointes* in 55 patients treated with procainamide for the suppression of inducible ventricular tachycardia (47[C]). Both were women in their sixties and in one case the QT interval was particularly prolonged to 600 ms after a dose of 4000 mg/day for 3 days. Neither case was fatal.

Immunological and hypersensitivity reactions   Procainamide-induced *lupus-like syndrome* is associated with a variety of antibodies, including antibodies to histones and histone—DNA complexes (SEDA-14, 152; SEDA-17, 226). This particularly affects the H2A-H2B dimer, especially when it is bound to DNA. The antibodies are of the IgG class. In a longitudinal study 31 patients, nine of whom stopped taking procainamide because of lupus-like syndrome, most of the patients with drug-induced lupus had IgG antibody to the (H2A-H2B)—DNA complex at the time of diagnosis (48[C]). In contrast, the patients who did not have lupus-like syndrome had

negligible concentrations of the antibody, although some of them had antibodies of the IgA and IgM classes. The authors concluded that chronic exposure to procainamide commonly produced autoantibodies with specificities for denatured epitopes on DNA and histones and for native regions on the (H2A-H2B)—DNA subunit of chromatin. However only in those who went on to develop lupus-like syndrome did the antibodies switch to the IgG class.

A case of *Achilles tendonitis* has been reported in a 63-year-old man with rheumatoid arthritis for many years who was treated with procainamide 1 g qds (49[C]). He also developed angio-edema, a pleural rub, tremor, and painful costochondritis, anemia, liver damage, pericarditis, and myasthenia gravis, all of which were attributed to the procainamide.

Propafenone *(SED-13, 465; SEDA-17, 226; SEDA-18, 206; SEDA-19, 196)*

The clinical pharmacology, pharmacological and therapeutic effects, adverse effects, and uses of propafenone been reviewed (50[R]), (51[R]).

In a study of the use of propafenone (13 mg/kg/day) in the prevention of paroxysmal atrial fibrillation in 102 patients, *nausea* (nine patients), *dizziness* (eight), and *headache* (five) were the most common adverse effects (52[C]). In all, adverse effects occurred in 27% of the patients taking propafenone and treatment was withdrawn in 3%. Although the ejection fraction was significantly reduced, there was no change in blood pressure or heart rate. Prodysrhythmic effects did not occur. Propafenone was more effective than placebo and less effective than sotalol, which however had more adverse effects.

Cardiovascular   In most studies, cardiovascular adverse effects are reported in a few patients. In a double-blind, placebo-controlled study of the effect of propafenone in 100 patients with either paroxysmal supraventricular tachycardia or atrial fibrillation/flutter, one patient developed a *ventricular dysrhythmia* and four developed *dyspnea* or *heart failure* (53[C]). In an open-label, randomized, parallel-group study in 335 patients with paroxysmal atrial fibrillation or paroxysmal supraventricular tachycardia and no history of heart disease, there was one case of ventricular tachycardia among one of the 103 patients being treated with propafenone. In addition, there were two cases of *atrioventricular block*, two of *bradycardia*, and two of *syncope* (46[C]). In a randomized study of the effects of propafenone in the treatment of atrial fibrillation of recent onset in 25 patients, there was one case of *bradycardia* with transient *hypotension* and one case of asymptomatic *sinus arrest* lasting 2 s (54[C]).

Nervous system In the study mentioned above of 100 patients treated with propafenone for paroxysmal dysrhythmias, the most common adverse effects were unspecified neuropsychiatric effects (53[C]). These accounted for 18 events during propafenone treatment compared with four events with placebo.

Propafenone had also been reported to have caused a *peripheral neuropathy* in a 41-year-old man who had taken 450 mg/day for about a year (55[c]). Although propafenone occasionally causes nervous system adverse effects (SEDA-10, 151), this seems to have been the first report of a peripheral neuropathy. The neuropathy resolved 6 months after withdrawal.

Quinidine *(SED-13, 466; SEDA-17, 227; SEDA-18, 207; SEDA-19, 196)*

In a randomized study of the effects of quinidine in 50 patients with persistent atrial fibrillation the commonest adverse effects were *gastrointestinal* (seven patients) (56[C]). There was *sinus bradycardia* in two patients and *worsening of congestive heart failure* in one. Four patients had *dysrhythmias*, three with torsade de pointes, and one with a sustained monomorphic ventricular tachycardia. In two patients torsade de pointes degenerated into ventricular fibrillation. In three of the four patients with dysrhythmias, the plasma quinidine concentration was well within the target range of 3−8 μg/ml. Quinidine withdrawal was required in 10 out of 14 patients with adverse effects, 25 in all having taken the drug.

Immunological and hypersensitivity reactions *Lupus-like syndrome* is rare in patients taking quinidine, but another case has been reported in a 79-year-old woman who took quinidine 324 mg 8-hourly for prevention of recurrence of atrial fibrillation (57[cr]). About 4 months later she developed a fever and tachycardia, a mild anemia, slight increases in liver enzyme activities, and later painful swelling of the fingers. The ANA titer was 1:20, with a speckled pattern, and antihistone antibodies were positive for the H2A-H2B dimer. The syndrome resolved on withdrawal of the drug and the administration of prednisone 10 mg/day for 5 days.

In another case, a 56-year-old man who took quinidine 324 mg five times a day for prevention of paroxysmal atrial fibrillation, developed an illness resembling *polymyalgia rheumatica* after about 2 months (57[cr]). The symptoms resolved with 24−48 h of withdrawal.

In a summary of 30 reported cases of quinidine-induced lupus-like syndrome various autoantibodies were documented (57[cr]). There were positive antihistone antibodies in five cases, positive anti-double-stranded DNA antibodies in four cases, and a positive Coombs' test in five cases. Serum complement (C3 and/or C4) was low in six cases. In most cases resolution of the syndrome occurred within 4 weeks of discontinuation, although in four cases it took 12−24 weeks, and in one case 104 weeks. The common clinical features were fever (10 cases), arthritis and/or arthralgia (25), myalgia (three), skin rashes (nine), hepatomegaly (four), splenomegaly (three), pleurisy or pleural effusion (six), and pericarditis (one). Renal involvement is rare in drug-induced lupus, and occurred in only two cases. There was neurological involvement in seven cases.

Lupus anticoagulant has been reported to be associated with the use of both quinine and quinidine (58[C]). All patients over 60 years old who had lupus anticoagulant detected over 21 months were reviewed. There were 31 in all, of whom 23 were taking cinchona alkaloids. Ten were taking quinine for night cramps, 11 were taking quinidine for dysrhythmias, and two were taking both. This was significantly higher than the incidence of the use of these drugs in 31 age- and sex-matched controls.

Four patients had features that could have been due to antiphospholipid syndrome: pulmonary emboli in two cases, a retinal artery thrombosis in one, and pulmonary embolus associated with thrombocytopenia and a facial rash in another.

REFERENCES

1. The Digitalis Investigation Group. The effect of digoxin on mortality and morbidity in patients with heart failure. New Engl J Med 1997; 336:525—33.

2. Van Veldhuisen DJ, Brouwer J, Man-in-t-Veld AJ, Dunselman PHJM, Boomsma F, Lie KI. Progression of mild untreated heart failure during six months follow-up and clinical and neurohumoral effects of ibopamine and digoxin as monotherapy. Am J Cardiol 1995;75:796—800.

3. Covit AB, Schaer GL, Sealey JE, Laragh JH, Cody RJ. Suppression of the renin-angiotensin system by intravenous digoxin in chronic congestive heart failure. Am J Med 1983;75:445—7.

4. Gheorghiade M, Hall VB, Jacobsen G, Alam M, Rosman H, Goldstein S. Effects of increasing maintenance dose of digoxin on left ventricular function and neurohormones in patients with chronic heart failure treated with diuretics and angiotensin-converting enzyme inhibitors. Circulation 1995;92:1801—7.

5. Duncker GIW, Kisters G, Grille W. Prospective, randomized, placebo-controlled, double-blind testing of colour vision and electroretinoram at therapeutic and subtherapeutic digitoxin serum levels. Ophthalmologica 1994;208:259—61.

6. Aronson JK, Ford AR. The use of colour vision measurement in the diagnosis of digoxin toxicity. Q J Med 1980;49:273—82.

7. Butler VP Jr, Odel JG, Rath E, Wolin MJ, Behrens MM, Martin TJ, Kardon RH, Gouras P. Digitalis-induced visual disturbances with therapeutic serum digitalis concentrations. Ann Intern Med 1995;123:676—80.

8. Magnani B, Malini PL. Cardiac glycosides: drug interactions of clinical significance. Drug Saf 1995;12:97—109.

9. Awni WM, Hussein Z, Cavanaugh JH, Granneman GR, Dube LM. Assessment of the pharmacokinetic interaction between zileuton and digoxin in humans. Clin Pharmacokinet 1995;29 Suppl 2:92—7.

10. Woolf A. Digitalis intoxication therapy with digoxin-specific antibody fragments. Clin Immunother 1995;4:312—30.

11. Anonymous. Digoxin-specific Fab therapy: an effective antidote for digoxin toxicity. Drugs Ther Perspect 1995;6:11—14.

12. Varriale P, Mossavi A. Rapid reversal of digitalis delirium using digoxin immune Fab therapy. Clin Cardiol 1995;18:351—2.

13. Kikura M, Lee MK, Safon RA, Bailey JM, Levy JH. The effects of milrinone on platelets in patients undergoing cardiac surgery. Anesth Analg 1995;81:44—8.

14. Vigreux P, Lemozit JP, Delay M, Bernadet P, Montastruc JL. Antiarrhythmic drug-induced side effects: a prospective survey of 300 patients. Thérapie 1995;50:413—18.

15. Tan HL, Hou CJY, Lauer MR, Sung RJ. Electrophysiologic mechanisms of the long QT interval syndromes and torsade de pointes. Ann Intern Med 1995;122:701—14.

16. Maruyama T, Ohe T, Kurita T, Aihara N, Shimizu W. Physiological and pathological responses of TU waves to class Ia antiarrhythmic drugs. Eur Heart J 1995;16:667—73.

17. Madsen CD, Pointer JE, Lynch TG. A comparison of adenosine and verapamil for the treatment of supraventricular tachycardia in the pre-hospital setting. Ann Emerg Med 1995;25:649—55.

18. Miyagawa M, Kumano S, Sekiya M, Watanabe K, Akutzu H, Imachi T, Tanada S, Hamamoto K. Thallium-201 myocardial tomography with intravenous infusion of adenosine triphosphate in diagnosis of coronary artery disease. J Am Coll Cardiol 1995;26:1196—201.

19. Claeys MJ, Vrints CJ, Krug B, Bosmans JM, Blockx PP, Bossaert LL, Snoeck JP. Adenosine technetium-99m sestamibi (SPECT) for the early assessment of jeopardized myocardium after acute myocardial infarction. Eur Heart J 1995; 16:1186—94.

20. Fukai T, Koyanagi S, Tashiro H, Ichiki T, Tsutsui H, Matsumoto T, Takeshita A. Adenosine triphosphate stress echocardiography in the detection of myocardial ischemia. Am J Card Imaging 1995;9:237—44.

21. Soricelli A, Postiglione A, Cuocolo A, De Chiara S, Ruocco A, Brunetti A, Salvatore M, Ell PJ. Effect of adenosine on cerebral blood flow as evaluated by single-photon emission computed tomography in normal subjects and in patients with occlusive carotid disease: a comparison with acetazolamide. Stroke 1995;26:1572—6.

22. Mulla N, Karpawich PP. Ventricular fibrillation following adenosine therapy for supraventricular tachycardia in a neonate with concealed Wolff-Parkinson-White syndrome treated with digoxin. Pediatr Emerg Care 1995;11:238—9.

23. Houltz E, Ricksten SE, Milocco I, Gustavsson T, Caidahl K. Effects of adenosine infusion on systolic and diastolic left ventricular function after coronary artery bypass surgery: evaluation by computer-assisted quantitative 2-D and Doppler echocardiography. Anesth Analg 1995;80:47—53.

24. Pennell DJ, Mavrogeni SI, Forbat SM, Karwatowski SP, Underwood SR. Adenosine combined with dynamic exercise for myocardial perfusion imaging. J Am Coll Cardiol 1995;25:1300—9.

25. O Keefe JH Jr, Bateman TM, Handlin LR, Barnhart CS. Four- versus 6-minute infusion protocol for adenosine thallium-201 single photon emission computed tomography imaging. Am Heart J 1995;129:482—7.

26. Podrid PJ. Amiodarone: reevaluation of an old drug. Ann Intern Med 1995;122:689—700.

27. Howard PA. Amiodarone for the maintenance of sinus rhythm in patients with atrial fibrillation. Ann Pharmacother 1995;29:596—602.

28. Ozdil E, Carlson TA, Massumi A. Use of amiodarone in the postmyocardial infarction patient. Tex Heart Inst J 1995;22:40—3.

29. Garguichevich JJ, Ramos JL, Gambarte A, Gentile A, Hauad S, Scapin O, Sirena J, Tibaldi M, Toplikar J. Effect of amiodarone therapy on mortality in patients with left ventricular dysfunction and asymptomatic complex ventricular arrhythmias: Argentine Pilot Study of Sudden Death and Amiodarone (EPAMSA). Am Heart J 1995;130:494—500.

30. Singh SN, Fletcher RD, Fisher SG, Singh BN, Lewis HD, Deedwania PC, Massie BM, Colling C, Lazzeri D. Amiodarone in patients with congestive heart failure and asymptomatic ventricular arrhythmia. New Engl J Med 1995;333:77—82.

31. Bates SE, Meadows B, Goldspiel BR, Denicoff A, Le TB, Tucker E, Steinberg SM, Elwood LJ. A pilot study of amiodarone with infusional doxorubicin or vinblastine in refractory breast cancer. Cancer Chemother Pharmacol 1995;35:457—63.

32. Hou ZY, Chang MS, Chen CY, Tu MS, Lin SL, Chiang HT, Woosley RL. Acute treatment of recent-onset atrial fibrillation and flutter with a tailored dosing regimen of intravenous amiodarone. A randomized, digoxin-controlled study. Eur Heart J 1995;16:521—8.

33. Kowey PR. A new treatment for catastrophic arrhythmias. Cardiovasc Rev Rep 1995;16:27—9.

34. Anonymous. Intravenous amiodarone. Med Lett Drugs Ther 1995;37:114—15.

35. Scheinman MM. Parenteral antiarrhythmic drug therapy in ventricular tachycardia/ventricular fibrillation: evolving role of class III agents—focus on amiodarone. J Cardiovasc Electrophysiol 1995;6:914—19.

36. Tran HT, Kluger J, Chow MSS. Focus on IV amiodarone: a new formulation for acute arrhythmia treatment. Formulary 1995;30:509—19.

37. Valle JM, Alvarez D, Antunez J, Valdes L. Bronchiolitis obliterans organizing pneumonia secondary to amiodarone: a rare aetiology. Eur Respir J 1995;8:470—1.

38. Collins P, Ferguson J. Narrow-band UVB (TL-01) phototherapy: an effective preventative treatment for the photodermatoses. Br J Dermatol 1995;132:956—63.

39. Tisdale JE, Follin SL, Ordelova A, Webb CR. Risk factors for the development of specific non-cardiovascular adverse effects associated with amiodarone. J Clin Pharmacol 1995;35:351—6.

40. Magee LA, Downar E, Sermer M, Boulton BC, Allen LC, Koren G. Pregnancy outcome after gestational exposure to amiodarone in Canada. Am J Obstet Gynecol 1995;172:1307—11.

41. El Allaf D, Schifflers E, Kormoss N. Cibenzoline in the prevention of recurrence of supraventricular arrhythmias. Acta Cardiol 1995;50:53—64.

42. Bru P, Cointe R, Paganelli F, Ricard P, Levy S. Intravenous cibenzoline in the management of acute supraventricular tachyarrhythmias. Cardiovasc Drugs Ther 1995;9:85—8.

43. Masuhara K, Ohno T, Hamaguchi K, Katoh K, Kashiwada K, Takahashi S, Tanaka V, Someya K, Ogata H. Relationship between the therapeutic effects or side-effects and the serum disopyramide or mono-*N*-dealkylated disopyramide concentration after repeated oral administration of disopyramide to arrhythmic patients. Int J Clin Pharmacol Res 1995;15:103—13.

44. Hallstrom AP, Anderson JL, Carlson M, Davies R, Greene HL, Kammerling JM, Romhilt DW, Duff HJ, Huther M. Time to arrhythmic, ischemic, and heart failure events: exploratory analyses to elucidate mechanisms of adverse drug effects in the Cardiac Arrhythmia Suppression Trial. Am Heart J 1995;130:71—9.

45. Greenberg HM, Dwyer EM Jr, Hochman JS, Steinberg JS, Echt DS, Peters RW. Interaction of ischaemia and encainide/flecainide treatment: a proposed mechanism for the increased mortality in CAST I. Br Heart J 1995;74:631—5.

46. Chimienti M, Cullen MT Jr, Casadei G. Safety of flecainide versus propafenone for the long-term management of symptomatic paroxysmal supraventricular tachyarrhythmias—report from the Flecainide and Propafenone Italian Study (FAPIS) Group. Eur Heart J 1995;16:1943—51.

47. Singh BN, Kehoe R, Woosley RL, Scheinman M, Quart B. Multicenter trial of sotalol compared with procainamide in the suppression of inducible ventricular tachycardia: a double-blind, randomized parallel evaluation. Am Heart J 1995;129:87—97.

48. Rubin RL, Burlingame RW, Arnott JE, Totoritis MC, McNally EM, Johnson AD. IgG but not other classes of anti-((H2A-H2B)-DNA) is an early sign of procainamide-induced lupus. J Immunol 1995;154:2483—93.

49. Sinatra BA. Acute resistant procainamide hydrochloride-induced lupus-like Achilles tendonitis: case report. J Neurol Orthop Med Surg 1995;16:227.

50. Capucci A, Boriani G. Propafenone in the treatment of cardiac arrhythmias: a risk-benefit appraisal. Drug Saf 1995;12:55—72.

51. Kishore AGR, Camm AJ. Guidelines for the use of propafenone in treating supraventricular arrhythmias. Drugs 1995;50:250—62.

52. Bellandi F, Dabizzi RP, Niccoli L, Cantini F. Propafenone and sotalol in the prevention of paroxysmal atrial fibrillation: long-term safety and efficacy study. Curr Ther Res Clin Exp 1995; 56:1154—68.

53. Cobbe SM, Rae AP, Poloniecki JD, Chong E, Balnave K, Moriarty A, Blackwood R, Cahill N, Cobbe S, Pye M, Sedgwick M, Cooper D, Flint J, Gould B, Hutchison S, Irvine N, Lewis P, O'Keefe B, Sanderson J et al. A randomized, placebo-controlled trial of propafenone in the prophylaxis of paroxysmal supraventricular tachycardia and paroxysmal atrial fibrillation. Circulation 1995;92:2550—7.

54. Baroffio R, Tisi G, Guzzini F, Milvio E, Annoni P. A randomised study comparing digoxin and propafenone in the treatment of recent onset atrial fibrillation. Clin Drug Invest 1995;9:277—83.

55. Galasso PJ, Stanton MS, Vogel H. Propafenone-induced peripheral neuropathy. Mayo Clin Proc 1995;70:469—72.

56. Hohnloser SH, Van De Loo A, Baedeker F. Efficacy and proarrhythmic hazards of pharmacologic cardioversion of atrial fibrillation: prospective comparison of sotalol versus quinidine. J Am Coll Cardiol 1995;26:852—8.

57. Alloway JA, Salata MP. Quinidine-induced rheumatic syndromes. Semin Arthritis Rheum 1995;24:315—22.

58. Bird MR, O'Neill AI, Buchanan RRC, Ibrahim KMA, Des Parkin J. Lupus anticoagulant in the elderly may be associated with both quinine and quinidine usage. Pathology 1995;27:136-9.

A.P. Maggioni, M.G. Franzosi and R. Latini

18 β-Adrenoceptor antagonists and antianginal drugs

β-ADRENOCEPTOR ANTAGONISTS (SED-13, 491; SEDA-17, 234; SEDA-18, 213; SEDA-19, 201)

ORGANS AND SYSTEMS

Cardiovascular Like other antidysrhythmic drugs, sotalol has a *negative inotropic effect*. Among 37 patients with atrial fibrillation, after electrical cardioversion (when atrial stunning is prominent) sotalol ($n = 17$) had a more negative inotropic effect than placebo ($n = 20$) (1[C]). However, this effect was temporary, since echocardiograms showed that there was no difference between sotalol and placebo in terms of myocardial contractility 1 month later. This effect can prejudice long-term maintenance of sinus rhythm after cardioversion.

Sotalol had *prodysrhythmic effects* in seven (10%) of 71 children (mean age 7.3 years) with various supraventricular and ventricular dysrhythmias, detected by surface ECG and serial Holter monitoring (2[C]). Prodysrhythmia required withdrawal of sotalol in four children: one with sino-atrial block, two with complex ventricular dysrhythmias, and one with recurrent syncope due to torsade de pointes. No other factors (such as electrolyte imbalance or concomitant medications) predisposing to these dysrhythmias were found. These prodysrhythmic effects of sotalol are consistent with similar reports in adults (SED-13, 493; SEDA-13, 149; SEDA-16, 191).

Respiratory Topical β-blockers given for the treatment of glaucoma may be absorbed systemically and cause *bronchospasm* especially among elderly people, even if they have no history of reversible airways disease. A randomized comparison of topical betaxolol, a cardioselective β-adrenoceptor antagonist, and dipifevrine, a sympathomimetic, has been carried out in 80 patients aged over 60 years who had no history of reversible airways disease and who were already using timolol. There was significant improvement in exercise tolerance, forced expiratory volume, and mean peak flow rate in both groups. The use of topical β-blockers for life is not a low-risk strategy. Ophthalmologists should consider alternatives, and if none is suitable, should preferably use cardioselective drugs (3[C]).

Skin and appendages Two reports have suggested that β-adrenoceptors have a role in pigmentation.

Of 548 patients with vitiligo, seven developed rapid *worsening of depigmentation* within 3 months of starting β-blocking therapy for hypertension. The drugs used were atenolol and metoprolol, neither of which has any partial agonist (intrinsic sympathomimetic) activity (4[C]).

Three cases of *periocular cutaneous pigmentary changes* have been described in patients using topical betaxolol for glaucoma: two patients developed periocular cutaneous hypopigmentation and one hyperpigmentation (5[c]). The first two cases may have been examples of Koebner-induced vitiligo, caused by selective toxic effect on melanocytes of betaxolol (or of an excipient in the formulation). The authors suggested that the case of hyperpigmentation might have stemmed from the same toxic effect. The skin changes resolved on withdrawal; all three patients refused to undertake rechallenge.

Musculoskeletal The occurrence of *muscle cramps* has been evaluated in 78 patients with essential hypertension treated with β-blockers with and without partial agonist activity (6[C]). The patients were randomized to receive pindolol or carteolol (drugs with partial agonist activity) or propranolol, metoprolol, or aretinolol (drugs without partial agonist activity) for 3 months each in a crossover design. Cramps occurred in 27 patients taking pindolol and in 32 taking carteolol. No muscle cramps occurred during treatment with propranolol or aretinolol, while two patients suffered cramps while taking metoprolol. Serum CK and CK-MB activities increased significantly during treatment with pindolol and carteolol, but did not change during treatment with the drugs without partial agonist activity. There was no correlation between the severity of muscle cramps and CK activity. The association of β-blockers with partial agonist activity and increased CK-MB activity suggests that β-blockers with partial agonist activity can cause myocardial cell injury.

Leg cramps have been attributed to dilevalol in a study of 114 patients aged over 65 who were randomized to receive bendrofluazide or dilevalol for essential hypertension (7[C]). Both drugs caused equivalent reductions in blood pressure, but pre-existing leg cramps worsened by 27% in patients treated with dilevalol, and by 6% in those treated with bendrofluazide.

Use in pregnancy The effects of β-adrenoceptor antagonists in pregnancy-induced hypertension have been evaluated in two studies. In the first study 51 women with pregnancy-induced hypertension were randomly allocated to hydralazine, hydralazine plus propranolol, or hydralazine plus pindolol (8[C]). All three regimens significantly reduced blood pressure. None of the women developed eclampsia during pregnancy or delivery. However, there were more adverse effects (palpitation, dizziness, and headache) in the women treated with hydralazine alone than in those treated with the combination of hydralazine plus a β-blocker. Mean birth weight and blood glucose at birth were significantly lower in the babies whose mothers had taken hydralazine plus propranolol compared with the other two groups. These findings suggest that β-adrenoceptor antagonists without partial agonist activity reduce uteroplacental blood flow in pregnancy-induced hypertension, resulting in *worse fetal development*.

In the second study 104 women with pregnancy-induced hypertension were randomized to labetalol or methyldopa (9[C]). Labetalol was quicker and more effective in controlling blood pressure and caused fewer adverse effects. Furthermore, the rate of cesarean section for uncontrolled pregnancy-induced hypertension was significantly lower with labetalol. However, a case of neonatal low-output congestive heart failure has been reported after a large prenatal dose of labetalol (300 mg) for pre-eclampsia (10[C]). The baby improved steadily after infusion of glucagon, which is the agent of first choice for the treatment of β-blocker toxicity, since it stimulates β-adrenoceptors and is less likely than direct β-adrenoceptor agonists (such as isoproterenol) to cause dysrhythmias.

INDIVIDUAL β-ADRENOCEPTOR ANTAGONISTS

Carvedilol *(SED-13, 504; SEDA-19, 202)*

A reversible case of *renal failure* has been reported in a randomized clinical trial of carvedilol versus placebo in 56 patients with severe chronic congestive heart failure (11[C]).

Celiprolol *(SED-13, 505)*

In 171 hyperlipidemic hypertensive patients celiprolol had significantly more favorable effects on serum lipids than metoprolol (12[C]). There were no changes in plasma fibrinogen concentrations with celiprolol or metoprolol.

NITRATE DERIVATIVES *(SED-13, 506; SEDA-17, 237; SEDA-18, 214; SEDA-19, 203)*

Isosorbide-5-mononitrate

Nadolol has been compared with isosorbide-5 mononitrate plus nadolol in a multicenter randomized clinical trial in the prophylaxis of variceal bleeding in 96 patients with cirrhosis and esophageal varices (13[C]). The combination did not increase the risk of renal failure or the development of ascites.

CALCIUM ANTAGONISTS *(SED-13, 509; SEDA-17, 237; SEDA-18, 215; SEDA-19, 203)*

℞ *The cardiovascular safety of calcium antagonists*

The issue of the cardiovascular safety of calcium antagonists has been widely debated following the publication of three articles: (a) a case-control study on the occurrence of myocardial infarction in hypertensive patients treated with a short-acting calcium antagonist (14[Cr]); (b) a meta-analysis of 16 randomized secondary prevention trials of nifedipine in patients with coronary heart disease (15[CR]); (c) a prospective cohort study in hypertensive elderly patients of the comparative risks of mortality with calcium antagonists, ACE-inhibitors, or β-blockers (16[Cr]).

In the first study, 623 hypertensive patients in the Group Health Co-operative of Puget Sound who had sustained a first myocardial infarction were matched with 2032 randomly selected hypertensive controls from the same care organization (14[Cr]). Among individuals without cardiovascular disease (335 cases and 1395 controls) the risk ratio for myocardial infarction was increased by about 60% among users of calcium antagonists with or without diuretics. In a second analysis, among patients taking a calcium antagonist or a β-blocker (384 cases and 1108 controls), the use of calcium antagonists compared with β-blockers was associated with about a 60% increase in the adjusted risk of myocardial infarction. While high dosages of β-blockers were associated with a reduced risk of myocardial infarction, high dosages of calcium antagonists were associated with an increased risk. The accompanying editorial commented that these results, although not conclusive and possibly confounded by indication, raised the possibility that calcium antagonists might be harmful (17[cr]).

Further evidence against nifedipine has been produced by a meta-analysis of secondary prevention trials (15[CR]). The purpose of this study was to assess the effect of the dosage of nifedipine on the mortality risk of patients with coronary heart disease and to review the mechanisms by which this adverse effect might occur.

Overall, among 8350 patients with a history of myocardial infarction, angina, or unstable angina, the use of short-acting nifedipine was associated with a significant increase in total mortality (risk ratio 1.16; 95% CI 1.01−1.33). The increase was dose related: for daily nifedipine doses of 30−50, 60, and 80 mg the risk ratios for total mortality were 1.06, 1.18, and 2.83, respectively. The reflex increase in sympathetic activity that short-acting calcium antagonists induce has been suggested to be the underlying mechanism of the proischemic, negative inotropic, and dysrhythmogenic effects of these compounds. The authors stressed the lack of adequate documentation of long-term safety of calcium antagonists, and the need for well-designed, large-scale clinical trials.

The prospective cohort study (16[Cr]) followed 906 hypertensive elderly patients for 4 years to determine whether elderly patients with hypertension treated with calcium antagonists and ACE inhibitors had a higher risk of mortality than those treated with β-blockers. With respect to β-blockers, the relative risks (95% CI) for mortality were short-acting nifedipine 1.7 (1.1−2.7), diltiazem 1.3 (0.8−2.1), verapamil 0.8 (0.4−1.4), and ACE-inhibitors 0.9 (0.6−1.4). The authors concluded that even if selective factors influencing the use of specific drugs in high-risk patients could not be completely discounted, the results showed a significantly reduced survival of elderly hypertensive patients treated with nifedipine compared with β-blockers.

These papers have been extensively discussed (17[r])−(20[r]). Major arguments against the first study (14[Cr]) were: (a) that selection bias could have resulted from the fact that calcium antagonists were used for hypertensive patients whose concomitant disorders also required a calcium antagonist; (b) the possible existence of a confounding bias, for which the study was not controlled (20[cr]). The meta-analysis (15[CR]) has also been widely criticized. One of the accompanying editorials (19[cr]) stated that there are grave defects in the dossier and that the allegations focus on short-acting nifedipine, so that even if correct, they cannot be applied to other calcium antagonists; the accusation of a dose-related increase in mortality rests on a biased selection of data chosen for the meta-analysis; and several of the me-

chanisms suggested for the proposed adverse effects are unlikely. The controversy is not over, and more data and publications are expected. At present, the widespread use of calcium antagonists (in particular the short-acting dihydropyridines, such as nifedipine) should await the results of further randomized trials.

Overdosage   The widespread use of calcium antagonists increases the possibility of accidental or deliberate self-poisoning in adults and children. Although only a few cases have been described (SED-13, 514; SEDA-16, 198), these drugs account for a high proportion of deaths in cases of overdosage associated with cardiovascular drugs. Factors that increase the risk of death include the dosage, the use of modified-release formulations, the presence of concomitant diseases, and the time elapsed from ingestion to intervention. In a review of the reported cases of calcium antagonist poisoning the presenting symptoms have been described and their management discussed (21[R]).

It has recently been reported that the half-life of verapamil was prolonged after overdose in a 59-year-old man (22[c]). The authors suggested that this was due to rate-limiting prolongation of the rate of absorption and, therefore, that repeated administration of activated charcoal should be routine in such cases, even if an ordinary-release formulation has been taken.

INDIVIDUAL CALCIUM ANTAGONISTS

Amlodipine *(SED-13, 515; SEDA-17, 239; SEDA-18, 215)*

The safety profile of amlodipine, in dosages of 2.5—10 mg daily, is similar to that of other dihydropyridines, *headache* and *peripheral edema* being the most frequent adverse events (23[c]), (24[c]). In an open, cross-over comparison of amlodipine 5 mg daily and modified-release nifedipine 20 mg daily in 426 hypertensive patients, amlodipine was better tolerated: the withdrawal rate because of adverse effects was 4.5% for amlodipine and 11.7% for nifedipine (25[c]).

In a comparison of the effects of amlodipine, atenolol, and their combination on is-chemia during treadmill testing and 48-h ambulatory monitoring, adverse events requiring withdrawal were 14.6% in the patients randomized to atenolol and 2% in the amlodipine group, among whom one patient withdrew because of a feeling of pressure at the base of the throat (26[C]).

In a study of the effects of amlodipine in 35 hypertensive patients with renal impairment, serum creatinine concentration was increased slightly in four of the patients (27[c]).

Diltiazem *(SED-13, 515; SEDA-18, 215; SEDA-19, 203)*

Liver   In a multicenter, double-blind, crossover comparison of two formulations of diltiazem, modified-release and plain, 41 patients with stable angina pectoris were randomized. The frequency and seriousness of the adverse events did not differ between the two groups. However, during 18 days of treatment with modified-release diltiazem a 55-year-old man without known liver disease developed fatigue, dyspepsia, increasing nausea, abdominal pain, and increased activities of hepatic enzymes. The symptoms resolved by 2 weeks after withdrawal and ultrasonography of the liver and gallbladder showed nothing abnormal (28[c]).

Skin and appendages   Adverse cutaneous effects are uncommon with diltiazem (SED-13, 516; SEDA-14, 164; SEDA-16, 197, SEDA-18, 215). A 60-year-old man developed *erythema multiforme* within 4 days of diltiazem therapy, followed by an increase in hepatic enzymes. The hepatic enzymes returned to normal after withdrawal and the erythema progressively disappeared (29[c]).

Felodipine *(SED-13, 516; SEDA-17, 239)*

Felodipine has been compared with enalapril in a double-blind randomized trial for 16 weeks in 46 patients with heart failure of NYHA class II or III (30[Cr]). There were similar improvements in quality of life and tolerability in the two groups, the only statistically significant difference being an increase in *peripheral edema* with felodipine.

Two once-a-day modified-release formulations, felodipine ER and nifedipine CR, have been compared in a double-blind, cross-over study in 41 hypertensive patients (31[cr]). The treatments had similar effects.

Felodipine (2.5—10 mg bd) has been given to 132 patients with NYHA class II or III heart failure for 12 weeks in a multicenter, double-blind, placebo-controlled randomized trial (32[Cr]). The effects of felodipine on exercise tolerance and ejection fraction were similar to those of placebo; however, felodipine significantly reduced blood pressure. The two adverse events that were more common with felodipine than placebo were *peripheral edema* without weight gain (23%) and *worsening symptoms of heart failure* requiring withdrawal (8%).

Isradipine *(SEDA-17, 239; SEDA-18, 215; SEDA-19, 203)*

The efficacy and tolerability of isradipine have been reviewed (33[R]). Its adverse reaction profile is qualitatively similar to that of other calcium antagonists; isradipine seems to be better tolerated as monotherapy than in combination with ACE inhibitors, β-blockers, or diuretics. The incidence of adverse reactions is independent of age.

Isradipine (5 mg bd) has been given orally for 3 weeks to 54 hypertensive pregnant women in a placebo-controlled, double-blind, randomized trial (34[CR]). Overall, treatment did not reduce blood pressure, but it did so in the subgroup without proteinuria. Isradipine was as safe as placebo in mothers and fetuses, there was no tocolytic effect, and the outcome of pregnancy was unaffected.

Nicardipine *(SEDA-17, 239; SEDA-18, 215; SEDA-19, 204)*

Nicardipine can be administered intravenously, with several indications, including control of blood pressure intraoperatively in response to tracheal intubation and in the postoperative phase (35[R]). Nicardipine should have limited negative inotropic effects, and excessive hypotension seems to be rare after intravenous infusion or bolus administration. However, clinical experience is insufficient to define the benefit/risk profile of intravenous nicardipine.

Nifedipine *(SED-13, 516; SEDA-18, 216; SEDA-19, 204)*

Liver Potentially, calcium antagonists should reduce the hepatic venous pressure gradient in patients with cirrhosis. However, verapamil and nicardipine have not had beneficial effects on portal pressure in clinical studies, and the results with nifedipine are controversial. The effects of nifedipine on splanchnic hemodynamics have been studied in 10 control subjects and 13 patients with cirrhosis and portal hypertension using hepatic venous catheterization and pulsed Doppler ultrasound (36[C]). Nifedipine significantly increased the hepatic venous pressure gradient and portal vein blood flow. The increase in portal vein blood flow was related to splanchnic arterial vasodilatation. The authors concluded that nifedipine should be used with caution in patients with chronic liver disease, since it may *increase the risk of variceal hemorrhage* in patients with less advanced varices.

Endocrine, metabolic The results of studies of the metabolic effects of nifedipine have been divergent, with both improvement and impairment of glucose metabolism. The metabolic effects of nifedipine have been compared with those of furosemide in a double-blind crossover study in 23 patients with hypertension; both drugs caused *abnormalities in glucose metabolism* (37[C]). Nifedipine caused a significant increase in glycosylated hemoglobin and in steady-state insulin concentration during hyperinsulinemic clamp, probably representing a fall in insulin clearance. The effects on glucose metabolism were related to the occurrence of tachycardia, suggesting that sympathetic nervous activation could be involved.

Use in pregnancy A non-randomized comparison of the hemodynamic effects of oral nifedipine and intravenous dihydralazine in 20 pregnant women with severe pre-eclampsia has shown similar reductions in arterial blood pressure and systemic vascular resistance, and similar rises in heart rate and cardiac output (38[C]). Pulmonary capillary wedge pressure fell significantly less with nifedipine than with dihydralazine. In patients treated with nifedipine there were no signs of fetal distress, whereas with dihydralazine the fetal cardiotocogram showed reduced variability and late deceleration in five cases. Two patients treated with nifedipine complained of mild headache and eight treated with dihydralazine complained of severe headache, accompanied in seven of them by nausea and vomiting. The authors concluded that from the hemodynamic point of view nifedipine seems to be useful in the treatment of hypertensive emergencies in pregnancy.

The results of several studies have suggested that nifedipine is at least as effective for tocolysis as ritodrine, terbutaline, or magnesium sulfate, with fewer maternal adverse effects (SEDA-18, 216; (39^R)). A retrospective study on the treatment of preterm labor in 61 women with oral nifedipine compared with intravenous ritodrine has confirmed a lower incidence of maternal adverse effects in nifedipine-treated patients and has suggested that nifedipine is more successful in postponing delivery than ritodrine, with a better perinatal outcome (40^C).

Nimodipine *(SEDA-17, 240)*

High intravenous doses of nimodipine (2—4 mg/h) reduced vasospasm in 11 patients with subarachnoid hemorrhage and signs of vasospasm before starting treatment (41^{cr}). Drug infusion under strict control of arterial pressure and cerebral flow with transcranial Doppler only caused minor reductions in blood pressure. In 87 consecutive similar patients, intravenous nimodipine in a maximum dose of 2 mg/h caused *hypotension* (mean arterial pressure below 75 mmHg for longer than 30 min) in 26 patients (42^{Cr}). However, hypotension occurred in only five cases during maintenance oral dosing. The authors considered the risk of hypotension with intravenous nimodipine unacceptable, and they therefore suggested that nimodipine be given orally from the start; intubated patients can receive nimodipine through a nasogastric tube.

High-dose nimodipine (180—270 mg/day) has been given to 10 patients with depressive episodes and without cardiovascular disorders (43^{cr}). There were no serious adverse effects; mild orthostatic hypotension occurred in three patients and gastrointestinal symptoms in two.

A randomized, placebo-controlled, double-blind trial of nimodipine (30 mg qds) was prematurely stopped after 149 patients had been enrolled because of excess mortality on the active treatment (8/75 vs. 1/74 deaths on nimodipine and placebo, respectively) (44^{Cr}). Excess mortality was due to an increased incidence of major surgical bleeding (10 vs. 2 on nimodipine and placebo, respectively): this is the first report of this adverse event with a calcium antagonist.

Nisoldipine *(SEDA-17, 240)*

The effects of age and liver failure have been studied in 17 hypertensive patients and seven patients with cirrhosis or chronic active hepatitis who took nisoldipine (5 mg/day) for 1—4 weeks (45^{cr}). One of the patients with liver disease developed fluid retention, worsening of ascites, and weight gain. The duration of treatment in the elderly was too short (1 week) to obtain a reliable estimate of the incidence of adverse reactions, which were in any case insignificant.

A new modified-release formulation of nisoldipine (Coat Core) has been tested in a randomized, double-blind, placebo-controlled trial of efficacy and safety in 312 out-patients with chronic stable angina for 2 weeks in daily doses of 20, 40, and 60 mg (46^{Cr}). Adverse reactions consisted mainly of *headache* and *fluid retention* and were clearly dose-related. *Cardiac ischemic events* (changes in anginal pattern or myocardial infarction) that were considered serious by the investigator occurred in two patients taking placebo (2.6%), none taking nisoldipine 20 mg, six (8%) taking 40 mg, and two (2.4%) taking 60 mg. Treatment was withdrawn because of adverse reactions in 21 patients in all.

Verapamil *(SEDA-15, 194)*

Endocrine, metabolic Verapamil has been reported to *increase serum prolactin concentrations*. A patient with verapamil-induced hyperprolactinemia, whose management was complicated by the presence of a pituitary microadenoma, as seen on magnetic resonance imaging, has been described, highlighting the importance of obtaining a drug history in patients with hyperprolactinemia (47ᶜ).

A 74-year-old man with impotence had increased prolactin and low testosterone concentrations. He underwent extensive testing to rule out a pituitary tumor. Magnetic resonance imaging showed a 6-mm lesion consistent with a pituitary microadenoma that had remained unchanged for 6 months. Verapamil was withdrawn and within 1 month the prolactin concentration fell to within the reference range. The pituitary lesion was not responsible for the increase in prolactin, but rather complicated the identification of a drug-induced disorder. The initial failure to identify the hyperprolactinemic effect of verapamil may have resulted in unnecessary radiological procedures in this patient.

Prolactin secretion by pituitary lactotrophic cells is controlled primarily by tonic inhibition by prolactin inhibitory factor (dopamine) and by stimulatory factors, including thyrotropin-releasing hormone and vasoactive intestinal peptide, each of which requires calcium for its release. However, the mechanism by which calcium antagonism with verapamil alters the release of prolactin is unknown. Moreover, hyperprolactinemia is not associated with the use of other calcium antagonists, such as nifedipine or diltiazem. Verapamil may increase dopaminergic activity by blocking calcium channels in the cell membranes of neurones in the tuberoinfundibular tract, rather than in the lactotrophic cell membrane itself, where dopamine receptor antagonists are thought to act.

REFERENCES

1. Pollak A, Falk RH. Aggravation of postcardioversion atrial dysfunction by sotalol. J Am Coll Cardiol 1995;25:665—71.

2. Pfammatter JP, Paul T, Lehmann C, Kallfelz HC. Efficacy and proarrhythmia of oral sotalol in pediatric patients. J Am Coll Cardiol 1995; 26:1002—7.

3. Diggory P, Cassels-Brown A, Vail A, Abbey LM, Hillman JS. Avoiding unsuspected respiratory side-effects of topical timolol with cardioselective or sympathomimetic agents. Lancet 1995;345:1604—6.

4. Schallreuter KU. β-adrenergic blocking drugs may exacerbate vitiligo. Br J Dermatol 1995;132:168—9.

5. Arnoult L, Bowman ZL, Kimbrough RL, Stewart RH. Periocular cutaneous pigmentary changes associated with topical betaxolol. J Glaucoma 1995;4:263—7.

6. Imai Y, Watanabe N, Hashimoto J, Nishiyama A, Sakamura H, Sekino H, Omata K, Abe K. Muscle cramps and elevated serum creatine phosphokinase levels induced by β-adrenoceptor blockers. Eur J Clin Pharmacol 1995;48:29—34.

7. Slovick DI, Fletcher AE, Daymond M, Mackay EM, VandenBurg MV, Bulpitt CJ. Quality of life and cognitive function with a diuretic compared with a beta blocker: a randomized controlled trial of bendrofluazide versus dilevalol in elderly hypertensive patients. Cardiol Eld 1995;3:139—45.

8. Paran E, Holzberg G, Mazor M, Zmora E, Insler V. β-Adrenergic blocking agents in the treatment of pregnancy-induced hypertension. Int J Clin Pharmacol Ther 1995;33:119—23.

9. El-Qarmalawi AM, Morsy AH, Al-Fadly A, Obeid A, Hashem M. Labetalol vs. methyldopa in the treatment of pregnancy-induced hypertension. Int J Gynecol Obstet 1995;49:125—30.

10. Stevens TP, Guillet R. Use of glucagon to treat neonatal low-output congestive heart failure after maternal labetalol therapy. J Pediatr 1995;127:151—3.

11. Krum H, Sackner-Bernstein JD, Goldsmith RL, Kukin ML, Schwartz B, Penn J, Medina N, Yushak M, Horn E, Katz SD, Levin HR, Neuberg GW, DeLong G, Packer M. Double-blind, placebo-controlled study of the long-term efficacy of carvedilol in patients with severe chronic heart failure. Circulation 1995;92:1499—506.

12. Johnston GD, Vyssoulis G, Feely J, Holden RD, Radley DR. Effect of celiprolol and metoprolol on lipids, fibrinogen and airways function in hyperlipidaemic hypertensives: a randomised double-blind long-term parallel group trial. J Hum Hypertens 1995;9:123—9.

13. Merkel C, Gatta A, Donada C, Enzo E, Marin R, Amodio P, Torboli P, Angeli P, Cavallarin G, Sebastianelli G, Susanna S, Mazzaro C, Beltrame P, and the GTIP. Long-term effect of nadalol or nadolol plus isosorbide-5-mononitrate on renal function and ascites formation in patients with cirrhosis. Hepatology 1995;22:808—13.

14. Psaty BM, Heckbert SR, Koepsell TD, Siscovick DS, Raghunthan TE, Weiss NS, Rosendaal FR, Lemaitre RN, Smith NL, Wahl PW, Wagner EH, Furberg CD. The risk of myocardial infarction associated with antihypertensive drug therapies. J Am Med Assoc 1995;274:620—5.

15. Furberg CD, Psaty BM, Meyer JV. Nifedipine dose-related increase in mortality with coronary heart disease. Circulation 1995;92:1326—31.

16. Pahor M, Guralnik JM, Corti MC, Foley DJ, Carbonin P, Havlik RJ. Long-term survival and use of antihypertensive medications in older person. J Am Geriatr Soc 1995;43:1191—7.

17. Horton R. Spinning the risks and benefits of calcium antagonists. Lancet 1995;346:586—7.

18. Yusuf S. Calcium antagonists in coronary artery disease and hypertension. Time for reevaluation? Circulation 1995;92:1079—82.

19. Opie LH, Messerli FH. Nifedipine and mortality. Grave defects in the dossier. Circulation 1995;92:1068—72.

20. Messerli FH. Case-control study, meta-analysis, and bouillabaisse: putting the calcium antagonist scare into context. Ann Int Med 1995;123:888—9.

21. Lip GYH, Ferner RE. Poisoning with antihypertensive drugs: calcium antagonists. J Hum Hypertens 1995;9:155—61.

22. Buckley CD, Aronson JK. Prolonged half-life of verapamil in a case of overdose: implications for therapy. Br J Clin Pharmacol 1995;39:680—3.

23. Ezekowitz MD, Hossack K, Mehta JL, Thadani U, Weidler DJ, Kostuk W, Awan N, Grossman W, Bommer W. Amlodipine in chronic stable angina: results of a multicenter double-blind crossover trial. Am Heart J 1995;129:527—35.

24. Omvik P, Herland OB, Thaulow E, Eide I, Midha R, Turner RR. Evaluation and quality-of-life assessment of amlodipine and enalapril in patients with hypertension. J Hum Hypertens 1995;9 Suppl I:S17—S24.

25. Detry L-MR, Block P, De Backer G, Degaute JP, Six R. Patient compliance and therapeutic coverage: comparison of amlodipine and slow release nifedipine in the treatment of hypertension. Eur J Clin Pharmacol 1995;47:477—81.

26. Davies RF, Habibi H, Klinke WP, Dessain P, Nadeau C, Phaneuf DC, Lepage S, Raman S, Herbert M, Foris K, O'Linden W, Buttars JA. Effect of amlodipine, atenolol and their combination on myocardial ischemia during treadmill exercise and ambulatory monitoring. J Am Coll Cardiol 1995;25:619—25.

27. Saruta T, Kanno Y, Hayashi K, Suzuki H. Renal effects of amlodipine. J Hum Hypertens 1995;9 Suppl. I:S11—S16.

28. Boman K, Saetre H, Karlsson LG, Ritter B, Marsell R, Wingman H, Lövheim, Michaeli EW, Löfdahl P, Olsson SOR. Antianginal effect of conventional and controlled release diltiazem in stable angina pectoris. Eur J Clin Pharmacol 1995;49:27—30.

29. Avila JR. Elevation of hepatic enzymes after cutaneous reaction caused by diltiazem. Ann Pharmacother 1995;29:317—8.

30. de Vries RJM, Queré M, Lok DJA, Sijbring P, Bucx JJJ, van Veldhuisen DJ, Dunselman PHJM. Comparison of effects on peak oxygen consumption, quality of life and neurohormones of felodipine and enalapril in patients with congestive heart failure. Am J Cardiol 1995;76:1253—8.

31. Carrol J, Shamiss A, Zevis D, Levi J, Rosenthal T. Twenty-four-hour blood pressure monitoring during treatment with extended-release felodipine versus slow-release nifedipine: cross-over study. J Cardiovasc Pharmacol 1995;26:974—7.

32. Littler WA, Sheridan DJ. Placebo controlled trial of felodipine in patients with mild to moderate heart failure. Br Heart J 1995;73:428—33.

33. Brogden RN, Sorkin EM. Isradipine. An update of its pharmacodynamic and pharmacokinetic properties and therapeutic efficacy in the treatment of mild to moderate hypertension. Drugs 1995;49:618—49.

34. Wide-Svensson DH, Ingemarsson I, Lunell NO, Forman A, Skajaa K, Lindberg B, Lindeberg S, Marsàl K, Andersson KE. Calcium channel blockade (isradipine) in treatment of hypertension in pregnancy: a randomized placebo-controlled study. Am J Obstet Gynecol 1995;173:872—8.

35. Tobias JD. Nicardipine: applications in anesthesia practice. J Clin Anesth 1995;7:525—33.

36. Ota K, Shijo H, Kokawa H, Kubara K, Kim T, Akiyoshi N, Yokoyama M, Okumura M. Effects of nifedipine on hepatic venous pressure gradient and portal vein blood flow in patients with cirrhosis. J Gastroenterol Hepatol 1995;10:198—204.

37. Lind L, Berne C, Pollare T, Lithell H. Metabolic effects of anti-hypertensive treatment with nifedipine or furosemide: a double-blind, crossover study. J Hum Hypertens 1995;9:137—41.

38. Visser W, Wallenburg HCS. A comparison between the haemodynamic effects of oral nifedipine and intravenous dihydralazine in patients with severe pre-eclampsia. J Hypertens 1995;13:791—5.

39. Ray D, Dyson D. Calcium channel blockers. Clin Obstet Gynecol 1995;38:713—21.

40. van Dijk KGJ, Dekker GA, van Gaijn HP. Ritodrine and nifedipine as tocolytic agents: a preliminary comparison. J Perinat Med 1995;23:409—15.

41. Zygmunt SC, Delgado-Zygmunt TJ. The haemodynamic effect of transcranial Doppler-guided high-dose nimodipine treatment in established vasospasm after subarachnoid haemorrhage. Acta Neurochir 1995;135:179—85.

42. Porchet F, Chioléro R, de Tribolet N. Hypotensive effect of nimodipine during treatment for aneurysmal subarachnoid haemorrhage. Acta Neurochir 1995;137:62—9.

43. Walden J, Fritze J, Van Calker D, Berger M, Grunze H. A calcium antagonist for the treatment of depressive episodes: single case reports. J Psychiatr Res 1995;29:71—6.

44. Wagenknecht LE, Furberg CD, Hammon JW, Legault C, Troost BT. Surgical bleeding: unexpected effect of a calcium antagonist. Br Med J 1995;310:776—7.

45. Davidsson GK, Edwards JS, Davidson C. The effect of age and liver disease on the pharmacokinetics of the calcium antagonist, nisoldipine. Curr Med Res Opin 1995;13:285—97.

46. Glasser SP, Ripa S, Garland T, Weiss R, Nademanee K, Singh S, Bittar N. Antianginal and antiischemic efficacy of monotherapy extended-release nisoldipine (Coat Core) in chronic stable angina. J Clin Pharmacol 1995;35:780—4.

47. Dombrowski RC, Romeo JH, Aron DC. Verapamil-induced hyperprolactinemia complicated by a pituitary incidentaloma. Ann Pharmacother 1995;29:999—1001.

R. Verhaeghe

19   Drugs acting on the cerebral and peripheral circulations

DRUGS USED IN THE TREATMENT OF ARTERIAL DISORDERS OF THE BRAIN AND LIMBS *(SED-13, 537; SEDA-17, 234; SEDA-18, 219; SEDA-19, 206)*

Cyclandelate *(SED-13, 538)*

Cyclandelate, which mainly appears to act as a calcium antagonist in smooth muscle, is in general a safe drug, since major adverse effects have not been reported at daily doses of 1.6 g. This has once more been demonstrated in a double-blind cross-over study in which 1.2 and 1.6 g of cyclandelate were compared with 120 and 160 mg of propranolol for 8 weeks each as prophylaxis for migraine. The study started with a placebo run-in phase of 4 weeks. Adverse effects were mild and as common with placebo as with both active treatments (1[c]).

Flunarizine *(SED-13, 537; SEDA-15, 198)*

The calcium antagonist flunarizine is used in many countries for vertigo and migraine and in some countries for peripheral arterial disease as well. Its main adverse effects are *somnolence*, *sedation*, *fatigue*, and *drowsiness* during the first few days in up to 10% of patients. A dosage of 20 mg/day or more, instead of the recommended 10 mg, may cause *drowsiness*, increasing *sweating*, *peripheral edema*, and *fatigue*. *Parkinsonism*, *tardive dyskinesia*, and *depression* have been described in a number of mostly elderly patients taking flunarizine.

Clinical studies of the antiepileptic efficacy of flunarizine have been equivocal. There is large individual variability in the clearance of flunarizine, and so in a recent study the dosage was adjusted in each patient to achieve a plasma concentration of 60 ng/ml (2[c]): the percentage reduction from baseline seizure rate was modest (mean, 24%), although significantly greater than with placebo (mean, 6%). The investigators of one participating center extended the data in their patients with an open rising-dose phase after the placebo-controlled double-blind study (3[c]): the individually determined dosage to achieve a concentration of 60 ng/ml was increased every 8—12 weeks in three to six equal increments up to a maximum dose of 2.5—2.7 times the initially determined dose. The initial dose varied from 10 to 60 mg/day and the highest open-label dosage achieved varied from 25 to 130 mg/day. All but two of the 16 patients experienced some of the well-known adverse effects of flunarizine at the initial dose, *somnolence* being the most frequent complaint (nine out of 16). As the dosage was increased, adverse events became more prominent and often led to drug discontinuation. Higher dosages of flunarizine did not improve seizure control. This study illustrates again that higher dosages than 10 mg/day are poorly tolerated.

Nicotinic acid derivatives *(SED-13, 540, 1329; SEDA-17, 439; SEDA-18, 382; SEDA-19, 206)*

Nicotinic acid (niacin) is a potent vasodilator, but its clinical use as an effective and inexpensive lipid lowering agent currently far exceeds its use for vascular disease of the brain or limbs. The major drawback in the use of niacin is associated with poor tolerance (*flushing* and *palpitation*) and toxicity (*worsening of control of diabetes*, *exacerbation of peptic ulcer disease*, *gout*, *hepatitis*). A recent survey in a single clinic showed that over 40% of 133 patients given niacin in regular or modified-release tablets over a 5-year period eventually discontinued treatment because of intolerable adverse effects (4[C]). However, different figures have been obtained in clinical research. For instance, in a cross-over comparison with lovastatin, niacin was administered for 16 weeks to renal transplant patients with persistent hyperlipidemia despite dietary treatment: two-thirds of the patients developed flushing but none interrupted treatment (5[C]).

Little has been published on the ocular adverse effects of niacin. This may be because the observed adverse effects are reversible and patients are rarely referred to ophthalmologists. In a retrospective survey using a suggestive questionnaire sent to patients taking medication for hyperlipidemia, those taking niacin were more likely to report symptoms of the *sicca syndrome, blurred vision*, and *eyelid edema* compared with those who had never taken niacin (6[R]). Two patients stopped taking niacin because of cystoid macular edema. Many complaints of blurred vision may be due to incipient macular edema, which is reversible and partly dose related, because symptoms not only resolve after drug withdrawal but also appear to respond to reducing the dosage. A few cases of advanced 'cystoid' macular edema have been reported in the older literature and took months to resolve once niacin was discontinued. The authors also hypothesized that the symptoms of the sicca syndrome, which are rarely spontaneously reported by patients taking niacin, are rather aggravation of existing sicca syndrome in patients with familial hypercholesterolemia, one possible explanation being that niacin may be secreted in tears, thereby irritating an already dry eye.

Vitamin E (α-tocopherol) *(SED-13, 542; SEDA-17, 441)*

It was suggested many years ago that vitamin E could be useful in patients with peripheral arterial disease, but the evidence is meagre and incomplete. Nowadays vitamin E is expected to have a role in the prevention of atherosclerosis, through inhibition of oxidation of low-density lipoprotein. The hypo-

thesis that oxidative modification of low-density lipoprotein contributes to the progression of atherosclerosis is supported by an impressive amount of in vitro and animal data. Some epidemiological studies have associated a high dietary intake or high serum concentrations of α-tocopherol with a reduced risk of cardiovascular events. Large intervention studies with clinical endpoints have tested the hypothesis that daily supplementation with a high dose of α-tocopherol may reduce ischemic vascular events. Now a trial in 2002 patients has shown a substantial reduction in non-fatal myocardial infarction, but not in cardiovascular deaths (7[C]). Daily administration of 400 and 800 IU of vitamin E was well tolerated, and only 11 patients stopped treatment because of *diarrhea, dyspepsia*, or a *rash*. Drop outs were equally distributed between placebo and the two treatment groups.

DRUGS USED IN THE TREATMENT OF MIGRAINE

Ergotamine *(SED-13, 543; SEDA-17, 171, 243; SEDA-18, 220; SEDA-19, 206)*

The main adverse effect of ergotamine is *arterial spasm*, leading to severe ischemia in the limbs or other vascular beds. A less well-known complication of the rectal use of ergotamine is *proctitis* and *perianal and rectal ulceration*, eventually leading to necrosis and stenosis of the rectum, occasionally referred to as 'anorectal ergotism'. Reduced blood flow to the rectal wall secondary to vasospasm locally induced by ergotamine suppositories is thought to be the cause. Rectovaginal fistula has been described as a complication of 10-year abuse of up to five ergotamine suppositories each day for migraine in a 39-year-old woman (8[C]).

Sumatriptan *(SEDA-17, 171; SEDA-19, 207)*

The most commonly experienced adverse effects of sumatriptan are mild and transient: sensations of *tingling, heaviness, pressure*, or *warmth*. A feeling of *pressure, tightness*, or *pain in the chest* is also frequently reported. However, in general, the pattern and incidence of these adverse events have not been different between drug and placebo in double-blind controlled studies.

Cardiovascular   A major concern is the possibility of arterial spasm in the coronary circulation, leading to serious cardiac complications. New reports of myocardial infarction linked with a first or later administration of sumatriptan continue to appear (9[c]), (10[c]), (11[c]).

Nervous system   Persistent neurological complications associated with sumatriptan therapy have not been documented. Fatal cerebellar infarction has now been described in a 39-year-old man who took 100 mg of sumatriptan for an acute attack of migraine. The next morning he felt drowsy and had slurred speech. He died 3 days later. The cerebellar infarct was diagnosed at autopsy and intra-cranial vasospasm was thought to be the likely mechanism (12[c]). It should be noted that stroke is also documented in patients with migraine, independently of drug treatment.

Drug induced headache appears to be a fairly frequent complication of headache therapy. This problem has now also been reported in five women who woke up with a constant dull pressure in their head after 8—20 months of chronic sumatriptan (ab)use (13[c]). Withdrawal of sumatriptan solved the problem.

Immunological and hypersensitivity reactions   Hypersensitivity reactions with sumatriptan are extremely rare. A 26-year-old woman was given a first subcutaneous injection of sumatriptan for an attack of migraine and 5 min later complained of burning in the throat. Seconds later her hands became markedly erythematous and swollen, followed by swelling of the lips. Urgent intravenous administration of adrenaline and diphenhydramine abated all signs of angioedema within 15 min (14[c]).

REFERENCES

1. Gerber WD, Schellenberg R, Thom M, Haufe C, Bölsche F, Wedekind W, Niederberger U, Soyka D. Cyclandelate versus propranolol in the prophylaxis of migraine. A double-blind placebo-controlled study. Funct Neurol 1995;10:27—35.

2. Pledger GW, Sackellares JC, Treiman DM, Pellock JM, Wright FS, Mikati M, Sahlroot JT, Tsay JY, Drake ME, Olson L et al. Flunarizine for treatment of partial seizures: results of a concentration-controlled trial. Neurology 1994; 44:1830—6.

3. Handforth A, Mai T, Treiman DM. Rising dose study of safety and tolerance of flunarizine. Eur J Clin Pharmacol 1995;49:91—4.

4. Gibbons LW, Gonzales V, Gordon N, Grundy S. The prevalence of side-effects with regular and sustained-release nicotinic acid. Am J Med 1995;99:378—5.

5. Lal SM, Hewett JE, Petroski GF, Van Stone JC, Ross G. Effects of nicotinic acid and lovastatin in renal transplant: a prospective, randomized, open-labeled crossover trial. Am J Kidney Dis 1995;25:616—22.

6. Fraunfelder FW, Fraunfelder FT, Illingworth DR. Adverse ocular effects associated with niacin therapy. Br J Ophthalmol 1995;79;54—6.

7. Stephens NG, Parsons A, Schofield PM, Kelly F, Cheeseman K, Mitchinson MJ, Brown MJ. Randomised controlled trial of vitamin E in patients with coronary disease: Cambridge Heart Antioxidant Study (CHAOS). Lancet 1996; 346:781—6.

8. Pfeifer J, Reissman P, Wexner SD. Ergotamine induced complex rectovaginal fistula. Dis Colon Rectum 1995;38:1224—6.

9. Kelly KM. Cardiac arrest following use of sumatriptan. Neurology 1995;45:1211—3.

10. O'Connor P, Gladstone P. Oral sumatriptan-associated transmural myocardial infarction. Neurology 1995;45:2274.

11. Mueller L, Gallagher RM, Ciervo CA. Vasospasm-induced myocardial infarction with sumatriptan. Headache 1996;36:329—31.

12. Jayamaha JE, Street MK. Fatal cerebellar infarction in a migraine sufferer whilst receiving sumatriptan. Intensive Care Med 1995;21:82—3.

13. Göbel H, Stolze H, Heinze A, Dworschak M. Easy therapeutical management of sumatriptan-induced daily headache. Neurology 1996;47:297—8.

14. Dachs R, Vitillo J. Angioedema associated with sumatriptan administration. Am J Med 1995;99:684—5.

Faiez Zannad

20 Antihypertensive drugs

GENERAL

Case-control studies in hypertension During the last 2 years intense controversy and debate have been generated by several case-control studies on the safety of antihypertensive agents, such as diuretics, calcium antagonists, and β-blockers. The debate has focused primarily on whether case—control studies are reliable tools for clinical and therapeutic management decision making. The soundest conclusion from this debate is that case—control studies are powerful tools for generating hypotheses, which should be properly tested by prospective randomized trials. Since the majority of these case—control studies concerned calcium antagonists, which are considered in another chapter, they will not be discussed here.

Major trials The HOT study is being conducted in accordance with the PROBE (Prospective, Randomised, Open, Blinded Endpoint) design. Two major aims are being addressed:

(1) To determine the optimal therapeutic goal in the treatment of hypertension, i.e. which of three target diastolic blood pressures (95, 90, or 85 mmHg) is preferable in order to achieve optimal protection against hypertension-induced cardiovascular morbidity and mortality.

(2) To evaluate the effects of a low dosage of aspirin (75 mg/day) versus placebo in the prevention of cardiovascular morbidity and mortality in hypertensive patients.

Altogether 19—193 patients have been recruited and randomized, making this the largest intervention study in hypertension to date. Data are now available after 1 year of follow up (1[C]). Antihypertensive treatment is begun with felodipine 5 mg od. Additional antihypertensive therapy is given in a stepwise protocol, in order to achieve the target blood pressure:

Step 1: felodipine 5 mg/day.
Step 2: felodipine 5 mg/day + low-dosage β-blocker or ACE inhibitor.
Step 3: felodipine 10 mg/day + low-dosage β-blocker or ACE inhibitor.
Step 4: felodipine 10 mg/day + high-dosage β-blocker or ACE inhibitor.
Step 5: Step 4 + hydrochlorothiazide or complement with low-dosage ACE inhibitor or β-blocker.

Over 80% of the patients reached the predetermined target blood pressure in each group. Adverse effects have been relatively few. Only ankle edema (2.6—2.9%) and cough (0.9—1.3%) have exceeded a frequency of 1%. Of all the patients recruited, 88% were still taking their medications 1 year later. The overall incidence of adverse effects was not different in the three target groups, suggesting that it was not affected by the extent of blood pressure lowering. However, the number of antihypertensive agents prescribed and the number of dose titration steps were associated with an increased incidence of adverse effects, from 5% on average at step 1 to 15% at step 5. Adverse effects did not vary according to gender but were slightly more common in the elderly (over 65 years) than in the young (under 65 years). The full results of the HOT study are expected to be available late in 1997.

Quality of life Within the field of cardiovascular disease, quality of life as an outcome measure has been most often investigated in mild to moderate hypertension. The major available data on quality-of-life assessment in antihypertensive drugs trials have been summarized (2[R]). The two scales most often used were the Psychological General Well Being (PGWB) scale and the General Health Questionnaire (GHQ) within the PCASEE model (Physical, Cognitive, Affective and Social indicators, Economic-social stressors or negative life events and Egofunction or personality problems). The most specific components were, of course, adverse effects which, with antihypertensive agents, were typically circulatory symptoms and sexual dysfunction. However, the affective and cognitive components also had different weights within subclasses of drugs. For instance, ACE inhibitors act on the affective component (depression and anxiety) and calcium antagonists on the cognitive component. Captopril and lisinopril had a mood-elevating effect compared with metoprolol, while enalapril did not. It was suggested that this difference could be explained by the fact that enalapril, unlike captopril and lisinopril, does not cross the blood—brain barrier, although there is no information on its active metabolite, enalaprilat.

In a new relatively large prospective trial called OCAPI (Optimisation du Choix d'un Antihypertensent de Première Intention) (3^C) the effects of a diuretic combination (altizide plus spironolactone), a β-blocker (bisoprolol), a calcium antagonist (verapamil), and an ACE inhibitor (enalapril) on subjective quality of life and clinical safety have been assessed in 653 patients with mild to moderate hypertension with follow-up for 1 year. There were no significant differences in minor adverse effects among the four groups, although *cough* was more common with the ACE inhibitor and *fatigue* with the β-blocker and the diuretics. There was a higher incidence of non-specific and unexpected major adverse effects in the diuretic and β-blocker groups. Quality of life improved overall in all subgroups, with no long-term statistically significant differences among subgroups, which, as emphasized by the authors, was in contrast with the results of several other previous reports. The weakness of the open-label design used in this study was presented as a positive feature by the authors, who claimed that an open trial performed in general practice would be more pragmatic, reflecting real life as closely as possible. Another statistical weakness was related to the unbalanced baseline characteristics of the patients in the four groups, although the authors claimed that adjustment for the baseline differences did

not substantially change the overall conclusions.

Urinary system   The results of a recent study have suggested that the risk of *renal cell cancer* may be increased among users of diuretics and other antihypertensive drugs (4^C). This was a multicenter study pooling six closely coordinated case-control studies around the world, providing the largest database on the role of antihypertensive agents in the development of renal cell cancer. The study was initiated in order to investigate the assertion from several previous case—control studies that an increased risk of renal cell cancer may be linked to diuretic use. A total of 1732 histologically confirmed cases and 2309 controls matched to cases by age and sex were interviewed. After adjustment for hypertension, the risk of using diuretics was reduced to unity, except among long-term users (15 years). The risk of using the non-diuretic antihypertensive drugs remained significantly increased after adjustment for blood pressure and increased further with duration of use. It is noteworthy that the study was restricted to antihypertensive agents regularly in use before 1987, which included β-blockers, calcium antagonists, central sympatholytic agents, and ACE inhibitors. Excess risk was not restricted to any specific type of antihypertensive drug and no trend was observed with estimated lifetime consumption of any particular type of drug. Several cautious methodological adjustments were used. However, hypertension in itself also seemed to be moderately related to an increased risk of renal cell cancer; the authors could not rule out potential misclassifications and recognised the difficulty of distinguishing an effect of treatment from an effect of its indication.

ANGIOTENSIN-CONVERTING ENZYME INHIBITORS *(SED-13, 546; SEDA-17, 218; SEDA-18, 223; SEDA-19, 210)*

Despite continuously increasing use of ACE inhibitors, very few reports of adverse effects have been published during the past 2 years. This may be related to the very good tolerability of these agents, as well as their long record of extensive worldwide use, making newly recognized adverse effects unlikely. Large databases from recent large intervention trials have provided valuable information on the rates of the most common adverse effects. In the Studies Of Left Ventricular Dysfunction (SOLVD) adverse effects related to the long-term use of enalapril have been thoroughly investigated (5[C]). A total of 6797 patients with left ventricular dysfunction (ejection fraction of 0.35 or less) were randomized to enalapril or placebo. During 40 months average follow-up, 28% reported adverse effects with enalapril compared with 16% with placebo. *Hypotension* (15 vs. 7.1%), *uremia* (3.8 vs. 1.6%), *cough* (5.0 vs. 2.0%), *fatigue* (5.8 vs. 3.5%), *hyperkalemia* (1.2 vs. 0.4%), and *angioedema* (0.4 vs. 0.1%) were all reported significantly more often with enalapril. Adverse effects resulted in discontinuation of blinded therapy in 15% of the enalapril group compared with 8.6% in the placebo group.

Respiratory *Cough* is probably the most common cause of withdrawal of ACE inhibitors. Bradykinin has previously been incriminated as the most likely contributing factor in this setting, but the evidence for this has not been definitive. The concentration of substance P in sputum induced by hypertonic saline was significantly higher in nine patients with ACE inhibitor-induced cough than in five patients without cough 1 month after stopping enalapril (17 fmol/ml sputum vs. 0.9) (6[C]). Although this does not conclusively prove that substance P is the only cause of this adverse effect, this finding certainly supports the suspicion that the mechanism of ACE inhibitor-induced cough may be more complicated than just an increase in bradykinin concentrations.

Immunological and hypersensitivity reactions The incidence of *angioedema* during treatment with ACE inhibitors in black and white Americans has been compared in a retrospective cohort study. This study was particularly informative, because of the large number of patients and the large extent of drug exposure (43 989 and 114 448 personyears exposure in blacks and whites, respectively). The incidence of angioedema in blacks was three- to four-fold higher than in whites

(3.3—4.6 per 1000 person-years). Angioedema tended to occur earlier in black patients and more commonly after a first exposure than during long-term exposure. Adjustment for concurrent use of diuretics and antibiotics was allowed for. The authors were not able to account for various possible confounders, such as underlying medical diseases. They did not suggest a mechanistic explanation for their findings (7[C]).

ANGIOTENSIN II RECEPTOR ANTAGONISTS *(SED-13, 549; SEDA-19, 214)*

Inhibition of the renin-angiotensin system by ACE inhibitors has proved efficacious in the treatment of hypertension, cardiac failure, secondary prevention after myocardial infarction, and kidney protection in diabetic nephropathy. The development of specific antagonists to subtype 1 of the angiotensin II receptor (AT_1) has recently provided a new tool for inhibiting the renin-angiotensin system. Experimental data and preliminary clinical experience have suggested that the efficacy of AT_1 receptor antagonists in the treatment of hypertension is similar to that of ACE inhibitors. However, the two drug categories also have potential differences, because of their different mechanisms of action. Since they have an action that is exclusively targeted at angiotensin II, the AT_1 receptor antagonists should lack the effects of ACE inhibitors that are mediated through the accumulation of bradykinin and other peptides. Furthermore, since a significant amount of angiotensin II may be generated by enzymes other than ACE, namely the chymases, AT_1 receptor antagonists may achieve more complete blockade of the effects of angiotensin than the ACE inhibitors do. Nevertheless, whether these differences are clinically important is still being investigated.

Cough, a particular class-specific adverse effect of the ACE inhibitors, has been related to accumulation of bradykinin and substance P, which does not occur with AT_1 receptor antagonists. Thus, these agents may have the advantage of producing less or no cough (8[R]).

The first attempt at blocking the AT_1 receptor with the peptide analogues of angiotensin II resulted in the discovery of saralasin, an antagonist that lacked oral activity and had partial agonist properties. Losartan is the first agent in the new class of orally active AT_1 receptor antagonists. It is now widely available, and significant experience of its clinical use is accruing. Other similar agents or agents with slightly different receptor affinity and binding kinetics, such as valsartan, irbesartan, candesartan, and bosentan, will soon be available for clinical use in hypertension. Many more are undergoing clinical development. All are also being considered for the treatment of other diseases (heart failure, diabetic nephropathy, other forms of glomerulopathy, restenosis after coronary angioplasty, and atherosclerosis).

Losartan *(SEDA-19, 214)*

Losartan and other AT_1 receptor antagonists being developed are phenyltetrazole-substituted imidazoles. Losartan is 30 000 times more selective for subtype 1 of the AT receptors than for subtype 2, whose function is still unknown. Losartan has no intrinsic agonist properties. It is partly metabolized (14%) to an active metabolite, E-3174, which is a more potent AT_1 receptor antagonist, has a longer half-life, and appears to bind more avidly to the receptor, resulting in insurmountable antagonism. In preclinical studies, losartan reduced the blood pressure in a variety of animal models of hypertension, caused left ventricular hypertrophy to regress, and improved end-organ damage. In humans, several clinical studies have shown that 50—100 mg od has a significant antihypertensive effect, comparable to other antihypertensive agents, including ACE inhibitors. As expected, the blood pressure-lowering effect is increased by combining losartan with a thiazide diuretic. Clinical studies in congestive heart failure are still limited, but the results suggest that losartan may have favorable hemodynamic actions. Long-term effects on symptoms, exercise tolerance, morbidity, and mortality are planned. Moreover, a long-scale outcome trial (LIFE study) is under way to determine the effects of losartan on morbidity and mortality in patients with hypertension (8[R]).

Losartan appears to be extremely well tolerated. In about 2900 hypertensive patients treated in double-blind trials, the most frequently reported adverse effects were *headache* (14%), *upper respiratory infection* (6.5%), *dizziness* (4%), *weakness/fatigue* (3.8%), and *cough* (3.1%). All of these adverse effects were equally reported with placebo. Only dizziness was considered 'drug related', more often in losartan-treated (2.4%) than placebo-treated (1.3%) patients. Dry cough was more frequent with ACE inhibitors (8.8%) than with losartan (3.1%) or placebo (2.1%) in comparative trials. There were no effects of age, sex, or ethnic origin on the safety profile of losartan (9[R]), (10[C]).

Cardiovascular   A single case of losartan-induced *angina pectoris and myocardial ischemia* has been reported (11[c]).

A 67-year-old man with a history of coronary artery bypass surgery who had been free from angina since surgery was given losartan 50 mg od for hypertension. He complained of typical angina about 2 h after taking losartan, consistently every day for 6 days, until losartan was withdrawn. The angina was specifically relieved by sublingual glyceryl trinitrate. His only other medication was aspirin 325 mg/day. His blood pressure during treatment was 160/94 mmHg, but it was not stated whether this blood pressure was measured during an episode of angina or at another time. Withdrawal was followed by relief of symptoms. A single-dose rechallenge produced the same angina symptoms along with typical electrocardiographic signs of myocardial ischemia, both of which resolved after sublingual glyceryl trinitrate. Over the next month, he remained asymptomatic and his blood pressure was controlled with captopril.

Although the temporal association very strongly supports a cause and effect relation in this case, the mechanism is unclear. A significant drop in blood pressure at the time of peak effect cannot be ruled out, since the blood pressure during the episodes of angina was not reported. The author suggested that an excess rise in plasma catecholamines may have been the cause of the angina, and losartan has certainly been reported to increase plasma catecholamine concentrations (12[R]).

Respiratory   In a Scandinavian trial, in which 407 hypertensive patients were enrolled and randomized for 12 weeks to either losartan 50 mg/day or enalapril 20 mg/day, specific symptoms, including *cough*, were determined using a symptom questionnaire (13[C]). Dry cough occurred in 12% (enalapril) versus 1.0% (losartan) as a spontaneously reported discomfort and 15 versus 3.0% as a clinical adverse effect.

In one study the incidence of cough produced by losartan was compared with the incidence with the ACE inhibitor lisinopril and with hydrochlorothiazide in 135 hypertensive patients with previous ACE inhibitor-induced cough. Cough was detected by self-administered questionnaire. It was reported significantly less often with losartan (29%) than with lisinopril (72%) and at a similar incidence as hydrochlorothiazide (34%) (14[C]).

Nervous system   *Migraine* has been reported in association with losartan.

A 50-year-old woman with no personal or family history of migraine developed clinical features of migraine 6 h after starting to take losartan 50 mg od for essential hypertension (15[c]). She experienced sensations of colored light, scintillating spots, wavy lines, and severe throbbing headache, accompanied by vomiting, photophobia, and severe anxiety. She also complained of weakness and pain in the left side of her body and face and numbness in both hands and around her mouth. There was severe flushing around her face and neck. Losartan was discontinued and there were no sequelae on the following day. The authors did not state the duration of the symptoms and physical examination was not performed during the symptoms. She was then given enalapril 20 mg/day, which was well tolerated and controlled her blood pressure. Two weeks later, she was rechallenged with one dose of losartan 50 mg and her complaint of severe migraine recurred. She had taken no other medications and had not used alcohol or tobacco.

This is an isolated case report occurring after a single dose of losartan. However, the temporal association during challenge and re-challenge, although in unblinded conditions, argues a possible causal relation.

DRUGS THAT ACT ON THE SYMPATHETIC NERVOUS SYSTEM *(SED-13, 550; SEDA-17, 253; SEDA-18, 226; SEDA-19, 214)*

CENTRALLY ACTING DRUGS *(SED-13, 550; SEDA-17, 253; SEDA-18, 226)*

Clonidine *(SED-13, 551; SEDA-17, 253; SEDA-18, 226)*

Nervous system   The effect of clonidine on sleep has been prospectively investigated in hypertensive men using a double-blind, randomized, crossover design (vs. atenolol) and polygraphic sleep recordings (16[C]). A single dose of 150 μg was given at 18:00 h. Clonidine significantly reduced sleep latency and strikingly reduced both rapid eye movement (REM) sleep time and the percentage of REM sleep. The authors concluded that clonidine had a marked hypnotic effect comparable to that of some sedative medications. In contrast, atenolol had no such effect.

POST-SYNAPTIC α_1-ADRENOCEPTOR ANTAGONISTS *(SED-13, 552; SEDA-17, 254; SEDA-19, 215)*

Doxazosin *(SEDA-19, 215)*

In a review of the clinical pharmacology and therapeutic uses of doxazosin, reports of its tolerability included an update from previously unpublished pooled data on file (17[R]). In patients treated for hypertension ($n = 339$ vs. 336 treated with placebo), adverse effects were essentially the same as those reported in patients being treated for benign prostate hyperplasia ($n = 665$ vs. 300 treated with placebo). *Dizziness* (19 vs. 9% and 16 vs. 9%) and *fatigue* (12 vs. 6% and 8 vs. 2%) were significantly more often reported than with placebo (figures for patients with hypertension and benign prostate hyperplasia respectively, vs. placebo). However, *somnolence* was reported significantly versus placebo only in hypertensive patients (5 vs. 1%) and only in patients with benign prostate hyperplasia were the following adverse effects reported significantly versus placebo: *hypotension* (17 vs. 0%), *edema* (2.7 vs. 0.7%), and *dyspnea* (2.6 vs. 0.3%).

REFERENCES

1. Hansson L, Zanchetti A. The hypertension optimal treatment (HOT) study: 12-month data on blood pressure and tolerability. With special reference to age and gender. Blood Pressure 1995;4:313–19.

2. Bech P. Quality of life measurements for patients taking which drugs? The Clinical PCASEE perspective. Pharmacoeconomics 1995;7:141–51.

3. Boissel JP, Collet JP, Lion L, Ducruet T, Moleur P, Luciani J, Milon H et al and the OCAPI Study Group. A randomized comparison of the effect of four antihypertensive monotherapies on the subjective quality of life in previously untreated asymptomatic patients: field trial in general practice. J Hypertens 1995;13:1059–67.

4. McLaughlin JK, Ho Chow W, Mandel JS, Mellemgaard A, McCredie M, Lindblad P, Schlehofer B, Pommer W, Niwa S, Adami HO. International renal-cell cancer study. VIII. Role of diuretics, other antihypertensive medications and hypertension. Int J Cancer 1995;63:216–21.

5. Kostis JB, Shelton B, Gosselin G, Goulet C, Hood WB, Kohn RM, Kubo SH et al. Adverse effects of enalapril in the Studies of Left Ventricular Dysfunction (SOLVD). Am Heart J 1996;131:350–5.

6. Tomaki M, Ichinose M, Miura M, Hirayama Y, Kageyama N et al. Angiotensin converting enzyme (ACE) inhibitor-induced cough and substance P. Thorax 1996;51:199–201.

7. Burkhart GA, Brown NJ, Griffin MR, Ray WA, Hammertrom T, Weiss S. Angiotensin converting enzyme inhibitor-associated angioedema: higher risk in blacks than whites. Pharmacoepidemiol Drug Saf 1996;5:149–54.

8. Johnston CI. Angiotensin receptor antagonists: focus on losartan. Lancet 1995;346:1403–7.

9. Goldberg AI, Dunlay MC, Sweet CS. Safety and tolerability of losartan potassium, an angiotensin II receptor antagonist, compared with hydrochlorothiazide, atenolol, felodipine ER, and angiotensin converting enzyme inhibitors for the treatment of systemic hypertension. Am J Cardiol 1995;75:793–5.

10. Gradman AH, Arcuri KE, Goldberg AI, Ikeda LS, Nelson EB, Snavely DB, Sweet CS. A randomized, placebo-controlled, double-blind, parallel study of various doses of losartan potassium compared with enalapril maleate in patients with essential hypertension. Hypertension 1995;25:1345–50.

11. Ahmad S. Losartan and angina pectoris. Tex Heart Inst J 1995;22:347–8.

12. Goldberg MR, Bradstreet TE, McWilliams EJ, Tanaka WK, Lipert S, Bjornsson TD et al. Biochemical effects of losartan, a nonpeptide angiotensin II receptor antagonist, on the renin-angiotensin-aldosterone system in hypertensive patients. Hypertension 1995;25:37–46.

13. Tikkanen I, Omvik P, Jensen HA, for the Scandnavian Study Group. Comparison of the angiotensin II antagonist losartan with the angiotensin converting enzyme inhibitor enalapril in patients with essential hypertension. J Hypertens 1995;13:1343–51.

14. Ramsay LE, Yeo WW, on behalf of The Losartan Cough Study Group. ACE inhibitors, angiotensin II antagonists and cough. J Hum Hypertens 1995;9:S51–4.

15. Ahmad S. Losartan and severe migraine. J Am Med Assoc 1995;274:1266–7.

16. Danchin N, Genton P, Atlas P, Anconina J, Leclere J, Cherrier F. Comparative effects of atenolol and clonidine on polygraphically recorded sleep in hypertensive men: a randomized, double-blind, crossover study. Int J Clin Pharmacol Ther 1995;33:52–5.

17. Fulton B, Wagstaff AJ, Sorkin EM. Doxazosin. An update of its clinical pharmacology and therapeutic applications in hypertension and benign prostatic hyperplasia. Drugs 1995;49:295–320.

Gordon T. McInnes

21

Diuretics

GENERAL

In hypertension appropriately low dosages of diuretics provide protection against the major cardiovascular causes of death. This extends to regression of left ventricular mass in patients with left ventricular hypertrophy (1[C]), (2[C]). Furthermore, resistance to antihypertensive therapy is most commonly caused by inadequate diuretic therapy. An erstwhile critic of diuretics (SED-13, 558) has commented, "Therefore, I believe that diuretics will continue to be a cornerstone of antihypertensive therapy in the future" (3[R]).

Risk versus benefit Circumstantial evidence from randomized trials and case—control studies can be taken to suggest an association between diuretics and sudden death, perhaps mediated by dysrhythmias secondary to depletion of potassium and magnesium (4[R]). However, the evidence cited for the dysrhythmogenic effects of diuretic-induced hypokalemia does not withstand careful scrutiny (SED-13, 562; SEDA-12, 182; SEDA-13, 184; SEDA-15, 179), and there is no heterogeneity between the results of randomized trials in which non-potassium-sparing or potassium-sparing diuretics were used. The trial evidence for increased numbers of sudden deaths hinges on findings from a largely discredited post-hoc subgroup analysis of data from the Multiple Risk Factor Intervention Trial (MRFIT) (SEDA-18, 229) and the results of case-control studies. Such studies are undermined by non-randomized allocation to treatment, and their limitations have been discussed previously (SED-13, 559; SEDA-18, 229). Nevertheless, it is prudent to use thiazides in low dosages in the management of hypertension, in order to avoid unnecessary metabolic effects (SED-13, 563).

Data from the prospective observational Gothenburg study suggest that metabolic changes during long-term treatment with antihypertensive drugs (predominantly β-blockers and thiazides) are not associated with increased risks of coronary heart disease (5[C]). In 686 middle-aged men, diabetes mellitus, raised serum cholesterol, and raised serum triglycerides at the outset were significant predictors of coronary heart disease. However, of within-study metabolic variables, only serum cholesterol was significantly and independently associated with coronary heart disease. Thiazide diuretics have only marginal effects on serum cholesterol in the long term (SED-13, 566; SEDA-17, 265; SEDA-18, 233; SEDA-19, 219). These results challenge the view that metabolic changes related to diuretics have a major impact on prognosis in treated hypertensives. The role of drug-associated diabetic mellitus may have been greatly exaggerated. Nevertheless, this was not a randomized trial, and confidence intervals for risk estimates were wide. Its advantage was the length of follow-up (15 years), which may have been long enough to ensure that changes in the pattern of risk factors had an eventual impact on morbidity, given that the time over which coronary heart disease develops is substantial.

An observational study suggested that diuretic treatment was associated with increased morbidity and mortality in patients with diabetes mellitus (SEDA-16, 219), although a retrospective subset analysis of data from the Systolic Hypertension in the Elderly Program (SHEP) offered no support for this suggestion (6[C]). In 583 older non-insulin-dependent diabetic patients and 4149 non-diabetic subjects treated with a chlorthalidone-based regimen or placebo, the 5-year cardiovascular disease rate was reduced by 34% by active treatment, regardless of diabetic status; absolute risk reduction was twice as great in diabetic subjects. Therefore, low dosage diuretic-based treat-

Side Effects of Drugs, Annual 20
J.K. Aronson, ed.

ment is effective in preventing cardiovascular disease events, cerebral and cardiac, in both non-insulin-dependent diabetes mellitus and in non-diabetic older patients with isolated systolic hypertension; there was also a favourable trend for all-cause mortality in non-insulin-dependent diabetes mellitus.

Some studies have shown worsening of ventricular dysrhythmias with diuretic treatment, but many others have not (SED-13, 562; SEDA-12, 182; SEDA-13, 184; SEDA-15, 179; SEDA-17, 261; SEDA-18, 230). In African-American men with moderate to severe hypertension, hydrochlorothiazide 25—50 mg bd for at least 4 weeks did not worsen ventricular dysrhythmias or signal-averaged electrocardiographic variables (7[C]). Despite the use of hydrochlorothiazide in very high dosages, ventricular dysrhythmogenicity was not enhanced in these high-risk patients. However, the findings were somewhat weakened by the study design, with a fixed sequence of placebo and hydrochlorothiazide.

Endocrine, metabolic *Glucose metabolism (SED-13, 565; SEDA-17, 265; SEDA-18, 233; SEDA-19, 220)* Uncritical reviewers consider that the value of diuretics in the treatment of hypertension is diminished by adverse metabolic effects, such as impaired glucose tolerance, making diabetes mellitus a contraindication (8[R]). In a population study there was an independent effect on diabetic risk of antihypertensive drugs (not restricted to diuretics) in 5453 elderly patients (9[C]). The results of such studies must be interpreted with caution, since they are not designed to study the observed association and may be confounded by indication, i.e. patients with more severe hypertension or who are at increased risk of diabetes are more likely to be treated. Although insulin resistance may result from treatment with thiazides in high dosages, and because thiazides may promote the development of non-insulin-dependent diabetes mellitus in predisposed patients, the therapeutic implications of these observations remain unclear (10[R]).

Hydrochlorothiazide 12.5 mg/day or lisinopril 20 mg/day had little or no untoward effect on glucose or insulin metabolism in 28 obese patients with hypertension (11[C]). Although there was some deterioration with the thiazide, neither drug was associated with changes in insulin-mediated glucose disposal. This observation in obese (insulin-resistant) patients contrasts sharply with earlier claims that conventional dosages of thiazides reduce insulin sensitivity (SEDA-15, 216). However, this small study had a low power to detect differences between the treatment groups.

In a thoughtful review (12[R]), Harper et al. have concluded that little information is available on the short-term and long-term effects of thiazides in diabetes mellitus; many reviewers too readily extrapolate from findings in non-diabetic subjects. Low dosages of thiazides, while effectively reducing blood pressure, have much less impact on the metabolic process, including peripheral insulin resistance. Since the maximal antihypertensive effect of thiazides may not be achieved for 4—6 weeks, frustrated prescribers may increase the dosage prematurely, increasing the risk of adverse metabolic effects (8[R]). In practice, many patients require more than one antihypertensive drug to achieve a therapeutic effect and thiazides are rational partners for all other agents. Treatment with diuretics is invariably required in diabetic nephropathy, to reduce fluid overload and blood pressure. As there is now good evidence that low-dosage thiazides are effective and without detrimental effects on glycemic control and insulin resistance, a strong argument can be made for their continued use in diabetes mellitus. These drugs are inexpensive, safe, and well-tolerated, and have been proven to reduce cardiac and cerebrovascular events.

Serum lipids (SED-13, 566; SEDA-17, 264; SEDA-18, 232; SEDA-19, 219) The changes in serum lipids with thiazides and thiazide-like diuretics (such as metolazone and indapamide) are considered by some to be of clinical significance (13[R]) and sufficient to discourage their use in hypertension (8[R]). Diuretic-induced changes in VLDL cholesterol and triglycerides are thought to be secondary to hyperinsulinemia and to hypersecretion of cortisol, growth hormone, and catecholamines, which in turn promote a rise in serum insulin. Catecholamines also increase hepatic cholesterol production and release.

In a subset of hypertensive patients from a previously published study (SEDA-15, 216), randomized to hydrochlorothiazide in a relatively high dosage or to captopril, neither drug altered lipoprotein core composition after 5 months treatment, but both drugs had small effects on lipoprotein surface lipid composition that were confined to the HDL_2 cholesterol subfraction [14C]. The clinical significance of these findings is unknown.

A meta-analysis of published work has shown that indapamide had no adverse effects on lipids, while the effects of thiazides were dose-dependent; even low dosages of thiazides adversely affected lipids [15C]. However, these results depended critically on the definition of low-dosage thiazides, a dosage equivalent to hydrochlorothiazide 25 mg/day, which is probably too high by current standards. There was also considerable heterogeneity between the results of the studies included, raising doubts about the validity of the meta-analysis. A meta-analysis is scientifically less rigorous than a randomized trial and depends on the quality of individual studies. The one published randomized comparison of indapamide and thiazides on lipid concentrations showed equivalent effects (SEDA-14, 185; SEDA-15, 216). Further direct comparisons are needed. In a small study in 28 obese hypertensive subjects [11c], hydrochlorothiazide 12.5 mg/day was associated with little or no untoward effects on lipoprotein metabolism.

It is questionable whether the size of the effect of low-dosage thiazides on serum lipids is sufficient to influence cardiovascular risk. The temptation to use higher dosages in hypertension should be resisted. It is also unknown whether the use of antihypertensive drugs that are lipid neutral or that induce a more favourable lipid profile will be more beneficial in preventing coronary heart disease. There is a need for continued reappraisal of conventional antihypertensive treatment, taking into account all identified coronary heart disease risk factors.

Mineral and fluid balance   *Potassium balance (SED-13, 562; SEDA-17, 218; SEDA-18, 229; SEDA-19, 218)* Reduction of the serum potassium concentration from 4.2 to 3.7 mmol/l with hydrochlorothiazide 50—100 mg/day for at least 4 weeks in 45 black hypertensive patients with moderate to severe left ventricular hypertrophy was not associated with worsening of ventricular dysrhythmias [7C]. Patients with left ventricular hypertro-

phy have a high risk of malignant ventricular dysrhythmias, but this finding suggests that even unnecessarily high dosages of thiazides and consequently large changes in plasma potassium concentration are not associated with an increased risk.

The risk of hyperkalemia during treatment with spironolactone in combination with an ACE inhibitor has been examined in two studies [16C], [17C]. In RALES (Randomised Aldactone Evaluation Study) 214 patients aged 26—83 years with symptomatic congestive heart failure were treated for 12 weeks with placebo or spironolactone (12.5, 25, 50, or 75 mg/day) in addition to an ACE inhibitor and a loop diuretic; some were also taking digoxin [16C]. The incidences of hyperkalemia (serum potassium over 5.5 mmol/l) in the respective groups were 5, 5, 13, 20, and 25%; predictors of hyperkalemia were long-acting ACE inhibitors, ACE inhibitor dosage, and baseline increases in serum creatinine and potassium concentrations. In a similar but much smaller study ($n = 42$), four of 28 patients who took spironolactone 50—100 mg/day in addition to an ACE inhibitor developed a serum potassium concentration greater than 5.5 mmol/l, and the lack of significant effect probably reflected the small sample size [17C]. There was no association between ventricular ectopic activity and plasma potassium concentration. These findings reinforce earlier warnings of the risk of combining potassium-sparing diuretics with ACE inhibitors (SEDA-13, 577; SEDA-18, 236).

Magnesium balance (SED-13, 564; SEDA-17, 262; SEDA-18, 230) In 42 patients with heart failure treated with conventional therapy (including loop diuretics), spironolactone significantly reduced urinary magnesium excretion, increased plasma magnesium concentration, and reduced the frequency of ventricular dysrhythmias on 24-h ambulatory electrocardiography [17C]; the reduction in ectopic activity correlated with the increase in plasma magnesium ($r = -0.41$). The findings in RALES [16C] suggest a dose-dependent effect of spironolactone on serum magnesium concentration during the first few weeks of treatment but not later. The increase in plasma magnesium concentration with the addition of spironolactone should not be taken to imply that other diuretics cause magnesium depletion.

Urinary system Long-term (2-year) treatment with indapamide 2.5 mg/day and hydrochlorothiazide 50 mg/day had equivalent antihypertensive effects in 28 patients with impaired renal function (18[C]). Creatinine clearance increased by 29% with indapamide and fell by 17% with hydrochlorothiazide, suggesting that indapamide may be superior in patients with impaired renal function and moderate hypertension. However, the dosage of hydrochlorothiazide may have been excessive, and baseline mismatching raises the possibility that a regression effect contributed to the findings.

In a population-based case-control study of 440 patients with renal cell carcinoma, the spouses of an additional 151 patients, and 691 controls, the risk of renal cell carcinoma increased with the use of diuretics or other drugs that lower blood pressure, especially among those with no history of hypertension (19[C]). The highest risk was among those who had taken diuretics for 10 years or more (odds ratio, OR, 1.8, 95% confidence interval 1.3—2.8); with other antihypertensive drugs the OR was 2.0 (1.2—3.3). Adjustment for hypertension reduced the OR associated with diuretics to the non-significant value of 1.4 (0.8—2.2). These findings suggest a small effect on the risk of renal cell carcinoma associated with hypertension and the use of diuretics, but it is difficult to disentangle the separate effects, because of potential misclassification of highly-correlated events. Further large-scale studies are required, with more detailed documentation of drug use and in people who have regular blood pressure measurements.

Sexual function *(SED-13, 567; SEDA-17, 267; SEDA-18, 235; SEDA-19, 221)* In SHEP, problems with sexual function were more common in patients treated with a chlorthalidone-based regimen than in those treated with placebo (6[C]); the increased incidence was seen both in patients with diabetes (12 and

7%, respectively) and in non-diabetics (7.6 and 6.5%, respectively). The difference was entirely in men: diabetics 21 and 10%, non-diabetics 16 and 14%. Impotence was particularly common in diabetic men, who are likely to have difficulties with sexual function because of autonomic dysfunction. In this small subset, the excess risk over placebo was about 10%. This relatively low incidence is in keeping with earlier reports in the general hypertensive population (SED-13, 567) and should not act as a deterrent to the use of thiazides in elderly patients with non-insulin-dependent diabetes mellitus.

Risk factors An uncritical review (20[R]) has perpetuated many of the myths concerning the adverse effects of diuretics in elderly people, implying that postural hypotension is a major problem, that diuretic-induced hypokalemia and hypomagnesemia are more marked and associated with a high risk of cardiac dysrhythmias and sudden death, and that diuretic-induced hypokalemia provokes glucose intolerance. These misconceptions have been refuted (SED-13, 560; SEDA-17, 267). However, the review is accurate in pointing out that while abnormalities of glucose, lipid, and uric acid are common after diuretics in elderly people, the clinical effects are small and do not seem to worsen cardiovascular risks. Reducing the dosage lessens the risks of adverse effects.

In a comparison of bendrofluazide 2.5—5 mg daily and dilevalol in 114 elderly patients (21[C]), bendrofluazide had a satisfactory effect on quality of life (health status index) owing to increased social participation and symptomatic well-being. Although there was no evidence that patients taking bendrofluazide were aware of any cognitive impairment, improvement in psychomotor performance in the dilevalol group was not observed in the diuretic group, suggesting abolition of a learning effect. Previous work has suggested an adverse effect of bendrofluazide on psychomotor performance in healthy volunteers (SEDA-18, 234). Cognitive impairment with bendrofluazide deserves further study.

INDIVIDUAL COMPOUNDS

Carbonic anhydrase inhibitors

Acetazolamide *(SED-13, 571; SEDA-19, 222)*

Acetazolamide has been reported to precipitate pustular psoriasis.

A 28-year-old man with a 20-year history of generalized pustular psoriasis developed psoriatic arthritis and glaucoma; acetazolamide precipitated pustular lesions and widespread erythema (22[C]). The clinical features improved after restriction of acetazolamide and the administration of oral etretinate. Readministration of acetazolamide led to the appearance of generalized pustules within 24 h. Histological examination confirmed pustular psoriasis; patch and lymphocyte stimulation testing for acetazolamide were negative. Nevertheless, an allergic reaction to acetazolamide was considered the likely explanation.

Uveitis may be a complication of psoriasis, and acetazolamide is widely used for the treatment of glaucoma secondary to uveitis. Caution should be exercised when giving acetazolamide to patients with psoriasis-induced uveitis.

It is likely that compromised ciliary vasculature may result in increased sensitivity to aqueous suppressants, leading to profound hypotony, choroidal detachment, and hemorrhage.

A 78-year-old white man with vascular disease developed ocular hypotony, bullous ciliochoroidal detachments, and suprachoroidal hemorrhage secondary to treatment with acetazolamide and betaxolol, which resolved on withdrawal (23[c]).

The relative contributions of acetazolamide and betaxolol in this case are not clear.

Methazolamide

Two Japanese-American women developed clinical features which satisfied the criteria for Stevens-Johnson syndrome during methazolamide treatment (24[c]). Methazolamide is a sulfonamide derivative, the most common group of drugs associated with Stevens-Johnson syndrome.

Loop diuretics

Furosemide (frusemide) *(SED-13, 571)*

A 5-month-old infant with trisomy 21 (Down's syndrome) and complete atrioventricular block developed pyrexia of unknown origin, and was exhaustively investigated over a 7-week period (25[c]). The fever ceased abruptly when furosemide was withheld. After 72 h without fever, heart failure worsened and furosemide was resumed; after the first dose a temperature of 39°C was recorded. Substitution of furosemide with chlorothiazide resulted in resolution of fever within 24 h and there was no recurrence. Adverse drug experience files of the United States Food and Drug Administration contain 20 possible cases of fever associated with furosemide. In these patients, either other drugs were given concomitantly or patients were not rechallenged. Furosemide should be considered as a possible cause in the differential diagnosis of persistent fever.

Thiazide diuretics *(SED-13, 567)*

Skin and appendages *(SED-13, 569; SEDA-17, 266; SEDA-18, 234; SEDA-19, 220)* Two patients who developed lupus-like skin lesions while taking thiazide diuretics had circulating anti-SSA/Ro antibodies and antinuclear antibodies (26[c]). A further patient developed unequivocal antinuclear antibody (ANA) positivity while taking hydrochlorothiazide (27[c]). The ANA pattern was homogeneous, the pattern most commonly found in drug-induced lupus. It normalized when hydrochlorothiazide was withdrawn and returned on rechallenge. This case offers strong evidence that hydrochlorothiazide can induce ANA production. Antihistamine antibodies and clinical evidence of systemic lupus erythematosus (SLE) did not develop. Patients with suspected thiazide-induced lupus-like syndrome or photosensitivity should have tests to detect the presence of circulating antinuclear and anti-SSA/Ro antibodies. This approach would also help elucidate whether photosensitivity is an early sign of drug-induced lupus in thiazide-treated patients. Only pharmacoepidemiological studies can demonstrate if hydrochlorothiazide induces SLE, or at least ANA production, in the general population. In the meantime, a doctor confronted with a patient taking hydrochlorothiazide and with a significant ANA titer should consider withdrawal of the diuretic only if signs and symptoms of SLE develop and an alternative effective drug can be substituted.

Interactions *(SED-13, 569; SEDA-17, 268)* In a randomized, double-blind, parallel-group study, tenidap sodium, a novel antiarthritic cytokine modulating drug, reduced the anti-hypertensive efficacy of bendrofluazide and hydrochlorothiazide in 23 middle-aged to elderly patients with mild to moderate hypertension (28[C]). Mean increases in supine and erect blood pressure were 5.9/3.0 and 6.5/6.8 mmHg, respectively. Only the increase in erect blood pressure was statistically significant, but the 95% confidence intervals did not exclude a substantial effect, equivalent to that seen with a conventional non-steroidal anti-inflammatory drug.

Potassium-sparing diuretics

Spironolactone *(SED-13, 575)*

Liver   Hepatotoxicity from spironolactone is extremely rare.

A 74-year-old man with no history of liver or biliary disease or blood transfusion and daily alcohol consumption <30 g, presented with jaundice after 7 weeks of monotherapy with spironolactone 50 mg/day for leg edema (29[c]). Ultrasound of the biliary tree was normal and infective hepatitis was ruled out by serological tests. Liver biopsy showed cholestasis with hepatocyte damage and focal tubular necrosis. All liver function abnormalities were corrected 3 months after stopping spironolactone.

The sequence of events and absence of liver disorders in this case strongly suggests spironolactone-induced liver disease.

Interactions *(SED-13, 576, 577)*   A 55-year-old man with alcoholic cirrhosis and portal hypertension treated with spironolactone 100 mg/day developed severe metabolic acidosis accompanied by severe hyperkalemia (serum potassium 8.0 mmol/l) and a normal anion gap 1 month after the introduction of cholestyramine 8 g tds for pruritus (30[c]). Discontinuation of both drugs and treatment with sodium bicarbonate restored normal metabolic status. Cholestyramine could result in anion exchange of chloride for bicarbonate in the small bowel, predisposing to hyperchloremic acidosis; this, together with spironolactone, contributes to development of life-threatening hyperkalemia. Careful surveillance is required if cholestyramine is prescribed with spironolactone.

Acute renal failure after strenuous exercise has been reported as a consequence of concomitant therapy with hydrochlorothiazide 50 mg/day and triamterene 75 mg/day for hypertension in a 37-year-old black man who was also taking ibuprofen 800—2400 mg/day for osteoarthritis (31[c]). Renal biopsy showed acute tubular necrosis and nephrosclerosis. Mild diuretics cause volume depletion, and triamterene may cause acute renal failure secondary to crystalluria, tubular obstruction, interstitial nephritis, and nephrolithiasis. Triamterene also increases plasma renin activity and renal vascular resistance, with a compensatory increase in renal prostaglandins. All of these factors reduce renal blood flow and potentiate renal damage due to exercise and non-steroidal anti-inflammatory drugs. Although exercise-induced acute renal failure is uncommon, this complication should be considered in patients taking triamterene with drugs that inhibit prostaglandin synthesis.

REFERENCES

1.   Carey PA, Sheridan DJ, de Cordoue A, Guez D. Effect of indapamide on left ventricular hypertrophy in hypertension: a meta-analysis. Am J Cardiol 1996;77:17B—19B.
2.   Tan SA, Berk LS, Tan LG. Indapamide regresses, but transdermal clonidine does not regresses, left ventricular hypertrophy in hypertensive diabetic patients. Am J Cardiol 1996;77:20B—22B.
3.   Kaplan NM. Diuretics: cornerstone of antihypertensive therapy. Am J Cardiol 1996;77:3B—5B.

4.   Grobbee DE, Hoes AW. Non-potassium-sparing diuretics and risk of sudden cardiac death. J Hypertens 1995;13:1539—45.

5.   Samuelssen O, Pennert K, Andersson O, Beglund G, Hedner T, Persson B, Wedel H, Wilhelmsen L. Diabetes mellitus and raised serum triglyceride concentration in treated hypertension-are they of prognostic importance? Observational study. Br Med J 1996;313:660—3.

6.   Curb JD, Pressel SL, Cutler JA, Savage PJ, Applegate WB, Black H, Camel G, Davis BR, Frost PH, Gonzalez N, Guthrie G, Oberman A, Rutan GH, Stamler J. Effect of diuretic-based antihypertensive treatment on cardiovascular disease risk in older diabetic patients with isolated systolic hypertension. J Am Med Assoc 1996;276:1886—92.

7.   Narayan P, Papademetriou V. Effect of hydrochlorothiazide therapy on cardiac arrhythmias in African-American men with systemic hypertension and moderate to severe left ventricular hypertrophy. Am J Cardiol 1996;78:886—9.

8.   Suter PM, Vetter W. Metabolic effects of antihypertensive drugs. J Hypertens 995;13 Suppl 4:S11—S17.

9.   Stolk RP, Hoes AW, Pols HAP, Hofman A, de Jong PTVM, Lamberts SWJ, Grobbee DE. Insulin, hypertension and antihypertensive drugs in elderly patients: the Rotterdam Study. J Hypertens 1996;14:237—42.

10.   Krentz AJ. Insulin resistance. Br Med J 1996;313:1385—9.

11.   Reaven GM, Clinkingbeard C, Jeppessen J, Maheux P, Pei D, Foote J, Hollenbeck CB, Chen Y-DI. Comparison of the hemodynamic and metabolic effects of low-dose hydrochlorothiazide and lisinopril treatment in obese patients with high blood pressure. Am J Hypertens 1995; 8:461—6.

12.   Harper R, Atkinson AB, Bell PM. Should we use thiazide diuretics in hypertensive patients with non-insulin-dependent diabetes mellitus? Q J Med 1996;89:477—82.

13.   Madu EC, Reddy RC, Madu AN, Anyaogu C, Harris T, Fraker TD. Review: the effects of antihypertensive agents on serum lipids. Am J Med Sci 1996;312:76—84.

14.   Bagdade JD, Buchanan WF, Pollare T, Lithell H. Effects of hydrochlorothiazide and captopril on lipoprotein lipid composition in patients with essential hypertension. Eur J Clin Pharmacol 1996;49:355—9.

15.   Ames RP. A comparison of blood lipid and blood pressure responses during the treatment of systemic hypertension with indapamide and with thiazides. Am J Cardiol 1996;77:12B—16B.

16.   The RALES Investigators. Effectiveness of spironolactone added to an angiotensin-converting enzyme inhibitor and a loop diuretic for severe congestive heart failure. (The Randomized Aldactone Evaluation Study (RALES).) Am J Cardiol 1996;78:902—7.

17.   Barr CS, Lang CC, Hanson J, Arnott M, Kennedy N, Struthers AD. Effects of adding spironolactone to an angiotensin-converting enzyme inhibitor in chronic congestive heart failure secondary to coronary artery disease. Am J Cardiol 1995;76:1259—65.

18.   Madkour H, Gadallah M, Riveline B, Plante GE, Massry SG. Indapamide is superior to thiazide in the preservation of renal function in patients with renal insufficiency and systemic hypertension. Am J Cardiol 1996;77:23B—25B.

19.   Chow W-H, McLaughlin JK, Mandel JS, Wacholder S, Niwa S, Fraumeni JF. Risk of renal cell cancer in relation to diuretics, antihypertensive drugs, and hypertension. Cancer Epidemiol Biomarkers Prev 1995;4:327—31.

20.   Baglin A, Boulard J-C, Hanslik T, Prinseau J. Metabolic adverse reactions to diuretics. Clinical relevance to elderly patients. Drug Saf 1995; 12:161—7.

21.   Slovik DI, Fletcher AE, Daymond M, MacKay EM, VandenBurg MV, Bulpitt CJ. Quality of life and cognitive function with a diuretic compared with a beta-blocker: a randomized controlled trial of bendrofluazide versus dilevalol in elderly hypertensive patients. Cardiol Eld 1995; 3:139—45.

22.   Kuroda K, Kojima T, Tanabe E, Fujita M, Shinkai H. Pustular psoriasis precipitated by acetazolamide. J Dermatol 1995;22:784—7.

23.   Machon P, Barton K, Ionides A, Hitchings RA. Ciliochoroidal detachment after aqueous suppressant therapy. J Glaucoma 1995;4:344—5.

24.   Flack AJ, Smith RE, Fraunfelder FT. Stevens-Johnson syndrome associated with methazolamide treatment reported in two Japanese-American women. Ophthalmology 1995;102:1677—80.

25.   Clegg HW, Riopel DA. Furosemide-associated fever. J Pediatr 1995;126:817—18.

26.   Brown CW, Deng J-S. Thiazide diuretics induce cutaneous lupus-like adverse reaction. Clin Toxicol 1995;33:729—33.

27.   Rich MW, Eckman JM. Can hydrochlorothiazide cause lupus? J Rheumatol 1995;22:1001.

28.   Rapeport WG, Grimwood VC, Korlipara K, Grillage MG. James I, Anderton JL, Selfridge DI. The effect of tenidap on the anti-hypertensive efficacy of thiazide diuretics in patients treated for mild to moderate hypertension. Br J Clin Pharmacol 1995;39:51S—55S.

29.   Renkes P, Gaucher P, Tréchot P. Spironolactone and hepatic toxicity. J Am Med Assoc 1995;273:376—7.

30.   Zapater P, Alba D. Acidosis and extreme hyperkalemia associated with cholestyramine and spironolactone. Ann Pharmacother 1995;29:199—200.

31.   Sanders LR. Exercise-induced acute renal failure associated with ibuprofen, hydrochlorothiazide, and triamterene. J Am Soc Nephrol 1995; 5:2020—3.

Gijsbert B. van der Voet and Frederik A. de Wolff

22 Metals

Aluminium (aluminum) *(SED-13, 583; SEDA-17, 273; SEDA-18, 240; SEDA-19, 223)*

Aluminium metabolism and toxicity, including its possible role in Alzheimer's disease have been recently reviewed (1[R]).

The effectiveness of a cartridge with immobilized desferrioxamine has been tested to treat aluminium overload in six dialysis patients (2[C]). Using this device the time needed for treating aluminium overload with intravenous desferrioxamine will be greatly shortened and its toxic effects reduced. The oral chelator deferiprone (L1) appears to be as effective as desferrioxamine in iron and aluminium removal and has low toxicity (3[r]).

Nervous system A 16-year-old boy developed *headache* and *vomiting* and 3 months later *memory impairment*, *epileptic seizures*, permanent right-sided *myoclonic jerks*, and *speech disorder* with dysarthric and aphasic components (4[c]). He later became bed-ridden and developed further speech disorders and ultimately mutism. The MRI scan was normal, but an EEG showed diffuse slowing, predominantly in the left hemisphere, and pseudoperiodic bursts of high-voltage slow waves. Aluminium intoxication was diagnosed and related to a metallic foreign body (a piece of a metallic mast from a small ship toy) which had injured his neck when he was 9 months old; the object was in the first thoracic vertebral body and an extremity had penetrated the subarachnoid space. The aluminium concentration in the CSF was 3.8 μg/l. The object was removed and therapy involved lumbar drainage and later intravenous desferrioxamine.

Aluminium toxicity has been reported after bladder irrigation with alum for hemorrhagic cystitis (5[c]). A teenage girl with acute lymphoblastic leukemia developed *mental changes*, *speech disturbances*, *coarse tremor*, and an *abnormal EEG* after intravesical 1% alum irrigation and administration of aluminium-containing antacids. Serum aluminum concentrations were slightly increased (14—22 μg/l), and bone-marrow biopsy specimens showed aluminium deposition on staining by Krueger's method. All the abnormalities resolved after a 9-week course of desferrioxamine.

Of five men who had pulmonary aluminosis due to exposure to aluminum in pyrotechnic flake powders during the late 1940s, two still survived (6[c]). One developed a *dementia with motor disturbances*, which was not consistent with Alzheimer's dementia. He had a very high concentration of aluminium in his cerebrospinal fluid. The other man was not demented and had a normal aluminium concentration in the cerebrospinal fluid.

Skin and appendages Aluminium causes histological changes at injection sites that stain with hematoxylin and eosin (7[c]). Among four cases, one had a *sclerosing lipogranuloma-like reaction* with unlined cystic spaces containing crystalline material. Another case presented as a large symptomatic subcutaneous swelling which microscopically showed diffuse and widespread involvement of the subcutaneous tissues by a *lymphoid infiltrate* with prominent lymphoid follicles.

Antimony *(SED-13, 838; SEDA-19, 223)*

Respiratory system Antimonate ore caused *chronic bronchitis* in 16 of 100 miners exposed (8[c]). The chronic bronchitis was characterized by a mild slow course with ventilation disturbances. There were no cases of pneumoconiosis.

Mutagenic, teratogenic, and carcinogenic

Side Effects of Drugs, Annual 20
J.K. Aronson, ed.

effects The mutagenic, teratogenic and carcinogenic effects of antimony have been reviewed; if they exist at all, they are not very important (9[R]). In man antimony trisulfide may possibly be carcinogenic, although studies with pure antimony compounds need to be performed to clarify the issue.

Bismuth *(SED-13, 585; SEDA-17, 274; SEDA-18, 240; SEDA-19, 223)*

Bismuth is still used as tripotassium dicitratobismuthate in dual, triple, and quadruple therapies for eradication of *Helicobacter pylori* (10[C]).

Urinary system Bismuth *nephrotoxicity* has been reported in a 16-year-old girl who had nausea, vomiting, and dizziness for 4—5 days and oliguria for 2 days (11[c]). She had taken up to 10—15 tablets of tripotassium dicitratobismuthate containing a total amount of 3—4.5 g of bismuth. Blood urea and serum creatinine were increased and there was proteinuria and erythrocytes in the urine. Acute tubular necrosis was observed on biopsy. The nephrotoxicity was reversible.

Chromium

Skin and appendages The risk of *allergic contact dermatitis* of the hand caused by chromium among 913 house construction workers and 707 concrete element prefabrication workers has been studied by questionnaire and clinical examination (12[C]). The prevalence of allergic contact dermatitis was reduced compared with an earlier study. Apparently lowering the water-soluble chromium content of cement by the addition of ferrous sulfate during the production process may have reduced the number of cases.

Tumor-inducing effects A prospective cohort study has been conducted to examine the health hazards of chromium plating, with a follow-up period over 16 years (13[C]). A group of chromium platers ($n = 623$) was compared with a non-plater group ($n = 567$). In the chromium plating group the risk of chronic hepatitis or liver cirrhosis was significantly increased and there was a trend toward statistical significance for the risk of *lung cancer*.

As part of a high-risk notification project of workers from four of seven facilities producing chromium compounds from chromite, a mortality study has been performed using retrospective data (14[C]). The overall risk for *lung cancer* was increased significantly despite cessation of exposure. The risk of *nasal cavity/sinus cancer* was also significantly increased. The increased risk of lung cancer after cessation of exposure emphasizes the need for developing early detection tests for lung cancer.

Copper *(SED-13, 587; SEDA-18, 241; SEDA-19, 224)*

The discovery that the gene for Wilson's disease encodes a copper-transporting ATPase has greatly improved our understanding of the pathophysiology of this disorder and copper metabolism in humans (15[R]). The abundance of disease-specific mutations and their location at multiple sites across the genome have limited molecular diagnosis to kindred of known patients, and confirm the necessity for screening by well-proven clinical and biochemical means. Chelation therapy with penicillamine, trientine, and recently tetrathiomolybdate, and therapy with zinc salts are still in use for Wilson's disease. Although gene therapy is on the horizon, the ability to treat this disorder effectively in this way awaits further characterization of the gene product and more efficient methods for gene delivery to all hepatocytes in the liver.

Skin and appendages A man with *green hair* has been described (16[c]). The cause was exogenous deposition of copper from domestic tap water with a high copper concentration. The discoloration disappeared promptly after the use of a shampoo containing penicillamine.

Genital system A meta-analysis of studies performed between 1965 and 1992, involving data on thousands of insertions of intrauterine contraceptive devices (IUCDs), has been conducted to determine whether the presence of the tailstring is associated with increased rates of pelvic inflammatory disease among copper IUCD users (17[C]). There was no difference in the rate of pelvic inflammatory disease among users of IUCDs with or without a tail, or among users of copper IUCDs with different tailstring materials. These findings support the hypothesis that the presence of a IUCD tailstring does not increase the rate of pelvic inflammatory disease.

In another study, 422 women aged 17—42 years have been evaluated (18[C]). There was no correlation between the duration of use of the Copper-T200 intrauterine device and percent positivity for *Chlamydia trachomatis* antigen. Although milder genital tract symptoms and signs were more common in woman with chlamydial cervicitis, clinical pelvic inflammatory disease was uncommon (0.5%). Pelvic inflammatory disease was not related to use of the Copper-T200 but to chlamydial cervicitis in this group of women with low risk sexual behaviour.

Gallium *(SED-13, 588; SEDA-19, 224)*

A phase II trial of gallium nitrate for patients with recurrent or metastatic non-squamous cell carcinoma of the cervix has been conducted in 26 patients aged 30—74 years (19[C]). Two patients had a complete response, one had a partial response, 13 had stable disease, and 10 had worsening disease. Gallium nitrate has modest activity in these patients. The major toxic effects were *nausea*, *vomiting*, and *anemia*.

Gold *(SED-13, 588; SEDA-17, 274; SEDA-18, 241; SEDA-19, 224)*

Adverse effects of gold continue to be reported mainly in relation to the use of gold salts in patients with rheumatoid arthritis, although occupational exposure is occasionally reported.

Nervous system   *Tremor* has been attributed to gold therapy (20[c]).

A 57-year old woman with active rheumatoid arthritis (arthritis, subcutaneous nodules histologically consistent with rheumatoid arthritis, anemia, and positive latex and ANA tests) was given sodium aurothiomalate, which was stopped after the second injection because of a mild skin rash. About 1 week later she developed a severe Parkinsonian tremor, initially in her left hand and the next day in the right hand. The tendon reflexes were normal and there was neither ataxia nor motor nor sensory changes. She was given steroids and improved: the tremor disappeared, apart from a degree of intention tremor. The appearance of the tremor shortly after the skin rash (which followed the gold injection) raised the possibility of a delayed (hypersensitivity) reaction.

Hematological   In a review of experience in 390 patients treated with slow-acting antirheumatic drugs at three adjacent rheumatology units in London, hematological adverse reactions were infrequent (21[C]).

Gastrointestinal   A 6-month, double-blind, parallel, randomized placebo-controlled, multicenter trial of auranofin has been conducted in 231 children with juvenile rheumatoid arthritis, about 80% of whom had polyarticular disease (22[C]). The efficacy of auranofin was slightly higher than that of placebo. *Diarrhea* was the most common adverse effect.

In a 28-year-old woman with juvenile-onset rheumatoid arthritis, treated with auranofin for almost 10 years, who developed *diarrhea*, biopsies of the distal duodenum showed partial villous atrophy with variation of villous/crypt ratio and architecture and increased inflammatory cells in the lamina propria (23[c]). These results were consistent with a malabsorption syndrome. Treatment consisted of withdrawal of the auranofin, while other medication was continued. The diarrhea settled, there was a 3-kg weight gain, and a repeat duodenal biopsy showed improvement.

A woman with classic rheumatoid arthritis, treated with parenteral sodium aurothiomalate for 10 years, developed *obstructive sialadenitis* caused by local compression on the excretory ducts of the parotid glands due to deposits of gold in the intraparotid lymphoid tissues (24[c]). She had swelling of both parotid glands on eating and computed tomography images showed accumulation of high density spots.

Urinary system   In 20 patients with drug-induced *membranous glomerulonephritis*, renal injury was produced by gold salts in six cases (25[C]). This drug-induced glomerulonephritis ran a benign course after drug withdrawal.

The prevalence of *microalbuminuria* has been evaluated in 65 patients with rheumatoid arthritis compared with 51 control subjects (26[C]). Treatment with gold and penicillamine increased the risk.

Skin and appendages   Chrysiasis is a distinctive permanent *pigmentation of light-exposed skin* resulting from the administration of parenteral gold salts. Chrysiasis developed in 31 of 40 Caucasian patients with rheumatoid arthritis treated with intramuscular sodium aurothiomalate (27[C]). Visible changes develop above a threshold equivalent to 20 mg/kg total gold administration, and their severity depends on cumulative dose. Focal aggregates are deposited in the reticular and papillary dermis in amounts that correlate with the degree of pigmentation. Characteristically the periorbital region is affected by mauve discoloration, which intensifies and deepens into a blue/slate-grey color, extending to the face, neck, and upper limbs. Although chrysiasis develops insidiously and patients may be unaware of the changes, positive identification is important in order to avoid misdiagnosis and medical mismanagement, and to give appropriate reassurance. Prevention is difficult, but reduced exposure to sunlight may help.

A case of chrysiasis in a 54-year-old Australian woman was confirmed by light microscopy, transmission electron microscopy, and radiographic microanalysis (28[c]). The condition developed after a relatively low dose of gold (aurothiomalate 50 mg/week for 8 weeks then 50 mg on alternate weeks; total cumulative dose 1.05 g). It was proposed that chrysiasis developed because of exposure to intense UV light.

A group of 13 patients with rheumatoid arthritis developed mucocutaneous adverse effects within 20 weeks of beginning of gold therapy (29[C]). Adverse effects were managed by temporary withdrawal of gold until adverse effects resolved and resumption of treatment using 50% of the usual dosage. When adverse effects recurred the dosage was reduced by a further 50%. The minimum effective dose of intramuscular gold is not known. Doses and dosage intervals should be individualized for optimal benefits and tolerability.

After intradermal testing with sodium aurothiomalate, five of eight patients developed skin papules at the test sites (30[C]). The papules persisted up to 20 months and histology showed *pseudolymphoma* of B and T cell type containing follicular structures and occasional small granulomata. Thus, sodium aurothiomalate seemed to accumulate in tissue macrophages, leading to constant immunological activation with lymphoid proliferation and a histiocytic response.

A 53-year-old woman with rheumatoid arthritis developed myasthenia gravis after 6 months of therapy with D-penicillamine; she was given gold instead and 12 months later developed *pemphigus vulgaris* (31[c]). This is the first reported case of gold-induced pemphigus in rheumatoid arthritis.

A 24-year-old man presented with a cutaneous eruption that was clinically consistent with *lichen planus* (32[c]). He had discrete, pruritic, violaceous, planar papules on the forearms, shins, and ankles, as well as fine reticulated plaques on the buccal mucosa. A skin biopsy of a lesion on the lower leg showed hyperkeratosis, focal hypergranulosis, and an inflammatory mononuclear cell infiltrate at the dermal—epidermal junction that also contained a few eosinophils. The patient had regularly consumed a gold-containing cinnamon schnapps (Goldschlager; Schmid and Gassler, Lausanne, Switzerland) for about 1 year, and after he stopping drinking it the pruritic eruption gradually cleared and the gold concentrations in his blood and urine fell.

Contact allergy to sodium aurothiosulfate and sodium aurothiomalate was established by skin testing in a 52-year-old woman with rheumatoid arthritis for 3 years in whom gold therapy was planned (33[c]). An intramuscular test dose of gold sodium aurothiomalate induced a flare-up of previously positive epicutaneous and intradermal test reactions, with a histological and immunohistochemical picture compatible with an allergic contact dermatitis. Since gold allergy is frequent, the cutaneous adverse effects of gold therapy ('gold dermatitis') may be explained by such an immune reaction.

Occupational contact dermatitis to gold is uncommon, since gold is relatively insoluble. In one case allergic contact dermatitis to gold was confirmed by patch testing with sodium aurothiosulfate in petrolatum (34[c]). Occupational contact dermatitis in the gold industry can be reduced by providing workers with more protective gear and better ventilation.

Immunological and hypersensitivity reactions   A clinical and immunological study has been performed in 22 patients with rheumatoid arthritis who developed subnormal serum immunoglobulin concentrations as a consequence of gold treatment (35^C). There were mild *deficiencies of single immunoglobulin isotypes* or severe deficiencies affecting two or three isotypes. Gold-induced antibody deficiency may be more common than is usually recognized.

To assess possible associations between human leukocyte antigens (HLA) and the achievement of remission during gold treatment, HLA typing was performed in 67 patients with rheumatoid arthritis with a gold-induced remission and in 25 control patients in whom gold had been ineffective (36^C). HLA typing was not helpful in predicting the therapeutic response to parenteral gold.

Tumor-inducing effects   In a comparison of 305 patients with rheumatoid arthritis exposed to Proresid® and 305 patients exposed to sodium aurothiomalate there was no increase in the risk of total malignancies in either group (37^C). Looking at separate tumors there was an increased risk of *lymphoma* and *leukemia* only in the gold-treated patients.

Iron *(SED-13, 595; SEDA-17, 277, SEDA-18, 242; SEDA-19, 225)*

Intravenous iron dextran has been evaluated in 537 patients undergoing dialysis (38^C). The most common adverse reactions included *itching, dyspnea or wheezing, chest pain, nausea, hypotension, angio-edema, dyspepsia, diarrhea, flushing, headache, cardiac arrest*, and *myalgia*. Serious adverse reactions appear to be uncommon in these patients; however, in 27 patients with adverse reactions in this series, cardiac arrest occurred in one case and hospitalization was required in three cases for serious adverse effects.

Rusty-colored peritoneal dialysate fluid was observed after intravenous administration of iron dextran to a patient with peritonitis being treated with vancomycin and rifampicin (39^c). The discoloration gradually cleared over 24 h.

The authors postulated that a combination of iron and rifampicin had caused the discoloration.

Iron dextran, iron gluconate, and iron saccharate are the iron formulations that are generally given to renal patients (40^C). Possible adverse effects are *anaphylactic reactions* due to preformed antibodies to dextran or vascular reactions due to unbound iron. Intravenous iron saccharate does not cause oversaturation of transferrin iron binding. This may explain in part the minimal adverse effects observed during intravenous administration of iron saccharate.

Respiratory   *Acute bronchial necrosis* occurred in two patients who required pulmonary resection (41^c).

A 59-year-old woman consulted a physician after she had inhaled a ferrous sulphate tablet (Tardyferon). After extraction of the tablet a necrotic inflammatory process of the mucosa of the right distal bronchus was observed. Four days later a second bronchoscopic examination showed inflammatory lesions of the right intermediate bronchus with patchy necrosis of the mucosa. Nine days after the first consultation collapse of the lower lobe was seen, with hemoptysis sufficient to cause hypovolemic shock. There was a polypoid mass and ulceration in the bronchial posterior zone. Five hours later the patient died in cardiac arrest.

A 54-year-old man with a history of neonatal hypoxia and subsequent spastic paraplegia developed vigorous coughing that produced a cupful of blood. He had a hiatus hernia with chronic blood loss and iron deficiency anemia, and for this reason was taking Tardyferon iron tablets and had inhaled one. Bronchoscopy showed total occlusion of the left lower bronchus by a polypoid mass covered with greenish brown necrotic material. After lobectomy the patient recovered.

Nervous system   The hypothesis that *akathisia* is related to alterations in iron metabolism has led to the suggestion that iron supplementation might be a useful therapeutic intervention for patients with akathisia (42^R). However, the rationale for iron supplementation in the treatment of akathisia is relatively weak, and there are potentially adverse long-term consequences.

Liver   There is growing evidence that normal or only mildly increased amounts of iron in liver can be damaging, particularly when combined with other hepatotoxic factors, such as alcohol, porphyrogenic drugs, or chronic viral hepatitis (43[R]). Iron enhances the pathogenicity of micro-organisms, adversely affects the function of macrophages and lymphocytes, and enhances fibrogenic pathways, all of which may increase hepatic injury due to iron itself or to iron and other factors. Blood-letting is enjoying a therapeutic renaissance based on the current understanding of the toxic effects of iron.

Gastrointestinal Iron protein succinylate is an iron derivative for oral use, providing protein-bound iron (44[C]). It has been evaluated in 1800 patients and compared with other oral iron compounds (iron sulphate and iron-polystyrene sulfonate). Iron protein succinylate was more slowly absorbed than divalent iron, resulting in better gastrointestinal tolerability.

In a multicenter trial in 174 patients iron protein succinylate was compared with iron sulfate in the treatment of iron deficiency anemia (45[C]). General tolerability was good with both treatments, but iron protein succinylate caused fewer gastrointestinal symptoms than iron sulfate.

In 40 women aged 20—35 years with iron deficiency anemia during or immediately after pregnancy, oral liquid ferrous gluconate was compared with ferrous gluconate and ferrous sulphate tablets and liquid ferric protein succinylate (46[C]). Liquid ferrous gluconate was more effective and gastrointestinally better tolerated.

Iron tablets cause histopathologically distinctive lesions in mucosal biopsies of the stomach and esophagus (47[c]). In a histological study of three esophageal lesions and six gastric lesions there was heavy iron accumulation within ulcer granulation tissue, in the connective tissue and blood vessels of the mucosal lamina propria, and within glandular and squamous epithelia. The appearance was distinctive and similar to that seen after overdosage.

Skin and appendages Skin cruptions have been described in two patients taking iron.

A 36-year-old woman developed a generalized exanthematous pustular eruption (48[c]). She had taken ferrous fumarate (Ferrum®) combined with other medications, because of anemia due to cancer of the uterine cervix and probably idiopathic thrombocytopenic purpura, and after 15 days developed a skin rash on both thighs spreading gradually over her whole body. Physical examination showed diffuse or various-sized patches of erythema and miliary papules. In addition, erosions, hemorrhagic vesicles, and miliary pustules were seen on the waist and both thighs. Ferrous fumarate was withdrawn and she was given methylprednisolone. Two days later, the rash and fever began to resolve; the rash completely disappeared in 2 weeks.

A 54-year-old man developed erythema and lichenification on sun-exposed areas after taking sodium ferrous citrate (Ferromia®) orally for anemia for 2 weeks, in combination with various other drugs (49[c]). A screening phototest showed increased photosensitivity. The authors suggested that iron or the transferrin iron complex (diferric transferrin) may be a photosensitizer. After withdrawal the photosensitivity normalized.

Tumor-inducing effects Iron, when bound to certain ligands, can cause free radical-mediated tissue damage and become carcinogenic (50[r]).

The risk of *colorectal cancer* due to consumption of oral iron has been prospectively studied in 14 407 patients (51[C]). Iron may confer an increased risk of colorectal cancer, and the localization of risk may be attributable to the mode of epithelial exposure. It seems that luminal exposure to oral iron increases the risk proximally, whereas an increased serum iron concentration increases the risk distally.

Manganese *(SED-13, 1001; SEDA-19, 225)*

Manganese toxicity in relation to exposure has been recently reviewed (52[R]). Occupational exposure and exposure to formulations used in parenteral nutrition (53[C]), (54[C]) remain important sources. Manganese seems to increase erythropoietin (55[C]) and serum lysozyme (56[C]) in occupationally exposed workers engaged in the production of iron-manganese alloys.

Nervous system A high degree of chronic manganese exposure produces *dystonic rigidity* and *proximal tremor*. The late effects of asymptomatic exposure are uncertain. In 59 Chilean miners with past exposure in the mines, hand tremor has been studied (57[C]). Chronic asymptomatic manganese exposure resulted in detectable late-life movement abnormalities.

Endocrine, metabolic   In 31 workers occupationally exposed to manganese dust for 14.5 years in a ferroalloy-producing plant the correlation between prolactin and manganese in blood and in urine was studied in samples collected at least 48 h after the last exposure (58[C]). In the manganese-exposed workers there was an *increase in serum prolactin*, which correlated with manganese in both the blood and urine, suggesting impairment of tonic inhibition by tubero-infundibular dopaminergic neurones.

Risk factors   *Chronic liver disease* is associated with manganese overload. Patients with cirrhosis ($n = 11$) had significantly higher blood manganese concentrations than 11 controls (59[C]). Semiquantitative scores of T1-weighted signal hyperintensity on MRI in the patients with cirrhosis correlated with blood manganese concentration.

Mercury *(SED-13, 598; SEDA-17, 278; SEDA-19, 225)*

Most reports of mercury toxicity, with compounds such as thiomersal and mercurochrome, are related to *allergic skin reactions*. The significance of thiomersal (thimerosal, mercurithiosalicylate), an organic mercury compound, as a hidden sensitizer for mucocutaneous reactions has been reviewed (60[R]).

A 44-year-old man took 83 mg/kg of thiomersal and developed *gastritis, renal failure, dermatitis, gingivitis, delirium, coma, polyneuropathy, and respiratory failure* (61[c]). Complete recovery followed symptomatic treatment plus gastric lavage and administration of the oral chelating agents dimercaptopropane sulfonate and dimercaptosuccinic acid.

Discussion of the effects of mercury in dental amalgams continues without a clear evaluation of the risks, and cases of toxicity, mostly neurotoxicity, continue to be published. Various aspects of the toxicity of methyl mercury have recently been reviewed (62[R]). The use of chelation (meso-2,3-dimercaptosuccinic acid) in patients with motor neurone disease to eliminate mercury (and lead) may open new therapeutic approaches (63[c]).

Nervous system   While shaking a mercury thermometer, a 35-year-old nurse plunged it into her left hand (64[c]). Elementary mercury infiltrated the soft tissues of her palm. The diffusely distributed mercury particles could not be completely removed surgically. Three-and-a-half years later she developed progressive weakness of the legs over a few weeks. She had moderate *muscle weakness*, most pronounced in the lower limbs, slight *cerebellar ataxia*, and *muscle fasciculation* in the thigh; her deep tendon reflexes were increased and Babinski's sign was abnormal on the left; her cranial nerves and sensation were normal. Mercury and lead concentration in blood, urine, and hair were not raised. Amyotrophic lateral sclerosis was diagnosed and followed by a treatment with chelation (dimercaptosuccinic acid) which was not successful. The authors speculated that pre-existing or genetically determined motor dysfunction could be aggravated by exogenous mercury. Chelation treatment should be started soon after exposure to mercury to prevent accumulation and irreversible damage.

Neuropsychological follow up in a patient with chronic elemental mercury intoxication showed reversible *impairment of neuropsychological function* if prompt removal from the toxic environment was accomplished, together with proper medical treatment (65[c]).

Urinary system   The effects of exposure to elemental mercury on the nervous system and the kidneys have been studied in three groups of workers exposed to different amounts of mercury (66[c]). There were no differences across the groups with respect to either motor nerve conduction velocity or tremor frequency spectra of physiological tremors. In contrast, N-acetyl-β-D-glucosaminidase (NAG) was significantly increased in the group with the highest exposure and correlated strongly with the concentration of mercury in urine. This rise in NAG was considered transient and not an early indicator of developing renal dysfunction.

Skin and appendages   The allergenic effects of mercury, particularly organic compounds such as thiomersal, have been reviewed, with discussion of the contribution of preventive vaccinations to the occurrence of allergy (67[R]). The authors suggested that the number of sensitized persons will increase because of routine vaccination of health service workers and medical students against viral hepatitis.

The incidence and causes of allergy to thiomersal has been studied in 685 patients (68[C]). Allergy to thiomersal was diagnosed in 39 patients, including 25 women and 14 men. Vaccination of health service workers against viral hepatitis as well as immunotherapy with pollen formulations containing thiomersal (Catelet, Biomed, Poland) were the main causes of allergy. Allergy to thiosalicylic acid was not observed and two patients reacted positively to mercuric chloride.

Photodermatitis from systemic or topical piroxicam has been known for years. Patients, 63 in all, with an erythemato-edematous and sometimes vesicular patch test to thimerosal, were tested for different allergens (69[C]). In patients with piroxicam photosensitivity, frequent patch test reactions to thiomersal were found, mainly in those sensitized to the thiosalicylate component. It was proposed that skin lesions were due to a photoproduct of piroxicam.

A 5-year-old boy with previous skin intolerance to mercurochrome (merbromin) developed a severe *allergic contact dermatitis* of both feet when wearing new polyvinyl chloride (PVC) boots (70[c]). Within a few days he developed a mercury exanthem involving both legs, groins, and sides of the trunk. Patch tests showed strong reactions to organic and inorganic mercury compounds, in particular mercurous chloride (HgCl2), which was identified in the boots using atomic absorption spectrophotometry and polarography. New hidden sources of mercury in consumer goods may represent potential sources of danger, if its use is not more strictly regulated.

Immunological and hypersensitivity reactions Lymphocyte counts (T cells, T helper cells, T suppressor cells, and NK cells) have been determined in the peripheral blood of 81 men with a history of occupational exposure to metallic mercury vapors and in 36 men without exposure (71[C]). There were *increases in the T helper cell count and the T helper/T suppressor ratio*, which may have been immunological indicators of exposure to mercury vapors.

Miscellaneous Subcutaneous injection by gunshot of elemental mercury resulted in subsequent *granuloma* formation in a 19-year-old man with an 8-month history of a tender enlarging mass in his left antecubital fossa while on active military service (72[c]). Surgical removal of mercury from a presumed mercury tipped bullet was undertaken but was incomplete, and the patient declined further operative intervention as he remained asymptomatic. Chelation therapy was not instituted, while serum and urine mercury was monitored and was detectable for 6 years after presentation.

Nickel *(SED-13, 599)*

Respiratory A high rate of toxic *pneumosclerosis* resulting from extrinsic alveolitis has been observed in workers engaged in hydrometallurgic nickel production (73[C]). Pathogenesis of the condition includes changes in lung surfactant, an imbalance between lipid peroxidation and antioxidant activity, immune disorders, and the formation of circulating immune complexes.

Gastrointestinal Histological and immunohistochemical studies of the gastrointestinal mucosa in 20 patients with contact allergic dermatitis to nickel with symptom recrudescence due to nickel in food ingested have suggested that sensitivity to nickel in food may be caused by a type IV immunological reaction in the gut (74[C]).

Skin and appendages In 700 Finnish adolescents aged 14—18 years, of whom 476 had a history of orthodontic treatment with metallic appliances, the frequency of *nickel sensitization* was 19% (75[C]). Nickel allergy was more frequent in girls than in boys, and more frequent in subjects with pierced ears than without. The results suggested that orthodontic treatment does not seem to increase the risk of nickel hypersensitivity, but rather that treatment with nickel-containing metallic orthodontic appliances before sensitization to nickel (ear piercing) may have reduced the frequency of nickel hypersensitivity.

An eight-year-old girl swallowed a Canadian 25 cent piece and 24 h later developed a scaly, red, papular skin rash (76[c]). The rash started initially over the nasal bridge, ear lobules, and behind both ears, areas where she had previously had well-documented contact dermatitis due to nickel in the metallic frame of her spectacles and earrings. Within 12 h the rash had spread to the rest of her body and had become confluent, erythematous, and pruritic in many areas; on the fourth day she had developed vesicles on her fingers. At endoscopy markedly erythematous patches were observed, with mild friability and a thin exudate in the gastric body. Biopsies showed moderate acute duodenitis with highly reactive epithelium and an increase in lymphocytes and plasma cells in the mucosa. After removal of the coin she used a topical steroid ointment for another 24 h and the rash rapidly resolved.

Tumor-inducing effects   Mortality patterns in a cohort of 284 nickel platers have been re-examined (77[C]). There was only weak evidence that nickel plating is associated with an excess risk of *stomach cancer*. This cohort of nickel platers does not seem to have experienced any discernible risk of occupational lung cancer. Other studies of nickel platers rather than nickel/chromium platers would be useful.

Selenium *(SED-13, 600; SED-19, 226)*

Nervous system   The incidence of *amyotrophic lateral sclerosis*, a disease previously associated with a high selenium environment, has been studied in 5182 residents of an area in Italy over a period of 9 years (78[C]). They had accidentally been exposed to drinking water with a high selenium content. The findings confirmed a possible association between overexposure to environmental selenium and amyotrophic lateral sclerosis.

Tumor-inducing effects   The possible role of selenium in *oral cancer* has been reviewed (79[R]). A plasma selenium concentration in the reference range may represent a form of chemoprevention of carcinogenesis. The concept of chemoprevention of carcinogenesis with inhibitory chemical compounds is particularly appropriate to head and neck squamous cell cancer control, because the inci-

dence of a second primary tumor in surviving patients with oral cancer is very high.

Silver *(SED-13, 600; SEDA-19, 226)*

The effect of an intranasal vasoconstrictor (oxymetazoline), with or without silver nitrate cautery, has been studied in the treatment of epistaxis in 60 patients, 11 of whom required a combination of oxymetazoline with silver nitrate cautery (80[C]). Pharmacological management was adequate in 50 of the patients, and nasal packing was avoided.

Nervous system   A schizophrenic patient developed argyria from chronic and excessive ingestion of anti-smoking pills containing silver (81[c]). *Seizures* developed after he had taken the pills for 40 years. There was an extremely high concentration of silver in the serum. This case provides support for the hypothesis that silver may cause seizures as a result of systemic poisoning.

Titanium *(SEDA-19, 226)*

In an effort to predict which slipped capital femoral epiphysis fixation devices might cause fewer retrieval problems, 27 consecutive implant-retrieval procedures have been reviewed (82[r]). Problems occurred with both stainless steel and titanium devices if implanted for over 1 year. A retrieved titanium screw showed evidence of osseointegration (direct bone contact at over 90% of the interface) using back-scattered image scanning electron microscopic analysis.

Zinc *(SED-13, 601)*

Liver   Excess hepatic copper and zinc has been reported in six native Canadian children, aged 22 months to 8 years, with severe *chronic cholestatic liver disease* (83[C]). The excess copper may have been due to the cholestatic liver disease, but the excess zinc was unexplained. It has been suggested that a genetic disorder of metal metabolism may have been involved (84).

Gastrointestinal   In children with severe zinc deficiency, *diarrhea* is common and responds quickly to zinc supplementation. In 937 children with diarrhea, aged 6—35 months, zinc supplementation zinc supplementation resulted in clinically important reductions in the duration and severity of diarrhea (85[C]).

Bacitracin zinc, bacitracin, or neomycin have been used prospectively to treat 82 patients infected with the protozoon *Giardia lamblia* (86[C]). Final cure rates were highest for bacitracin zinc, and adverse effects were limited to *nausea, abdominal discomfort, and diarrhea in a small number of patients.*

REFERENCES

1. Yokel RA, Golub MS, editors. Research issues in aluminum toxicity. J Toxicol Environ Health (Special Issue) 1996;48:527—686.

2. Anthone S, Ambrus CM, Kohli R, Anthone R, Stadler A, Stadler I, Vladutiu A. Treatment of aluminum overload using a cartridge with immobilized desferrioxamine. J Am Soc Nephrol 1995;6:1271—7.

3. Kontoghiorghes GJ. New concepts of iron and aluminium chelation therapy with oral L1 (deferiprone) and other chelators. A review. Analyst 1995;120:845—51.

4. Hoang-Xuan K, Perrotte P, Dubas F, Philippon J, Poisson FM. Myoclonic encephalopathy after exposure to aluminum. Lancet 1996; 347:910—11.

5. Kanwar VS, Jenkins JJ, Mandrell BN, Furman WL. Aluminum toxicity following intravesical alum irrigation for hemorrhagic cystitis. Med Pediatr Oncol 1996;27:64—7.

6. Sjögren B, Ljunggren KG, Almkvist O, Frech W, Basun H. A follow-up study of five cases of aluminosis. Int Arch Occup Environ Health 1996;68:161—4.

7. Culora GA, Ramsay AD, Theaker JM. Aluminium and injection site reactions. J Clin Pathol 1996;49:844—7.

8. Lobanova EA, Ivanova LA, Pavlova TA, Prosina II. Kliniko-pathogeneticheskie osobennosti pri vozdeistvii antimonitovykh rud na organizm rabotaiushchikh. (Clinical and pathogenetic features of exposure of workers to antimonate ore.) Med Tr Prom Ekol 1996;4:12—15.

9. Leonard A, Gerber GB. Mutagenicity, carcinogenicity and teratogenicity of antimony compounds. Mut Res 366:1—8.

10. De Boer WA, Driessen WMM, Tytgat GNJ. Only four days of quadruple therapy can effectively cure *Helicobacter pylori* infection. Aliment Pharmacol Ther 1995;9:633—8.

11. Akpolat I, Kahraman H, Akpolat T, Kandemir B, Cengiz K. Acute renal failure due to overdose of colloidal bismuth. Nephrol Dial Transplant 1996;11:1890—1.

12. Roto P, Sainio H, Reunala T, Laippala P. Addition of ferrous sulfate to cement and risk of chromium dermatitis among construction workers. Contact Dermatitis 1996;34:43—50.

13. Itoh T, Takahashi K, Okubo T. Mortality of chromium plating workers in Japan—a 16-year follow-up study. Sangyo Ika Daigaku Zasshi 1996;18:7—18.

14. Rosenman KD, Stanbury M. Risk of lung cancer among former chromium smelter workers. Am J Ind Med 1996;29:491—500.

15. Schilsky ML. Wilson's disease: genetic basis of copper toxicity and natural history. Semin Liver Dis 1996;16:83—95.

16. Munkvad S, Weismann K. Kobberinduceret gront har. Behandlung med en penicillaminshampoo. (Copper-induced green hair. Treatment with a penicillamine-containing shampoo.) Ugeskr Laeger 1996;158:3791—2.

17. Ebi KL, Piziali RL, Rosenberg M, Wachob HF. Evidence against tailstrings increasing the rate of pelvic inflammatory disease among IUD users. Contraception 1996;53:25—32.

18. Palayekar V, Joshi JV, Hazari KT, Shah RS, Chitlange SM. Chlamydia trachomatis detected in cervical smears from Copper-T users by DFA test. Adv Contracept 1996;12:145—52.

19. Malfetano JH, Blessing JA, Homesly HD. A phase II trial of gallium nitrate (NSC 15200) in nonsquamous cell carcinoma of the cervix: a Gynecologic Group study. Am J Oncol Cancer Clin Trials 1995;18:495—7.

20. Machtey I. Neurological signs in RA patients receiving gold. Br J Rheumatol 1996;35:804.

21. Comer M, Scott DL, Doyle DV, Huskisson EC, Hopkins A. Are slow-acting anti-rheumatic drugs monitored too often? An audit of current clinical practice. Br J Rheumatol 1995;34:966—70.

22. Giannini EH, Brewer EJ, Kuzmina N, Shaikov A, Wallin B. Auranofin in the treatment of juvenile rheumatoid arthritis. Results of the USA—USSR double blind, placebo-controlled trial. Arthritis Rheum 1996;33:466—76.

23. Cook NJ, Owen ET, Donlon JB. A further possible cause of diarrhoea caused by oral gold. Br J Rheumatol 1995;34:395—6.

24. Zuazua JS, De La Fuente AM, Rodriguez JC, Carcia GB, Rodriguez AP. Obstructive sialadenitis caused by intraparotid deposits of gold salts: a case report. Oral Surg Oral Med Oral Pathol Oral Radiol Endodont 1996;81:649—51.

25. Popishil 'IuA. Patogistologicheskie i ul'trasfrukturnye osobennosti medikamentoznogo membranoznogo glomerulonefrita. (Pathohistologic and ultrastructural features of drug-induced membranous glomerulonephritis.) Arkh Patol 1996; 58:52—6.

26. Moller-Pedersen L, Nordin H, Svensson B,

Bliddal H. Microalbuminuria in patients with rheumatoid arthritis. Ann Rheum Dis 1995; 54:189—92.

27. Smith RW, Leppard B, Barnett NL, Millward-Sadler GH, McCrae F, Crawley MID. Chrysiasis revisited: a clinical and pathological study. Br J Dermatol 1995;133:671—8.

28. Fleming CJ, Salisbury EL, Kirwan P, Painter DM, Barnetson RS. Chrysiasis after low-dose gold and UV light exposure. J Am Acad Dermatol 1996;34:349—51.

29. Klinkhoff AV, Teufel A. How low can you go? Use of very low dosage of gold in patients with mucocutaneous reactions. J Rheumatol 1995;22:1657—9.

30. Kalimo K, Rasanen L, Aho H, Maki J, Mustikkamki UP, Rantala I. Persistent pseulolymphoma after intradermal gold injection. J Cutaneous Pathol 1996;23:328—34.

31. Ciompi ML, Martchetti G, Bazzichi L, Puccetti L, Agelli M. d-Penicillamine and gold salt treatments were complicated by myasthenia and pemphigus, respectively, in the same patient with rheumatoid arthritis. Rheumatol Int 1995;15:95—7.

32. Russell MA, King LE, Boyd AS. Lichen planus after consumption of a gold-containing liquor. New Engl J Med 1996;334:603.

33. Moller H, Larsson A, Bjorkner B, Bruze M, Hagstam A. Flare-up at contact allergy sites in a gold-treated rheumatic patient. Acta Dermatol Venereol 1996;76:55—8.

34. Tan E, Delaney TA. Occupational contact dermatitis to gold. Australas J Dermatol 1996; 37:218—19.

35. Snowden N, Dietch DM, Teh LS, Hilton RC, Haeney MR. Antibody deficiency associated with gold treatment: natural history and management in 22 patients. Ann Rheum Dis 1996;55:616—21.

36. Ten Wolde S, Dijkmans BAC, Van Rood JJ, Claas FHJ, De Vries RRP, Hazes JMW, Van Riel PLCM, Van Gestel A, Breedveld FC. Human leucocyte antigen phenotypes and gold-induced remissions in patients with rheumatoid arthritis. Br J Rheumatol 1995;34:343—6.

37. Bendix G, Bjelle A, Holmberg E. Cancer morbidity in rheumatoid arthritis patients treated with Proresid® or parenteral gold. Scand J Rheumatol 1995;24:79—84.

38. Fishbane S, Ungurueanu VD, Maesaka JK, Kaupke CJ, Lim V, Wish J. The safety of intravenous iron dextran in hemodialysis patients. Am J Kidney Dis 1996;28:529—34.

39. Carter TB, Garris AG, Ullian ME. Rusty peritoneal dialysis fluid after intravenous administration of iron dextran. Am J Kidney Dis 1996;27:147—50.

40. Sunder-Plassmann G, Horl WH. Safety of intravenous injection of iron saccharate in haemodialysis patients. Nephrol Dial Transplant 1996;11:1797—802.

41. Babatasi G, Massetti M, Galateau F, Mosquet B, Khayat A, Evrard C. Bronchial necrosis induced by inhalation of an iron tablet. J Thorac Cardiovasc Surg 1996;112:1397—9.

42. Gold R, Lenox RH. Is there a rationale for iron supplementation in the treatment of akathisia? A review of the evidence. J Clin Psychiatry 1995;56:476—83.

43. Bonkovsky HL, Banner BF, Lambrecht RW, Rubin RB. Iron in liver diseases other than hemochromatosis. Semin Liver Dis 1996;16:65—82.

44. Kopcke W, Sauerland MC. Meta-analysis of efficacy and tolerability data on iron protein succinylate in patients with iron deficiency anemia of different severity. Arzneim-Forsch (Drug Res) 1995;45:1211—16.

45. Najean Y, Acuto G, Scotti A. Multicentre double-blind clinical trial of iron protein succinylate in comparison with iron sulfate in the treatment of iron deficiency anaemia. Clin Drug Invest 1995;10:198—207.

46. Casparis D, Del Carlo P, Branconi F, Grossi A, Merante D, Gafforio L. Efficacia e tolerabilita del gluconato ferroso orale liquido nell'anemia da carenza da ferro in gravidanza e nell'immediato post-partum: confronto con altre formulazioni liquide o solide contenenti ferro bivalente o trivalente. Minerva Ginecol 1996;48:511—18.

47. Eckstein RP, Symons P. Iron tablets cause histopathologically distinctive lesions in mucosal biopsies of the stomach and esophagus. Pathology 1996;28:142—5.

48. Ito A, Nomura K, Hashimoto I. Pustular drug eruption induced by ferrous fumarate. Dermatology 1996;192:294—5.

49. Kawada A, Hiruma M, Noguchi H, Kimura M, Ishibashi A, Banba H, Marshall J. Photosensitivity due to sodium ferrous citrate. Contact Dermatitis 1996;34:77.

50. Okada S. Iron-induced tissue damage and cancer: the role of reactive oxygen species-free radicals. Pathol Int 1996;46:311—32.

51. Wurzelmann JI, Silver A, Schreinemacheis DM, Sandler RS, Everson RB. Iron intake and the risk of colorectal cancer. Cancer Epidemiol Biomarkers Prev 1996;5:503—7.

52. Mergler D. Manganese: the controversial metal. At what levels can deleterious effects occur? Can J Neurol Sci 1996;23:93—4.

53. Beath SV, Gopalan S, Booth IW. Manganese toxicity and parenteral nutrition. Lancet 1996; 347:1773—4.

54. Forbes A, Jawhari A. Manganese toxicity and parenteral nutrition. Lancet 1996;347:1774.

55. Misiewicz A. Stezenie erytropoetyny w surowicy krwi pracownikow narazonych na dzialanie manganu. (Concentrations of erythropoietin in the serum of workers exposed to manganese.) Przegl Lek 1995;52:538—40.

56. Misiewicz A. Wplyw srodowiska zawodowego zawierajacego mangan na zachowanie sie lizozymu w surowicy krwi. (The effect of occupational exposure to manganese on serum lysozyme activity.) Przegl Lek 1995;52:535—7.

57. Hochberg F, Miller G, Valenzuela R, McNelis

S, Crump KS, Covington T, Valdivia G, Hochberg B, Trustman JW. Late motor deficits of Chilean manganese miners: a blinded control study. Neurology 1996;47:788—95.

58. Mutti A, Bergamaschi E, Alinovi R, Lucchini R, Vettori MV, Franchini I. Serum prolactin in subjects occupationally exposed to manganese. Ann Clin Lab Sci 1996;26:10—17.

59. Hauser RA, Zesiewicz TA. Manganese and chronic liver disease. Mov Disord 1996;11:589.

60. Van 'T Veen AJ, Van Joost T. Bron en praktische betekenis van allergie voor thiomersal, een organische kwikverbinding. (Source and clinical significance of allergy for thiomersal, an organic mercury compound.) Ned Tijdschr Geneeskd 1996;140:297—300.

61. Pfab R, Muckter H, Roider G, Zilker T. Clinical course of severe poisoning with thiomersal. J Toxicol Clin Toxicol 1996;34:453—60.

62. Cranmer J, editor. Methylmercury. Neurotoxicology (Special Issue) 1995;16:577—730.

63. Louwerse ES, Buchet JP, Van Dijk MA, De Jong VJMB, Lauwerijs RR. Urinary excretion of lead and mercury after oral administraion of meso-2,3-dimercaptosuccinic acid in patients with motor neurone disease. Int Arch Occup Environ Health 1995;67:135—8.

64. Schwarz S, Husstedt I, Bertram HP, Kuchelmeister K, Amyotrophic lateral sclerosis after accidental injection of mercury. J Neurol Neurosurg Psychiatry 1996;60:698.

65. Hua MS, Huang CC, Yang YJ. Chronic elemental mercury intoxication: neuropsychological follow-up case study. Brain Inj 1996;10:377—84.

66. Boogaard PJ, Houtsma AT, Journee HL, Van Sittert NJ. Effects of exposure to elemental mercury on the nervous system and the kidneys of workers producing natural gas. Arch Environ Health 1996;51:108—15.

67. Kiec-Swierczynska M. Rtec jako czynnik alergizujacy. (Mercury as an allergic factor.) Med Pr 1996;47:77—81.

68. Kiec-Swierczynska M. Uczulajace dzialanie mertiolatu (prparat odkzzajacy) na podstawie materialu Instytutu Medycyny Pracy w Lodzi. (Allergic reaction to merthiolate (a disinfectant) based on material from the Occupational Medicine Institute in Lodz.) Med Pr 1996;47:125—31.

69. Stingeni L, Lapomarda V, Lisi P. What risk of piroxicam photodermatitis in thimerosal-positive patients? Contact Dermatitis 1996;34:60—1.

70. Koch P, Nickolaus G. Allergic contact dermatitis and mercury exanthem due to mercury chloride in plastic boots. Contact Dermatitis 1996; 34:405—9.

71. Moszczynski P, Rutowski J, Slowinski S, Bem S, Jakus-Stoga D. Effects of occupational exposure to mercury vapors on T-cell and NK-cell populations. Arch Med Res 1996;27:503—7.

72. Bradberry SM, Feldman MA, Braithwaite RA, Shortland-Webb W, Vale JA. Elemental mercury-induced skin granuloma: a case report and review of the literature. J Toxicol Clin Toxicol 1996;34:209—16.

73. Artiunina GP. Toksicheskii pnevmoskleroz i al'veolit u rabochikh gidrometallurgicheskogo proizvodstva nikelia. (Toxic pneumosclerosis and alveolitis in workers engaged in the hydrometallurgic production of nickel.) Med Tr Prom Ekol 1996;(3):22—5.

74. Di Gioacchino M, Masci S, Cavallucci E, Pavone G, Andreassi M, Gravante M, Pizzicannella G, Boscolo P. Modificazioni immuno-istopatologiche della mucosa gastro-intestinale in pazienti con allergia da contatto al nichel. (Immunohistopathologic changes in the gastrointestinal mucosa in patients with nickel contact allergy.) G Ital Med Lav 1995;17:33—6.

75. Kerosuo H, Kullaa A, Kerosuo E, Kanerva L, Hensten-Pettersen A. Nickel allergy in adolescents in relation to orthodontic treatment and piercing of ears. Am J Orthod Dentofacial Orthop 1996;109:148—54.

76. Mahdi G, Israel DM, Hassall E. Nickel dermatitis and associated gastritis after coin ingestion. J Pediatr Gastroenterol Nutr 1996;23:74—6.

77. Pang D, Burges DC, Sorahan T. Mortality study of nickel platers with special reference to cancers of the stomach and lung, 1945—1993. Occup Environ Med 1996;53:714—17.

78. Vinceti M, Guidetti D, Pinotti M, Rovesti S, Merlin M, Vescovi L, Bergomi M, Vivoli G. Amyotrophic lateral sclerosis after long-term exposure to drinking water with high selenium content. Epidemiology 1996;7:529—32.

79. Carinci F, Felisatti P. Selenio e carcinoma orale. Revisione della letteratura. (Selenium and oral cancer. Review of the literature.) Minerva Stomatol 1996;45:345—8.

80. Krempl GA, Noorily AD. Use of oxymetazoline in the management of epistaxis. Ann Otol Rhinol Laryngol 1995;104:704—6.

81. Ohbo Y, Fukuzako H, Takeuchi K, Takigawa M. Argyria and convulsive seizures caused by ingestion of silver in a patient with schizophrenia. Psychiatry Clin Neurosci 1996;50:89—90.

82. Lee TK, Haynes RJ, Longo JA, Chu JR. Pin removal in slipped capital femoral epiphysis: the unsuitability of titanium devices. J Pediatr Orthop 1996;16:49—52.

83. Phillips MJ, Ackerley CA, Superina RA, Roberts EA, Filler RM, Levy GA. Excess zinc associated with severe progressive cholestasis in Cree and Ojibwa-Cree children. Lancet 1996; 347:866—8.

84. Scheinberg H, Sternlieb I. Excess zinc associated with cholestasis. Lancet 1996;347:1331.

85. Sazawal S, Black RE, Bhan MK, Bhandari N, Sinha A, Jalla S. Zinc supplementation in young children with acute diarrhea in India. New Engl J Med 1995;333:839—44.

86. Andrews BJ, Panitescu D, Jipa GH, Vasile-Bugarin AC, Vasiliu RP, Ronnevig JR. Chemotherapy for giardiasis: randomized clinical trial of bacitracin, bacitracin zinc, and a combination of bacitracin zinc with neomycin. Am J Trop Med Hyg 1995;52:318—21.

R.H.B. Meyboom

23 Metal antagonists

PENICILLAMINE AND RELATED COMPOUNDS

(SED-13, 605; SEDA-17, 281; SEDA-18, 245; SEDA-19, 229)

One of the reasons for the diversity of adverse effects of metal-chelating drugs, such as penicillamine, deferiprone, and deferoxamine, is that metals such as iron, copper, and zinc are constituents of many physiological proteins (see Table 1) (1[R]).

Penicillamine

Because of its adverse effects and moderate efficacy penicillamine is losing its place in the management of rheumatoid arthritis (2[R]). Also a large observational study in Spain has shown a high discontinuation rate in patients using penicillamine compared with other disease-modifying antirheumatic drugs, especially in women and patients over 65 years (3[CR]). Mucocutaneous reactions were the most frequent reason for discontinuation.

The results of a long-term follow-up study of combination drug therapy have been described in 169 patients with rheumatoid arthritis, including penicillamine in 25 patients (4[cR]). The mean follow-up period was 7 years. Although overall toxicity of combination therapy was lower than expected, no details for specific drugs were provided.

Respiratory Pulmonary involvement is one of the extra-articular manifestations of rheumatoid arthritis and includes pleurisy, parenchymal nodules, interstitial involvement, and vasculitis. In addition, *obliterating bronchiolitis* may occur, either as part of rheumatoid arthritis or related to its treatment (5[R]). The majority of reported cases of rheumatoid arthritis with obliterating bronchiolitis have in-

volved penicillamine. However, other drugs (mainly parenteral gold) have also been implicated. The clinical presentation is acute, with cough, shortness of breath, and other non-specific respiratory complaints. The prognosis is often poor. Chest radiographs show hyperinflation or, less commonly, patchy interstitial disease. Pulmonary function tests generally show obstruction and reduced CO diffusion capacity, but a minority have evidence of a restrictive process or of mixed obstructive and restrictive disease. The histological findings are generally restricted to the small airways. Two separable but overlapping groups have been described: acute and chronic cellular bronchiolitis with less conspicuous scarring, and constrictive bronchiolitis, with histology varying from fibrotic and inflammatory lesions to complete small airway obliteration.

Nervous system A further case has been described of *myasthenia gravis* probably caused by penicillamine.

A 54-year-old woman with rheumatoid arthritis took penicillamine 600 mg/day for 6 months (6[c]). The reaction presented with bilateral ptosis, diplopia, nasal speech, and respiratory difficulties. Anti-acetylcholine receptor antibodies and antinuclear antibodies (speckled pattern) were positive; there was no thymus enlargement. Penicillamine was withdrawn and she recovered within a couple of months (now using corticosteroids). Later her rheumatoid arthritis was treated with gold sodium thiomalate. After 12 months this treatment was complicated by pemphigus, necessitating the withdrawal of gold.

The development of two different autoimmune reactions in this case illustrates the complex interactions that may occur between sulfhydryl compounds and the immunological system in patients with rheumatoid arthritis.

Hematological The pattern of causes of acute *agranulocytosis* in 30 patients collected over 11 years has been compared with the pattern in a similar study in the same hospital

Table 1.   *Review of metal-containing proteins (1^R)*

Iron	Copper	Zinc
Aconitase	Ascorbate oxidase	Alcohol dehydrogenase
Catalase	Amine (spermine) oxidase	Alkaline phosphatase
Cyclo-oxygenase	Ceruloplasmin	Carbonic anhydrase
Cytochromes	Cytochrome C oxidase	Carboxypeptidase
Ferrotoxins	Dopamine beta-hydroxylase	Insulin
Hemoglobin	Superoxide dismutase	Metallothionein
Lipoxygenase reductase	(cytosolic)	Superoxide dismutase
Myoglobin	L-tryptophan oxygenase	
Peroxidases	Tyrosinase	
Proline hydroxylase	Uricase	
Ribonucleotide reductase		
Tryptophan hydroxylase		
Tyrosine hydroxylase		

in the preceding decade (7^{CR}). In 25 patients the likely causative drug was identified and in the remaining five the cause was not found; in only one case was penicillamine implicated. A major finding was that in a decade the incidence of noramidopyrine-associated agranulocytosis had fallen from 38% (16/42) to 17 (5/30).

A third case report of *sideroblastic anemia* probably caused by penicillamine has underlined the importance of vigilance when anemia develops in a patient using penicillamine (8^c). In this patient, a 50-year-old man with rheumatoid arthritis, anemia was discovered after he had taken penicillamine 500 mg/day for 2 months. Penicillamine was continued for another 7 months until profound anemia requiring blood transfusion developed, and a bone-marrow aspirate showed a hypocellular marrow with markedly reduced erythropoiesis, gross dyserythropoiesis, and 24% ringed sideroblasts. The patient recovered when penicillamine was withdrawn and pyridoxine was added. It is not clear, however, whether ibuprofen, the other drug used, was also withdrawn or not.

In another study, *pancytopenia* developed in two of 178 patients taking penicillamine (3^c).

On the other hand, the cost-effectiveness of regular blood samples monitoring in patients taking penicillamine or other 'slow-acting antirheumatic drugs' has been disputed (9^R).

Urinary system Microalbuminuria is common in patients with rheumatoid arthritis (10^{CR}). This may reflect either rheumatoid nephropathy or *renal injury* caused by drugs,

in particular penicillamine or gold. The distinction between primary and iatrogenic renal injury may, however, be difficult to make. Subclinical renal involvement may not be revealed by routine laboratory tests such as serum creatinine. Whatever the cause, the long-term renal prognosis in patients with arthritis and microalbuminuria requires clarification in longitudinal studies.

Skin and appendages In a large observational study *mucocutaneous reactions* (for example rash, stomatitis) were the most frequent reason for discontinuing penicillamine (3^{CR}).

Hypersensitivity and immunological reactions Current knowledge of the pathology of drug-induced *lupus-like syndrome* has been reviewed (11^R). With penicillamine therapy autoantibodies develop in a high proportion of patients without clinical disease.

Bucillamine

Most experience with bucillamine has so far come from Japan. In a 16-week study of bucillamine (daily dose range 100—600 mg) in 36 Korean patients with rheumatoid arthritis two patients had serious adverse reactions: *agranulocytosis* with high fever after 3 weeks in one and *nephrosis* in the other (12^c). Two other patients had mild proteinuria. In addition, *pruritus* occurred in 22% of patients, a *rash* in 19%, *stomatitis* in 8%, *anorexia or nausea* in 12%, *epigastric discomfort or pain* in 18%, and *increased aminotransferases* in 6%. One patient had a *change in taste*. There were altogether three drop-outs because of adverse effects (8%).

OTHER METAL ANTAGONISTS

Deferoxamine (desferrioxamine) *(SED-13, 619; SEDA-17, 286; SEDA-18, 249; SEDA-19, 232)*

In 21 children the liberation of 'catalytic iron' in acute myeloid leukemia appeared to aggravate the adverse effects of high-dose methotrexate chemotherapy (13[C]). This finding suggests that the toxicity of chemotherapy might be reduced by the co-administration of iron chelators.

The efficacy and adverse effects of deferoxamine in a single high dose (30—40 mg/kg) and a low dose (500 mg in 100 ml of 0.9% saline) have been compared in 22 hemodialysis patients, as a test for aluminium storage (14[CR]). After a high dose, nine patients had adverse effects, mainly *nausea, itching*, and *dizziness*, compared with only one patient with a *headache* after the low dose. The authors concluded that the low-dose deferoxamine test is safe and reasonably sensitive and specific.

Skin and appendages In a study of 18 patients with bone-marrow transplantation for thalassemia, deferoxamine accelerated the clearance of iron deposits (15[CR]). Deferoxamine 40 mg/kg was infused subcutaneously over 12 h, six nights a week, for a median of 9 months. Ascorbic acid supplementation was not given. Local reactions, with *pruritus, erythema*, and *swelling*, were common (frequency not stated), but dilution of the deferoxamine solution reduced the frequency. In one patient, however, deferoxamine had to be withdrawn because of severe local reactions with fever.

Special senses Deferoxamine can cause ocular adverse effects (SED-13, 620). A series of 17 patients with hemolytic anemia, age range 5—25 years, was studied prospectively for ocular adverse effects of deferoxamine (16[C]). The standard dosage was 40 mg/kg/day (route not entirely clear, but probably by subcuta-

neous infusion). *Lens opacities* were found in 41%, *changes in the retinal pigment epithelium* in 35%, *tortuosity of retinal vessels* in 24%, *dilatation and sheathing of retinal vessels* in 18%, *defects in color vision* in 29%, and *abnormal dark adaptation* in 18%. Regular ophthalmological monitoring is indicated during the use of deferoxamine.

Deferiprone

The pharmacology and toxicology of deferiprone have been reviewed (1[R]). Deferiprone is an α-ketohydroxypyridine compound with metal-chelating properties. It is absorbed within minutes after oral administration and reaches maximum blood concentrations within 1 h. It is eliminated with a half-life of 1—2 h and is almost completely undetectable in blood within 5—7 h (after a single dose). Deferiprone is mostly metabolized to a glucuronide conjugate that reaches maximum blood concentrations within 1—1.5 h. Deferiprone, its iron complex, and its glucuronide conjugate are detectable in the urine, and in most instances the total amount of all three accounts for almost 100% of the dose. Deferiprone is not excreted in the feces. However, there is much interindividual variation in its metabolism. The order of metal binding by deferiprone at pH 7.4 is Fe > Cu > Al > Zn (see Table 2). The iron binding constant is higher than those of deferoxamine and diethylenetriaminepentaacetic acid (DTPA).

Deferiprone has a concentration-dependent affinity for iron. Three molecules of deferiprone bind one molecule of iron, whereas deferoxamine binds iron in a 1:1 ratio. For this reason, deferiprone must be present in very high concentrations, close to toxic concentrations, to be effective (17[R]). Deferiprone dissociates from iron when its concentration in body fluids falls to the concentration achieved just a few hours after oral administration

Table 2. *Metal stability constants of chelators in clinical use (1[R])*

Ion	Deferiprone	Deferoxamine	DTPA
Fe^{3+}	35.0	30.6	28.6
Cu^{2+}	19.6	14.0	21.0
Ni^{2+}	12.1	10.0	20.2
Co^{3+}	11.7	11.0	19.0
Zn^{2+}	13.5	11.1	18.4

(18[r]). Deferiprone is effective in excreting iron in iron storage diseases and aluminium in hemodialysis patients (1[R]).

Since the controversy discussed in SEDA-18 (p. 250), the position of deferiprone as a therapeutic agent seems to have been clarified (1[R]). Experience in 21 patents who took deferiprone 75 mg/kg/day orally for a mean period of 3.1 years has been reported (19[CR]). *Joint pain* developed in three patients, as has previously been described (SEDA-18, 251; SEDA-19, 231). One patient had *increased alanine aminotransferase activity*, falling after withdrawal. There were no cases of leukopenia, lupus-like syndrome, or changes in antinuclear antibodies. In a combined report of 84 patients derived from four different centers, probably including the patients in the study of Olivieri et al. (19[CR]), deferiprone had to be withdrawn in three patients because of *agranulocytosis*, in four because of severe *nausea*, in two because of *arthritis*, and in one because of *persistent liver dysfunction* (20[CR]). Less severe suspected adverse effects not requiring withdrawal were *transient increases in liver enzymes* ($n = 37$), *arthropathy* ($n = 17$), *zinc deficiency* ($n = 12$), *neutropenia* ($n = 4$), and moderate *nausea* ($n = 3$).

The results of a trial with deferiprone (75 mg/kg/day) in 20 children with either β-thalassemia or hemoglobin E-β thalassemia have been reported (21[C]). *Nausea* and occasional *vomiting* occurred in six patients (30%), and six patients complained of *joint pain* and *restriction of joint movement* (hip, knee, shoulder, ankle, and/or fingers), associated with swelling and warmth in three and necessitating withdrawal in five. All of these patients were negative for LE cells, antinuclear factor, and anti-double-stranded DNA. One of the patients developed *agranulocytosis* with fever and a prominent *gingival infection* after taking deferiprone for 11 months; the bone-marrow showed the picture of maturation arrest and the neutrophil count normalized within 7 days of stopping deferiprone.

It may be concluded that the use of deferiprone is indicated in patients with iron or aluminium storage who are unable or unwilling to use deferoxamine (17[R]), (19). In addition, the administration of shorter cycles of deferiprone administration, rather than continuous treatment, may improve compliance and reduce the incidence of toxic effects (22[c]). However, there is still debate about whether deferiprone is associated with a lupus-like syndrome and antinuclear antibodies (SEDA-18, 251; (23[CR])).

Dimercaptopropanesulfonate *(SED-13, 625)*

Sodium dimercaptopropane sulfonic acid, 300 mg/day orally for 5 days, was given to 10 men with occupational mercury intoxication (24[c]). In one patient a *macular erythematous rash* developed 3 days later and spontaneously resolved in the next few days.

In a 21-year-old man treated with dimercaptopropanesulfonate for acute poisoning with bismuth (tripotassium dicitratobismuthate), mild *nausea* was the only adverse effect, and it occurred after both oral and intravenous administration (25[c]).

Dimercaptosuccinic acid *(SED-13, 628)*

Dimercaptosuccinic acid, 10 mg/kg 8-hourly for 5 days followed by 10 mg/kg 12-hourly, has been given orally to 28 children with mild to moderate lead poisoning (26[c]). The only adverse effect was an episode of granulocytopenia (neutrophil count $0.752 - 10^9/l$).

Edetic acid derivatives *(SED 13, 626; SEDA-17, 288; SEDA-18, 251)*

In a study of the use of $^{117m}Sn^{4+}$-diethylenetriaminepentaacetic acid (DTPA) for palliative pain reduction in 15 patients with bone metastases, there were no myelotoxic or other adverse effects (27[c]).

DTPA is used to link the β-emitting radioisotope ^{90}Y to a monoclonal antibody (BrE3) against an epitope of the human milk fat globule. This combination is used in the treatment of advanced breast carcinoma. In a study in nine patients, administration of ^{90}Y-DTPA—BrE3 complex was associated with transient and uncomplicated *thrombocytopenia* in four patients and *leukopenia* in two patients (28[c]).

Trientine (triethylamine tetramine dihydrochloride) *(SED-13, 627; SEDA-17, 289; SEDA-18, 252)*

Long-term treatment of Wilson's disease with trientine has been evaluated in 19 patients, of whom 13 completed the study, with a mean observation time of 8.5 years (29[CR]). In two patients there was *neurological deterioration* early during treatment, permanent in one and transient in the other. These findings suggest that trientine may (as is known with penicillamine) initially worsen neurological manifestations of Wilson's disease, presumably by the mobilization and redistribution of copper. In two other patients trientine was associated with serious *colitis* (with concomitant *duodenitis* in one), raising the suspicion of a possible causal relation.

REFERENCES

1. Kontoghiorghes GJ. New concepts of iron and aluminium chelation therapy with oral L1 (deferiprone) and other chelators. A review. Analyst 1995;120:845—51.

2. Conaghan PG, Brooks P. Disease-modifying antirheumatic drugs, including methotrexate, gold, antimalarials, and D-penicillamine. Curr Opin Rheumatol 1995;7:167—73.

3. De La Mata J, Blanco FJ, Gomez Reino JJ. Survival analysis of disease modifying antirheumatic drugs in Spanish rheumatoid arthritis patients. Ann Rheum Dis 1995;54:881—5.

4. McCarty DJ, Harman JG, Grassanovich JL, Qian C, Klein JP. Combination drug therapy of seropositive rheumatoid arthritis. J Rheumatol 1995;22:1636—45.

5. Anaya JM, Diethelm L, Ortiz LA, Gutierrez M, Citera G, Welsh RA, Espinoza LR. Pulmonary involvement in rheumatoid arthritis. Semin Arthritis Rheum 1995;24:242—54.

6. Ciompi ML, Marchetti G, Bazzichi L, Puccetti L, Agelli M. D-Penicillamine and gold salt treatments were complicated by myasthenia and pemphigus, respectively, in the same patient with rheumatoid arthritis. Rheumatol Int 1995;15:95—7.

7. Paitel JF, Stockemer V, Dorvaux V, Witz F, Guerci A, Lederlin P. Drug-induced agranulocytosis. Clinical study about 30 patients and etiological evolution between 2 decades. Rev Méd Interne 1995;16:495—9.

8. Kandola L, Swannell AJ, Hunter A. Acquired sideroblastic anaemia associated with penicillamine therapy for rheumatoid arthritis. Ann Rheum Dis 1995;54:529—30.

9. Comer M, Scott DL, Doyle DV, Huskisson EC, Hopkins A. Are slow-acting anti-rheumatic drugs monitored too often? An audit of current clinical practice. Br J Rheumatol 1995;34:966—70.

10. Moller-Pedersen L, Nordin H, Svensson B, Bliddal H. Microalbuminuria in patients with rheumatoid arthritis. Ann Rheum Dis 1995;54:189—92.

11. Price EJ, Venables PJW. Drug-induced lupus. Drug Saf 1995;12:283—90.

12. Kim SY, Lee IH, Bae SC, Yoo DH. Preliminary trial of the efficacy of bucillamine in Korean patients with rheumatoid arthritis. Clin Drug Invest 1995;9:284—90.

13. Carmine TC, Evans P, Bruchelt G, Evans R, Handgretinger R, Niethammer D, Halliwell B. Presence of iron catalytic for free radical reactions in patients undergoing chemotherapy: implications for therapeutic management. Cancer Lett 1995;94:219—26.

14. Janssen MJA, Van Boven WPL. Efficacy of low-dose desferrioxamine for the estimation of aluminium overload in haemodyalysis patients. Pharm World Sci 1996;18:187—91.

15. Giardini C, Galimberti M, Lucarelli G, Polchi P, Angelucci E, Baronciani D, Gaziev D, Erer B, La Nasa G, Barbanti I, Muretto P. Desferrioxamine therapy accelerates clearance of iron deposits after bone marrow transplantation for thalassaemia. Br J Haematol 1995;89:868—73.

16. Dennerlein JA, Lang GE, Stahnke K, Kleihauer E, Lang GK. Ocular findings in desferrioxamine therapy. Ophthalmologie 1995;92:38—42.

17. Nathan DG. An orally active iron chelator. New Engl J Med 1995;332:953—4.

18. Nathan DG. Deferiprone in iron overload. New Engl J Med 1995;333:599.

19. Olivieri NF, Brittenham GM, Matsui D, Berkovitch M, Blendis LM, Cameron RG, McClelland RA, Liu PP, Templeton DM, Koren G. Iron-chelation therapy with oral deferiprone in patients with thalassemia major. New Engl J Med 1995;332:918—22.

20. Al-Refaie FN, Hershko C, Hoffbrand AV, Kosaryan M, Olivieri NF, Tondury P, Wonke B. Results of long-term deferiprone (L1) therapy: a report by the International Study Group on Oral Iron Chelators 1995;91:224—9.

21. Adhikari D, Basu Roy T, Biswas A, Chakraborty ML, Bhattacharya B, Maitra TK, Basu AK, Chandra S. Efficacy and safety of oral iron chelating agent deferiprone in beta-thalassemia and hemoglobin E-beta thalassemia. Indian Pediatr 1995;32:855—61.

22. Adhikari D. Deferiprone in iron overload. New Engl J Med 1995;333:598.

23. Mehta J, Singhal S, Mehta BC, Adhikari D, Hoffbrand AV, Wonke B, Nathan DG. Deferi-

prone in iron overload. New Engl J Med 1995;333:597—9.

24.   Torres Alanis O, Garza Ocanas L, Pineyro Lopez A. Evaluation of urinary mercury excretion after administration of 2,3-dimercaptol-propane sulfonic acid to occupationally exposed men. J Toxicol Clin Toxicol 1995;33:717—20.

25.   Stevens PE, Moore DF, House IM, Volans GN, Rainford DJ. Significant elimination of bismuth by haemodialysis with a new heavy-metal chelating agent. Nephrol Dial Transplant 1995; 10:696—8.

26.   Besunder JB, Anderson RL, Super DM. Short-term efficacy of oral dimercaptosuccinic acid in children with low to moderate lead intoxication. Pediatrics 1995;96:683—7.

27.   Atkins HL, Mausner LF, Srivastava SC, Meinken GE, Cabahug CJ, D Alessandro T. Tin-117m(4+)-DTPA for palliation of pain from osseous metastases: a pilot study. J Nucl Med 1995;36:725—9.

28.   Schrier DM, Stemmer SM, Johnson T, Kasliwal R, Lear J, Matthes S, Taffs S, Dufton C, Glenn SD, Butchko G, Ceriani RL, Rovira D, Bunn P, Shpall EJ, Bearman SI, Purdy M, Cagnoni P, Jones RB. High-dose [90]Y Mx-diethylenetriaminepentaacetic acid (DTPA)-BrE-3 and autologous hematopoietic stem cell support (AHSCS) for the treatment of advanced breast cancer: a phase I trial. Cancer Res 1995;55: 5921s—5924s.

29.   Dahlman T, Hartvig P, Lofholm M, Nordlinder H, Loof L, Westermark K. Long-term treatment of Wilson's disease with triethylene tetramine dihydrochloride (trientine). Q J Med 1995;88:609—16.

Pam Magee

24 Antiseptic drugs and disinfectants

ALDEHYDES *(SED-13, 644; SEDA-17, 293; SEDA-19, 235)*

Formaldehyde

The amino acid-formaldehyde condensate taurolidine has been studied as an antiendotoxic agent in 49 patients with septic shock; three patients became hypotensive and one experienced pain on injection (1ᶜ).

Glutaraldehyde

Glutaraldehyde is an ideal agent for the decontamination of flexible and other heat-sensitive endoscopes. However, it is irritant and sensitizes the skin and respiratory tract. Environmental contamination can take place and sensitization to glutaraldehyde among endoscopy nurses has led to a search for alternative disinfectants (2ʳ).

CATIONIC SURFACTANTS

Benzalkonium chloride *(SEDA-17, 542)*

Benzalkonium chloride is a quaternary ammonium disinfectant. Its adverse effects when used as a preservative in eye-drops have been extensively reported.

In a study to establish a set of contact allergens present in eye-drops, which could precipitate allergic conjunctivitis, benzalkonium chloride was found to be one of the most common allergens (3ᶜ).

Benzalkonium chloride, used as a preservative in ear-drops, has been identified as a common cause of allergic contact dermatitis

in patients with otitis. However, in a study designed to identify allergy due to topical medications in chronic otitis externa and chronic otitis media, benzalkonium elicited hardly any allergic reactions (4ᶜ).

Benzalkonium chloride is also used as a preservative in nasal sprays. In a randomized, double-blind, parallel study in 20 volunteers, 10 received oxymetazoline nasal spray with benzalkonium chloride and the others used oxymetazoline nasal spray without preservative, each three times a day for 30 days (5ᶜ). In those who used oxymetazoline with benzalkonium chloride, nasal stuffiness and mucosal swelling were significantly more common than in those who used oxymetazoline only. Benzalkonium chloride in oxymetazoline nasal spray therefore accentuates the severity of rhinitis medicamentosa in healthy volunteers.

In a similar study with 4 weeks of pre-treatment and then 10 days of rechallenge, oxymetazoline nasal spray in combination with benzalkonium chloride had a long-term adverse effect on the nasal mucosa, with increased nasal stuffiness and mucosal swelling after the 10 days (6ᶜ).

CHLORHEXIDINE *(SED-13, 651; SEDA-17, 293; SEDA-18, 255; SEDA-19, 235)*

Chlorhexidine is a bisbiguanide, the acetate, gluconate, and hydrochloride of which are all used as disinfectants.

Anaphylaxis to chlorhexidine is rare, although it has been reported after cystoscopy or urinary catheterization (SEDA-18, 225; SEDA-19, 235). However, a report of six cases of severe allergic reactions attributed to the chlorhexidine in lidocaine jelly used

Side Effects of Drugs, Annual 20
J.K. Aronson, ed.

before instrumentation of the urethra suggests that this serious adverse reaction is under-reported (7[c]). These patients had positive skin tests to chlorhexidine gluconate and negative tests to lidocaine and latex. An age-matched control group of five patients who had previously been exposed to chlorhexidine gluconate without problems were also tested intradermally with chlorhexidine; all had a negative response.

Both chlorhexidine and cetrimide, a quaternary ammonium disinfectant, are toxic to endothelial and epithelial cells, and contact with the eyes should be avoided. After the accidental use of solutions of these disinfectants to irrigate the eye during cataract surgery, immediate corneal edema occurred, in turn resulting in bullous keratopathy (8[c]).

IODOPHORS *(SED-13, 655; SEDA-17, 294; SEDA-18, 256)*

Povidone-iodine

Endocrine, metabolic Hypothyroidism has been reported with povidone-iodine antiseptics in neonates (SEDA-19, 235). However, in a study of more than 3000 new-borns who received a 2.5% ophthalmic solution of povidone-iodine to prevent ophthalmia neonatorum, no clinical thyroid disorders developed (9[c]).

Transient hyperthyrotropinemia occurred in neonates whose mothers had been exposed to povidone-iodine as a skin disinfectant during and after labour (10[c]). The urinary iodine concentrations in the neonates correlated with those in the maternal breast milk. It is recommended that the use of povidone-iodine be avoided during and after labor, particularly if the mother breast-feeds.

Special senses It has been suggested that povidone-iodine is potentially toxic to the corneal endothelium. The FDA recommends flushing the eye with saline after the preoperative use of a 5% solution of povidone-iodine (11[r]).

Immunological and hypersensitivity reactions Severe systemic adverse reactions have been reported with the lavage or instillation of povidone-iodine into wounds or body cavities (SED-13, 655; SEDA-14, 297; SED-17, 294; SEDA-18, 256). However, in a case report of anaphylaxis from povidone-iodine the disinfectant was used only to cleanse the vulva, vagina, and cervix (12[c]).

A 25-year-old white woman was referred for abortion from a clinic where she had had an anaphylactic reaction during a termination 2 years before, attributed to lidocaine. She also reported previous periorbital edema and hives from sulfonamides. While taking an oral contraceptive, she developed both pseudotumor cerebri and a large hepatic adenoma; a lidocaine skin sensitivity test was negative at the time of adenoma resection and a knee operation. Latex condoms had never caused allergic symptoms. The vulva, vagina, and cervix were cleansed with povidone-iodine solution, and menstrual aspiration proceeded uneventfully, with the use of a 7-mm flexible plastic cannula syringe without cervical dilatation or any anesthetic agent. Periorbital edema, generalized pruritus, and hives over her abdomen and arms developed 10—15 min later. Facial and acrocyanosis, dyspnea, sweating, and faintness followed. Respiration was slightly labored and rapid. Radial pulses were thready, but carotid pulses were strong. Her blood pressure was 88—100/50—60 mmHg. Despite oxygen and intravenous diphenhydramine, her respiratory distress continued 1.5 h after the procedure, but she responded immediately and favorably to adrenaline. A week later she felt well, but an allergist found signs of mild obstructive airway disease and gave her prednisolone. Two weeks later, prick tests were negative with latex and a 1:10 dilution of the same povidone-iodine solution, but at full strength povidone-iodine caused urticaria and generalized pruritus. Adrenaline, terfenadine, cimetidine, and a pirbuterol acetate inhalant aerosol produced complete recovery.

REFERENCES

1.   Willatts SM, Radford S, Leiterman M. Effect of the antiendotoxic agent taurolidine in the treatment of sepsis syndrome: a placebo-controlled double-blind trial. Crit Care Med 1995;23:1033—9.

2.   Fraise AP Disinfection in endoscopy. Lancet 1995;34:787—8.

3.   Rudzki E, Kecik T, Portacha L, Rebondel P, Peak M. Incidence of hypersensitivity to antibiotics and conservants in eye drops. Klin Oczna 1995;97:66—7.

4.   Ginkel CJW, Branitzes TD, Huizing EH. Allergy due to topical medications in chronicotitis externa and chronic otitis media. Clin Otolaryngol 1995;20:326—8.

5.   Graf P, Hallen H, Juto JE. Benzalkonium choride in a decongestant nasal spray aggravates rhinitis medicamentosa in healthy volunteers. Clin Exp Allergy 1995;25:395—400.

6.   Hallen H, Graf P. Benzalkonium chloride in nasal decongestive sprays has a long-lasting adverse effect on the nasal mucosa in healthy volunteers. Clin Exp Allergy 1995;25:401—5.

7.   Yong P, Parker FC, Foran S. Severe allergic reactions and intra-urethral chlorhexidine gluconate. Med J Aust 1995;162:257—8.

8.   VanRiz G, Beekhuis WH, Eygink CA, Geerards AJM, Remeijer L, Pels EL. Toxic keratopathy due to the accidental use of chlorhexidine, cetrimide and cialit. Doc Ophthalmol 1995;90:7—14.

9.   Rotta AT. Povidone-iodine to prevent ophthalmia neonatum. New Engl J Med 1995;333:126—7.

10.   Koga Y, Sano H, Kikukawa Y, Ishigouoka T, Kawamura M. Effect on neonatal thyroid function of povidone-iodine used on mothers during perinatal period. J Obstet Gynaecol 1995;21:581—5.

11.   Starr MB, Lally JM. Antimicrobial prophylaxis for ophthalmic surgery. Surv Ophthalmol 1995;39:485—501.

12.   Waran KD, Mansick RA. Anaphylaxis from povidone-iodine. Lancet 1995;345:1506.

T. Midtvedt

25 Penicillins, cephalosporins, other β-lactam antibiotics, and tetracyclines

T. Midtvedt

℞ Antibiotic resistance: new strategies

In the last 12—15 years there has been an alarming increase in bacterial resistance to antibiotics, resulting in the emergence of a serious threat to global public health (1[R])—(5[R]). In fact, the development of resistance is the most serious of all adverse effects to antibiotics. The need for new strategies is obvious, as has been underlined several times in these volumes (SEDA-12, 206; SEDA-16, 273; SEDA 19, 237). It should be clearly recognized that all use of antimicrobial agents creates the same problems, which can all too easily spread to another sections of the front. A specific veterinarian or marine resistance mechanism does not exist; all resistance mechanisms can be used by any microbe.

The latest alarm has come from Japan, where vancomycin-resistant Staphylococcus aureus is now an reality, and may very soon pose a major problem all over the world. Obviously, we may be close to the end of the antibiotic road.

What can we do? We can of course still reduce the total consumption of antibiotics, we can still create proper guidelines for the marketing and use of existing antibiotics, and we can still in several ways inform and educate prescribers and patients. The sad fact is that far more needs to be done.

One way to go may be to continue investigations of 'old' agents. As recently noted (6[R]), the discovery and successful development of currently used antibiotics led to termination of interest in other antibiotic classes discovered during the 1960s and 1970s. These underex-ploited agents include avilomycins, everninomycins, indolomycin, kirromycins, lankacidins, pleuromutilins, and sideromycins. At least some of these agents appear to have structures and modes of action that are distinct from the antibiotics in current use, suggesting that cross-resistance with agents already on the market may be minimal. However, some derivatives within these groups (avilomycins and pleuro-mutilins) have already been used in animal husbandry (7[R]), (8[R]). It goes without saying that this may have led to the selection of resistant environmental isolates that could serve as a source of resistance determinants in human pathogens, thereby compromising the therapeutic potential of new avilomycin and pleuro-mutilin analogs in human medicine. 'Ecological shadows' following the use of antibiotics are a sad reality in nature (SEDA-19, 237).

The pharmaceutical industry is still travelling along the old road, i.e. developing new derivatives within existing groups of antibiotics; this is best exemplified by the β-lactams. To counter the problem of enzymatic inactivation of various β-lactams, an enormous number of partly enzyme-stable analogs have been developed and marketed (penicillins, cephalosporins, carbapenems, monobactams, etc). So far, the microbes have always overcome these challenges by making more potent β-lactamases. Somebody should tell the pharmaceutical industry that this is probably not the best way to go.

Development of combination products containing an antibiotic and a specific inhibitor that protects the antibiotic from enzymatic inactivation is another way that industry is going. It has been used with some success in combating microbial β-lactamases, but can probably be extended to other areas as well. Bacterial

Side Effects of Drugs, Annual 20
J.K. Aronson, ed.

efflux pump inhibitors have been discovered, but their properties demonstrated to date seem to be insufficiently attractive to warrant development (9ᴿ).

However, these examples are all from the old road. As recently underlined, the present strategy depends principally on the synthesis of new analogs related to known antibiotics to create structural modifications that thwart the 'resistance phenotype' (10ᴿ).

An alternative approach is to seek structurally novel antibiotics that inhibit new molecular targets. Such agents are unlikely to be susceptible to existing mechanisms of resistance, because of their structural novelty and unique modes of action. One new area could be to search for agents that act against gene products expressed primarily or exclusively during infection. The strategy and tactics in this search, as well as some promising preliminary results, have recently been commented on (10ᴿ), (11ᴿ).

Summarizing these exciting topics, it should be underlined that targeting functions that are expressed in vivo may lead to narrow-spectrum agents, because the target can be highly specific for each pathogen. As a consequence, the introduction of such drugs will require the development of rapid and accurate methods for microbial diagnostics. In addition to minimizing the selection of resistant isolates, these new types of drugs may have the advantage of not disturbing the normal microflora in or on the patient and in the environment. If true, their ecological shadows should be negligible.

In spite of the urgent need for novel drugs, it is reasonable to assume that it will be some years before any such new agent is available for routine clinical use. In the meantime, we shall be faced with increasing microbial resistance to current antimicrobial agents.

PENICILLINS *(SED-13, 693; SEDA-17, 298; SEDA-18, 262; SEDA-19, 239)*

Co-administration of penicillins with β-lactamase inhibitors   One way of protecting the β-lactam structure in penicillins is the co-administration of a β-lactamase inhibitor, such as clavulanic acid, sulbactam, or tazobactam (a penicillanic acid sulfone structurally related to sulbactam). The most commonly used combinations are ampicillin–sulbactam, amoxycillin–clavulanic acid (co-amoxiclav), ticarcillin–clavulanic acid, and piperacillin–tazobactam. All these β-lactamase inhibitors themselves have adverse profiles (SEDA-17, 296), which have not yet been satisfactorily elucidated. In a review of piperacillin–tazobactam it has been clearly stated that "information provided in clinical investigations was usually poorly detailed, describing overall incidence rates with few details concerning the actual adverse events" (12ᴿ).

It is generally assumed that maintenance of a critical ratio between the β-lactam and the inhibitor is essential for optimum bactericidal activity. However, in a recent investigation of the combinations piperacillin–tazobactam and piperacillin–sulbactam it was shown that the most important factor was maintenance of a critical concentration of inhibitor necessary to suppress β-lactamase activity sufficiently (13ᶜ). This critical concentration will vary depending on the host organism, the amount and type of β-lactamase produced, the specific inhibitor used in the combination, and the pharmacokinetics of the inhibitor. Clearly, additional studies are required, until these combinations have been fully evaluated.

It is also wise to remember that these β-lactamase inhibitors may have adverse effects in *altering microbial sensitivity to antibiotics*. For example, clavulanic acid binds to penicillin-binding protein (PBP) 3, giving rise to abnormal physiological properties of the cell wall (14ᶜ). At least in *Pseudomonas aeruginosa*, PBP 3 is thought to be the primary target for expanded-spectrum and fourth-generation cephalosporins, and increased production of PBP 3 results in reduced sensitivity to these antibiotics (15ᶜ). Whether and to what extent possible cell-wall alterations induced by the inhibitors may alter the effect of these new cephalosporins should be investigated.

CEPHALOSPORINS *(SED-13, 711; SEDA-17, 298; SEDA-18, 263; SEDA-19, 242)*

New cephalosporins—a waste of time and money?   The pipeline for new cephalosporins is more full than ever before. Accepting an arbitrary classification into a system of generations, Periti has recently summarized the properties of 19 third-generation and 10 fourth-generation derivatives (16ᴿ). However, there might be several more derivatives around (17[R]). The so-called fourth-generation drugs feature a methoxyimylaminothiazole moiety at position 7-β of the cephem ring and contain a positively charged quaternary nitrogen at position 3. According to Periti, "they represent attempts to maintain the activity of the third generation, which is now compromised by the rapid development of mutant, plasmid-encoded TEM β-lactamases, and by their ineffectiveness against strains of *Enterobacter cloacae* and *Pseudomonas aeruginosa*, because of derepressed chromosomal β-lactamases that somewhat limit their clinical success" (16[R]).

The claim is that these new compounds may have better activity than the third generation against Gram-negative organisms, especially the Enterobacteriaceae, and good activity against *Pseudomonas aeruginosa*, while maintaining or partially increasing their Gram-positive activity, compared with the third generation. However, the warning signals are already there. Development of novel resistance is already foreseen (17[R]) and doubts have been expressed "whether or not fourth-generation cephalosporins will provide adequate therapy for patients infected with extended-spectrum β-lactamase-producing Enterobacteriaceae" (18[C]). There is certainly not a market for 10 new fourth-generation cephalosporins. Some companies will lose a lot of money.

CARBAPENEMS *(SED-13, 720)*

Carbapenems are β-lactam antibiotics with a broad antibacterial spectrum. They have been widely investigated in the past, and imipenem/cilastatin, biapenem, meropenem, and panipenem/betamipron are currently in clinical use or under trial. Imipenem has to be given with cilastatin in order to reduce its renal hydrolysis. Similarly, panipenem is given with betamipron, an organic ion transport inhibitor (19[C]).

Nervous system   Many antibiotics, especially some β-lactams, are often associated with an increased risk of *seizures* (SEDA-19, 238; SEDA-18, 261). Imipenem has a convulsant potency similar to benzylpenicillin, ceftezole, and aztreonam. In fact, the occurrence of sei-

zures in children treated with imipenem/cilastatin for meningitis has been reported as being high as 33% (20[C]). In a preliminary survey from the manufacturer, it was stated that seizures had occurred in 15 of 256 with meningitis treated with meropenem and 21 of 252 patients treated with a cephalosporin. The mechanisms of the differences in proconvulsant properties between imipenem/cilastatin and meropenem have not yet been satisfactorily worked out. The lack of a 1-β-methyl group and/or the basic side-chain at position C-2 of the carbapenem nucleus may account for the incidence of seizures seen with imipenem in animals (21[C]). In contrast, the low degree of proconvulsant activity seen with meropenem in animal models as well as in clinical trials may be related to the fact that this molecule is β-1 methylated at C-1 and does not have a free amino group in the C-2 side-chain. However, whatever the mechanisms might be, clinicians should not forget that meropenem may cause seizures in patients with meningitis.

Interactions   *Valproic acid* Serum concentrations of valproic acid have been measured in three patients who were taking panipenem/betamipron (22[c]). There was a marked reduction in serum concentrations of valproic acid in all three patients, and they returned to normal after withdrawal of panipenem/betamipron. The mechanisms of this interaction were not fully elucidated. Competition of valproic acid with panipenem/betamipron for plasma binding proteins was discussed, but considered unlikely. Based on additional investigations in one of the patients, it was suggested that panipenem/betamipron might accelerate the renal excretion of valproic acid.

Salicylates In general, adverse drug interactions occur in patients rather than microbes. However, in some recent reports, it has been stated that *Pseudomonas aeruginosa* showed increased phenotypic in vitro resistance to imipenem, panipenem, and biapenem (and to quinolones) in the presence of salicylate (23[R]), (24[R]). The antipseudomonal activity of the carbapenems was reduced in proportion to the concentration of salicylate. The clinical significance of these findings has yet to be elucidated. Interestingly, one of the carbapenems, meropenem, was still active against

Ps. aeruginosa in the presence of salicylate. Thus, in patients taking both a carbapenem and a salicylate, it might be wise to prefer meropenem if a carbapenem has to be given.

TETRACYCLINES *(SED-13, 725; SEDA-17, 298)*

Minocycline

Skin and appendages *Hyperpigmentation* with minocycline is well recognized (SEDA-17, 300) and the incidence varies from 0.35 to 4% (25[C]), (26[C]). However, the incidence may be even higher in some groups of patients, as has recently been reported (27[c]). Seven patients, aged 56—76 years, with cicatricial pemphigoid took minocycline 100 mg/day for 3—39 months, and six of them reported a marked symptomatic improvement within 2—3 months. However, troublesome hyperpigmentation developed in four of them; three developed lower leg hyperpigmentation, two conjunctival hyperpigmentation, and one perioral hyperpigmentation. The mechanisms of this hyperpigmentation are obscure. However, elderly people may be at greater risk of developing minocycline-associated hyperpigmentation and high dosages and/or prolonged treatment are also risk factors (28[C]). It has been claimed that elderly people are slower to clear minocycline degradation products within their dermal macrophages (29[C]), (30[C]).

The mechanisms responsible for suppression of blistering in patients with dystrophic epidermolysis bullosa are also unclear. One theory is that minocycline, as other tetracyclines, has anticollagenase activity (31[C]). Reduced breakdown of collagen should then give less antigen(s) for possible autoimmune reactions to take place and less deposition of immunoglobulins in the basement membranes of the skin and mucosae.

Special senses Of 40 adults with active rheumatoid arthritis who took minocycline (maximal oral dose 100 mg bd) for 26 weeks, 34 patients completed the course, and 21 had adverse effects; 18 cases were related to the gastrointestinal tract and 12 patients had *vestibular disturbances* (32[C]). There was no correlation between the serum concentration of minocycline and dizziness, but the authors stated that "dose adjustment in six patients reduced the vestibular dysfunction". Previously, a higher frequency of vestibular adverse effects in women has been ascribed to a higher serum concentration found in women (33[C]). However, in another investigation, the incidence of vestibular dysfunction in women taking minocycline 150 mg/day was the same as in women taking 200 mg/day, although the serum concentrations were significantly higher in the latter (34[C]). The mechanism of the vestibular dysfunction caused by minocycline is not known. However, the relatively high incidence of this adverse effect (12 of 34 patients) in patients taking prolonged minocycline therapy should be kept in mind.

Sexual function Many drugs can cause *gynecomastia* (35[C]), (36[C]) and minocycline can now be added to the list (37[c]).

A 15-year-old boy developed tender gynecomastia after taking minocycline for facial acne, without a preceding history. He had tender retroareolar swelling of the breast disc, but was otherwise clinically fit and his hormone values were all normal. Minocycline was withdrawn and the gynecomastia resolved within 2 weeks.

Between 1973 and 1993 the Committee on Safety of Medicines in the UK was notified about 754 cases of 1270 reactions possibly associated with minocycline; of these, six included reports of gynecomastia. The patients were aged 18—32 years, and no other causal factors were apparent. Obviously, minocycline can cause gynecomastia.

REFERENCES

1. Cannon J. Superbug. Nature's revenge. Why antibiotics can breed disease. London: Virgin Publishing Ltd, 1995:1—339.
2. Cohen ML. Epidemiology of drug resistance: implications for a post-antimicrobial era. Science 1992;257:1050—5.
3. Neu HC. The crisis in antibiotic resistance. Science 1992;257:1064—73.
4. Tenover FC, Hughes JM. The challenges of emerging infectious diseases. Development and spread of multiply-resistant bacterial pathogens. J Am Med Assoc 1996;275:300—4.
5. Tomasz A. Multiple-antibiotic-resistant pathogenic bacteria. A report on the Rockefeller University Workshop. New Engl J Med 1994; 11330:1247—51.
6. Zahner H. Fidler H-P. The need for new antibiotics: possible ways forward. In: Hunter PA, Darby GK, Russel NJ, editors. Fifty Years of Antimicrobials: Past Perspectives and Future Trends. Fifty-third Symposium of the Society for General Microbiology. Cambridge: Cambridge University Press, 1995.
7. Donnelly JP, Voss A, Witte W, Murray BE. Does the use in animals of antimicrobial agents, including glycopeptide antibiotics, influence the efficacy of antimicrobial therapy in humans? J Antimicrob Chemother 1996;37:389—92.
8. Piddock LJV. Does the use of antimicrobial agents in veterinary medicine and animal husbandry select antibiotic-resistant bacteria that infect man and compromise antimicrobial chemotherapy? J Antimicrob Chemother 1996;38:1—3.
9. Coleman K, Athalye M, Clancey A, Davison M, Payne DJ, Perry CR, Chopra I. Bacterial resistance mechanisms as therapeutic targets. J Antimicrob Chemother 1994;33:1091—116.
10. Chopra I, Hodgson J, Metcalf B, Poste G. The search for antimicrobial agents effective against bacteria resistant to multiple antibiotics. Antimicrob Agents Chemother 1997;41:497—503.
11. Chopra I, Hodgson J, Metcalf B, Poste G. New approaches to the control of infections caused by antibiotic-resistant bacteria. An industry perspective. J Am Med Assoc 1996; 275:401—3.
12. Bryson HM, Brogden RN. Piperacillin/tazobactam. A review of its antibacterial activity, pharmacokinetic properties and therapeutic potential. Drugs 1994;47:506—35.
13. Lister PD, Prevan AM, Sanders CC. Importance of β-lactamase inhibitor pharmacokinetics in the pharmacodynamics of inhibitor-drug combinations: studies with piperacillin-tazobactam and piperacillin-sulbactam. Antimicrob Agents Chemother 1997;41:721—7.
14. Severin A, Severina E, Tomasz A. Abnormal physiological properties and altered cell wall composition in *Streptococcus pneumoniae* grown in the presence of clavulanic acid. Antimicrob Agents Chemother 1997;41:504—10.
15. Liao X, Hancock REW. Susceptibility to β-lactam antibiotics of *Pseudomonas aeruginosa*. Antimicrob Agents Chemother 1997;41:1158—61.
16. Periti P. Introduction: cephalosporin generations. J Chemother 1996;8 Suppl 2:3—6.
17. Watanabe NA. Newer antipseudomonal cephalosporins. J Chemother 1996;8 Suppl 2:48—56.
18. Sanders CC. In vitro activity of fourth generation cephalosporins against Enterobacteriaceae producing extended-spectrum β-lactamases. J Chemother 1996;8 Suppl 2:57—62.
19. Shimada K. New antimicrobial agent series XLVI: panipenem/betamipron. Jpn J Antibiotics 1994;47:219—44.
20. Wong VK, Wright HT, Ross LA, Mason WH, Inderlied CB, Kim KS. Imipenem/cilastatin treatment of bacterial meningitis in children. Pediatr Infect Dis J 1991;10:122—5.
21. Hikida M, Masukawa Y, Nishiki K, Inomata N. Low neurotoxicity of LJC 10,627, a novel 1-β-methylcarbapenem antibiotic: inhibition of β-aminobutyric acid A, benzodiazepine and glycine receptor binding in relation to lack of central nervous system toxicity in rats. Antimicrob Agents Chemother 1993;37:199—202.
22. Nagai K, Shimizu T, Togo A, Takeya M, Yokomizo Y, Sakata Y, Matsuishi T, Kato H. Decrease in serum levels of valproic acid during treatment with a new carbapenem, panipenem/betamipron. J Antimicrob Chemother 1997;39:295—6.
23. Shimada J, Kawahara Y. Overview of a new carbapenem, panipenem/betamipron. Drugs Exp Clin Res 1994;20:241—5.
24. Sumita Y, Fukasawa M. Transient carbapenem resistance induced by salicylate in *Pseudomonas aeruginosa* associated with suppression of outer membrane protein D2 synthesis. Antimicrob Agents Chemother 1993;37:2743—6.
25. Bok LB. Practical experience with minocycline. In: Cullen SI, editor. Focus on Acne Vulgaris. Roy Soc Med Int Congr Symp Ser 1985; 95:83—6.
26. Velasco JE, Miller AE, Zaias N. Minocycline in the treatment of venereal disease. J Am Med Assoc 1972;220:1323—5.
27. Poskitt L, Wojnarowska F. Minimizing cicatricial pemphigoid orodynia with minocycline. Br J Dermatol 1995;132:784—9.
28. Basler RSW. Minocycline therapy for acne. Arch Dermatol 1979;115:1391.
29. Basler RSW. Minocycline-related hyperpigmentation. Arch Dermatol 1985;121:606—8.
30. Gordon G, Sparano BM, Iatropoulos MJ. Hyperpigmentation of the skin associated with minocycline therapy. Arch Dermatol 1985;121:618—23.
31. White JE. Minocycline for dystrophic epidermolysis bullosa. Lancet 1989;i:966.

32. Kloppenburg M, Mattie H, Douwes N, Dijkmans BAC, Breedveld FC. Minocycline in the treatment of rheumatoid arthritis: relationship of serum concentrations to efficacy. J Rheumatol 1995;22:611—16.

33. Fanning WL, Gump DW, Sofferman RA. Side effects of minocycline: a double-blind study. Antimicrob Agents Chemother 1977;11:713—17.

34. Gump DW, Ashikaga T, Fink TJ, Radin AM. Side effects of minocycline: different dosage regimens. Antimicrob Agents Chemother 1977;12:643—6.

35. Carlson HE. Gynecomastia. New Engl J Med 1980;303:795—9.

36. Wilson JD, Aiman J, MacDonald PC. The pathogenesis of gynecomastia. Adv Intern Med 1980;25:1—32.

37. Davies JP, Price-Thomas JM. Gynaecomastia in association with minocycline. Br J Clin Pract 1995;49:179.

S.H. Khoo and T. Walley

26   Miscellaneous antibacterial drugs

AMINOGLYCOSIDE ANTIBIOTICS *(SED-13, 744; SEDA-17, 304; SEDA-18, 268; SEDA-19, 245)*

℞ *Once daily dosage regimens* *(SEDA-18, 268; SEDA-19, 245)*

Aminoglycosides remain a cornerstone of therapy against serious Gram-negative infections, despite their narrow therapeutic index and potential for nephrotoxicity and ototoxicity. The pharmacokinetics of aminoglycosides vary considerably among patients, and may also change substantially during drug therapy. Although therapy can be optimized in the majority, conventional therapy carries the burden of drug toxicity, the cost of monitoring treatment, and the need for frequent administration. We have previously discussed the arguments for and against once-daily regimens (SEDA-19, 245), but this mode of administration can potentially reduce all these problems.

Plasma concentrations *In a study of the requirements for dosage modification in once-daily and thrice-daily regimens, patients with serious infections were randomized to receive once-daily gentamicin (4 mg/day, n = 69), the same daily dose of gentamicin in three divided doses (n = 46), or once-daily netilmicin (5.5 mg/kg, n = 59) (1ᶜ). Dosage adjustments based upon first trough and/or peak serum concentrations were required in 6, 78, and 12% of the patients, respectively. Second trough and peak concentrations were significantly higher with thrice-daily gentamicin, while serum concentrations remained constant with once-daily gentamicin or netilmicin. Once-daily regimens*

may reduce the frequency of administration but will not obviate the need for drug monitoring, since nephrotoxicity also developed with once-daily treatment.

Efficacy *Although once-daily regimens are undoubtedly easier to use, their efficacy is still being studied. Most studies to date have shown little or no differences in cure rates between once-daily and conventional regimens. In a study of adults with suspected or proven Gram-negative infections who were randomized to receive gentamicin once-daily doses (4.5 mg/kg/day; n = 48) versus thrice-daily doses (1.5 mg/kg/day; n = 52) there was a significantly higher clinical cure rate with once-daily dosing (88 vs. 69%), with a similar but not statistically significant difference in microbiological cure rate (86 vs. 74%) (2ᶜ). Nephrotoxicity was not observed, but ototoxicity developed in three patients on thrice-daily dosing. In another study once-daily netilmicin (300 mg/day, n = 50) was compared with the same daily dose in two divided doses (n = 46) (3ᶜ). There were no differences in cure rates either clinical (94 vs. 95%) or bacteriological (89 vs. 92%). There was also no difference in the incidence of nephrotoxicity or ototoxicity.*

Comparative nephrotoxicity of different aminoglycosides *Not all aminoglycosides have equivalent nephrotoxicity. For example, amikacin may be associated with less nephrotoxicity, owing to differences in binding to tubular cells (see below). Studies with conventional dosage regimens have suggested that netilmicin is less nephrotoxic than gentamicin. However, similar studies are required using gentamicin in potentially less nephrotoxic once-daily regimens. In one such prospective randomized study once-daily gentamicin (4 mg/kg/day, n = 54) has been compared with once-daily netilmicin (5.5 mg/kg/day, n = 52)*

(4^C). Clinical cure rates were comparable (93 vs. 92%), as were the rates of nephrotoxicity (6.9% for gentamicin vs. 15% for netilmicin, P = 0.15) and ototoxicity (of the 15 patients in each treatment group who had audiometry before treatment, about half had some evidence of ototoxicity after each treatment). Although no large differences emerged, this study did not have the power to detect smaller but nevertheless clinically significant differences in toxicity.

Optimum doses *In one of the largest recent studies, clinical experience with a once-daily regimen of gentamicin has been evaluated in 2184 adult patients at one institution (5^C). A pilot study suggested that an initial daily dose of 7 mg/kg was required to achieve peak gentamicin concentrations of around 20 μg/ml (10 times the MIC of their most troublesome pathogen, Pseudomonas aeruginosa). This is higher than previous once-daily regimens of 4–5 mg/kg (equivalent to the total daily dose of conventional regimens). The same fixed dose was used, but a nomogram was constructed to allow the dosage interval to be determined after a random concentration measurement at 6–14 h after infusion (instead of peak or trough concentrations). The median daily dose was 450 mg. Gentamicin was given every 24 h in 77% of the patients, every 36 h in 15%, every 48 h in 6%, and at longer intervals in 2%. Nephrotoxicity developed in 1.2% (compared with historical rates of 3–5%), and three patients developed ototoxicity. The number of requests for serum gentamicin concentration measurements was reduced by about 40%. This study has confirmed the cost-saving implications of once-daily dosing but has suggested that doses higher than commonly used may be required to achieve favourable MIC:peak serum concentration ratios.*

Use in children *Once-daily gentamicin (4.5 mg/kg/day, n = 26) has been compared with the same amount of drug administered in three divided doses (n = 24) in an open randomized study of 50 children aged 3 months to 16 years with moderately serious Gram-negative bacterial infections (6^C). As expected, serum trough gentamicin concentrations were significantly lower and peak concentrations significantly higher in the once-daily group. There were similar cure rates (89 vs. 92%) and fre-*

quency of ototoxicity (two children in each group); nephrotoxicity was not seen. Experience with once-daily regimens is limited in children, and this study, although small, has contributed useful data.

Nephrotoxicity in obstructive jaundice Experimental data have demonstrated that gentamicin nephrotoxicity is increased in biliary obstruction. The increased susceptibility to renal damage in patients with obstructive jaundice may be related to hyperbilirubinemia, or else to endotoxemia, renal ischemia induced by circulating bile salts, disturbances of coagulation, abnormalities of prostaglandin metabolism, or hemodynamic and body fluid disturbances (7^R). It has been noted in previous retrospective reviews that pre-treatment serum bilirubin was higher in patients who developed aminoglycoside nephrotoxicity. Three groups of in-patients have been examined in a prospective study: those with extrahepatic jaundice receiving gentamicin or tobramycin ($n = 84$); those with extrahepatic jaundice receiving other antibiotics ($n = 81$), and those without cholestasis receiving aminoglycosides ($n = 72$) (8^C). The incidence of nephrotoxicity was 32% in jaundiced patients given aminoglycosides versus 11% in jaundiced patients given other antibiotics, and 5.6% in non-icteric patients given aminoglycosides, a highly significant difference. Although the incidence of aminoglycoside nephrotoxicity in jaundiced patients was related both to bilirubin concentrations and initial steady-state concentrations of the aminoglycoside, multivariate analysis showed that the most significant variable for the development of nephrotoxicity was the serum bilirubin. Thus, the serum bilirubin concentration represents a distinct and independent risk factor for the development of aminoglycoside-related nephrotoxicity.

Special senses The mechanism of aminoglycoside ototoxicity has been extensively investigated. Both vestibular and auditory dysfunction occur, presumably as a result of destruction of hair cells in the vestibular and cochlear organs. In populations in which aminoglycosides have been widely used, it has been noted that individuals susceptible to drug-induced ototoxicity appear to be clustered within certain families. Subsequent genetic studies have now shown that certain mutations of mitochondrial DNA, which affect the small ribosomal RNA (rRNA) in humans (and which is inherited maternally), are associated with increased susceptibility to aminoglycoside ototoxicity (9^C). These mutations may make the mitochondrial rRNA more structurally similar to its bacterial counterpart.

Research has also focused on the use of topical aminoglycosides in treating otitis media and externa. Various commercially available topical formulations were instilled directly into the middle ear space of guineapigs (10). The average cochlear hair cell loss was 66% for Cortisporin otic solution (containing polymyxin B, neomycin, and hydrocortisone) and 6.5% for gentamicin ophthalmic solution, compared with 1% for ofloxacin, benzalkonium, and saline.

Gentamicin has been used in the treatment of intractable tinnitus in Menière's disease. In a study of 69 such patients who received intratympanic injections of gentamicin there was significant relief from tinnitus but there was hearing loss of over 10 dB in 26% of the patients (who tended to be older) (11^C). However in a further 36% patients, hearing was improved by over 10 dB.

Loading dose in neonates The benefit of loading 26 critically ill neonates of more than 48 weeks gestational age with an initial dose of gentamicin (4 mg/kg; $n = 13$) has been assessed in a prospective randomized comparison with the standard regimen ($n = 13$) of 2.5 mg/kg every 12, 24, or 48 h, based on serum creatinine concentrations (12^C). Outcomes were defined as the time taken to reach a therapeutic peak serum concentration, as well as the occurrence of concentrations within the toxic range (trough below 2 μg/ml, peak above 10 μg/ml). There was no difference between the regimens in the frequency of toxic concentrations. Since none of the patients had positive blood cultures or was septic on follow up, clinical outcomes could not be assessed. The authors concluded that therapeutic concentrations could be achieved more rapidly in neonates of less than 34 weeks gestation with the administration of a loading dose, whereas older neonates generally achieved these concentrations after the first dose with conventional regimens.

Amikacin *(SED-13, 752)*

There are limited data supporting the view that amikacin is less nephrotoxic than other aminoglycosides, possibly because of a lower binding affinity to proximal tubular cells or a reduced potential to induce phospholipidosis. In a detailed study 30 premature infants were treated within 24 h of birth with amikacin (10 mg/kg), gentamicin (2.5 mg/kg), or netilmicin (2.5 mg/kg) (10 babies in each group) at dosage intervals that were determined by body weight and peak/trough concentrations of drug (13^C). Serial determinations of plasma creatinine, fractional urinary excretion of sodium, magnesium, phosphate, and uric acid, and urinary excretion of calcium were assessed before, during, and after treatment. There were abnormalities in fractional excretion of sodium and urinary calcium excretion in those given gentamicin (who also had abnormalities of fractional excretion of magnesium) and netilmicin; these abnormalities were reversed 2 days after discontinuation of therapy. Plasma creatinine rose in eight neonates but became normal after 10 days. Aminoglycoside therapy, which may be lifesaving in critically ill premature infants, may nevertheless be associated with electrolyte disturbances that must be closely monitored during therapy.

Tobramycin *(SED-13, 751)*

Urinary system Renal tubular damage during therapy with tobramycin (5 mg/kg/day) plus cefotaxime (150 mg/kg/day) has been assessed in 33 neonates by measuring urinary excretion of adenosine deaminase binding protein (14^C). There were no differences from age-matched healthy babies in creatinine clearance or electrolyte disturbances, although urinary adenosine deaminase binding protein and subsequently urinary β_1- and β_2-microglobulins were increased in treated neonates. The authors' reliance on these proteins as measures of drug-induced tubular toxicity may need re-evaluation in the light of evidence that other markers (such as *N*-acetyl-β-

glycosaminidase) may be raised during serious infections.

In animals calcium antagonists, such as verapamil and nitrendipine, protect against aminoglycoside-induced nephrotoxicity, possibly by acting as competitive inhibitors of drug absorption in the renal proximal tubule, or blocking the influx of calcium in the proximal tubule, preventing aminoglycoside-induced mitochondrial damage. The effect of verapamil in reducing gentamicin nephrotoxicity has recently been investigated (15[C]). Gentamicin was given intravenously every 8 h to a total of 19 doses (with dosage adjusted to maintain peak serum concentrations of 5.5 mg/l and trough concentrations of 0.5 mg/l) to 15 healthy volunteers, of whom six were also given modified-release oral verapamil (180 mg 12-hourly) starting 2 days before gentamicin and continuing for 4 days after stopping it. Although there were no differences between the two groups of patients in gentamicin exposure or AUC, verapamil significantly reduced 24-h urinary excretion of alanine aminopeptidase, which was used as a marker of nephrotoxicity. Clearly, premedication with calcium antagonists is not feasible in the majority of individuals, and these drugs are not without adverse effects of their own. Further trials are required before any conclusions on clinical benefit can be reached.

Hypersensitivity and immunological reactions A hypersensitivity reaction developed in an 18-year-old patient with cystic fibrosis given intravenous tobramycin for a chest infection, who had had an anaphylactoid reaction to intravenous tobramycin 5 years before (associated with skin test positivity to tobramycin, gentamicin, and amikacin), which had been followed by a subsequent (and apparently successful) desensitization program with intravenous tobramycin (16[c]). Desensitization had subsequently been maintained with nebulized tobramycin, which had been stopped 6 months before his latest presentation. On this occasion he once again developed an anaphylactoid reaction to the drug.

Unusual routes of administration

Wound irrigation Although the efficacy of peroperative wound irrigation with aminogly-

cosides has yet to be firmly established in prospective comparative trials, they are frequently used during intra-abdominal and thoracic surgery. Depending on the amount of drug used and the nature of the operation, it is likely that significant amounts of the drug are absorbed. This potential problem has recently been highlighted in the light of a report (17[c]). Surgical debridement of an infected wound site after coronary bypass grafting in a 61-year-old man was followed by topical irrigation with kanamycin (7.2 g/day) as well as systemic treatment with tobramycin (5 mg/kg/day). Tobramycin peak and trough concentrations at steady state were higher than expected, and this was attributed to the fluorescent polarization immunoassay used, which cross-reacted with kanamycin. Apparent tobramycin concentrations were reduced after withdrawal of kanamycin. However, the role of kanamycin in causing a possibly spurious rise in tobramycin concentrations was far from proven, since vancomycin was also used and may have affected tobramycin excretion through nephrotoxicity. In addition, a more specific assay for tobramycin gave trough concentrations that were only slightly lower than those found with the less specific assay. Clinicians should be aware of the possibility of systemic absorption after wound irrigation with aminoglycosides, particularly if it is prolonged.

Ear-drops Prolonged use of aminoglycoside-containing ear-drops in patients with chronic otitis externa and media may result in contact dermatitis. In a study of 34 patients with chronic otorrhea, delayed skin hypersensitivity was elicited by patch testing (18[c]). There were positive patch tests to neomycin and framycetin each in 35% of patients, to neomycin in 29%, to gentamicin in 26%, and to colistin in 23%. There may have been some degree of cross-reactivity between these drugs. No data were presented on prior exposure to these agents or any correlation with dermatitis.

Ophthalmic formulations Collagen corneal shields pre-soaked with antibiotics are used as a means of delivering drug to the cornea and anterior chamber of the eye. The use of a gentamicin-impregnated shield in an 80-year-old man after cataract surgery was associated with loss of visual acuity and fundoscopic appearances of macular infarction (19[c]). Gentamicin has previously been found to damage the primate retina, particularly by macular infarction, and amikacin can have a similar effect; a subconjunctival injection of tobramycin has also previously resulted in macular infarction (SEDA-19, 245). This potentially devastating consequence suggests that care must be exercised when contemplating instillation of aminoglycosides directly into the eye.

Allergic contact dermatitis causing conjunctivitis and blepharitis has been reported with ophthalmic topical tobramycin (20[c]).

Inhalation   Tobramycin is extensively used in cystic fibrosis because of its good effect on *Pseudomonas* organisms. Used as an adjunct to intravenous antibiotics in acute infections, it may lower sputum colony counts. Aerosolized antibiotics over prolonged periods may improve lung function and reduce hospital admissions, but carry the potential risk of drug toxicity and resistance. In a review of clinical studies it was concluded that there was no evidence for nephrotoxicity or ototoxicity (21[R]), although long-term toxicity studies at higher dosages are awaited.

LINCOSAMIDES *(SED-13, 756; SEDA-19, 245)*

Nervous system   Clindamycin, either alone or in combination with neuromuscular blocking drugs or aminoglycosides, has previously been associated with neuromuscular blockade. A 58-year-old woman who was accidentally overdosed with 2400 mg (40 mg/kg) of clindamycin during anesthesia (with tubocurarine and succinylcholine induction) developed prolonged neuromuscular blockade, unresponsive to intravenous calcium or anticholinesterases (edrophonium and neostigmine), and requiring assisted ventilation for 11 h (22[c]). It seems likely that the large dose of clindamycin used in this case produced sustained neuromuscular blockade in the absence of non-depolarizing relaxants and after full recovery from succinylcholine.

Gastrointestinal   The propensity of clindamycin and lincomycin to cause pseudomembranous colitis and *Clostridium difficile*-associated diarrhea is undisputed. With diminishing use of this drug, the majority of cases are now associated with broad-spectrum penicillins and cephalosporins (23[r]), although the relative risk for *Clostridium difficile*-associated diarrhea remains higher with clindamycin and lincomycin than with cephalosporins (70 and 40 times, respectively) (24[r]).

Skin and appendages   Toxic epidermal necrolysis has been described in a 50-year-old insulin-dependent diabetic man who received clindamycin (300 mg 8-hourly) (25[c]). On the seventh day, he developed flu-like symptoms, fever, and an erythematous rash, associated with sloughing of 30% of the body surface after a further 4 days (when Nikolsky's sign became positive). He was given 32 mg of oral methylprednisolone and eventually made a full recovery.

Hypersensitivity and immunological reactions   Although the risk of drug hypersensitivity is increased in patients with AIDS, clindamycin hypersensitivity has been considered a relatively rare occurrence, despite its widespread use, with rash developing in around 9% of patients. However, in a retrospective survey of 50 patients with AIDS recruited in a European multicenter study of treatment for *Toxoplasma* encephalitis the incidence of rash in 26 patients given pyrimethamine plus clindamycin was 58% compared with 75% in those given pyrimethamine plus sulfadiazine, a non-significant difference (26[C]). Treatment was initially continued throughout the duration of hypersensitivity, and was tolerated in all patients taking pyrimethamine plus clindamycin, but had to be discontinued in half of those taking pyrimethamine plus sulphadiazine. Stevens-Johnson syndrome developed in two patients and fatal toxic epidermal necrolysis in one. Thus, the continuation of treatment despite a rash was more likely to succeed with pyrimethamine plus clindamycin but was potentially hazardous with pyrimethamine plus sulphadiazine.

Successful desensitization has been described in a 35-year-old woman who developed a generalized rash after 12 days of treatment with clindamycin (600 mg 6-hourly) and pyrimethamine for AIDS-associated cerebral toxoplasmosis; the rash resolved after withdrawal of clindamycin (27[c]). Subsequent oral rechallenge was performed (without pre-treatment with steroids or antihistamines), starting with three doses of 20 mg on day 1, 40 mg on day 2, 80 mg on day 3, and so on, until a dose of 600 mg four times a day was achieved on day 7. A transient rash lasting 5 h developed after the second dose of 600 mg. She remained free of adverse reactions for the duration of follow-up (13 months).

Topical formulations   Bacterial vaginosis is the commonest cause of discharge in women of childbearing age, and occurs when organisms such as *Mycoplasma hominis*, *Gardnerella vaginalis*, and other anerobic bacteria replace lactobacilli in the vaginal fluid. Conventional treatment is with oral antibiotics, such as metronidazole or clindamycin, although topical antibiotic therapy has been advocated. In one study, women with bacterial vaginosis were randomized to receive either topical clindamycin cream 2% ($n = 107$) or placebo ($n = 114$) for 3 days (28[C]). Clindamycin had a beneficial effect (improvement in symptoms, normalization of vaginal fluid and pH, cytology, and Gram stain), but relapse occurred in 25% of women at 1 month of follow-up. There were no significant differences in adverse effects (local irritation, diarrhea) between the groups. However, before this can be recommended, comparisons with oral antibiotics are required, particularly with reference to the high relapse rates seen.

MACROLIDES *(SED-13, 734; SEDA-17, 307; SEDA-18, 269; SEDA-19, 246)*

Erythromycin

Cardiovascular   In addition to the recognised risk of ventricular dysrhythmias when erythromycin and terfenadine are combined, cardiac toxicity of erythromycin on its own has also been described. Erythromycin has Class IA-like antidysrhythmic properties, causing an increase in atrial and ventricular refractory periods. The risks associated with high-dose intravenous administration have been highlighted (29[c]).

A 32-year-old woman with insulin-dependent diabetes and systemic lupus erythematosus was given erythromycin (1 g 6-hourly by intravenous infusion over 30—60 min) for lobar pneumonia. She had no previous history of cardiac disease and an echocardiogram showed an ejection fraction of 53%. She developed ventricular fibrillation and torsade de pointes 60 h after the start of treatment, associated with hypokalemia, and requiring electrical cardioversion. On days 5 and 6, she developed hypotension with QTc prolongation, a reduced cardiac output (ejection fraction 20%), and later bradycardia, followed by ventricular bigeminy and torsade de pointes again; on this occasion, her serum electrolyte concentrations were normal. Each episode of dysrhythmia, QTc prolongation, and myocardial dysfunction occurred 1—1.5 h after erythromycin infusion and resolved after withdrawal.

Serum erythromycin concentrations in this case were in excess of the therapeutic range and the timing of adverse effects corresponded with expected peak concentrations, leading the authors to conclude that cardiac toxicity was probably dose-dependent.

Hypotension without evidence of any dysrhythmia has been documented in a seriously ill patient receiving intravenous erythromycin (30[c]). A 55-year-old man with a community-acquired pneumonia complicated by respiratory failure requiring mechanical ventilation had transient episodes of hypotension with each intravenous dose of erythromycin (1 g every 6 h, given over 1 h via a central line). This effect was not abolished by premedication with diphenhydramine, but after withdrawal of erythromycin inotropic support was no longer necessary. No dysrhythmias or QT interval prolongation were documented. The patient subsequently died of multiorgan failure.

Immunological and hypersensitivity reactions   A 27-year-old woman developed urticaria 30 min after taking a single dose of erythromycin (31[c]). An identical episode had occurred 3 years before. Erythromycin-specific IgE was detected in her serum by radioimmunoassay.

Stevens-Johnson syndrome developed in a 64-year-old man who took erythromycin stearate for non-specific upper respiratory tract symptoms (32[c]). After four doses of 250 mg, he developed a fever and typical lesions in the mouth and conjunctivae and on the lips. He was treated with prednisolone and recovered rapidly.

Interactions Many clinically significant drug interactions with erythromycin occur because it inhibits CYP3A4, leading to reduced metabolism of other drugs. Newer semisynthetic 14- and 16-membered ring macrolides, such as clarithromycin, dirithromycin, and roxithromycin, have a variable effect on drug-metabolizing enzymes, but azithromycin, a member of the new azalide class of antibiotics, appears to have fewer interactions.

Antihistamines The association of ventricular dysrhythmias with co-administration of erythromycin and terfenadine is thought to be due to inhibition of CYP3A4 by erythromycin The cardiotoxicity of antihistamines is not a class effect, since cetrizine at up to six times the recommended dose has not been found to prolong the QTc interval. A double-blind crossover study of the potential interaction between erythromycin and loratidine in 24 healthy volunteers (33[c]) showed that the AUCs of loratidine and its metabolite descarboethoxyloratidine were increased by 40 and 46%, respectively, by erythromycin, but with no discernible effect on the QTc interval. Similar studies have shown that erythromycin increases concentrations of astemizole (34[R]). Pending further data, these combinations should be avoided.

Benzodiazepines Erythromycin may increase concentrations of midazolam and triazolam by inhibition of CYP3A4, and dosage reductions of 50% have been proposed if concomitant therapy is unavoidable (34[R]).

Carbamazepine Previous case reports and pharmacokinetic studies have shown that erythromycin inhibits the metabolism of carbamazepine (which is metabolized by CYP3A4) and can potentiate its toxicity. Erythromycin may also directly inhibit the conversion of carbamazepine to its epoxide. Two new case reports have again drawn attention to this problem (35[c]).

Lethargy, vomiting, and dehydration developed in a 3-year-old girl who was taking carbamazepine after four doses of oral erythromycin (50 mg/kg/day); carbamazepine concentrations, having been in the target range, were greatly increased (over 3.5 times the upper limit). After withdrawal of erythromycin the carbamazepine concentration returned to within the target range.

A 9-year-old boy who was taking carbamazepine developed lethargy, disorientation, and seizures 5 days after starting erythromycin (50 mg/kg/day); his serum carbamazepine concentration (previously acceptable) increased, but returned to within the target range after withdrawal of erythromycin.

If co-administration of erythromycin and carbamazepine cannot be avoided, a dosage reduction of carbamazepine of around 25% should be considered, with careful monitoring of drug concentrations (34[R]).

Cyclosporin Serum concentrations of cyclosporin are increased five-fold after 2—14 days of treatment with erythromycin (34[R]). This may be due to erythromycin-induced inhibition of CYP3A4. Blood cyclosporin concentrations must be monitored closely if erythromycin is used.

Digoxin Erythromycin may increase digoxin concentrations and cause toxicity (34[R]). About 10% of patients carry *Eubacterium lentum* as part of their bowel flora; this organism hydrolyses digoxin in the gut, and the antimicrobial effect of erythromycin may result in reduced metabolism and consequently increased availability of digoxin.

HMG CoA reductase inhibitors Rhabdomyolysis with or without renal impairment has been reported in patients taking both erythromycin and lovastatin (36[R]). The exact mechanism is unknown, but lovastatin is extensively metabolized by CYP3A4 and its metabolism may therefore be inhibited by erythromycin. The manufacturers have advised in the package insert that careful monitoring is required when these two drugs are given together. There are no data for any pharmacokinetic interaction with simvastatin, pravastatin, or fluvastatin, but in the case of simvastatin the major route of metabolism is by CYP3A4 and the potential for an adverse interaction exists.

Theophylline Erythromycin may increase theophylline concentrations by 20—25% and cause toxicity, although there is considerable variation among individuals (34[R]).

Warfarin Warfarin concentrations are modestly increased by erythromycin (by about

14%), with a corresponding rise in the prothrombin time (around 8%) (34[R]).

New macrolides/azalides

Since their introduction, the new macrolides and azalides have been increasingly used in children, and comparisons have been made with more conventional antibiotics in acute otitis media and bacterial pharyngitis. In adults and children these drugs have recently been used against an expanding range of organisms and infections, including: *Helicobacter pylori* (see below); *Neisseria gonorrheae* (37[R]); *Chlamydia trachomatis* (38[R]); *Chlamydia pneumoniae* and *Mycoplasma pneumoniae* (39[C]); non-gonococcal urethritis (40[C]); AIDS-associated *Mycobacterium avium* complex (MAC) infection (41[R]) and non-AIDS-associated MAC infection (42[C]); and in antimalarial prophylaxis (43[C]). In the cases of *Helicobacter pylori* and *Mycobacterium avium* (see also Chapter 30), clarithromycin is of established benefit and now forms part of standard regimens in many institutions. Long-term administration in the case of MAC raises issues relating to unknown toxicity, cost, and resistance.

Eradication of *Helicobacter pylori*   Clarithromycin is a regular part of many new regimens for the eradication of *Helicobacter pylori*, usually with a proton pump inhibitor or a histamine H$_2$ receptor antagonist, and often with a nitroimidazole antibiotic as well. Comparisons between regimens with clarithromycin or amoxycillin have produced conflicting results. In one study there were similar rates of efficacy and adverse effects (clarithromycin 500 mg bd versus amoxycillin 1 g bd, *n* = 25 each) (44[C]), but in another there was similar efficacy but an excess of minor adverse effects with clarithromycin 500 mg tds (diarrhea in 3/25 and altered taste in 5/25 compared with no cases of either with amoxycillin 500 mg tds) (45[C]). The authors of the second paper recommended that clarithromycin should not replace amoxycillin in such regimens, because of its relative expense as well as its more frequent adverse effects.

Azithromycin has also been the subject of such trials. In a comparison of two 14-day regimens (bismuth and tetracycline with azithromycin 250 mg either bd or tds) (*n* = 30), the eradication rate was superior with the higher dosage of azithromycin (83 vs. 28%). The higher eradication rate is similar to what would be anticipated with a regimen of metronidazole, bismuth, and tetracycline (46[C]). However, the rate of adverse effects was substantially higher with high-dose azithromycin (including diarrhea, stomatitis, and dysgeusia), and the authors concluded that these regimens were not acceptable.

The search for the most effective and best tolerated regimen for the eradication of *Helicobacter pylori* is of enormous commercial as well as medical interest and will undoubtedly continue for some time to come. Some well-designed large trials of different regimens are urgently needed.

Azithromycin

Azithromycin (34[R]), (47[R]), (48[R]) is the first of the azalide class of antimicrobials, and is synthesized by the addition of a methylated nitrogen group at the 9a position on the aglycone ring of erythromycin. Azithromycin does not inhibit CYP3A4 and thus has a significantly different pharmacokinetic and adverse interaction profile from erythromycin and many of the other new macrolides. It has excellent antimicrobial activity against a broad spectrum of infections (including atypical infections) and penetrates well into bronchial mucosa, gynecological tissue, the prostate, and phagocytic cells, maintaining high concentrations for several days.

Use in children   So far, use of the new macrolides has been limited in children, but experience is now growing. In a multicenter study of 484 children, aged 6 months to 12 years, with otitis media there were comparable efficacy and toxicity between a 3-day course of azithromycin (10 mg/kg, od) and a 10-day course of co-amoxiclav (40 mg/kg/day, in three divided doses) (49[C]). Clinical response rates were similar (93 vs. 94%, although azithromycin-treated children responded slightly more quickly), as was the rate of adverse events (4.5% with azithromycin vs. 8.3% with co-amoxiclav), which in the case of azithromycin comprised mainly gastrointestinal adverse effects (nausea, vomiting, diarrhea, and abnormal liver function in those over 2 years of age) or rash. All patients randomized to receive azithromycin completed therapy, but treatment was stopped in patients who took co-amoxiclav, because of adverse effects.

The safety of azithromycin has been compared to that of clarithromycin in an open prospective study of 153 children with otitis media (50[C]). The drugs were equally effective. Minor adverse effects occurred in 13% of children taking clarithromycin and 14% taking azithromycin: these effects included diarrhea and abdominal pain.

Phase II/III clinical trials in the US have yielded data on 1928 children aged 6 months to 15 years who received azithromycin for infections that included acute otitis media ($n = 1150$) and streptococcal pharyngitis ($n = 754$) (51[C]). Most patients received a 5-day course of azithromycin (5—12 mg/kg once daily). There were adverse effects in 190 patients (9.9%): diarrhea (3.1%), vomiting (2.5%), abdominal pain (1.9%), loose stools (1%), and rash (2.5%). In three comparisons with co-amoxiclav, the overall incidence of adverse effects was significantly lower with azithromycin (7.7 vs. 29%), with discontinuation rates of 0.3 vs. 3.6%. However, the incidence of adverse effects was significantly greater with azithromycin than with penicillin V in comparisons in patients with streptococcal pharyngitis (13 vs. 6.7%). In conclusion, it appears that the safety and tolerability of azithromycin was similar in children as in previous studies of adults.

Interactions   As discussed above, the cardiotoxicity of erythromycin plus terfenadine is thought to be due to increased concentrations of terfenadine caused by inhibition of CYP3A4 by erythromycin. The potential interaction of azithromycin with terfenadine has been evaluated in a randomized placebo-controlled study in 24 patients (12 in each group) who received terfenadine plus azithromycin or terfenadine plus placebo (52[C]). Azithromycin did not alter the pharmacokinetics of the active carboxylate metabolite of terfenadine or the effect of terfenadine on the QTc interval.

There are no clinically significant interactions of azithromycin with cimetidine, theophylline, carbamazepine, zidovudine, or warfarin (34[R]).

Clarithromycin

Cardiovascular   Thrombophlebitis occurred in four cases with intravenous clarithromycin when it was given inappropriately as a rapid bolus injection instead of as a short infusion; the manufacturer has apparently received other reports of similar reactions, even with infusions, but the incidence seems to be considerably lower than seen with erythromycin (53[c])

Nervous system   Patients with AIDS are particularly susceptible to adverse drug reactions, not only because of increased hypersensitivity but also because of low body weight, the need for prolonged drug therapy, and the potential for interactions with many other medications that are required. A myasthenic syndrome has been described in a 28-year-old man with AIDS being treated for cerebral toxoplasmosis with clarithromycin (2 g/day) (54[c]). His complaints of nausea, dizziness, progressive loss of strength, and difficulty in swallowing and opening his eyes started shortly after he started to take clarithromycin, and settled 6 h after withdrawal and treatment with pyridostigmine. A similar syndrome occurs with erythromycin, and is thought to relate to inhibition of the presynaptic release of acetylcholine.

Psychiatric   Two patients (aged 21 and 33 years) with late-stage AIDS had acute psychoses shortly after taking clarithromycin (2 g/day) for *Mycobacterium avium* complex bacteremia (55[c]). In both cases, the psychosis resolved on withdrawal, but recurred on rechallenge. In one case, treatment with azithromycin was well tolerated.

Mania has also been reported in a 77-year-old man who was HIV-negative 6 days into treatment with clarithromycin (1 g/day) for a soft tissue infection; his mental state resolved on withdrawal (56[c]).

A 53-year-old Canadian lawyer taking long-term fluoxetine and nitrazepam developed a frank psychosis 1—3 days after starting to take clarithromycin (500 mg/day) for a chest infection (57[c]). His symptoms resolved with discontinuation of all three drugs, and did not recur with erythromycin or when fluoxetine and nitrazepam were restarted in the absence of antibiotics. The symptoms may have been due to a direct effect of clarithromycin or else its inhibition of hepatic cytochrome P450 metabolism, leading to fluoxetine toxicity.

Visual hallucinations developed in a 56-year-old man with chronic renal failure and underlying aluminium intoxication maintained on peritoneal dialysis (58[c]). The symptoms developed 24 h after starting clarithromycin (500 mg 12-hourly) for a chest infection, and resolved completely 3 days after stopping the antibiotic. Although there is no evidence that neuropsychiatric complications of macrolides develop more readily in uremic patients, several factors may predispose towards these adverse effects, such as reduced drug clearance, altered plasma protein binding, different penetration of drug across the blood—brain barrier, or an increased propensity for drug interactions.

Liver With increasing use of clarithromycin for infections such as *Mycobacterium avium* complex, for which high dosages are given over prolonged periods, previously unreported adverse effects have come to light. To date, at least nine cases of hepatotoxicity have been described in HIV-negative patients taking clarithromycin (1—2 g/day) for chronic lung disease due to *Mycobacterium* avium or *Mycobactcrium abscessus* (59[c]), (60[c]). The pattern of liver enzyme abnormality was primarily cholestatic, and the patients were typically elderly (all but one aged over 60), or of low weight. Only three patients were symptomatic, and liver function abnormalities resolved on withdrawal. Subsequent rechallenge was successful in four patients, unsuccessful in one, and not performed in four. There was some dispute as to whether toxicity was dose-related or not, but it seems prudent to recommend that elderly patients should receive an initial daily dose of 1 g in this disease setting.

Gastrointestinal Pseudomembranous colitis has been reported in two women (aged 77 and 78 years) with duodenal ulceration who took clarithromycin (1.5 g/day) plus omeprazole for the treatment of *Helicobacter pylori* infection (61[c]). After initial improvement in symptoms, both women had *Clostridium difficile*-associated diarrhea, despite treatment with vancomycin and metronidazole. Both died in hospital, although their deaths do not seem to have been directly related to the pseudomembranous colitis. The authors advocated caution in the use of clarithromycin in elderly patients, but this was disputed by the manufacturers, who pointed out that one of the patients had received other antibiotics that are well recognised to cause pseudomembranous colitis, making the role of clarithromycin less certain. They suggested that the incidence of pseudomembranous colitis seemed to be no higher than for other broad-spectrum antibiotics (62[r]).

Studies in elderly patients with non-tuberculous mycobacterial infections have shown a high incidence of adverse effects with high dosages of clarithromycin (1000 mg 12-hourly), predominantly bitter taste, nausea, vomiting, CNS symptoms, and abnormal liver function tests (47[R]). A reduction in dosage to 500 mg 12-hourly greatly improved tolerability.

Interactions Most drug interactions with clarithromycin can be attributed to the fact that, like many other macrolides, it inhibits CYP3A4. The following list includes important interactions.

Antihistamines The co-administration of clarithromycin and terfenadine should be avoided, particularly in patients with electrolyte abnormalitics or pre-existing cardiac disease. Prospective electrocardiographic and pharmacokinetic studies have shown increased concentrations of terfenadine with evidence of cardiographic abnormalities, such as QTc interval prolongation. There are no published data on interactions with loratidine or astemizole.

Anti-retroviral drugs Several studies have shown that co-administration of clarithromycin and zidovudine reduces the AUC of zidovudine at steady state by about 12% (possibly as a result of a reduction in zidovudine absorption) (34[R]). However, if the drugs are taken at least 2 h apart, the pharmacokinetics of zidovudine are unaffected. One study of 12 HIV-positive patients did not show any statistically significant difference in concentrations of didanosine when clarithromycin was added (63[C]).

Antituberculous drugs Given that many macrolides inhibit CYP3A4 and that rifabutin and rifampicin are potent inducers of P450 cytochrome enzymes, including CYP3A4, the potential for interaction between these two classes of compounds is considerable. In one study of rifabutin or rifampicin (600 mg/day) plus clarithromycin (500 mg 12-hourly) the mean serum concentrations of clarithromycin fell from 5.4 to 0.7 µg/ml with rifampicin, and 2.0 µg/ml with rifabutin (64[C]). Mean serum concentrations of the major metabolite 14-hydroxyclarithromycin were unaffected. A previous study (the DATRI study) of clarithromycin with rifabutin (300 mg/day) showed that the AUC of clarithromycin fell by 50% and the AUC of 14-hydroxyclarithromycin increased by 40% (35[R]). These effects occurred within 2 weeks of adding rifabutin.

Preliminary data from the DATRI study have also suggested that rifabutin concentrations may be increased by clarithromycin, but the clinical significance of this is unknown. High rates of adverse events due to rifabutin were seen in 26 patients given rifabutin in multidrug regimens that included clarithromycin (500 mg 12-hourly; $n = 15$) or azithromycin (600 mg od; $n = 11$) (65[C]). Each patient had taken the macrolide for about 4 months before the addition of rifabutin (600 mg/day). A total of 77% of patients had some adverse effect, and 54% had multiple adverse effects. Over half (58%) required dosage adjustment of rifabutin as a result of an adverse event; these were mainly hematological (50%; leukopenia 31%, thrombocytopenia 15%), gastrointestinal symptoms (42%), myalgia/arthralgia (19%), hyperpigmentation (15%), hepatotoxicity (12%), and uveitis (8%).

The interactions between clarithromycin and rifampicin or rifabutin are very likely to be clinically relevant, given the magnitude of reductions in clarithromycin concentrations, and may argue for the use of higher dosages of clarithromycin in combination therapy for *Mycobacterium avium* complex infection.

Carbamazepine The metabolism of carbamazepine (which binds to CYP3A4) may be inhibited by macrolides such as erythromycin (see above). Carbamazepine toxicity, with dizziness, lethargy, and nystagmus, developed in a 17-year-old boy 2 days after he started to take clarithromycin (500 mg/day) (35[c]). His serum carbamazepine concentration (previously acceptable) rose but returned to within the target range after withdrawal of clarithromycin.

Theophylline Studies by the manufacturer have shown that theophylline concentrations increase by around 20% when it is given with clarithromycin. This suggests that a clinically important interaction may develop. Close monitoring of theophylline concentrations is advised during therapy with clarithromycin.

Dirithromycin

The good sputum penetration and anti-*Haemophilus* activity of the new macrolides makes them suitable for use in infective exacerbations of chronic bronchitis. In a single-blind multicenter comparison of clarithromycin (250 mg 12-hourly for 7 days) with dirithromycin (500 mg od for 5 days) in 212 patients with acute infective exacerbation of chronic bronchitis there were no differences in clinical (95 vs. 99%) or bacteriological (93 vs. 96%) response rates (66[C]). Adverse events (mainly gastrointestinal) occurred in 13% of those taking dirithromicin and 16% of those taking clarithromycin, necessitating withdrawal of drug in 1.9 and 4.6%, respectively.

Interactions Animal and banked human liver experiments suggest that dirithromycin does not bind to CYP3A4, and thus would not be expected to affect the metabolism of other drugs to the same extent as erythromycin; further studies are awaited to confirm this finding. Dirithromycin produced a slight fall in steady-state plasma concentrations of theophylline by increasing its clearance, but the magnitude of change was unlikely to be clinically significant.

Roxithromycin

The safety of roxithromycin in children has been reviewed, based on data from two open trials involving 477 children with respiratory or soft tissue infections (67[R]). The overall rate of drug-related adverse events was 4.2%; they were mostly gastrointestinal and mild to moderate in severity; only six children (1.3%) had adverse events sufficiently severe to warrant drug withdrawal.

Interactions   Roxithromycin does not interact with theophylline, warfarin, or carbamazepine (34[R]). There is probably no clinically significant interaction with cyclosporin (34[R]), despite a previous report that inhibition of the renal clearance of roxithromycin by cyclosporin prolonged the half-life and reduced the clearance rate of roxithromycin (SEDA-17, 308).

GLYCOPEPTIDES *(SED-13, 757; SEDA-17, 311; SEDA-19, 251)*

Vancomycin

Cardiovascular   A 13-day-old girl was given vancomycin 150 mg in error over 20 min; within 10 min she was cyanotic, had stopped breathing, and had no heart sounds (68[c]). Cardiopulmonary resuscitation was successful and she made a full recovery. Since her cardiac rhythm was not recorded during this episode, the authors' diagnosis of cardiac arrest was uncertain, and this episode could conceivably have been due to an anaphylactoid response. The authors reviewed four previous reports of similar possible cardiotoxicity, and pointed out that three of the previous cases were also in very young children.

Gastrointestinal   Antibiotic-associated diarrhea may develop with any antibacterial agent. Case reports have implicated vancomycin as a rare cause of *Clostridium difficile*-associated diarrhea. Diarrhea developed in a 60-year-old man on chronic hemodialysis after 20 doses of parenteral vancomycin (250 mg at each time of dialysis) (69[c]). Although culture for *Clostridium difficile* was not performed, latex agglutination was positive for *Clostridium difficile* toxin. Seven other cases of antibiotic-associated diarrhea with vancomycin have been described, in association with *Clostridium difficile*. This paradoxical association, although very uncommon, should be considered in patients who develop diarrhea during vancomycin therapy.

Urinary system   Nephrotoxicity remains the major adverse effect that limits the use of vancomycin (SEDA-19, 252). However, it has been argued that vancomycin is not nephrotoxic if used properly as a single agent (70[R]). The argument is that the nephrotoxicity of vancomycin was due to impurities in earlier formulations, and that current reports relate to patients taking other nephrotoxic drugs, especially aminoglycosides. If this were so, there would be no need to monitor plasma concentrations in most patients, unless the patients had renal disease, was elderly, or was taking other nephrotoxic drugs. This view has been supported by others (71[C]), although one case report has suggested that acute renal failure can be caused by vancomycin alone (72[c]).

Skin and appendages   Two further reports of linear IgA dermatosis in patients taking vancomycin have been published since last year's review (SEDA-19, 252).

A 72-year-old woman developed a bullous eruption on her palms, soles, and conjunctivae a day after receiving vancomycin (intravenously and via a cecostomy tube) for staphylococcal sepsis (73[c]). Immunofluorescence of the skin biopsy showed linear IgA deposition along the basement membrane. The lesions cleared over the next 2 weeks after withdrawal of vancomycin.

A blistering eruption developed in the skin and buccal mucosa of a 79-year-old man after 8 days of vancomycin therapy for an infected leg ulcer (74[c]). Biopsy showed linear IgA deposition along the basement membrane. The lesions cleared spontaneously within 2 days of withdrawal.

Monitoring drug therapy   Debate continues on optimizing vancomycin therapy by monitoring serum drug concentrations. Saunders has suggested that if the trough concentration is below 15 mg/l in adults, the peak concentration after infusion is unlikely to exceed 40 mg/l, a concentration that is widely accepted as being safe; measuring only trough concentrations should therefore be adequate (SEDA-19, 252; (75[C])). Saunders has also suggested that maintaining trough concentrations at 5—12 mg/l will ensure therapeutic concentrations.

Both of these assertions have been contested (71[C]), (76[C]), (77[r]). Central to the debate is our lack of knowledge about the relation between serum concentrations and toxicity or efficacy, and suggestions that currently available formulations of vancomycin are not nephrotoxic at all (70[R]). There is no good evidence that transiently high peak concentrations are associated with ototoxicity (78[r]) or that keeping concentrations below 40 mg/l minimizes toxicity. Most guidelines have set targets for peak and trough concentrations on a fairly arbitrary basis, and it can be argued that such guidelines need to take into account special groups of patients in whom pharmacokinetic variation may occur (for example, children, elderly people, patients with pre-existing renal impairment, and patients taking other nephrotoxic drugs, such as aminoglycosides), as well as the penetration of the drug to the site of infection (for example, in endocarditis), and the target organism (e.g. methicillin-resistant *Staphylococcus aureus*). Unlike aminoglycosides, the bactericidal effect of vancomycin depends on the duration of exposure as well as the concentration, and regimens should maximize the total time during which concentrations are above the MIC of the organism. There is therefore an argument for using continuous infusions of vancomycin, aiming to maintain serum concentrations at around 20—30 mg/l (77[r]), (78[r]).

The relations between vancomycin concentrations and both nephrotoxicity and clinical response to therapy have been assessed in adults ($n = 45$ and 31, respectively) admitted with community-acquired Gram-positive bacteremia (79[C]). Retrospective analysis confirmed the nephrotoxic potential of vancomycin, particularly with trough concentrations over 20 mg/l. The authors concluded that the recommendation of some that trough concentrations be below 10 mg/l is too restrictive, particularly for serious Gram-positive infections such as endocarditis, and suggested that concentrations of 10—20 mg/l are well tolerated and associated with a better response. However, patients receiving aminoglycosides as well are likely to be more susceptible to toxicity and may not tolerate these concentrations.

For the present, the wisest course to follow is probably that recommended by Saunders (80[r]), who accepts the lack of any evidence relating peak concentrations to toxicity or outcome, but who argues that on the basis of previous experience, we should continue to monitor plasma vancomycin concentrations in patients on long-term therapy, but that we need only measure the trough and not the peak.

Monitoring in children Paired serum vancomycin concentrations have been assessed in 68 preterm neonates (81[C]). Four babies with trough concentrations below 15 mg/l had peak concentrations above 40 mg/l; all four had gestational ages of below 30 weeks. In 38 infants who had trough concentrations between 5 and 12 mg/l (the proposed target trough concentrations), two had peaks over 40 mg/l; both had compromised renal function (one was in hypovolemic shock). Thus, peak concentration measurements are probably still required in neonates of under 30 weeks gestation or with renal impairment.

Teicoplanin

Teicoplanin has a higher volume of distribution into tissues than vancomycin, and is considered less toxic when used to treat serious Gram-positive infections, thus obviating the need for routine drug monitoring (82[R]). In a prospective study 56 patients with suspected or proven severe Gram-positive infections were randomized to receive vancomycin (1 g 12-hourly intravenously) or teicoplanin (200—400 mg/day intravenously or intramuscularly) (83[C]). Clinical and bacteriological cure rates were similar, but vancomycin was associated with significantly greater toxicity (16 vancomycin, seven teicoplanin), predominantly histamine-associated reactions (15, including two cases of red man syndrome, SEDA-17, 312), and nephrotoxicity (five with vancomycin compared with one with teicoplanin). In relation to the debate about the nephrotoxicity of vancomycin, four of the five vancomycin patients who developed nephrotoxicity were receiving netilmicin at the time, some with amphotericin as well.

Other major advantages of teicoplanin are the requirement for once-daily dosing and the possibility of intramuscular administration. This make teicoplanin suitable for out-patient treatment of infective episodes (for example, infected indwelling catheters (84[C]) and chronic osteomyelitis (85[C])) in combination with other antibiotics.

The efficacy of teicoplanin, either alone or in combination with other antibiotics (usually aminoglycosides or rifampicin), has been assessed in the treatment of bacterial endocarditis in 115 patients in a multicenter study (86[C]). The patients were not randomized into treatment groups, which may have influenced the results. In native valve endocarditis, there were high cure rates in both groups, although combination therapy resulted in an higher overall cure rate (93 vs. 85%), particularly for *Staphylococcus aureus* (84 vs. 50%). There were similar cure rates for prosthetic valve endocarditis (75 vs. 79%), although *Staphylococcus aureus* infections again appeared to respond better to combination therapy. Adverse events were reported in 24% of patients, most often skin reactions, fevers/chills, and abnormalities of liver function. Adverse events leading to withdrawal of therapy occurred in 8.7% patients, predominantly rash, abnormal liver transaminases, cholestatic hepatitis, and hematuria. Seven patients (10%) had rises in serum creatinine concentration; all but one of these were also receiving aminoglycosides.

REFERENCES

1. Prins JM, Koopmans RP, Buller HR, Kuijper EJ, Speelman P. Easier monitoring of aminoglycoside therapy with once daily dosing. Eur J Clin Microbiol Infect Dis 1995;14:531—55.
2. Raz R, Adawi M, Romano S. Intravenous administration of gentamicin once daily versus thrice daily in adults. Eur J Clin Microbiol Infect Dis 1995;14:88—91.
3. Karachalios GN, Georgiopoulos AN, Kintziou H, Mitsoga C. Efficacy and safety of once-daily versus twice daily netilmicin in patients with acute urinary tract infections. Curr Ther Res Clin Exp 1995;56:1169—74.
4. Tange RA, Dreschler WA, Prins JM, Buller HR, Kuijper EJ, Speelman P. Ototoxicity and nephrotoxicity of gentamicin vs netilmicin in patients with serious infections. A randomised clinical trial. Clin Otolaryngol Allied Sci 1995;20:118—23.
5. Nicolau DP, Freeman CD, Belliveau PP, Nightingale CH, Ross JW, Quintiliani R. Experience with a once daily aminoglycoside program administered to 2184 adults. Antimicrob Agents Chemother 1995;39:650—5.
6. Elhanan K, Sipovich L, Raz R. Gentamicin once-daily versus thrice-daily in children. J Antimicrob Chemother 1995;35:327—32.
7. Fogarty BJ, Parks RW, Rowlands BJ, Diamond T. Renal function in obstructive jaundice. Br J Surg 1995; 82: 877—84.
8. Lucena MI, Andrade RJ, Cabello MR, Hidalgo R, Gonzalez-Correa JA, Sanchez de la Cuesta F. Aminoglycoside-associated nephrotoxicity in extrahepatic obstructive jaundice. J Hepatol 1995;22:189—96.
9. Bacino C, Prezant TR, Bu X, Fournier P, Fischel-Ghodsian N. Susceptibility mutations in the mitochondrial small ribosomal RNA. Pharmacogenetics 1995;5:165—72.
10. Barlow DW, Duckert LG, Kreig S, Gates GA. Ototoxicity of topical otomicrobial agents. Acta Otolaryngol 1994;115:231—5.
11. Kaasinen S, Pyykko I, Ishikazi H, Aalto H. Effect of intratympanically administered gentamicin on hearing and tinnitus in Menière's disease. Acta Otol Laryngol 1995;520 Suppl:184—5.
12. Semchuk WM, Sevchuk YM, Sankaran K, Wallace SM. Prospective, randomized, controlled evaluation of a gentamicin loading dose in neonates. Biol Neonate 1995;67:13—20.
13. Giapros VI, Andronikou S, Cholevas VI, Papadopolou ZL. Renal function in premature infants during aminoglycoside therapy. Pediatr Nephrol 1995;9:163—6.
14. Gordjani N, Burghard R, Muller D, Mathai H, Mergehenn G, Leititis JU, Brandis M. Urinary excretion of adenosine deaminase binding protein in neonates treated with tobramycin. Pediatr Nephrol 1995;9:419—22.
15. Kazeriad DJ, Wojcik GJ, Nix DE, Goldfarb AL, Schentag JJ. The effect of verapamil on the nephrotoxic potential of gentamicin as measured by urinary enzyme excretion in healthy volunteers. J Clin Pharmacol 1995;35.196—201.
16. Schretlen-Doherty JS, Troutman WG. Tobramycin-induced hypersensitivity reaction. Ann Pharmacother 1995;29:704—6.
17. Hernandez JE, Kerns FT, Teague AC. Aminoglycoside toxicity after sternal wound irrigations. Ann Thorac Surg 1995; 61:772.
18. van Ginkel CJ, Bruintjes TD, Huizing EH. Allergy due to topical medications in chronic otitis externa and chronic otitis media. Clin Otolaryngol 1995;20:326—8.
19. Kanter ED, Brucker AJ. Aminoglycoside macular infarction in association with gentamicin-soaked collagen corneal shield. Arch Ophthalmol 1995;113:1359—60.
20. Caraffini S, Assalve D, Stingeni L, Lisi P. Allergic contact conjunctivitis and blepharitis from tobramycin. Contact Dermatitis 1995;32:186—7.
21. Touw DJ, Brimicombe RW, Hodson ME, Heijerman HGM, Bakker W. Inhalation of antibiotics in cystic fibrosis. Eur Respir J 1995; 8:1594—604.
22. Al Ahdal O, Bevan DR. Clindamycin induced

neuromuscular blockade. Can J Anaesth 1995; 42: 614−7.

23. Soto J. Clindamycin and pseudomembranous colitis. Lancet 1995;346:249.

24. Riley TV, Golledge CL. Clindamycin and pseudomembranous colitis. Lancet 1995;346:639.

25. Paquet P, Schaaf-Lafontaine N, Pierard GE. Toxic epidermal necrolysis following clindamycin treatment. Br J Dermatol 1995; 132:665−6.

26. Caumes E, Bocquet H, Guermonprez G, Rogeaux O, Bricaire F, Katlama C, Gentilini M. Adverse cutaneous reactions to pyrimethamine/sulfadiazine and pryimethamine/clindamycin in AIDS patients with toxoplasmic encephalitis. Clin Infect Dis 1995;21:656−8.

27. Marcos C, Sopena B, Lune I, Gonzalez R, de la Fuente J, Martinez-Vazquez C. Clindamycin desensitization in an AIDS patient. AIDS 1995;9:1201−2.

28. Ahmed-Jushuf IH, Shahmanesh M, Arya OP. The treatment of bacterial vaginosis with a 3 day course of 2% clindamycin cream: results of a multicentre, double blind, placebo-controlled trial. Genitourin Med 1995;71:254−6.

29. Orban Z, MacDonald LL, Peters MA, Guslits B. Erythromycin-induced cardiac toxicity. Am J Cardiol 1995;75:859−61.

30. Brown GR. Erythromycin-induced hypotension. Ann Pharmacother 1995;29:934−5.

31. Pascual C, Crespo JF, Quiralte J, Lopez C, Wheeler G, Martin Esteban M. In-vitro detection of specific IgE antibodies to erythromycin. J Allergy Clin Immunol 1995;95:668−71.

32. Pandha HS, Dunn PJ. Stevens-Johnson syndrome associated with erythromycin therapy. NZ Med J 1995;108:13.

33. Brannan MD, Reidenberg P, Radwanski E, Shneyer L, Lin CC, Cayen MN, Affrime MB. Loratidine administered concomitantly with erythromycin: pharmacokinetic and electrocardiographic evaluations. Clin Pharmacol Ther 1995; 58:269−78.

34. Amsden GW. Macrolides versus azalides: a drug interaction update. Ann Pharmacother 1995;29:906−17.

35. Stafstrom CE, Nohria V, Loganbill H, Nahouraii R, Boustany RM, DeLong GR. Erythromycin-induced carbamazepine toxicity: a continuing problem. Arch Pediatr Adolesc Med 1995; 149:99−101.

36. Garnett WR. Interactions with hydroxymethylglutaryl-coenzyme A reductase inhibitors. Am J Health Syst Pharm 1995;52:1639−45.

37. Moran JS, Levine WC. Drugs of choice for the treatment of uncomplicated gonococcal infections. Clin Infect Dis 1995;20 Suppl 1:S47−65.

38. Weber JT, Johnson RE. New treatments for *Chlamydia trachomatis* genital infection. J Infect Dis 1995;20 Suppl 1:S66−71.

39. Block S, Hedrick J, Hammerschlag MR, Cassell GH, Craft JC. *Mycoplasma pneumoniae* and *Chlamydia pneumoniae* in pediatric community acquired pneumonia: comparative efficacy and safety of clarithromycin vs erythromycin ethylsuccinate. Pediatr Infect Dis J 1995;14:471−7.

40. Stamm WE, Hicks CB, Martin DH, Leone P, Hook EW 3rd, Cooper RH, Cohen MS, Batteiger BE, Workowski K, McCormack WM, et al. Azithromycin for empirical treatment of the nongonococcal urethritis syndrome in men: a randomized double-blind study. J Am Med Assoc 1995;274:545−9.

41. Chin DP, Hopewell PC. How to treat bacteraemic *Mycobacterium avium* complex disease. Lancet 1995;346:920−1.

42. Dautzenberg B, Piperno D, Doit P, Truffot-Pernot C, Chauvin JP. Clarithromycin in the treatment of *Mycobacterium avium* lung infections in patients without AIDS. Chest 1995; 107:1035−40.

43. Anderson SL, Berman J, Kuschner R, Wesche D, Magill A, Wellde B, Schneider I, Dunne M, Schuster BG. Prophylaxis of *Plasmodium falciparum* malaria with azithromycin administered to volunteers. Ann Intern Med 1995;123:771−3.

44. Labenz J, Stolte M, Domain C, Bertrams J, Borsch J. High dose omeprazole plus amoxicillin or clarithromycin cures *Helicobacter pylori* infection in duodenal ulcer disease. Digestion 1995; 56: 14−20.

45. Katelaris PH, Patchett SE, Zhang ZW, Domizio P, Farthing MJG. A randomized prospective comparison of clarithromycin versus amoxycillin in combination with omeprazole for eradication of *Helicobacter pylori*. Aliment Pharmacol Ther 1995;9:205−8.

46. Al-Assi M, Genta R, Karttunen T, Cole R, Graham D. Azithromycin triple therapy for *Helicobacter pylori* infection: azithromycin, bismuth and tetracycline. Am J Gastroenterol 1995; 90: 403−5.

47. Schlossberg D. Azithromycin and clarithromycin. Med Clin N Am 1995;79:803−15.

48. Hoepelman IM, Schneider MME. Azithromycin: the first of the tissue selective azalides. Int J Antimicrob Agents 1995;5:145−67.

49. Principi N. Multicentre comparative study of the efficacy and safety of azithromycin compared with amoxicillin/clavulanic acid in the treatment of paediatric patients with otitis media. Eur J Clin Microbiol Infect Dis 1995;14:669−76.

50. Ramet J, on behalf of the Belgium Paediatrician Clarithromycin Work Group. Comparative safety and efficacy of clarithromycin and azithromycin suspensions in the short course treatment of children with acute otitis media. Clin Drug Invest 1995;9:61−6.

51. Hopkins SJ, Williams D. Clinical tolerability and safety of azithromycin in children. Pediatr Infect Dis J 1995;14 Suppl:S67−71.

52. Harris S, Hilligross DM, Colangelo PM, Eller M, Okerholm R. Azithromycin and terfenadine: lack of drug interaction. Clin Pharmacol Ther 1995;58:310−14.

53. Cousins D, Upton D. Beware bolus clarithromycin. Pharm Pract 1996;4:443−5.

54. Pijpers E, van Rijswijk EN, Takx-Kohlen B, Schrey G. A clarithromycin-induced myasthenic syndrome. Clin Infect Dis 1996;22:175−6.

55. Nightingale SD, Koster FT, Mertz GJ, Loss SD. Clarithromycin-induced mania in two patients with AIDS. Clin Infect Dis 1995;20:1563—4.

56. Cone LA, Sneider RA, Nazemi R, Dieterich EJ. Mania due to clarithromycin therapy in a patient who was not infected with human immunodeficiency virus. Clin Infect Dis 1996;22:595—6.

57. Pollak PT, Sketris IS, MacKenzie SL, Hewlett TJ. Delirium probably induced by clarithromycin in a patient receiving fluoxetine. Ann Pharmacother 1995;29:486—8.

58. Steinman MA, Steinman TI. Clarithromycin-associated visual hallucinations in a patient with chronic renal failure on continuous ambulatory peritoneal dialysis. Am J Kidney Dis 1996; 27:143—6.

59. Brown BA, Wallace RJ, Griffith DE, Girard W. Clarithromycin-induced hepatotoxicity. Clin Infect Dis 1995;20:1073—4.

60. Yew WW, Chau CH, Lee J, Leung CW. Clarithromycin-induced hepatotoxicity. Clin Infect Dis 1995;20:1074.

61. Teare JP, Booth JC, Brown JL, Martin J, Thomas HC. Pseudomembranous colitis following clarithromycin therapy. Eur J Gastroenterol Hepatol 1995;7:275—7.

62. Englishby VL. Case reports of death associated with pseudomembranous colitis and clarithromycin. Eur J Gastroenterol Hepatol 1995; 7:811.

63. Gillum JG, Bruzzese VL, Israel DS, Kaplowitz LG, Polk RE. Effect of clarithromycin on the pharmacokinetics of 2,3-dexoyinosine in patients who are seropositive for human immunodeficiency virus. Clin Infect Dis 1996;22:716—17.

64. Wallace RJ, Brown BA, Griffith DE, Girard W, Tanaka K. Reduced serum levels of clarithromycin in patients treated with multidrug regimens including rifampin or rifabutin for *Mycobacterium avium-M. intracellulare* infection. J Infect Dis 1995;171:747—50.

65. Griffith DE, Brown BA, Girard WM, Wallace RJ Jr. Adverse events associated with high-dose rifabutin in macrolide-containing regimens for the treatment of *Mycobacterium avium* complex lung disease. Clin Infect Dis 1995;21:594—8.

66. Hosie J, Quinn P, Sides G. A comparison of 5 days of dirithromycin and 7 days of clarithromycin in acute bacterial exacerbation of chronic bronchitis. J Antimicrob Chemother 1995;36: 173—83.

67. Begue P, Astruc J. The overall safety of oral roxithromycin in pediatric clinical studies. Infection 1995;23 Suppl 1:S25—7.

68. Boussemart T, Cardona J, Berthier M, Chevrel J, Oriot D. Cardiac arrest associated with vancomycin in a neonate. Arch Dis Child Fetal Neonatal Ed 1995;73:123.

69. Schenfield LA, Pote HH Jr. Diarrhea associated with parenteral vancomycin therapy. Clin Infect Dis 1995;20:1578—9.

70. Cunha BA. Vancomycin. Med Clin North Am 1995;79:817—31.

71. MacGowan A, Lovering A, White L, Reeves D. Why monitor peak vancomycin concentrations? Lancet 1995;345:645.

72. Frimat L, Hestin D, Hanesse B, Cao-Huu T, Kessler M. Acute renal failure due to vancomycin alone. Nephrol Dial Transplant 1995;10:550—1.

73. Richards SS, Hall S, Yokel B, Whitmore SE. A bullous eruption in an elderly woman. Vancomycin-associated linear IgA dermatosis (LAD). Arch Dermatol 1995;131:1447—51.

74. Geissman C, Beylot-Barry M, Doutre MS, Beylot C. Drug-induced linear IgA bullous dermatosis. J Am Acad Dermatol 1995;32:296.

75. Saunders N. Why monitor peak vancomycin concentrations? Lancet 1994;344:1748—50.

76. Collyns TA, Oppenheim BA. Why monitor peak vancomycin concentrations? Lancet 1995; 345:645.

77. Wysocki M, Thomas F, Wolff M. Why monitor peak vancomycin concentrations? Lancet 1995;345:646.

78. Duffull SB, Begg EJ. Why monitor peak vancomycin concentrations? Lancet 1995;345:646.

79. Zimmermann AE, Katona BG, Plaisance KI. Association of vancomycin serum concentrations with outcomes in patients with Gram-positive bacteremia. Pharmacotherapy 1995;15:85—91.

80. Saunders N. Why monitor peak vancomycin concentrations? Lancet 1994;345:647.

81. de Hoog M, Mouton JW, van den Anker JN. Why monitor peak vancomycin concentrations? Lancet 1995;345:646.

82. Shea KW, Cunha BA. Teicoplanin. Med Clin North Am 1995;79:833—44.

83. Neville LO, Brumfitt W, Hamilton-Miller JMT, Harding I. Teicoplanin vs vancomycin for the treatment of serious infections: a randomised trial. Int J Antimicrob Agents 1995;5:187—93.

84. Ketley NJ, Kelsey SM, Newland AC. Teicoplanin and oral ciprofloxacin as outpatient treatment of infective episodes in patients with indwelling central venous catheters and haematological malignancy. Clin Lab Haematol 1995;17:71—4.

85. Graninger W, Wenisch C, Weisinger E, Menschik M, Karimi J, Presterl E. Experience with outpatient intravenous teicoplanin therapy for chronic osteomyelitis. Eur J Microbiol Infect Dis 1995;14:643—7.

86. Lewis PJ, Martino P, Mosconi G, Harding I. Teicoplanin in endocarditis: a multicentre, open European study. Chemotherapy 1995;41:399—411.

27

Antifungal drugs

AMPHOTERICIN *(SED-13, 774; SEDA-17, 319; SEDA-18, 278; SEDA-19, 257)*

Formulations of amphotericin

Evidence continues to appear that amphotericin formulated in lipid emulsion may cause less *renal damage* than standard formulations (1[R]), (2[R]), (3[CR]).

Of 20 patients with neutropenia with hematological malignancies and proven or suspected fungal infections, 10 were given amphotericin (0.1 mg/ml) in 5% dextrose and 10 amphotericin (1 mg/ml) in a 20% lipid emulsion, in each case over a period of 1 h (4[C]). Clinical tolerance (in terms of fever, shaking chills, nausea, blood pressure, pulse rate) was comparable. However, the difference between the initial and the final serum urea concentration was greater in those given amphotericin in dextrose (29 mmol/l) than in those given the lipid emulsion (20 mmol/l); the same was true for serum creatinine (124 vs. 85 μmol/l). There were no differences in antifungal efficacy.

In 60 patients undergoing bone-marrow or stem cell transplantation, of whom 34 had had a previous course of conventional amphotericin, liposomal amphotericin was used to treat documented or suspected fungal infections (5[C]). Adverse effects with conventional amphotericin had included: increasing serum creatinine concentrations (*n* = 26) and clinical adverse effects (*n* = 4). Liposomal amphotericin was well tolerated in 57 patients. There were adverse effects in three cases, requiring withdrawal in one. In eight patients creatinine concentrations fell, having increased during therapy with conventional amphotericin.

In six patients with invasive fungal infections who received large cumulative doses (22—74 g) of amphotericin lipid complex over

21—121 (mean 54) weeks, mean (range) serum creatinine concentrations at the start of therapy were 88 (35—168) μmol/l, and at the end of therapy 133 (88—177) μmol/l (6[C]). During therapy, only two patients had serum creatinine concentrations of 177 μmol/l or more, with transient peak serum concentrations of 248 and 309 μmol/l. Several patients required replacement therapy with oral or intravenous potassium. None had amphotericin-associated adverse effects necessitating withdrawal.

A colloidal dispersion of amphotericin in cholesteryl sulfate in a 1:1 ratio, has been given to 168 patients with documented or presumed systemic mycoses in an open-label study in dosages as high as 6 mg/kg/day (mean cumulative dose 4 g) (7[C]). All the patients had responded incompletely to treatment with conventional amphotericin for at least 7 days, had amphotericin-induced nephrotoxicity, had pre-existing renal impairment, or had experienced other amphotericin-related treatment-limiting adverse effects. There was a complete clinical response or improvement in 48 (49%) of the 97 patients who could be evaluated, after a mean treatment duration of 18.5 days. Adverse effects were evaluated in all 168 patients; even at the highest dosage, amphotericin in colloidal dispersion caused little renal toxicity: the mean change in serum creatinine concentration from baseline was −2 μmol/l. Hypokalemia developed in eight patients (5%).

When 20 patients with proven or suspected fungal infections were treated with amphotericin lipid complex 5 mg/kg/day for 1—25 days, six patients died because of fungal infection (three) or underlying disease (three); one was not evaluable; 13 were cured or improved (8[C]). Except for hypokalemia in five patients there were no systemic adverse effects.

Amphotericin by inhalation

In 18 patients given amphotericin by inhalation on 132 occasions, four stopped treat-

Side Effects of Drugs, Annual 20
J.K. Aronson, ed.

ment because of *nausea* and *vomiting*, believed to be due to the inhaled amphotericin (9[C]). There were nine cases of clinically significant *bronchospasm*, defined by a fall in peak flow rate of 20% or more, nine cases of worsening cough, and three of worsening *dyspnea*; in none of these cases was treatment withdrawn.

Of 115 patients with prolonged neutropenia after chemotherapy for acute myeloid leukemia, acute lymphoblastic leukemia/high-grade non-Hodgkin's lymphoma, or solid tumors undergoing autologous stem cell transplantation, 65 were randomized to receive prophylactic aerosol inhalations of amphotericin (10 mg bd) and 50 to no prophylaxis (10[C]). There were no serious adverse effects from amphotericin, but *coughing* (54%), *bad taste* (51%), and *nausea* (37%) caused early withdrawal in 15 courses (23%).

Amphotericin by bladder irrigation

In a randomized comparison of amphotericin by bladder irrigation (50 mg/l over 24 h or 50 mg/l for 7 days) and oral fluconazole (200 mg/day for 7 days) in 53 patients with urinary candidiasis, eradication rates at 24 h and 5—9 days after therapy were 82 and 75% respectively with the 1-day amphotericin regimen; 94 and 79% respectively with the 7-day amphotericin regimen; and 83 and 77% respectively with fluconazole (11[C]). The only adverse effect of amphotericin was a *feeling of bladder fullness* in one patient.

Cardiovascular   In six of 90 children given intravenous amphotericin the *heart rate fell* acutely during the infusion on days 3—7 after the start of therapy (12[C]). The mean heart rate fell from 104 (range 96—114) to 62 (48—72). The authors suggested that care should be taken when giving amphotericin to children with underlying heart conditions or in patients who are already receiving drugs that slow the heart rate.

Hematological   Among 40 liver transplant recipients who received liposomal amphotericin there were two cases of transient *thrombocytopenia* attributed to the amphotericin, which was otherwise well tolerated (13[C]).

Risk factors   Dosage and the rate and duration of infusion may influence the risk of adverse reactions to amphotericin.

Dosage In 427 consecutive patients with candidemia the mortality rate (34%) was reduced by both low-dose amphotericin (500 mg or less; 13%) and high-dose amphotericin B (over 500 mg; 15%), but there were fewer adverse effects with the low dose (40 vs. 55%) (14[C]).

Rate of infusion It has been suggested that rapid infusion of amphotericin in dextrose should be avoided, at least during the start of therapy, when infusion-related reactions tend to be most problematic, and in patients with cardiovascular disease, renal dysfunction, and potassium disorders, because of the potential risk of cardiac dysrhythmias (15[R]). There is, however, some evidence that tolerance to infusion-related reactions develops during therapy.

Duration of infusion The effect of duration of infusion has been studied in 25 consecutive patients with bone-marrow transplants for leukemia who received 162 prophylactic infusions and 169 treatment infusions of amphotericin via a central line (16[C]). Before each infusion all received parenteral diphenhydramine 25 mg and hydrocortisone 25 mg. There were no differences between 2-h infusions ($n = 166$) and 4-h infusions ($n = 165$) in the incidence and severity of infusion-related adverse effects, including overall events (29 vs. 25%), chill scores (8 vs. 7%), nausea and vomiting (7 vs. 12%), fever (3 vs. 2%), systolic hypotension (6 vs. 2%), and diastolic hypotension (5 vs. 3%). Adverse events were significantly less common during prophylaxis than during treatment (22 vs. 32%).

In another study, in 50 patients with kala-azar, a 2-h infusion of amphotericin caused fewer infusion-related toxic effects (*shivering* and *fever*) than a 6-h infusion (17[C]). Rises in serum creatinine, falls in serum potassium, and impairment of appetite were the same in the two groups. There were no differences in clinical, parasitological, and eventual cure rates.

Mechanisms of amphotericin toxicity

The expression of cytokines may play an important role in mediating amphotericin-related acute toxicity in vivo. Six adult patients with acute leukemia, neutropenia, and suspected or documented systemic fungal infections were given conventional amphotericin, liposomal amphotericin, and amphotericin mixed in lipid emulsion on three consecutive days (18[C]). The formulations were given over 1–2 h. Plasma concentrations of tumor necrosis factor-α (TNF-α), interleukin-6 (IL-6) and interleukin-1 receptor antagonist (IL-1-RA) were measured during and after the infusions. There was clinical evidence of toxicity in four of the patients after conventional amphotericin and amphotericin in lipid emulsion, while only one patient reacted to liposomal amphotericin. Clinical toxicity was associated with increases in TNF-α plasma concentrations during two of four infusions of conventional amphotericin and three of four infusions of amphotericin in lipid emulsion. There were major increases in IL-6 during three of four infusions of conventional amphotericin and during all of the four infusions of amphotericin in lipid emulsion that were associated with clinical toxicity. Three of four infusions of conventional amphotericin and all four infusions of amphotericin in lipid emulsion accompanied by clinical toxicity were associated with major increases in plasma concentrations of IL-1-RA. Liposomal amphotericin was better tolerated than conventional amphotericin and amphotericin in lipid emulsion. Liposomal amphotericin also had the smallest effect on the cytokines. The severity of clinical symptoms did not correlate closely with absolute cytokine plasma concentrations.

Prevention of adverse effects

In 197 adults who received amphotericin during the first week of therapy, 282 (71%) developed at least one infusion-related adverse event during the first 7 days of therapy, most commonly *fever* (51%), *chills* (28%), *nausea* (18%), *headache* (9%), and *thrombophlebitis* (5%) (19[C]). The most common drugs that were used to prevent such effects included diphenhydramine, corticosteroids, paracetamol (acetaminophen), and heparin (given alone or in combination with these or other drugs). These pretreatment regimens were similar in efficacy to no pretreatment

in the prevention of the adverse effects. The authors concluded that empirical premedication for the infusion-related adverse effects of amphotericin could not be routinely advocated; instead, they recommended that patients should be treated when symptoms first occur and then premedicated for subsequent infusions.

AZOLE DERIVATIVES *(SED-13, 782; SEDA-17, 320; SEDA-18, 280; SEDA-19, 259)*

Contact sensitivity to imidazoles has been reviewed in the context of 15 patients (20[CR]). The imidazole derivatives most frequently reported to be allergenic are miconazole, econazole, tioconazole, and isoconazole. There is cross-reactivity between miconazole, econazole, and isoconazole; between sulconazole, miconazole, and econazole; and between isoconazole and tioconazole. The authors recommended that patients who are sensitive to phenylethylimidazoles (except ketoconazole) should be advised to use ketoconazole, clotrimazole, bifonazole, or perhaps flutrimazole, or a non-imidazole antifungal drug.

Bifonazole *(SEDA-15, 280)*

In a double-blind, randomized comparison of bifonazole 1% solution with flutrimazole 1% solution, applied once daily for 4 weeks, in 40 patients with dermatophytosis or cutaneous candidiasis, only 40% of those treated with bifonazole were judged to have received effective treatment (21[C]). In one case there was a *mild local reaction* and one patient had to abandon treatment because of *severe intolerance*.

In a similar comparison in 449 patients with fungal infections of the skin the rates of clinical and mycological cure after 4 weeks were 65% with bifonazole and 73% with flutrimazole (22[C]). The overall incidence of adverse effects (mainly mild local effects such as *irritation* or a *burning sensation*) was 5%.

Clotrimazole *(SED-13, 796; SEDA-18, 281; SEDA-19, 259)*

The use of corticosteroids in combination with antifungal agents to facilitate symptomatic relief in *tinea cruris* infection is controversial. In a randomized, single-blind multicenter parallel-group comparison of Lotrisone (clotrimazole 1%/betamethasone dipropionate 0.05% cream) and Nizoral (ketoconazole 2% cream) for 2 weeks in 198 patients with culture-confirmed *tinea cruris*, the combination of betamethasone dipropionate with clotrimazole provided effective disease management, with early relief of signs and symptoms (23[C]). Treatment-related adverse events occurred in 7.8% of Lotrisone-treated patients. *Reactions at the site of application*, *paresthesia*, and *pruritus* were the most frequently reported events; they were mild and none required withdrawal.

Fluconazole *(SED 13, 789; SEDA 17, 320; SEDA-18, 280; SEDA 19, 260)*

The use of fluconazole has been reviewed (24[R]). Serious adverse effects of fluconazole are rare; drug interactions can occur, but are less important than with itraconazole. The development of resistance is of concern with the triazoles, especially the emergence of fluconazole-resistant *Candida albicans* strains in AIDS patients on chronic suppressive treatment. The occurrence of fluconazole-resistant strains other than *Candida albicans* (*Candida krusei*) in hematological patients on prophylaxis with fluconazole should also be recognized.

The use of fluconazole in immunocompromised patients has also been reviewed (25[R]). Fluconazole is effective against oropharyngeal/esophageal candidiasis, either as treatment or secondary prophylaxis in patients with AIDS or as treatment or primary prophylaxis in neutropenia associated with cancer therapy. It also resolves symptoms in up to 60% of patients with cryptococcal meningitis and AIDS. Its major role is in maintenance therapy after induction with amphotericin. The incidence of adverse events is higher in patients with AIDS compared with HIV-negative patients, but the pattern of events is similar. The most frequent events are *gastrointestinal complaints*, headache, and skin rash. Rare *exfoliative skin reactions* and isolated instances of clinically overt *hepatic dysfunction* have occurred in patients with AIDS.

In 42 patients with AIDS who had endo-scopic evidence of white plaques or exudate in the esophagus and microscopic confirmation of fungal infection on biopsy or brushing specimens, fluconazole oral suspension (200 mg loading dose followed by 100 mg qds for 2 weeks after symptom resolution) caused adverse events that led to early withdrawal in five patients (*skin rash* in one, *nausea/vomiting* in two, *abnormal liver function tests* in two), all of whom had clinical and endoscopic cures (26[C]).

In a trial of fluconazole (800, 1200, 1600, or 2000 mg/day) in 39 cancer patients with presumed or proven mold infections, adverse effects included *abnormal liver function tests* (eight patients), *nausea and vomiting* (two), and *erythema multiforme* (one); *neurological toxicity* occurred in three patients taking 2000 mg/day (27[C]).

Endocrine, metabolic   In a randomized comparison of amphotericin by bladder irrigation (see above) and oral fluconazole (200 mg/day for 7 days) in 53 patients with urinary candidiasis, eradication rates at 24 h and 5–9 days after therapy were 83 and 77%, respectively, with fluconazole (11[C]). The only adverse effect of fluconazole was *hypoglycemia* in a patient who was also taking glyburide.

Liver   During 6 months of administration of oral fluconazole to 16 subjects none had any changes in liver function enzymes (28[C]).

Skin and appendages   In a multicenter retrospective survey of patients taking long-term fluconazole, 33 patients with various deep and superficial mycoses were identified who developed *alopecia* (29[C]). Of those, 29 (88%) had taken at least 400 mg/day of fluconazole for a mean of 7.1 months. Alopecia developed a median of 3 months after starting therapy and involved the scalp in all cases and other sites in about one-third of cases. Three patients required wigs because of extensive hair loss. Alopecia resolved within 6 months of withdrawal of fluconazole or reduction of the daily dose by at least 50%.

Interaction   Fluconazole had no effect on the pharmacokinetics of *didanosine* in 12 adults with HIV infection (30[C]).

Flutrimazole

In a double-blind, randomized comparison of flutrimazole 1% solution with bifonazole 1% solution, applied once daily for 4 weeks, in 40 patients with dermatophytosis or cutaneous candidiasis, 80% of those treated with flutrimazole were judged to have received effective treatment (21[C]). There were mild local reactions, such as *irritation*, *burning*, and *itching*, in seven patients.

In a similar comparison in 449 patients with fungal infections of the skin the rates of clinical and mycological cure after 4 weeks were 73% with flutrimazole and 65% with bifonazole (22[C]). The overall incidence of adverse effects (mainly mild local effects such as *irritation* or a *burning sensation*) was 5%.

Ketoconazole *(SED-13, 782; SEDA-17, 322; SEDA-18, 284)*

Adverse effects of topical ketoconazole are uncommon. For example, in 256 patients who used 2% ketoconazole cream once a day for *tinea pedis*, *tinea cruris*, or *tinea corporis*, only three reported *local irritant reactions* to ketoconazole, two of whom discontinued treatment (31[C]).

Endocrine, metabolic Ketoconazole has been used to treat patients with paraneoplastic Cushing's syndrome secondary to ectopic production of adrenocorticotropin (ACTH) by malignant neoplasms. In 15 such patients, aged 44−84 years, ketoconazole (400−1200 mg/day) improved hypokalemia, metabolic alkalosis, diabetes mellitus, and hypertension in the majority, and 10 had a hormonal response, with seven complete responses (32[C]). However, symptomatic *hypoadrenalism* definitely occurred in three patients and probably in one. The authors commented that because ketoconazole may impair the cortisol response to stress, replacement corticosteroids should be considered for patients with a hormonal response, and moderate- to high-dose corticosteroids should be given for any potential stresses.

Skin and appendages *Sticky skin* has been described in eight of 39 patients who were receiving oral ketoconazole (400 mg 8-hourly) and doxorubicin (20 mg/m² continuously for 24 h) for androgen-independent prostate cancer (33[C]). If this effect was drug-induced it is not clear whether it was attributable to the ketoconazole, or the doxorubicin, or a combination of the two. However, sticky skin has been reported in patients with psoriasis who are taking retinoids, and inhibition of retinoid metabolism by ketoconazole could have explained it (but see Interactions below).

Interactions Ketoconazole has been reported to inhibit the accelerated clearance of *all-trans-retinoic acid* during therapy with retinoic acid (SEDA-18, 284). However, this effect has not been confirmed in a study of 13 patients who took all-*trans*-retinoic acid for 14 days with and without oral ketoconazole (400 mg followed by 200 mg tds) (34[C]). There was a marked fall in plasma concentrations of all-*trans*-retinoic acid after 14 days, regardless of whether ketoconazole was given or not. This lack of effect was not due to inadequate plasma ketoconazole concentrations.

OTHER ANTIFUNGAL DRUGS

Amorolfine

Amorolfine is a broad-spectrum antifungal drug with in vitro activity against dermatophytes, yeasts, and molds. It is formulated as a lacquer for the treatment of onychomycosis. In small clinical trials conducted to date about a half of patients with mild disease not involving the nail matrix and predominantly dermatophyte infections have achieved mycological and clinical cure (35[R]). The efficacy of amorolfine appears to be greater in the fingernails than the toenails. Less than 2% of patients have experienced adverse events, all mild and localized to the site of application.

In a randomized open study, 194 patients with dermatophytosis (mostly of the toenails) either used amorolfine nail lacquer twice a week for 12 months, with or without concomitant griseofulvin therapy (500 mg bd) for the first 2 months, or took griseofulvin alone (500 mg bd for the first 2 months and 500 mg od for the remaining 10 months) (36[C]). The clinical cure and improvement rate (including intact lunulae/matrices) was 81% in the group using the combined treatment and 79% in those who took griseofulvin alone. The most commonly reported adverse events were *headache*, *nausea*, and *vomiting*, presumably due to the griseofulvin. In another study of 714 patients with onychomycosis without matrix involvement, amorolfine nail lacquer was applied once a week for 6 months (36^C). There was a clinical cure or improvement in 78% of all toenail mycoses, and in 84% of all fingernail mycoses; *local adverse events* probably or possibly related to the nail lacquer, mostly skin irritation, were reported in six patients (<1%).

Griseofulvin *(SED-13, 780; SEDA-18, 283)*

Urinary system Griseofulvin can rarely cause a *lupus-like syndrome*, and patients with pre-existing systemic lupus erythematosus are more prone to adverse skin reactions to griseofulvin (SED-13, 781). After treatment with griseofulvin a 16-year-old man developed nephrotic syndrome related to membranous glomerulopathy, with clinical and serological evidence of systemic lupus erythematosus (37^c). This seems to have been the first case of griseofulvin-exacerbated lupus in which nephrotic syndrome has been observed.

REFERENCES

1. Rho JP, Cupo JH. Efficacy and toxicity of amphotericin B liposomal and lipid formulations. J Pharm Technol 1995;11:99—104.

2. Van Burik JAH, Bowden RA. Standard antifungal treatment, including role of alternative modalities to administer amphotericin B. Baillière's Clin Infect Dis 1995;2:89—109.

3. Ng TTC, Denning DW. Liposomal amphotericin (AmBisome) therapy in invasive fungal infections: evaluation of United Kingdom Compassionate Use Data. Arch Intern Med 1995; 155:1093—8.

4. Pascual B, Ayestaran A, Montoro JB, Oliveras J, Estibalez A, Julia A, Lopez A. Administration of lipid-emulsion versus conventional amphotericin B in patients with neutropenia. Ann Pharmacother 1995;29:1197—201.

5. Kruger W, Stockschlader M, Russmann B, Berger C, Hoffknecht M, Sobottka I, Kohlschutter B, Kroschke G, Kroger N, Horstmann M, Kabisch H, Zander AR. Experience with liposomal amphotericin-B in 60 patients undergoing high-dose therapy and bone marrow or peripheral blood stem cell transplantation. Br J Haematol 1995;91:684—90.

6. Kline S, Larsen TA, Fieber L, Fishbach R, Greenwood M, Harris R, Kline MW, Tennican PO, Janoff EN. Limited toxicity of prolonged therapy with high doses of amphotericin B lipid complex. Clin Infect Dis 1995;21:1154—8.

7. Oppenheim BA, Herbrecht R, Kusne S. The safety and efficacy of amphotericin B colloidal dispersion in the treatment of invasive mycoses. Clin Infect Dis 1995;21:1145—53.

8. Oravcova E, Mistrik M, Sakalova A, Drgona L, Kollar T, Helpianska L, Ilavska I, Sorkovska D, Spanik S, Kukuckova E, Krcmery V Jr. Amphotericin B lipid complex to treat invasive fungal infections in cancer patients: report of efficacy and safety in 20 patients. Chemotherapy (Switzerland) 1995;41:473—6.

9. Dubois J, Bartter T, Gryn J, Pratter MR. The physiologic effects of inhaled amphotericin B. Chest 1995;108:50—3.

10. Behre GF, Schwartz S, Lenz K, Ludwig WD, Wandt H, Schilling E, Heinemann V, Link H, Trittin A, Boenisch O, Treder W, Siegert W, Hiddemann W, Beyer J. Aerosol amphotericin B inhalations for prevention of invasive pulmonary aspergillosis in neutropenic cancer patients. Ann Hematol 1995;71:287—91.

11. Fan-Havard P, O'Donovan C, Smith SM, Oh J, Bamberger M, Eng RHK. Oral fluconazole versus amphotericin B bladder irrigation for treatment of candidal funguria. Clin Infect Dis 1995;21:960—5.

12. Levy M, Domaratzki J, Koren G. Amphotericin-induced heart-rate decrease in children. Clin Pediatr 1995;34:358—64.

13. Tollemar J, Hockerstedt K, Ericzon BG, Jalanko H, Ringden O. Liposomal amphotericin B prevents invasive fungal infections in liver transplant recipients. A randomized, placebo-controlled study. Transplantation 1995;59:45—50.

14. Nguyen MH, Peacock JE Jr, Tanner DC, Morris AJ, Minh Ly Nguyen, Snydman DR, Wagener MM, Yu VL. Therapeutic approaches in patients with candidemia: evaluation in a multicenter, prospective, observational study. Arch Intern Med 1995;155:2429—35.

15. Gales MA, Gales BJ. Rapid infusion of amphotericin B in dextrose. Ann Pharmacother 1995;29:523—9.

16. Nicholl TA, Nimmo CR, Shepherd JD, Phillips P, Jewesson PJ. Amphotericin B infusion-related toxicity: comparison of two- and four-hour infusions. Ann Pharmacother 1995;29:1081—7.

17. Thakur CP, Sinha GP, Barat D, Singh RK. Two-hour versus six-hour administration of amphotericin B in the treatment of kala-azar. Int J Antimicrob Agents 1995;5:115—17.

18. Arning M, Kliche KO, Heer-Sonderhoff AH, Wehmeier A. Infusion-related toxicity of three different amphotericin B formulations and its relation to cytokine plasma levels. Mycoses 1995; 38:459—65.

19. Goodwin SD, Cleary JD, Walawander CA, Taylor JW, Grasela TH Jr. Pretreatment regimens for adverse events related to infusion of amphotericin B. Clin Infect Dis 1995;20:755—61.

20. Dooms Goossens A, Matura M, Drieghe J, Degreef H. Contact allergy to imidazoles used as antimycotic agents. Contact Dermatitis 1995; 33:73—7.

21. Del Palacio A, Cuetara S, Izquierdo I, Videla S, Delgadillo J, Boncompte E, Rodriguez Noriega A. A double-blind randomized comparative trial: flutrimazole 1% solution versus bifonazole 1% solution once daily in dermatomycoses. Mycoses 1995;38:395—403.

22. Alomar A, Videla S, Delgadillo J, Gich I, Izquierdo I, Forn J, Muntanola AA, Masoliver AA, Corominas AB, Montesinos EB, Bresca SB, Seuma JMC, Rodellas AC, Foraster CF, Marques JMG, Alava JG, Sariola CJ, Llach EL, Cardell CM, et al. Flutrimazole 1% dermal cream in the treatment of dermatomycoses: a multicentre, double-blind, randomized, comparative clinical trial with bifonazole 1% cream-efficacy of flutrimazole 1% dermal cream in dermatomycoses. Dermatology 1995;190:295—300.

23. Pariser RJ, Pariser DM, Caro E, Gomez C, Lazan DW, Martin S, Morman MR, Phillips JH III, Rosario R, Stewart D, Tucker SB. Clinical and mycological effect of clotrimazole/betamethasone dipropionate cream versus ketoconazole cream in patients with tinea cruris. J Dermatol Treat 1995;6:173—7.

24. Van't Wout JW. Therapeutic indications for new triazoles and potential emergence of resistance. Baillière's Clin Infect Dis 1995;2:111—26.

25. Goa KL, Barradell LB. Fluconazole. An update of its pharmacodynamic and pharmacokinetic properties and therapeutic use in major superficial and systemic mycoses in immunocompromised patients. Drugs 1995;50:658—90.

26. Laine L, Rabeneck L. Prospective study of fluconazole suspension for the treatment of oesophageal candidiasis in patients with AIDS. Aliment Pharmacol Ther 1995;9:553—6.

27. Anaissie EJ, Kontoyiannis DP, Huls C, Vartivarian SE, Karl C, Prince RA, Bosso J, Bodey GP. Safety, plasma concentrations, and efficacy of high-dose fluconazole in invasive mold infections. J Infect Dis 1995;172:599—602.

28. Smith SW, Sealy DP, Schneider E, Lackland D. An evaluation of the safety and efficacy of fluconazole in the treatment of onychomycosis. South Med J 1995;88:1217—20.

29. Pappas PG, Kauffman CA, Perfect J, Johnson PJ, McKinsey DS, Bamberger DM, Hamill R, Sharkey PK, Chapman SW, Sobel JD. Alopecia associated with fluconazole therapy. Ann Intern Med 1995;123:354—7.

30. Bruzzese VL, Gillum JG, Israel DS, Johnson GL, Kaplowitz LG, Polk RE. Effect of fluconazole on pharmacokinetics of 2',3'-dideoxyinosine in persons seropositive for human immunodeficiency virus. Antimicrob Agents Chemother 1995;39:1050—3.

31. Lester M. Ketoconazole 2 percent cream in the treatment of tinea pedis, tinea cruris, and tinea corporis. Cutis 1995;55:181—3.

32. Winquist EW, Laskey J, Crump M, Khamsi F, Shepherd FA. Ketoconazole in the management of paraneoplastic Cushing's syndrome secondary to ectopic adrenocorticotropin production. J Clin Oncol 1995;13:157—64.

33. Polsen JA, Cohen PR, Sella A. Acquired cutaneous adherence in patients with androgen-independent prostate cancer receiving ketoconazole and doxorubicin: medication-induced sticky skin. J Am Acad Dermatol 1995;32:571—5.

34. Lee JS, Newman RA, Lippman SM, Fossella FV, Calayag M, Raber MN, Krakoff IH, Hong WK. Phase I evaluation of all-trans retinoic acid with and without ketoconazole in adults with solid tumors. J Clin Oncol 1995;13:1501—8.

35. Anonymous. Amorolfine: topical therapy for mild onychomycosis. Drugs Ther Perspect 1995; 5:4—7.

36. Zaug M. Amorolfine nail lacquer: clinical experience in onychomycosis. J Eur Acad Dermatol Venereol 1995;Suppl 1:S23—S30.

37. Bonilla-Felix M, Verani R, Vanasse LG, Herbert A. Nephrotic syndrome related to systemic lupus erythematosus after griseofulvin therapy. Pediatr Nephrol 1995;9:478—9.

M. Pirmohamed and P.A. Winstanley

28   Antiprotozoal drugs

ANTIMALARIAL DRUGS
(SED-13, 799; SEDA-17, 325; SEDA-18, 286; SEDA-19, 262)

℞ *The current status of antimalarial drugs*

Reviews have appeared on current recommendations for the prevention and treatment of malaria (1[R]), the clinical pharmacology of antimalarial drugs (2[R]), and their benefit:risk ratio (3[R]).

Malaria has always been a major global health problem, but the situation is set to become disastrous in the near future because of widespread drug resistance, a lack of new drugs, and the combined effects of other diseases, poverty, war, and pressure of population on health budgets in developing countries. The main burden of mortality and morbidity will be borne by the two billion residents of endemic areas (predominantly in Africa), but malaria is also a major threat to the increasing numbers of travellers to the tropics, particularly those bound for areas where drug-resistance is widespread.

The use of chloroquine   Of the four species of parasite that infect man, Plasmodium falciparum causes the most severe illness, often fatal, and has developed resistance to many drugs. The area of highest risk for its acquisition is sub-Saharan Africa, but it may also be acquired in Southeast Asia, the Indian sub-continent, Oceania, and South America (1[R]). Strains that are resistant to chloroquine are widespread throughout the tropics, and multidrug resistance is particularly common in Southeast Asia. P. vivax, P. ovale, and P. malariae do not cause such severe illness. P. ovale and P. malariae retain sensitivity to chloroquine; although generally chloroquine-sensi-tive, some strains of P. vivax have developed resistance to chloroquine.

Nevertheless, because of its low cost chloroquine is still the most commonly used antimalarial drug in the world. Despite widespread resistance, chloroquine is still useful for uncomplicated malaria in semi-immune patients in sub-Saharan Africa (given orally in a dose of 25 mg/kg divided over 3 days). Chloroquine should not be used for severe malaria or for uncomplicated disease in non-immune patients, unless no alternative is available: drug failure may result in rapid death. Weekly chloroquine, usually in combination with proguanil (see below), is still used for the prophylaxis of malaria (1[R]).

When used in standard dosages for malaria prophylaxis or therapy, chloroquine is very safe. However, caution is required when it is given intravenously, since rapid infusion causes shock and dysrhythmias; it must be diluted and infused slowly to avoid cardiovascular toxicity. In the setting of deliberate self-poisoning chloroquine causes early cardiovascular collapse.

In developed countries hydroxychloroquine is used much more commonly than chloroquine, as a second-line drug for rheumatoid disease and in the treatment of chronic discoid lupus. Such second-line agents (which also include gold, penicillamine, sulphasalazine, azathioprine, and methotrexate) are usually given for aggressive disease after an (unsuccessful) trial of non-steroidal anti-inflammatory drugs. Comparisons have been made between the various second-line agents in terms of efficacy and toxicity, but rarely have sufficient power to reach definite conclusions; it seems likely that all are of comparable efficacy.

Chemoprophylaxis   Antimalarials cause a wide range of dose-dependent, idiopathic, and cumulative adverse effects, and these are of most concern in the setting of chemoprophylaxis, where the benefits of the drug must clearly outweigh its risks. This is mainly of concern to travellers (1[R]), since most residents of endemic areas cannot afford chemoprophylaxis. Prophylaxis is advisable in areas of intense transmission (see above), even for relatively short visits and even for subjects who may originally have come from the area (since malaria immunity may be lost without continuing exposure). However, in areas with a low risk of transmission, such as the Middle East, the traveller may be more at risk from the drug than from the disease. Drug selection is based on efficacy and toxicity data and the likelihood of infection in the individual patient. Avoidance of mosquito bites is essentially free from risk for most travellers and contributes greatly to protection. It is most important that the traveller should be aware that protection is not absolute, whatever precautions are taken.

Chloroquine-sensitive areas: In chloroquine-sensitive areas, or if the predominant malaria species is not P. falciparum, weekly chloroquine is still adequate.

Chloroquine-resistant areas: The whole of sub-Saharan Africa should be assumed to be a high-risk area for the transmission of chloroquine-resistant P. falciparum, but both P. malariae and P. ovale can be acquired, and these are chloroquine-sensitive. The two regimens in frequent use are weekly mefloquine (250 mg) or weekly chloroquine (300 mg of the base) plus daily proguanil (200 mg); however, some believe that mefloquine causes symptomatic adverse effects so often that it is unacceptable for chemoprophylaxis (see below).

Areas of multidrug resistance: In Southeast Asia the risk of transmission of P. falciparum is low, relative to Africa, but organisms may be multidrug resistant. Subjects at most risk include visitors to rural areas, particularly the Thai-Burmese border. Detailed specialist advice should be sought.

Pregnancy: Semi-immune patients lose much of their resistance to local strains of P. falciparum during pregnancy; this commonly results in massive sequestration of organisms in the placenta, causing maternal anemia, low birth-weight babies, pre-term delivery, and abortions; other malaria species can have the same effects. Thus, pregnant women in endemic areas are at high risk, and should take chemoprophylaxis, despite the risks of teratogenicity. Pregnant travellers should be dissu-

aded from taking holidays in areas of intense transmission, particularly during the first trimester. If travel is essential, pregnant travellers should avoid bites and take prophylaxis. Chloroquine and proguanil do not appear to be associated with increased risks of fetal malformations, although proguanil is an inhibitor of dihydrofolate reductase (mainly through its metabolite cycloguanil), and folic acid supplements (200–500 µg/day) should be used. Mefloquine is not recommended by its manufacturer for use in pregnancy, although it does not appear to cause an increase in fetal malformations. The use of antimalarial drugs in pregnancy has been recently reviewed (4[R]).

Chemotherapy of uncomplicated malaria Chloroquine is still used in most African countries, but widespread resistance has dictated the use of alternatives, particularly for children and pregnant women. Fansidar (pyrimethamine + sulfadoxine) is effective and relatively cheap and it may be given parenterally. However, concern remains over the speed of clinical improvement with this combination, its risk of toxicity, and its selection of drug-resistant parasites (5[C]). Pyronaridine (6[C]) has been shown to be effective in clinical trial in Africa, but logistics may yet limit its use (7[r]). In Southeast Asia, chloroquine and Fansidar are ineffective, and mefloquine or halofantrine (relatively expensive drugs) are used for uncomplicated disease. The worrying emergence of P. falciparum strains resistant to mefloquine and halofantrine, and the report that halofantrine can be cardiotoxic (SEDA-17, 328) are likely to alter the use of these drugs. The combination of atovaquone with proguanil has recently been shown to be efficacious (8[C]); this is likely to be expensive, but affordable in Southeast Asia. Artemisinin derivatives, which are generally regarded as therapy for severe malaria, may be given orally or rectally and are increasingly used in Southeast Asia for uncomplicated disease. These drugs seem remarkably safe, but in animal experiments they produce dose-related nervous system toxicity; whether these effects are relevant to man remains to be seen.

Established P. falciparum malaria is a medical emergency in non-immune patients, since it may rapidly become complicated. Cases imported into developed countries are no longer treated with chloroquine, because of fears of drug resistance. Fansidar, mefloquine, or halofantrine may all be given orally, and can be expected to produce a cure if the infection was acquired in Africa. Infections acquired in Southeast Asia are more difficult to treat: mefloquine and halofantrine are usually effective, but many clinicians would choose parenteral quinine, even for uncomplicated cases, despite the inconvenience of using it and its predictable uncomfortable adverse effects. Artemisinin derivatives may become available in the European Union in the future, but their use is likely to be restricted to severe disease.

The risks of P. falciparum infection have been particularly stressed, because it can kill. P. vivax, P. malariae, and P. ovale produce less severe illnesses and have not commonly become drug-resistant: chloroquine is still usually effective, and remains the treatment of choice. However, it should not be forgotten that P. vivax and P. ovale both have dormant stages (in the liver), which require treatment with an 8-aminoquinoline, like primaquine, for eradication. Primaquine is generally well tolerated, but it may cause hemolysis and methemoglobinemia, particularly in subjects with glucose-6-phosphate dehydrogenase (G6PD) deficiency.

Chemotherapy of severe malaria   Parenteral quinine remains the drug of first choice for severe malaria; it must be given with close attention to the rate of infusion, since rapid injection may cause hypoglycemia and cardiovascular adverse effects. Derivatives of artemisinin are showing promise as drugs with parasitological properties superior to those of quinine. However, recently completed large clinical trials in Southeast Asia and Africa have failed to demonstrate the anticipated lower mortality in patients given artemether instead of quinine.

Artemisinin and derivatives *(SED-13, 818; SEDA-17, 326; SEDA-18, 286; SEDA-19, 262)*

The chemistry, clinical pharmacology, toxicology, and clinical use of this class of drugs has recently been reviewed (9[R]).

Artemisinin is the name given to the active antimalarial drug isolated from a Chinese herbal remedy (called Qinghaosu), while artemether and artesunate are the most commonly used semi-synthetic derivatives of artemisinin; arteether, another derivative being developed by the World Health Organization, is very similar to artemether but is not yet generally available. All the derivatives are more potent than artemisinin and have longer shelf-lives, but are more expensive. Artemisinin is given orally or rectally, artemether orally or intramuscularly, and artesunate orally or by intravenous infusion.

Intramuscular artemether has been compared with intravenous quinine in three large clinical trials in severe falciparum malaria (10[C])–(12[C]), and a meta-analysis of the data is awaited. No serious adverse effects were seen. As anticipated, the rate of clearance of peripheral parasitemia was faster with artemether than quinine in all three trials. The Kenyan trial (in 160 children with cerebral malaria) reported an overall mortality of 16%, with no overall significant difference between the two treatments (10[C]). However, in a subgroup of children with respiratory distress, mortality was significantly higher in those treated with artemether (44 vs. 11%); the significance of this finding is unknown. In the Gambian trial (in 576 children with cerebral malaria), 21 and 22%, respectively, died after treatment with artemether and quinine (11[C]). Finally, in the Vietnamese trial (in 560 adults with severe malaria, not all of whom had cerebral malaria), there were 36 deaths in the artemether group (13%) and 47 in the quinine group (17%); patients randomized to artemether had a slower resolution of fever and longer stay in hospital (12[C]).

All the drugs in this class produce dose-dependent central nervous system toxicity in laboratory animals (13 and inhibit the growth of neuroblastoma cell lines (14), (15). However, human neurotoxicity is yet to be reported, and artemisinin derivatives seem to have a large therapeutic index.

Atovaquone *(SED-13, 828; SEDA-18, 286; SEDA-19, 266)*

Atovaquone is an antiprotozoal agent with activity against *P. falciparum* (16[c]), *Pneumocystis carinii*, and *Toxoplasma gondii*. It probably works by blocking electron transport at the cytochrome-bc1 complex of the respiratory chain, inhibiting pyrimidine synthesis. It will also be considered under the heading of *Pneumocystis carinii*.

Atovaquone and proguanil have synergistic effects (see below) against *P. falciparum*, and in an open trial atovaquone was superior to amodiaquine in the treatment of uncomplicated *P. falciparum* malaria in Gabon (8[C]). Significantly more patients on atovaquone/proguanil complained of nausea and abdominal pain, while amodiaquine was associated with complaints of pruritus, weakness, insomnia, and dizziness. Atovaquone/proguanil is likely to be relatively expensive and of most value in areas of multidrug resistance, including Southeast Asia.

Chloroquine and congeners *(SED-13, 801; SEDA-17, 327; SEDA-18, 286; SEDA-19, 262)*

Amodiaquine

Amodiaquine was never in such widespread use as chloroquine, mainly because it is more expensive. When it was appreciated, in about 1986, that it carries a high risk of agranulocytosis and hepatitis, it was withdrawn for chemoprophylaxis; indeed, enthusiasm for its use in treatment also waned, and in 1990 the WHO withdrew it from malaria control programs. More recently, faced with ever greater pressures from drug resistance, amodiaquine has been re-examined: the authors of a recent systematic review (17[R]) have supported the use of amodiaquine for *P. falciparum* malaria, but warned of cross-resistance with chloroquine. The adverse effects profile of amodiaquine, when used several times annually for malaria treatment, is unknown.

Amodiaquine or chloroquine have been randomly given to 158 Kenyan symptomatic outpatients with *P. falciparum* malaria (18[C]). Amodiaquine was significantly more effective in terms of the rate of parasite clearance and clinical amelioration. Overall, tolerance was better with amodiaquine than with chloroquine (in particular, cutaneous adverse effects were less frequent). There was no evidence of bone-marrow or gross hepatic toxicity, but the sample size was too small to estimate the

incidence of these life-threatening adverse effects during treatment.

Halofantrine *(SED-13, 820; SEDA-17, 327; SEDA-18, 287; SEDA-19, 263)*

The pharmacokinetics of halofantrine have been reviewed (19[r]). It is used to treat uncomplicated *P. falciparum* malaria and is not suitable for prophylaxis. Oral halofantrine has a very low systemic availability, but this is increased if it is taken with food. It prolongs the electrocardiographic corrected QT interval (SEDA-17, 328) and might therefore cause dysrhythmias. Even so, in areas of multidrug resistance, high dosages of halofantrine are now being used to ensure cure. In a comparison of halofantrine (three doses of 500 mg each at 4-h intervals on the first day, followed by 500 mg/day for 6 days; total dose 4.5 g) with quinine plus tetracycline, there was no difference in efficacy between the two regimens, but halofantrine was better tolerated (20[C]).

Proguanil and chlorproguanil

Proguanil is currently one of the commonest prophylactic antimalarial drugs in use. No new adverse effects to proguanil have been reported over the last year, and it has a reputation for safety even in overdose.

Chlorproguanil, a close structural analog of proguanil, is not currently in general use, although its use against pyrimethamine-resistant *P. falciparum* is being investigated.

To test the efficacy of chlorproguanil prophylaxis, 156 malaria-free Kenyan schoolchildren were given either chlorproguanil 7.5 mg/day, chlorproguanil 50 mg/week, proguanil 100 mg/day, or placebo (21[C]). After 169 days there was *P. falciparum* parasitemia in 92% of those taking placebo, 31% of those taking daily proguanil, 38% of those taking daily chlorproguanil, and 55% of those taking weekly chlorproguanil. No significant adverse effects were reported or observed.

Quinine and congeners *(SED-13, 814; SEDA-17, 329; SEDA-18, 288; SEDA-19, 265)*

Quinine and quinidine

Quinine is the drug of first-choice for complicated malaria in much of the world; in the USA intravenous quinine has been discontinued in favor of quinidine.

Cardiovascular Quinine may cause cardiac dysrhythmias.

A 71-year-old woman was given quinine (1.4 g; about 20 mg/kg) intravenously over 4 h, and then 600 mg 8-hourly (22[c]). After the third dose she developed ventricular fibrillation. Unbound quinine concentrations were unusually high (peaking at 9 mg/l) and constituted an unusually high fraction of the total quinine concentration. Plasma protein concentrations were within the ranges expected in severe malaria, and no explanation for the observations was offered.

More usually, quinine is safe in standard dosages. Electrocardiographic monitoring over 24 h has been performed in 53 patients (11 adults and 42 children) with severe *P. falciparum* malaria (23[c]). Nine patients (17%) died, five during the monitoring period and four afterwards. There were pauses lasting 2–3 s in three children, a single couplet in one child, and frequent supraventricular extra beats in another. In none of the patients who died could death be attributed to a cardiac dysrhythmia, and the authors were dubious of the value of routine cardiographic monitoring in this setting.

Quinidine, the diastereoisomer of quinine, is more potent than quinine against *P. falciparum*, but is also more cardiotoxic.

P. falciparum malaria was diagnosed in a woman visiting the USA from Nigeria (24[c]). Intravenous quinidine was given because her parasitemia was high. During the infusion, her QT interval was prolonged and she had an episode of supraventricular tachycardia. The infusion rate was reduced and the QT duration returned to normal; there were no further episodes of dysrhythmia.

Immunological and hypersensitivity reactions
Quinidine-induced lupus-like syndrome, antinuclear antibody-negative lupus-like syndrome, a polymyalgia rheumatica-like illness, muscle weakness, and isolated creatine phosphokinase elevation have all been reported. A further case of quinidine-induced lupus-like syndrome and another of a quinidine-induced

polymyalgia rheumatica have recently been reported (25[r]).

Risk factors The cardiographic effects of quinine have been studied in children under 2 years of age treated for severe *P. falciparum* malaria with a parenteral loading dose of 20 mg/kg of quinine dihydrochloride, followed by 10 mg/kg doses at 12-h intervals (26[c]). At 2 and 4 h after starting treatment, there was significant prolongation of the QRS interval compared with baseline (16 and 17% at 2 and 4 h, respectively), but not in a control group of nine older children (age range 2–10 years) who received the same intramuscular dosage regimen. Unbound and total quinine concentrations were not significantly correlated with changes in the QRS interval. These findings raise the possibility that young children are more susceptible to quinine toxicity than older children, and indicate the need for further evaluation of quinine dosage regimens in this age group.

Overdosage Quinine is held to be a relatively safe drug if dosage recommendations are followed. Overdosage, on the other hand, can be serious, as has been reported in five children, aged 14 months to 13 years, who were admitted for treatment of malaria and given quinine intravenously (27[c]). Four children developed a seizure, with recurrence in three; the fifth child suffered from headache, tinnitus, and visual anomalies. Four children rapidly developed hypotension followed by cardiac arrest. All had abnormal electrocardiograms. Retrospective inspection of the instructions given for quinine administration showed that they were not explicit and had been responsible for incorrect dilution of the drug. Four of the five children recovered completely. The fifth developed ventricular tachycardia followed by bradycardia that did not respond to resuscitation.

Mefloquine *(SED-13, 808; SEDA-17, 329; SEDA-18, 288; SEDA-19, 265)*

The therapeutic efficacy and toxicity of a combination of low-dose mefloquine (15 mg/kg) plus artesunate 10 mg/kg in one day have been compared with the high-dose mefloquine (25 mg/kg) in 552 patients with uncomplicated *P. falciparum* malaria on the Thai-Burmese border (28[C]). Gastrointestinal adverse effects and dizziness were more likely in the high-dose mefloquine monotherapy group. There were no adverse effects with artesunate.

Nervous system The apparently high incidence and severity of neuropsychiatric adverse reactions to mefloquine are causing some to doubt its advisability for malaria prophylaxis (29[r]). Its role in the treatment of established *P. falciparum* malaria, especially in Southeast Asia, is not in question (although resistance is fast developing). Central nervous system adverse effects of antimalarial drugs (including mefloquine) have recently been reviewed (30[R]).

TETRACYCLINES

The tetracyclines are covered in Chapter 25, but it is worth noting that they have antimalarial activity and are used for both prevention and treatment of *P. falciparum* malaria. In Southeast Asia, where quinine sensitivity seems to be declining, *P. falciparum* malaria can only be cleared after prolonged quinine treatment (for 7 days) if the drug is given alone; combining quinine with tetracycline reduces the length of the treatment course.

Doxycycline

Like other tetracyclines, doxycycline may be used for suppressive chemoprophylaxis and has causal prophylactic activity (i.e. it is active against the pre-erythrocytic stages of the parasite); doxycycline has the advantage of a relatively long half-life.

Doxycycline (100 mg/day) plus primaquine (7.5 mg/day) has been used as chemoprophylaxis in 53 soldiers during deployment to a high-transmission area of multidrug resistant *P. falciparum* (31[C]). It was generally well tolerated; the most common adverse effects were nausea, sunburn, and headache.

Gastrointestinal Doxycycline (in varying dosages) has also been used in 1500 soldiers as part of their malaria chemoprophylaxis (32[C]). Gastrointestinal upsets were common if doxycycline was not taken with food; photosensitization was also reported.

Enteric coating of doxycycline probably reduces the prevalence of gastrointestinal adverse effects (33[c]) but the effect of this formulation change on the cost of the drug was not discussed.

DRUGS USED FOR TOXOPLASMOSIS *(SEDA-17, 330; SEDA-18, 289; SEDA-19, 265)*

Treatment of toxoplasmosis

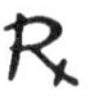

Toxoplasma gondii is a ubiquitous parasite that normally produces few symptoms in immune-competent hosts, and rarely requires treatment. The parasite causes major problems in three main settings: (a) transplacental spread, (b) retinal reactivation, and (c) reactivation (usually in the central nervous system) due to immune suppression or depletion.

Congenital toxoplasmosis *Congenital toxoplasmosis usually results from a newly-acquired acute infection (often asymptomatic); the risks to the fetus are highest in the first trimester and fall thereafter. The consequences range from abortion and severe brain damage to no apparent sequelae at all: specialist advice is essential to determine the likely prognosis. Treatment of the acutely infected woman reduces the incidence of fetal infection. Regimens include spiramycin, which may be used throughout pregnancy, or pyrimethamine/sulfadiazine: some experts are wary about the use of the latter combination in the first trimester of pregnancy.*

Ocular toxoplasmosis *Ocular toxoplasmosis may be regarded as a delayed form of congenital infection, since this is the route of transmission, but symptoms do not usually appear until the second, third, and fourth decades. Acute choroidoretinitis may present as pain and/or altered vision. Examination of the optic fundus usually reveals focal necrotizing retinitis. Pyrimethamine plus either sulfadiazine or clindamycin are the drugs of first choice.*

Infection in the immunocompromised host
Infection in the immunocompromised host usually results from reactivation of latent disease, and may complicate the use of immunosuppressive drugs, or disease-induced immunodeficiency. Toxoplasma encephalitis remains one of the commonest opportunistic infections of the central nervous system in late AIDS; however, secondary prophylaxis has reduced its incidence in Europe to around 4–12% (34^C). Co-trimoxazole is the prophylaxis of choice (see under Pneumocystis carinii pneumonia below), but pyrimethamine is an alternative (usually in combination with either dapsone or a sulfonamide). Treatment is given empirically if clinical and radiological features suggest the diagnosis; brain biopsy is reserved for patients who present diagnostic difficulty. Pyrimethamine plus sulfadiazine remains the drug combination of first choice, although it is far from satisfactory: response to therapy can take up to 15 days, some patients fail to respond, some relapse while on maintenance therapy, up to 60% develop adverse drug reactions, mainly to the sulfonamide, and latent infection is not eliminated. Various lincosamine and macrolide antibiotics have been used in combination with pyrimethamine, including clindamycin, azithromycin, spiramycin, roxithromycin, and clarithromycin. Most of the drugs used in the treatment of this condition (pyrimethamine, atovaquone, sulfadiazine, and clindamycin and other lincosamines/macrolides) are dealt with elsewhere.

Toxoplasma encephalitis *Pyrimethamine, 25 mg thrice weekly, has been evaluated in 335 patients as primary prophylaxis for Toxoplasma encephalitis in a double-blind, randomized clinical trial in late AIDS (in addition to prophylaxis against Pneumocystis carinii pneumonia) (35^c). Folinic acid (leucovorin) was co-administered only for hematological toxicity. There was a significantly higher death rate among patients receiving pyrimethamine (relative risk 2.5), even after adjusting for factors predictive of survival. This study also found that co-trimoxazole prophylaxis against Pneumocystis carinii pneumonia was protective against toxoplasmosis. The cause of the excess mortality in the pyrimethamine group was not clear, but was felt to be related to the drug's antifolate activity.*

Trimetrexate *Trimetrexate is a dihydrofolate reductase inhibitor, structurally related to methotrexate, but differing from it in that trimetrexate does not require uptake by the folate carrier transport system. Trimetrexate is being used for malignant disease and rheumatoid disorders, but also has efficacy against both Pneumocystis carinii pneumonia and Toxoplasma gondii (36^r). In Pneumocystis carinii pneumonia, trimetrexate probably has inferior efficacy to co-trimoxazole, but it is an alternative for patients who are allergic to first-line drugs. Its principal adverse effects are dose-dependent, and include gastrointestinal upset, fever, abnormal liver function, and hematological toxicity.*

DRUGS USED FOR PNEUMOCYSTIS CARINII PNEUMONIA *(SED-13, 822; SEDA-17, 330; SEDA-18, 289; SEDA-19, 266)*

Drug prophylaxis for *Pneumocystis carinii* is now well established. From the limited data available it has been estimated that initiation of prophylaxis before the onset of clinical AIDS will delay both the date of diagnosis of AIDS and the date of death by 9 months in North American men (37^r). The benefit is less if prophylaxis is started after the onset of AIDS, and probably also in developing countries. This has to be contrasted with the benefits of zidovudine, which has been estimated to delay death by about 12 months.

The drugs used for the treatment of and prophylaxis for *Pneumocystis carinii* pneumonia were reviewed in SEDA-18 (p. 289). There is no doubt that all of these drugs are toxic: one large study in 843 patients, in which three agents for prophylaxis were compared, showed that over half of the patients will develop severe adverse events (38^C) (Table 1). Unfortunately, the most efficacious drug (co-trimoxazole) (38^C), (39^c)–(41^c) also seems to be amongst the most toxic, particularly when compared with aerosolized pentamidine (41^c). For example, in a study in 367 patients with *Pneumocystis carinii* pneumonia, 40% of those taking co-trimoxazole had to discontinue therapy because of toxi-

Table 1. *Toxicity of three drug regimens used for prophylaxis of Pneumocystis carinii pneumonia (38[c])*

Toxicity	Co-trimoxazole (1.92 g/d)	Dapsone (100 mg/d)	Aerosolized pentamidine (300 mg/month)
Reduced neutrophil count	40%	34%	28%
Fever >40°C	25%	29%	19%
Reduced hemoglobin	20%	25%	21%
Severe nausea	14%	16%	9%
Rash	16%	9%	5%
Pancreatitis	2.9%	2.8%	2.2%

city, compared with 9% on aerosolized pentamidine. Rash (15 vs. 0.6%), nausea and vomiting (12 vs. 1.7%), and abnormalities of liver function tests (12 vs. 1.7%) were the most common adverse effects (41[c]). However, treatment failure occurred in fewer patients taking co-trimoxazole, although there was no difference in mortality between the two groups.

There is clear evidence to suggest that the dosage of co-trimoxazole in HIV-positive patients is positively correlated with the frequency of toxicity (SEDA-18, 290). This seems to have been confirmed by a study in 260 patients, in which 480 mg of co-trimoxazole was as efficacious as 960 mg for primary prophylaxis against *Pneumocystis carinii* pneumonia but less toxic (42[c]). However, during the treatment of microscopically confirmed *Pneumocystis carinii* pneumonia, where the high dosages used are associated with a high frequency of toxicity, the use of serum sulfamethoxazole concentration monitoring to achieve a target range of 150—200 μg/ml in 40 patients failed to improve either the efficacy or tolerability of the drug (43[c]).

Atovaquone (see also above)

The role of atovaquone in the treatment of *Pneumocystis carinii* pneumonia was reviewed in SEDA-19 (p. 266). Clinical experience with atovaquone is limited, its use in the treatment of severe *Pneumocystis carinii* pneumonia and in prophylaxis having been investigated in few studies (44[r]). In mild to moderate *Pneumocystis carinii* pneumonia, atovaquone is less effective than co-trimoxazole, and it is therefore reserved as a second-line agent (44[r])—(49[r]). Adverse events associated with atovaquone include rash, diarrhea, constipation, anemia, neutropenia, fever, and liver transaminase elevation (46[c]). Of these, only rash

has been shown to relate to plasma concentrations (46[c]).

Pentamidine *(SED-13, 823; SEDA-17, 331; SEDA-18, 291; SEDA-19, 267)*

Pentamidine is used in the treatment of *Pneumocystis carinii* pneumonia, trypanosomiasis, and cutaneous leishmaniasis. The pancreas is a major target organ for pentamidine toxicity, resulting in either dysglycemia (SEDA-19, 268) or acute pancreatitis; the role of pentamidine in causing pancreatitis has recently been confirmed by a case-control study that implicated its use in 12 of 44 patients with AIDS who developed pancreatitis (50[c]). Other target organs for pentamidine toxicity include the skin, kidneys, and lungs.

Co-trimoxazole (trimethoprim-sulfamethoxazole) *(SED-13, 826; SEDA-17, 332; SEDA-18, 290; SEDA-19, 268)*

Hypersensitivity reactions to co-trimoxazole

Hypersensitivity reactions to co-trimoxazole, which have largely been attributed to the sulfonamide component, have been the focus of recent research. The problem is of particular importance in HIV-positive patients, because of the increased frequency and severity of reactions (51[R])—(53[R]). However, hypersensitivity reactions are also seen in HIV-negative individuals; a recent survey showed that the use of co-trimoxazole is associated with a relative risk of 172 (95% confidence intervals 75—396) for the development of Stevens-Johnson syndrome or toxic epidermal necrolysis (Lyell's syndrome) (54[C]). Given the high risk of idiosyncratic toxicity associated with co-trimoxazole and the availability of safer and equally effective antibiotics (at least in HIV-negative pa-

tients), the licensing authority in the UK has now restricted its use to Pneumocystis carinii pneumonia (treatment and prophylaxis) and as a second-line antibacterial agent (55[R]). In effect, this means that the major use of co-trimoxazole in the UK is now going to be in HIV-positive patients (56[R]).

Hypersensitivity usually signifies that the reaction is immune mediated. With co-trimoxazole, evidence that this is so is mostly clinical (53[R]), although various recent laboratory studies have provided some supportive evidence. For example, circulating drug-specific T cells have been shown in three HIV-negative patients with a history of allergy to sulfamethoxazole (57[c]), (58[c]). Additionally, positive patch testing to sulfamethoxazole but not to trimethoprim has been reported in a 90-year-old woman with toxic epidermal necrolysis (59[c]). How such studies on cell-mediated immunity relate to the situation in HIV-positive patients is unclear at present, since (a) these patients are immunosuppressed with a reduction in the CD4+ cell count and (b) there is conflicting evidence on the relation between the CD4+ count and the risk of hypersensitivity. The latter has been compounded by another study (n = 236), which suggests that a higher CD4+ count confers protection (60[C]), which is in accordance with the results of one previous study (n = 130) (61[C]), but in conflict with another (n = 143) (62[C]). Moreover, there was no evidence of drug-specific cellular immunity (as determined by the lymphocyte proliferation test) in six HIV-positive patients with a history of skin rash to co-trimoxazole (63[c]). In the same study, anti-drug antibodies (i.e. humoral immunity) were demonstrated in all the patients with a history of hypersensitivity. However, these antibodies were also found in patients without a history of hypersensitivity, although the antibody titer was lower. Thus, the pathogenic role of anti-sulfamethoxazole antibodies in mediating cutaneous hypersensitivity reactions remains uncertain.

Given the superior efficacy of co-trimoxazole in the treatment of Pneumocystis carinii pneumonia, many clinicians have advocated

desensitization in patients with a history of hypersensitivity. Several such studies have been published over the last year (64[C])–(69[C]); the protocols used for desensitization were highly variable, as was the percentage of patients successfully desensitized. Clearly further research is needed in this area, not only to develop more uniform desensitization protocols, but also to investigate the actual mechanism of the desensitization.

Hematological A 42-year-old black HIV-positive woman developed hemolysis (with a 50% drop in hemoglobin over 24 h) after receiving only two doses of co-trimoxazole intravenously (960 mg/dose) (70[C]). She was given four units of blood and her hematological indices stabilized. The authors postulated that the reaction may have been caused by a deficiency of G6PD, although this unfortunately was not measured before she died (of an AIDS-related illness). They also postulated that glutathione deficiency, which has been reported in HIV-positive patients (71[c])–(75[c]), may have been a contributory factor. However, it is important to note that the issue of glutathione status in HIV-positive patients remains unresolved, earlier reports of glutathione deficiency not having been confirmed in more recent studies (76[c]), (77[c]).

Endocrine, metabolic A 50-year-old man with short bowel syndrome developed recurrent lactic acidosis following oral antibiotics (78[C]). The first episode of lactic acidosis developed after treatment with doxycycline, the second without any antibiotic exposure, and the third after 3 days of co-trimoxazole (dosage not stated). Stool cultures yielded *Lactobacillus acidophilus* resistant to the implicated antibiotics. The patient had also taken ciprofloxacin, but had not developed lactic acidosis; subsequent cultures showed that the organism was sensitive to this antibiotic. In order to avoid the overgrowth of resistant organisms in patients with short bowel syndrome, the authors suggested periodic stool culture, and specific antibiotic choices based on antimicrobial susceptibility testing.

REFERENCES

1. Bradley DJ, Warhurst DC. Malaria prophylaxis—guidelines for travelers from Britain. Br Med J 1995;310:709—14.

2. Winstanley PA. Antimalarial chemotherapy. Baillieres Clin Infect Dis 1995;2:293—308.

3. Nosten F, Price RN. New antimalarials—a risk-benefit analysis. Drug Saf 1995;12:264—73.

4. Phillips-Howard PA, Wood D. The safety of antimalarial drugs in pregnancy. Drug Saf 1996;14:131—45.

5. Watkins WM, Mosobo M. Treatment of *Plasmodium falciparum* malaria with pyrimethamine-sulfadoxine-selective pressure for resistance is a function of long elimination half-life. Trans R Soc Trop Med Hyg 1993;87:75—8.

6. Ringwald P, Bickii J, Basco L. Randomized trial of pyronaridine versus chloroquine for acute uncomplicated falciparum malaria in Africa. Lancet 1996;347:24—8.

7. Winstanley P. Pyronaridine—a promising drug for Africa. Lancet 1996;347:2—3.

8. Radloff PD, Philipps J, Nkeyi M, Hutchinson D, Kremsner PG. Atovaquone and proguanil for *Plasmodium falciparum* malaria. Lancet 1996;347:1511—4.

9. White NJ, editor. Artemisinin: proceedings of a meeting convened by the Wellcome Trust on 25—27 April 1993. Trans R Soc Trop Med Hyg 1994;88:S1—S65.

10. Murphy S, English M, Waruiru C, Mwangi I, Amukoye E, Crawley J, Newton C, Winstanley P, Peshu N, Marsh K. An open randomized trial of artemether versus quinine in the treatment of cerebral malaria in African children. Trans R Soc Trop Med Hyg 1996;90:298—301.

11. Vanhensbroek MB, Onyiorah E, Jaffar S, Schneider G, Palmer A, Frenkel J, Enwere G, Forck S, Nusmeijer A, Bennett S, Greenwood B, Kwiatkowski D. A trial of artemether or quinine in children with cerebral malaria. New Engl J Med 1996;335:69—75.

12. Hien TT, Day NPJ, Phu NH, Mai NTH, Chau TTH, Loc PP, Sinh DX, Chuong LV, Vinh H, Waller D, Peto TEA, White NJ. A controlled trial of artemether or quinine in Vietnamese adults with severe falciparum malaria. New Engl J Med 1996;335:76—83.

13. Brewer TG, Peggins JO, Grate SJ, Petras JM, Levine BS, Weina PJ, Swearengen J, Heiffer MH, Schuster BG. Neurotoxicity in animals due to arteether and artemether. Trans R Soc Trop Med Hyg 1994;88:33—6.

14. Fishwick J, McLean WG, Edward G, Ward SA. The toxicity of artemisinin and related compounds on neuronal and glial cells in culture. Chem-Biol Interact 1995;96:263—71.

15. Wesche DL, Decoster MA, Tortella FC, Brewer TG. Neurotoxicity of artemisinin analogs in vitro. Antimicrob Agents Chemother 1994;38:1813—19.

16. Chiodini PL, Conlon CP, Hutchinson DBA, Farquhar JA, Hall AP, Peto TEA, Birley H, Warrell DA. Evaluation of atovaquone in the treatment of patients with uncomplicated plasmodium-falciparum malaria. J Antimicrob Chemother 1995;36:1073—8.

17. Olliaro P, Nevill C, Lebras J, Ringwald P, Mussano P, Garner P, Brasseur P. Systematic review of amodiaquine treatment in uncomplicated malaria. Lancet 1996;348:1196—201.

18. Nevill CG, Verhoeff FH, Munafu CG, Tenhove WR, Vanderkaay HJ, Were JBO. A comparison of amodiaquine and chloroquine in the treatment therapy of falciparum malaria in Kenya. East Afr Med J 1994;71:167—70.

19. Karbwang J, Bangchang KN. Clinical pharmacokinetics of halofantrine. Clin Pharmacokin 1994;27:104—19.

20. Watt G, Loesuttiviboon L, Jongsakul K, Shanks GD, Ohrt CK, Karnasuta C, Schuster B, Fleckenstein L. Efficacy and tolerance of extended-dose halofantrine for drug-resistant falciparum malaria in Thailand. Am J Trop Med Hyg 1994;50:187—92.

21. Nevill CG, Lury JD, Mosobo MK, Watkins HM, Watkins WM. Daily chlorproguanil is an effective alternative to daily proguanil in the prevention of *Plasmodium falciparum* malaria in Kenya. Trans R Soc Trop Med Hyg 1994;88:319—20.

22. Bonington A, Davidson RN, Winstanley PA, Pasvol G. Fatal quinine cardiotoxicity in the treatment of falciparum malaria. Trans R Soc Trop Med Hyg 1996;90:305—7.

23. Bethell DB, Phuong PT, Phuong CXT, Nosten F, Waller D, Davis TME, Day NPJ, Crawley J, Brewster D, Pukrittayakamee S, White NJ. Electrocardiographic monitoring in severe falciparum malaria. Trans R Soc Trop Med Hyg 1996;90:266—9.

24. Bhavnani SM, Preston SL. Monitoring of intravenous quinidine infusion in the treatment of *Plasmodium falciparum* malaria. Ann Pharmacother 1995;29:33—5.

25. Alloway JA, Salata MP. Quinidine-induced rheumatic syndromes. Semin Arthritis Rheum 1995;24:315—22.

26. Vanhensbroek MB, Kwiatkowski D, Vandenberg B, Hoek FJ, Van Boxtel CJ, Kager PA. Quinine pharmacokinetics in young children with severe malaria. Am J Trop Med Hyg 1996;54:237—42.

27. Jacqzaigrain E, Bennasr S, Desplanques L, Peralma A, Beaufils F. Quinine overdose in children. Arch Ped 1994;1:14—19.

28. Luxemburger C, Terkuile FO, Nosten F, Dolan G, Bradol JH, Phaipun L, Chongsuphajaisiddhi T, White NJ. Single day mefloquine-artesunate combination in the treatment of multidrug-

resistant falciparum malaria. Trans R Soc Trop Med Hyg 1994;88:213−7.

29. Winstanley P. Mefloquine—the benefits outweigh the risks. Br J Clin Pharmacol 1996; 42:411−3.

30. Phillips-Howard PA, Terkuile FO. CNS adverse events associated with antimalarial agents—fact or fiction. Drug Saf 1995;12:370−83.

31. Shanks GD, Barnett A, Edstein MD, Rieckmann KH. Effectiveness of doxycycline combined with primaquine for malaria prophylaxis. Med J Aust 1995;162:306.

32. Shanks D, Roessler P, Edstein MD, Rieckmann KH. Doxycycline for malaria prophylaxis in australian soldiers deployed to United Nations missions in Somalia and Cambodia. Mil Med 1995;160:443−5.

33. Jarvinen A, Nykanen S, Paasiniemi L, Hirsjarvilahti T, Mattila J. Enteric coating reduces upper gastrointestinal adverse reactions to doxycycline. Clin Drug Invest 1995;10:323−7.

34. Leport C, Chene G, Morlat P, Luft BJ, Rousseau F, Pueyo S, Hafner R, Miro J, Aubertin J, Salamon R, Vilde JL, Blanc AP, Schmitt JL, Arlaud J, Estavoyer JM. Pyrimethamine for primary prophylaxis of toxoplasmic encephalitis in patients with human-immunodeficiency-virus infection—a double-blind, randomized trial. J Infect Dis 1996;173:91−7.

35. Jacobson MA, Besch CL, Child C, Hafner R, Matts JP, Muth K, Wentworth DN, Neaton JD, Abrams D, Rimland D, Perez G, Grant IH, Saravolatz LD, Brown LS, Deyton L. Primary prophylaxis with pyrimethamine for toxoplasmic encephalitis in patients with advanced human-immunodeficiency-virus disease—results of a randomized trial. J Infect Dis 1994;169:384−94.

36. Behbahani R, Moshfeghi M, Baxter JD. Therapeutic approaches for AIDS-related toxoplasmosis. Ann Pharmacother 1995;29:760−8.

37. Hoover DR. The effects of long-term zidovudine therapy and *Pneumocystis carinii* on HIV disease—a review of the literature. Drugs 1995; 49:20−36.

38. Bozzette SA, Finkelstein DM, Spector SA, Frame P, Powderly WG, He WL, Phillips L, Craven D, Vanderhorst C, Feinberg J. A randomized trial of 3 antipneumocystis agents in patients with advanced human-immunodeficiency-virus infection. New Engl J Med 1995;332:693−9.

39. Nielsen TL, Jensen BN, Nelsing S, Mathiesen LR, Skinhoj P, Nielsen JO. Randomized study of sulfamethoxazole-trimethoprim versus aerosolized pentamidine for secondary prophylaxis of *Pneumocystis carinii* pneumonia in patients with AIDS. Scand J Infect Dis 1995;27:217−20.

40. Antinori A, Murri R, Ammassari A, Deluca A, Lanzalone A, Cingolani A, Damiano F, Maiuro G, Vecchiet J, Scoppettuolo G, Tamburrini E, Ortona L. Aerosolized pentamidine, cotrimoxazole and dapsone pyrimethamine for primary prophylaxis of *Pneumocystis carinii* pneumonia

and toxoplasmic encephalitis. AIDS 1995; 9:1343−50.

41. Montgomery AB, Feigal DW, Sattler F, Mason GR, Catanzaro A, Edison R, Markowitz N, Johnson E, Ogawa S, Rovzar M, Udem SA, Eden E, Hyslop N, Cheung TW, Kessler H, Mildvan D, Giron JA, Ettinger N, Crumpacker C, Frame P, Steigbigel N, Vanderhorst C, Hirsch M, Lederman MM, Hewitt RG, Fallat R, Farber HW, Sacks HS, Eisman SA, Luce JM, Boylan T, Adams M, Feinberg J, Hopewell PC. Pentamidine aerosol versus trimethoprim-sulfamethoxazole for *Pneumocystis carinii* in acquired-immune-deficiency-syndrome. Am J Respir Crit Care Med 1995;151:1068−74.

42. Schneider MME, Nielsen TL, Nelsing S, Hoepelman AIM, Schattenkerk JKME, Vandergraaf Y, Kolsters AFP, Borleffs JCC, Danner SA, Vanleeuwen R, Frissen JPHJ, Weigel HM, Vanderende IME, Sprenger HG, Kauffmann RH, Kroon F, Meenhorst PL, Tennapel CHH, Schreij G, Tenkate RW, Juttmann JR, Koopmans PP. Efficacy and toxicity of 2 doses of trimethoprim-sulfamethoxazole as primary prophylaxis against *Pneumocystis carinii* pneumonia in patients with human-immunodeficiency-virus. J Infect Dis 1995;171:1632−6.

43. Joos B, Blaser J, Opravil M, Chave JP, Luthy R. Monitoring of cotrimoxazole concentrations in serum during treatment of *Pneumocystis carinii* pneumonia. Antimicrob Agents Chemother 1995;39:2661−6.

44. Hughes WT. The role of atovaquone tablets in treating *Pneumocystis carinii* pneumonia. J AIDS Hum Retrovirol 1995;8:247−52.

45. Spencer CM, Goa KL. Atovaquone—a review of its pharmacological properties and therapeutic efficacy in opportunistic infections. Drugs 1995;50:176−96.

46. Hughes WT, Lafon SW, Scott JD, Masur H. Adverse events associated with trimethoprim-sulfamethoxazole and atovaquone during the treatment of AIDS-related *Pneumocystis carinii* pneumonia. J Infect Dis 1995;171:1295−301.

47. White A, Lafon S, Rogers M, Andrews E, Brown N. Clinical experience with atovaquone on a treatment investigational new drug protocol for *Pneumocystis carinii* pneumonia. J AIDS Hum Retrovirol 1995;9:280−5.

48. Anonymous. Atovaquone and trimetrexate: useful second-line treatments for PCP. Drugs Ther Perspect 1995;6:1−5.

49. May JR, Williams DB. Formulary considerations for AIDS-associated illnesses: a focus on atovaquone. P and T 1995;20:283−92.

50. Cappell MS, Marks M. Acute pancreatitis in HIV-seropositive patients—a case-control study of 44 patients. Am J Med 1995;98:243−8.

51. Koopmans PP, Vanderven AJAM, Vree TB, Vandermeer JWM. Pathogenesis of hypersensitivity reactions to drugs in patients with HIV-infection-allergic or toxic. AIDS 1995;9:217−22.

52. Vanderven AJM, Koopmans PP, Vree TB,

Vandermeer JWM. Drug intolerance in HIV disease. J Antimicrob Chemother 1994;34:1—5.

53. Pirmohamed M, Park BK. Drug reactions in HIV infected patients. Postgrad Doctor 1995; 18:438—44.

54. Roujeau J-C, Kelly JP, Naldi L, Rzany B, Stern RS, Anderson T, Auquier A, Bastuji-Garin S, Correia O, Locati F, Mockenhaupt M, Paoletti C, Shapiro S, Shear N, Schopf E, Kaufman DW. Medication use and the risk of Stevens-Johnson syndrome or toxic epidermal necrolysis. New Engl J Med 1995;333:1600—7.

55. Anonymous. Revised indications for co-trimoxazole (Septrin, Bactrim, various generic preparations). Curr Probl Pharmacovig 1995;21:6.

56. Anonymous. Co-trimoxazole use restricted. Drug Ther Bull 1995;33:92—3.

57. Maurihellweg D, Bettens F, Mauri D, Brander C, Hunziker T, Pichler WJ. Activation of drug-specific CD4(+) and CD8(+) T-cells in individuals allergic to sulfonamides, phenytoin, and carbamazepine. J Immunol 1995;155:462—72.

58. Hertl M, Jugert F, Merk HF. CD8(+) dermal T-cells from a sulfamethoxazole-induced bullous exanthem proliferate in response to drug-modified liver-microsomes. Br J Dermatol 1995;132:215—20.

59. Klein CE, Trautmann A, Zillikens D, Brocker EB. Patch testing in an unusual case of toxic epidermal necrolysis. Contact Dermatitis 1995; 33:448—9.

60. Hennessy S, Strom BL, Berlin JA, Brennan PJ. Predicting cutaneous hypersensitivity reactions to cotrimoxazole in HIV-infected individuals receiving primary Pneumocystis carinii pneumonia prophylaxis. J Gen Intern Med 1995; 10:380—6.

61. Kennedy CA, Pimentel JA, Lewis DE, Anderson MD, Weiss PJ, Oldfield PC. Crossover of human immunodeficiency virus-infected patients from aerosolized pentamidine to trimethoprim-sulfamethoxazole: lack of hematologic toxicity and a relationship of side effects to CD4+ lymphocyte count. J Infect Dis 1993;168:314—7.

62. Carr A, Swanson C, Penny R, Cooper DA. Clinical and laboratory markers of hypersensitivity to trimethoprim-sulfamethoxazole in patients with Pneumocystis carinii pneumonia and AIDS. J Infect Dis 1993;167:180—5.

63. Daftarian MP, Filion LG, Cameron W, Conway B, Roy R, Tropper F, Diaz-Mitoma F. Immune response to sulfamethoxazole in patients with AIDS. Clin Diagn Lab Immunol 1995; 2:199—204.

64. Bachmeyer C, Salmon D, Guerin C, Barre C, Hazebroucq G, Sicard D, Sereni D. Trimethoprim-sulfamethoxazole desensitization in HIV-infected patients—an open study. AIDS 1995; 9:299—300.

65. Moreno JN, Poblete RB, Maggio C, Gagnon S, Fischl MA. Rapid oral desensitization for sulfonamides in patients with the acquired-immuno-deficiency-syndrome. Ann Allergy Asthma Immunol 1995;74:140—6.

66. Bissuel F, Cotte L, Crapanne JB, Rougier P, Schlienger I, Trepo C. Trimethoprim-sulfamethoxazole rechallenge in 20 previously allergic HIV-infected patients after homeopathic desensitization. AIDS 1995;9:407—8.

67. Gluckstein D, Ruskin J. Rapid oral desensitization to trimethoprim-sulfamethoxazole (TMP-SMZ)-use in prophylaxis for Pneumocystis carinii pneumonia in patients with AIDS who were previously intolerant to TMP-SMZ. Clin Infect Dis 1995;20:849—53.

68. Nguyen MT, Weiss PJ, Wallace MR. 2-day oral desensitization to trimethoprim-sulfamethoxazole in HIV-infected patients. AIDS 1995; 9:573—5.

69. Rudin C, Gunthard J, Zumsteg U. Successful desensitization to trimethoprim-sulfamethoxazole in a young infant with AIDS. Pediatr AIDS HIV Infect 1995;6:212—4.

70. Reinke CM, Thomas JK, Graves AH. Apparent hemolysis in an AIDS patient receiving trimethoprim/sulfamethoxazole: case report and literature review. J Pharm Technol 1995;11:252—62.

71. Eck H-P, Gmunder H, Hartmann M, Petzoldt D, Daniel V, Droge W. Low concentrations of acid-soluble thiol (cysteine) in the plasma of HIV-1 infected patients. Biol Chem Hoppe-Seyler 1989;370:101—8.

72. Buhl R, Holroyd KJ, Mastrangeli A, Cantin AM, Jaffe HA, Wells FB, Saltini C, Crystal RG. Systemic glutathione deficiency in symptom-free HIV-seropositive individuals. Lancet 1989;2: 1294—8.

73. de Quay B, Malinverni R, Lauterburg BH. Glutathione depletion in HIV-infected patients: role of cysteine deficiency and effect of oral N-acetylcysteine. AIDS 1992;6:815—9.

74. Staal FJT, Ela SW, Roederer M, Anderson MT, Herzenberg LA, Herzenberg LA. Glutathione deficiency and human immunodeficiency virus infection. Lancet 1992;339:909—12.

75. Staal FJT, Roederer M, Israelski DM, Bubp J, Mole LA, McShane D, Deresinski SC, Ross W, Sussman H, Raju PA, Anderson MT, Moore W, Ela SW, Herzenberg LA, Herzenberg LA. Intracellular glutathione levels in T-cell subsets decrease in HIV-infected individuals. AIDS Res Hum Retroviruses 1992;8:305—11.

76. Aukrust P, Svardal AM, Muller F, Lunden B, Berge RK, Ueland PM, Froland SS. Increased levels of oxidized glutathione in CD4+ lymphocytes associated with disturbed intracellular redox balance in human immunodeficiency virus type 1 infection. Blood 1995;86:258—67.

77. Pirmohamed M, Williams D, Tingle MD, Barry M, Khoo SH, O'Mahony C, Wilkins EGL, Breckenridge AM, Park BK. Intracellular glutathione in the peripheral blood cells of HIV-infected patients: failure to show a deficiency. AIDS 1996;10:501—7.

78. Coronado BE, Opal SM, Yoburn DC. Antibiotic-induced C-lactic acidosis. Ann Intern Med 1995;122:839—42.

29 Antiviral drugs

COMPOUNDS ACTIVE AGAINST DNA VIRUSES

Acyclovir *(SED-13, 872; SEDA-17, 337; SEDA-18, 299; SEDA-19, 273)*

In an open study of the efficacy of acyclovir in the treatment of adult varicella, 148 patients were treated with high-dose oral acyclovir (800 mg five times daily for 7 days). The most common adverse effect in this group (in 35% of patients) was mild *diarrhea* lasting one to four days. Other adverse reactions included *generalized urticaria* in one patient, resolving within 2 days after withdrawal, *vomiting* in three patients, and *abdominal pain, bloating,* and *nausea* in another three (1[c]).

Skin and appendages A case of possible acyclovir-induced *Stevens-Johnson* syndrome has been reported (2[C]).

A 41-year-old man infected with HIV-1 started to take oral acyclovir (400 mg bd) at his own request, because of reports claiming improved survival in HIV-infected patients taking acyclovir. During the year before presentation he had also been taking isoniazid (900 mg twice weekly) and rifampicin (600 mg twice weekly) for pulmonary tuberculosis, and co-trimoxazole (one tablet od) for *Pneumocystis carinii* pneumonia prophylaxis. In addition, he had taken fluconazole (100 mg od) for 4 months for oral candidiasis. One day after starting acyclovir he developed Stevens-Johnson syndrome, characterized by fever, necrotizing cutaneous macules over the face, trunk, and extremities, and mucosal involvement in the mouth. In addition, he developed a transient increase in the blood urea nitrogen concentration with proteinuria and microscopic hematuria, suggestive of accompanying glomerulonephritis. He recovered completely after withdrawal of all drugs. Acid-fast bacilli were found in the sputum, and he was given six antituberculous drugs, including isoniazid and rifampicin, without recurrence of the skin rash. Nor was there recurrence with subsequent rechallenge with co-trimox-

azole and fluconazole. Treatment with acyclovir was not restarted because it was believed to carry an unacceptable risk.

While Stevens–Johnson syndrome in this case may have been associated with one of the other drugs, or with the tuberculosis, the authors concluded that the temporal sequence of events after administration of acyclovir, the clinical improvement following withdrawal, and the lack of recurrence after reintroduction of all other previous medications, strongly suggested that it was associated with acyclovir.

Hematological A case of acyclovir-induced *neutropenia* has been reported in an infant treated with acyclovir for *Herpes simplex* encephalitis (3[CR]). The infant had repeated episodes of neutropenia while receiving intravenous or oral acyclovir (30 mg/kg/day), with improvement after withdrawal. Reintroduction of therapy, because of relapsing manifestations of *Herpes simplex* infection, repeatedly resulted in recurrence of neutropenia. The neutropenia did not recur after dosage reduction of oral acyclovir to 10 mg/kg/day.

Famciclovir *(SEDA-19, 273)*

Famciclovir is an oral form of penciclovir, a selective antiviral agent with activity against *Varicella zoster* virus, *Herpes simplex* virus types 1 and 2, and Epstein-Barr virus. After oral administration, famciclovir is well-absorbed (systemic availability 77%), with little intersubject variability, and is rapidly converted to penciclovir. This compares favorably with acyclovir, the absorption of which after oral administration is slow and incomplete, with a highly variable systemic availability of only 10–20%.

An integrated safety analysis of 1607 patients who had taken famciclovir for the treatment of *Herpes zoster* or genital herpes in clinical trials has shown that famciclovir is extremely well tolerated, with an adverse events profile similar to placebo (4[R]). *Headache, nausea*, and *diarrhea* were the most frequently reported adverse events in those taking both famciclovir and placebo. No laboratory abnormalities were consistently associated with famciclovir.

Sexual function Prolonged administration of high dosages of famciclovir has been associated with reversible, dose-dependent adverse effects on testicular function in rats and dogs. However, in a double-blind placebo-controlled trial in which 34 men with recurrent genital herpes took famciclovir 250 mg bd for 18 weeks, there were no significant effects on sperm production or function (5[r]).

Foscarnet *(SED-13, 873; SEDA-17, 338; SEDA-18, 300; SEDA-19, 274)*

Like ganciclovir, foscarnet is being used extensively for the treatment of cytomegalovirus infections, both in patients with AIDS and in other immunosuppressed patients. Its main treatment-limiting effects are *nephrotoxicity, abnormalities of ionized calcium*, and *penile ulceration*. An excellent review of the current management of cytomegalovirus disease in patients with AIDS, including the management of antiviral drug-related toxicity, has recently appeared (6[R]).

Ganciclovir *(SED-13, 873; SEDA-17, 339; SEDA-18, 301; SEDA-19, 275)*

Ganciclovir (dihydropropoxymethylguanine, DHPG) is a nucleoside analogue with activity against viruses of the herpes group. Together with foscarnet, it currently remains the mainstay of treatment for patients with cytomegalovirus (CMV) infection. An excellent review of the current management of cytomegalovirus disease in patients with AIDS, including the management of antiviral drug-related toxicity, has recently appeared (6[R]).

Neutropenia remains the major dose-limiting toxic effect of ganciclovir, and an absolute neutrophil count of below $500 \times 10^6/l$ occurs in over 15% of AIDS patients treated with monotherapy ganciclovir for CMV retinitis. The addition of granulocyte-macrophage col-

ony stimulating factor (GM-CSF, molgramostim) to standard ganciclovir monotherapy for HIV-related CMV retinitis reduces its hematological toxicity and allows closer adherence to the dosage schedule (7[C]). This approach had the additional advantage of allowing patients to take zidovudine concomitantly.

Although a small randomized study of concurrent or alternating combination therapy with ganciclovir and foscarnet for CMV retinitis in AIDS has provided evidence for greater antiviral and possibly clinical efficacy than historically known for either drug alone, severe neutropenia (absolute neutrophil count below $500 \times 10^6/l$) was observed in 32 patients (38%) (8[C]). This was more pronounced in those taking concurrent combination therapy (62%) than in those taking alternating treatment (19%). The neutropenia was easily controlled with adjunctive molgramostim.

In patients with HIV infection intravenous and oral ganciclovir have been compared for maintenance therapy of CMV retinitis, following successful induction therapy with intravenous ganciclovir (9[c]), (10[c]). Although not statistically significant, the incidence of severe neutropenia (absolute neutrophil count below $500 \times 10^6/l$) was higher in patients treated intravenously. In one study, anemia was significantly more frequent in patients on intravenous ganciclovir (9[c]). Sepsis was less frequent in the orally treated patients, which is what one would have expected, in view of the absence of permanent intravenous access in these patients.

In patients undergoing heart or liver transplantation, the prophylactic intravenous administration of ganciclovir for 4 or more weeks after transplantation has in general resulted in a reduced incidence of CMV disease. Tolerance has been acceptable, neutropenia being the most common toxic effect (11[c])−(13[c]). In the setting of bone-marrow transplantation, a strategy of pre-emptive therapy with ganciclovir (rather than prophylaxis) may shorten the duration of use of ganciclovir and thereby reduce the incidence of neutropenia. Pre-emptive therapy targets treatment at those patients who have evidence of active CMV replication, by demonstrating the presence of viral antigen in the blood or, more recently, viral DNA by polymerase chain reaction (14[c]), (15[r]).

Cidofovir

Cidofovir ([S]-1-[3-hydroxy-2-phosphonyl-methoxypropyl] cytosine), also known as HPMPC, is an acyclic nucleoside analogue with potent anti-CMV activity in vitro and in vivo. In patients with HIV infection it has been used for the treatment of CMV retinitis by both intraocular and intravenous administration. Intravitreal administration, although efficacious, may be associated with the development of *ocular hypotony* (decreased intraocular pressure) or *vitreitis* (16[c]). Cidofovir is eliminated via the kidneys, and the main toxic effect associated with intravenous administration is *nephrotoxicity*, which may be prevented by adequate hydration in conjunction with the preventive use of probenecid (17[R]).

Ribavirin *(SED-13, 876; SEDA-17, 339; SEDA-18, 301; SEDA-19, 275)*

Ribavirin is generally well tolerated. The only major toxic effect reported thus far is *hemolytic anemia*, which is generally mild and reversible on withdrawal.

Combination therapy with interferon-α and ribavirin has shown promise in 50 patients with hepatitis C infection refractory to or relapsing after monotherapy with interferon-α alone. Mild anemia, usually not necessitating dosage reduction of ribavirin, was seen in most patients during the 6 months of treatment (18[c]), (19[c]). The same was true in a pilot study of ribavirin monotherapy for 4 weeks in 24 patients with chronic active hepatitis B infection (20[c]).

COMPOUNDS ACTIVE AGAINST RNA VIRUSES

Didanosine (2′,3′-dideoxyinosine, ddI) *(SED-13, 875; SEDA-17, 340; SEDA-18, 302; SEDA-19, 276)*

The major toxic effects of didanosine are *pancreatic damage* and *peripheral neuropathy*, both clearly dose-related, as evidenced by two comparisons of the efficacy of high-dosage treatment (750 mg/day for patients over 60 kg) and low-dosage treatment (200 mg/day for patients under 60 kg) in late-stage HIV-infected people who were intolerant to or who progressed on zidovudine (21[cR]), (22[cR]). While there were no differences in survival or disease progression rates between the two dosages, both studies clearly showed increased incidences of pancreatitis (in some cases with a fatal outcome) and peripheral neuropathy in the high-dosage groups.

Lamivudine (2′-deoxy-3′-thiacytidine, 3TC) *(SED-13, 876; SEDA-19, 276)* Lamivudine is a nucleoside analogue, an inhibitor of HIV reverse transcriptase, which is used for the treatment of HIV infection in combination with other antiretroviral agents. Compared with most other nucleoside analogues, lamivudine is remarkably well tolerated. Its safety has been confirmed in a placebo-controlled, randomized comparison of the efficacy of lamivudine (150—300 mg bd) and zidovudine (200 mg tds) either alone or in combination in the treatment of HIV-1 infection in 366 patients (23[cR]). While all treatment regimens were generally well tolerated, gastrointestinal symptoms, most notably *nausea*, were the most common adverse reactions observed, although they were more frequent in those taking zidovudine. *Headache* was the second most common adverse effect, evenly distributed over the treatment groups. *Peripheral neuropathy* requiring dosage interruption was reported in one patient taking lamivudine. Hematological toxicity was not observed in patients taking lamivudine alone.

In a study of the efficacy of lamivudine (25, 100, or 300 mg/day for 12 weeks) in the treatment of chronic hepatitis B virus infections, lamivudine was similarly well tolerated in 32 patients (24[cR]). Only minor non-specific non-dose-related adverse reactions were observed. In addition, there were mild asymptomatic increases in serum levels of amylase, lipase, and creatine kinase, which in most cases resolved despite continuation of therapy. Treatment was interrupted in one patient taking the 25-mg dose, because of an abrupt increase in transaminases. A liver biopsy showed no changes compared with pre-treatment histology. Follow-up after withdrawal was not reported.

Ritonavir

Ritonavir is an inhibitor of the HIV-encoded proteinase, which has been licensed by the FDA for the treatment of HIV infections. The safety and efficacy of monotherapy with ritonavir (600—1200 mg/day) have been evaluated in two preliminary studies in 62 and 87 patients (25[cr]), (26[cr]). Ritonavir had potent antiretroviral effects, as shown by substantial reductions in plasma viremia and increases in CD4+ lymphocyte counts.

In these studies, the most common adverse events attributed to ritonavir were *nausea, diarrhea, headache, circumoral paresthesia,* and *altered taste sensation.* These effects were tolerated in most cases, requiring withdrawal in only a few patients. Laboratory abnormalities included reversible increases in hepatic transaminases, mainly during the first weeks of treatment, requiring withdrawal in some patients. In addition, there were frequent increases in triglyceride concentrations, and to a lesser extent cholesterol concentrations, persisting throughout the 32-week study period. In all cases, the ritonavir-related hypertriglyceridemia was asymptomatic and not associated with evidence of pancreatitis. Both laboratory abnormalities appeared to occur more frequently at the highest dosages (800—1200 mg/day). While the maximum tolerated dosage of ritonavir was determined in neither study, the authors of one of the studies concluded that nausea and of increases in hepatic transaminase concentrations suggested that the dosage of 600 mg bd approaches the maximum (26[cr]).

Rimantadine *(SED-13, 874; SEDA-18, 301)*

Rimantadine hydrochloride is the α-methyl derivative of amantadine. It is available as an alternative to amantadine for the prevention and treatment of influenza A virus infection in adults and for the prevention of influenza in children. Its major advantage is a lower risk of central nervous system effects, such as *light-headedness, difficulty in concentrating, nervousness,* and *insomnia,* which can be a significant problem with amantadine, particularly in older patients. An extensive review of the English-language literature published in 1966—94 has recently appeared and has confirmed that the most common adverse effects of rimantadine are on the central nervous system and the gastrointestinal tract (27[R]). Nervous system effects such as *dizziness, insomnia, depression, anxiety, irritability,* and *hallucinations* occurred in 3.2% of 439 children younger than 10 years of age and in 8.4% of 323 adults. In 598 elderly patients, nervous system adverse effects were more common with higher dosages (4.9% at 100 mg/day to 12.5% at 200 mg/day). Gastrointestinal effects, including *nausea, loss of appetite, diarrhea,* and *dry mouth,* occurred in 8.4% of children below 10 years of age, in 3.1% of adults, and in 2.9% of elderly patients taking 100 mg/day and 17.0% taking 200 mg/day (27[R]).

Saquinavir *(SEDA-19, 278)*

Saquinavir mesylate belongs to a new class of drugs (HIV-proteinase inhibitors) that have been developed for treating HIV infection. The HIV-encoded proteinase that they inhibit is responsible for cleaving the viral gag-pol precursor polyproteins into smaller viral structural proteins, necessary for the formation of mature and infectious viral particles. HIV-proteinase inhibition thus results in the formation of immature and non-infectious viral particles. As this effect occurs at a step in the virus life-cycle that occurs after integration of the HIV genome into the genome of the host-cell, HIV-proteinase inhibitors, unlike nucleoside analogues, are also active against chronically HIV-infected cells. A major drawback of the currently available formulation of saquinavir is its poor oral systemic availability (around 4%).

Preliminary results from three small European double-blind clinical trials and one larger American trial (AIDS Clinical Trials Group protocol 229) have been reported (28[r]). In the European studies the antiviral activity and immunological effects of saquinavir were evaluated in patients with early, intermediate, and advanced HIV-1 infection. In two of the studies, conducted in the UK and France, patients were randomized to various dosages of saquinavir monotherapy, whereas in the third study, conducted in Italy, treatment arms were included in which saquinavir and zidovudine were combined. In the UK study 49 antiretroviral-naive patients with few or no symptoms and CD4 cell counts below 500 × 106/l were randomized to receive 25, 75, 200, or 600 mg of saquinavir tds for 16 weeks (29ᶜ). Saquinavir was well tolerated; adverse events, including changes in laboratory measurements, were mild and most were thought to be unrelated to treatment. Based on the CD4-cell responses observed in these three studies, the best dose of saquinavir (600 mg tds) was selected for future trials, including the US AIDS Clinical Trials Group (ACTG) protocol number 229. In this randomized, double-blind, placebo-controlled phase II study, 302 patients with a CD4 cell count of 50—300 × 10⁶/l who had taken zidovudine for at least 4 months before were randomized to treatment with zidovudine (600 mg/day) plus zalcitabine (2.25 mg/day), zidovudine plus saquinavir (1800 mg/day), or triple therapy with zidovudine, zalcitabine, and saquinavir for 24 weeks, with the option of extending blinded treatment for another 12—32 weeks (30ᶜ). The three treatments were tolerated equally well, without evidence of any particular saquinavir-attributable adverse effects.

Stavudine (2′,3′-didehydro-3′-deoxythymidine, D4T)

The pyrimidine nucleoside analogue stavudine has been approved by the FDA for the treatment of HIV-1 infection in adults who have clinical progression or immunological deterioration while taking zidovudine, didanosine, or zalcitabine, or who are intolerant of these drugs. The approved dosage is 1.0 mg/kg/day.

Nervous system   The principal toxic effect of stavudine is *peripheral neuropathy*, with symptoms similar to the neuropathy associated with didanosine and zalcitabine (31ᴿ), (32ᴿ). Neuropathy has been reported to occur at 1—66 weeks after the start of therapy. While it seems to occur at all doses from 0.1 to 12.0 mg/kg/day, the frequency of neuropathy rises with increasing dosages: in phase I studies, dose-limiting peripheral neuropathy occurred in 23% of those taking 0.5—1.0 mg/kg/day, 53% at a dosage of 2.0 mg/kg/day, and 67% at dosages of 4.0—12.0 mg/kg/day.

In addition, the development of neuropathy seems to depend on the duration of treatment, with an increasing risk after 12 weeks of treatment. A prior history of neuropathy increases the risk of stavudine-induced neuropathy. After withdrawal, the symptoms usually resolve within 2 weeks, although they may persist for several months. In phase I and II trials, about half of the patients with neuropathy were able to tolerate prolonged treatment at a reduced dose.

Hematological   Modest dose-related *macrocytosis* without associated anemia may occur during treatment with stavudine (31ᴿ), (32ᴿ). *Anemia, neutropenia*, or *thrombocytopenia* have been reported in small numbers of patients taking stavudine, and there is no evidence that these abnormalities are dose-related.

Liver   Asymptomatic increases in hepatic transaminases, which are not clearly dose-related, may occur during treatment with stavudine, requiring dosage modification because of moderate or severe toxicity in about 10% of patients (31ᴿ), (32ᴿ).

Zalcitabine (dideoxycytidine, ddC) *(SED-13, 876; SEDA-17, 342; SEDA-18, 302)*

The most important adverse effect of zalcitabine is *peripheral neuropathy*. Patients with low baseline cobalamin concentrations, a history of heavy ethanol consumption, or a history of symptoms of peripheral nerve dysfunction are more likely to develop neuropathy during zalcitabine therapy (33ᴿ). These factors may be useful in distinguishing patients at higher risk of this adverse effect.

Zidovudine (AZT) *(SED-13, 875; SEDA-17, 343; SEDA-18, 303; SEDA-19, 278)*

Cardiovascular   A retrospective study in 137 children aged 4 months to 7 years has suggested that treatment of HIV-infected children with zidovudine may be associated with *cardiomyopathy* (34ᶜ). On average, children treated with zidovudine had reduced left ventricular function. Cardiomyopathy was 8.4 (95% CI 1.7—42) times more likely to develop in children who had previously used zidovudine than in children who had never been exposed to it. On the basis of these findings, it may be concluded that serial cardiac examination is warranted in children receiving zidovudine.

Hematological The most important dose-limiting adverse effects of zidovudine are hematological complications, including *macrocytic anemia* and *neutropenia*. A randomized study has shown that supplementation with vitamin B_{12} and folinic acid does not prevent or reduce zidovudine-induced myelosuppression (35^{CR}). While recombinant erythropoietin is useful in correcting zidovudine-induced anemia, some cases of anemia are associated with high serum erythropoietin concentrations and normocytic cells, indicating bone-marrow unresponsiveness to erythropoietin (36^R). Measuring baseline serum erythropoietin concentrations may help to predict the response to this very costly hormone supplementation.

Liver Another case of presumed zidovudine-induced massive *hepatic steatosis* and *lactic acidosis* with a fatal outcome has been reported in a 35-year-old woman (37^{CR}). Ultrastructural studies of the liver showed no morphological changes other than modest mitochondrial enlargement, suggesting mito-

chondrial toxicity. Since the patient was also taking long-term fluconazole, it is possible that an interaction between zidovudine and fluconazole, rather than zidovudine alone, may have been responsible.

Musculoskeletal Zidovudine-induced *myopathy* has been discussed previously (SEDA-14, 254; SEDA-15, 321; SEDA 18, 303; SEDA-19, 278), including the possible pathogenetic mechanisms. Histological, ultrastructural, biochemical, and molecular studies have suggested that the zidovudine-induced myopathy is caused by mitochondrial toxicity. Phosphorus magnetic resonance spectroscopy has been used to study the changes in phosphorylated metabolites (ATP, phosphocreatine, and inorganic phosphate) during exercise in 19 healthy volunteers, six untreated HIV-positive individuals, and nine zidovudine-treated patients with biopsy-proven myopathy (38^{CR}). Zidovudine altered the normal muscle energy metabolism in the patients with myopathy, suggesting that it reduces the maximal work output, and thus the maximal rate of mitochondrial ATP synthesis, in human muscle. In addition to the direct mitochondrial toxicity of zidovudine, it has been suggested that muscle damage may also be related to zidovudine-induced vascular dysfunction and resulting chronic muscle ischemia (39^{CR}).

REFERENCES

1. Choo DCA, Chew SK, Tan EH, Lim MK, Monteiro EH. Oral acyclovir in the treatment of adult varicella. Ann Acad Med Singapore 1995;24:316—21.

2. Fazal BA, Turett GS, Justman JE, Hall G, Telzak EE. Stevens-Johnson syndrome induced by treatment with acyclovir. Clin Infect Dis 1995;21:1038—1039.

3. Feder HM, Goyal RK, Krause PJ. Acyclovir-induced neutropenia in an infant with herpes simplex encephalitis: case report. Clin Infect Dis 1995;20:1557—9.

4. Saltzman R, Jurewicz R, Boon R. Safety of famciclovir in patients with herpes zoster and genital herpes. Antimicrob Agents Chemother 1994;38:2454—57.

5. Perry CM, Wagstaff AJ. Famciclovir. A review of its pharmacological properties and therapeutic efficacy in herpesvirus infections. Drugs 1995;50:396—415.

6. Jacobson MA. Current management of cyto-

megalovirus disease in patients with AIDS. AIDS Res Hum Retroviruses 1994;10:917—23.

7. Hardy D, Spector S, Polsky B, Crumpacker C, van der Horst C, Holland G, Freeman W, Heinemann MH, Sharuk G, Klystra J, Chown M. Combination of ganciclovir and granulocyte-macrophage colony-stimulating factor in the treatment of cytomegalovirus retinitis in AIDS patients. Eur J Clin Microbiol Infect Dis 1994;13 Suppl 2:34—40.

8. Jacobson MA, Kramer F, Bassiakos Y, Hooton T, Polsky B, Geheb H, O'Donnell JJ, Walker JD, Korvick JA, van der Horst C. Randomized phase I trial of two different combination foscarnet and ganciclovir chronic maintenance therapy regimens for AIDS patients with cytomegalovirus retinitis: AIDS Clinical Trials Group protocol 151. J Infect Dis 1994;170:189—93.

9. Drew WL, Ives D, Lalezari JP, Crumpacker C, Follansbee SE, Spector SE, Benson CA, Friedberg DN, Hubbard L, Stempien MJ, Shadman

A, Buhles W, for the Syntex Cooperative Oral Ganciclovir Study Group. Oral ganciclovir as maintenance treatment for cytomegalovirus retinitis in patients with AIDS. New Engl J Med 1995;333:615—20.

10. Danner SA. Intravenous versus oral ganciclovir: European/Australian comparative study of efficacy and safety in the prevention of cytomegalovirus retinitis recurrence in patients with AIDS. AIDS 1995;9:471—77.

11. Winston DJ, Wirin D, Shaked A, Busuttil RW. Randomised comparison of ganciclovir and high-dose acyclovir for long-term cytomegalovirus prophylaxis in liver-transplant recipients. Lancet 1995;346:69—74.

12. Winston DJ, Imagawa DK, Holt CD, Kaldas F, Shaked A, Busuttil RW. Long-term ganciclovir prophylaxis eliminates serious cytomegalovirus disease in liver transplant recipients receiving OKT3 therapy for rejection. Transplantation 1995;60:1357—60.

13. Aguado JM, Gomez-Sanchez MA, Lumbreras C, Delgado J, Lizasoain M, Otero JR, Rufilanchas JJ, Noriega AR. Prospective randomized trial of efficacy of ganciclovir versus that of anticytomegalovirus (CMV) immunoglobulin to prevent CMV disease in CMV-seropositive heart transplant recipients treated with OKT3. Antimicrob Agents Chemother 1995;39:1643—45.

14. Einsele H, Ehninger G, Hebart H, Wittkowski KM, Schuler U, Jahn G, Mackes P, Herter M, Klingebiel T, Löffler J, Wagner S, Müller CA. Polymerase chain reaction monitoring reduces the incidence of cytomegaloirus disease and the duration and side effects of antiviral therapy after bone marow transplantation. Blood 1995;86: 2815—20.

15. Goodrich JM, Zaia JA, Boeckh M, Bowden RA, Carrigan DR, Knox KK, Drobyski WR. Ganciclovir strategies after marrrow transplantation. Bone Marrow Transpl 1995;15:S156—61.

16. Kirsch LS, Arevalo JF, De Clercq E, Chavez de la Paz E, Munguia D, Garcia R, Freeman WR. Phase I/II study of intravitreal cidofovir for the treatment of cytomegalovirus retinitis in patients with the acquired immunodeficiency syndrome. Am J Ophthalmol 1995;119:466—76.

17. Lea AP, Bryson HM. Cidofovir. Drugs 1996;52:225—30.

18. Brillanti S, Miglioli M, Barbara L. Combination antiviral therapy with ribavirin and interferon — in interferon — relapsers and non-responders: Italian experience. J Hepatol 1995;23 Suppl 2:13—16.

19. Schvarcz R, Ando Y, Sönnerborg A, Weiland O. Combination treatment with interferon α-2b and ribavirin for chronic hepatitis C in atients who have failed to achieve sustained response to interferon alone: Swedish experience. J Hepatol 1995;23 Suppl 2:17—21.

20. Tong MJ, Hwang S-J, Lefkowitz M, Lee S-D, Co RL, Lo K-J. A pilot, open labelled, phase II study using oral ribavirin in the treatment of pa-tients with chronic active hepatitis B. Clin Diagn Virol 1995;3:377—85.

21. Jablonowski H, Arasteh K, Staszewski S, Ruf B, Stellbrink HJ, Schrappe M, Stoehr A, Haase W, Schomaker U, Von Eisenhart Rothe B, Thomis J, Stille W. A dose comparison study of didanosine in patients with very advanced HIV infection who are intolerant to or clinically deteriorate on zidovudine. AIDS 1995;9:463—9.

22. Alpha International Coordinating Committee. The Alpha trial: European/Australian randomized double-blind trial of two doses of didanosine in zidovudine-intolerant patients with symptomatic HIV disease. AIDS 1996;10:867—80.

23. Eron JJ, Benoit SL, Jemsek J, MacArthur RD, Santana J, Quinn JB, Kuritzkes DR, Fallon MA, Rubin M. Treatment with lamivudine, zido-vudine, or both in HIV-positive patients with 200 to 500 CD4+ cells per cubic millimeter. New Engl J Med 1995;333:1662—9.

24. Dienstag JL, Perrillo RP, Schiff ER, Bartholomew M, Vicary C, Rubin M. A preliminary trial of lamivudine for chronic hepatitis B infection. New Engl J Med 1995;333:1657—161.

25. Markowitz M, Saag M, Powderly WG, Hurley AM, Hsu A, Valdes JM, Henry D, Sattler F, La Marca A, Leonard JM, Ho DD. A preliminary study of ritonavir, an inhibitor of HIV-1 protease, to treat HIV-1 infection. New Engl J Med 1995;333:1534—1539.

26. Danner SA, Carr A, Leonard JM, Lehman LM, Gudiol F, Gonzales J, Raventos A, Rubio R, Bouza E, Pintado V, Aguado AG, De Lomas JG, Delgado R, Borleffs JCC, Hsu A, Valdes JM, Boucher CAB, Cooper DA. A short-term study of the safety, pharmacokinetics, and efficacy of ritonavir, an inhibitor of HIV-1 protease. New Engl J Med 1995;333:1528—33.

27. Wintermeyer SM, Nahata MC. Rimantadine: a clinical persective. Ann Pharmacother 1995; 29:299—310.

28. Pollard RB. Use of proteinase inhibitors in clinical practice. Pharmacotherapy 1994;14:21S—29S.

29. Kitchen VS, Skinner C, Ariyoshi K, Lane EA, Duncan IB, Burckhardt J, Burger HU, Bragman K, Pinching AJ, Weber JN. Safety and activity of saquinavir in HIV infection. Lancet 1995; 345:952—5.

30. Collier AC, Coombs RW, Schoenfeld DA, Bassett RL, Timpone J, Baruch A, Jones M, Facey K, Whitacre C, McAuliffe VJ, Friedman HM, Merigan TC, Reichman RC, Hooper C, Corey L. Treatment of human immunodeficiency virus infection with saquinavir, zidovudine, and zalcitabine. New Engl J Med 1996;334:1011—17.

31. Riddler SA, Anderson RE, Mellors JW. Anti-retroviral activity of stavudine (2′,3′-didehydro-3′-deoxythymidine, D4T). Antiviral Res 1995; 27:189—203.

32. Skowron G. Biologic effects and safety of sta-vudine: overview of phase I and II clinical trials. J Infect Dis 1995;171 Suppl 2:S113—S117.

33. Fichtenbaum CJ, Clifford DB, Powderly WG. Risk factors for dideoxynucleoside-induced toxic neuropathy in patients with the human immunodeficiency virus infection. J AIDS Hum Retrovirol 1995;10:169—74.

34. Domanski MJ, Sloas MM, Follmann DA, Scalise PP III, Tucker EE, Egan D, Pizzo PA. Effect of zidovudine and didanosine treatment on heart function in children infected with human immunodeficiency virus. J Pediatr 1995;127:137—46.

35. Falguera M, Perez-Mur J, Puig T, Cao G. Study of the role of vitamin B12 and folinic acid supplementation in preventing hematologic toxicity of zidovudine. Eur J Haematol 1995;55:97—102.

36. Kuehl AK, Noormohamed SE. Recombinant erythropoietin for zidovudine-induced anemia in AIDS. Ann Pharmacother 1995;29:778—9.

37. Olano JP, Borucki MJ, Wen JW, Haque AK. Massive hepatic steatosis and lactic acidosis in a patient with AIDS who was receiving zidovudine. Clin Infect Dis 1995;21:973—6.

38. Sinnwell TM, Sivakumar K, Soueidan S, Jay C, Frank JA, McLaughlin AC, Dalakas MC. Metabolic abnormalities in skeletal muscle of patients receiving zidovudine therapy observed by 31P in vivo magnetic resonance spectroscopy. J Clin Invest 1995;96:126—31.

39. Chariot P, Le Maguet F, Authier FJ, Labes D, Poron F, Gherardi R. Cytochrome c oxidase deficiency in zidovudine myopathy affects perifascicular muscle fibers and arterial smooth muscle cells. Neuropathol Appl Neurobiol 1995;21:540—7.

30 Drugs used in tuberculosis and leprosy

DRUGS USED IN TUBERCULOSIS *(SED-13, 880; SEDA-17, 351; SEDA-18, 309; SEDA-19, 282)*

GENERAL

Liver *Prediction of hepatotoxicity* Hepatotoxicity is consistently the most common serious adverse reaction in patients taking treatment for tuberculosis. In a case-control study of 60 patients in India, conducted in order to identify features predicting hepatotoxicity, the body mass index was significantly lower (17.2) in patients who experienced hepatotoxicity than in controls (19.5) (1[C]). A comparison between the two groups showed no significant differences in age, sex, alcohol consumption, chronic liver disease, hepatitis B virus carrier status, or acetylator status.

Skin *Acneiform eruptions* Acneiform eruptions in patients being treated for pulmonary tuberculosis have been studied prospectively in 774 patients in India (2[C]). Patients with pre-existing acne were excluded. Withdrawal and rechallenge were performed to identify the offending drug in 11 cases. Acneiform eruptions developed in only 11 cases (1.4%), including 0.5% of patients taking isoniazid, 1.5% of patients taking rifampicin and 0.6% of patients taking ethambutol. The authors concluded that acneiform eruptions rarely complicate tuberculosis treatment.

Risk factors *Adverse reactions in elderly patients with tuberculosis* The incidence of adverse reactions to drugs used in the treatment of tuberculosis is higher in elderly patients, who are more likely to have intercurrent illness and a lower lean body mass than younger patients. In two studies from Hong Kong in patients being treated for tuberculosis with rifampicin, the incidence of adverse reactions was higher with regimens containing rifampicin; furthermore, patients taking rifampicin had a higher steady-state plasma concentration of isoniazid (3[C]), (4[C]). However, if rifampicin was omitted there was an unsatisfactory rate of treatment failure. The authors concluded that the inclusion of rifampicin offered a better therapeutic response without significantly affecting the incidence of adverse reactions, provided that the patients were closely monitored and appropriate dosage reductions were made, especially in elderly patients with co-existing diseases.

Isoniazid

Overdosage Overdosage of isoniazid can cause acute *neurotoxicity*, which may present with seizures, metabolic acidosis, and coma. Seven cases in children aged 5—15 years have been reported from a single inner city hospital in New York between 1991 and 1993 (5[c]). Isoniazid 14—99 mg/kg was taken accidentally or in an attempt at self harm. Six of the patients presented with afebrile seizures. The specific antidote for acute isoniazid neurotoxicity, pyridoxine, was administered in five cases. Two patients with seizures unresponsive at first to anticonvulsants responded only after injection of pyridoxine. The diagnosis of acute isoniazid toxicity was confirmed by serum isoniazid concentrations in four cases.

Patients are usually symptomatic within 45 min of ingestion of an overdose of isoniazid, but symptoms may be delayed for up to 2 h, by which time peak absorption occurs.

With the resurgence of pulmonary tuberculosis the availability of isoniazid for accidental or deliberate self harm is increased. The possibility of acute isoniazid toxicity needs to be considered when a patient presents with seizures. Parenteral pyridoxine should be readily available in emergency facilities that serve communities in which isoniazid overdosage is likely.

℞ *Treatment and prophylaxis of Mycobacterium avium-complex infection*

Mycobacterium avium-complex (MAC) infection is rare, except in patients with AIDS, of whom over half are infected with Mycobacterium avium at post-mortem. This infection is a late event, becoming likely only in patients with CD4 counts of under 100. The clinical features are often nondescript, with nothing more definite than fever and weight loss. However, even in the absence of clinical organ involvement, the organism can be isolated from spleen, lymph nodes, liver, lung, bone-marrow, and (of most diagnostic value) from blood cultures. Histologically, Mycobacteria are often visible within macrophages, but granulomata may be absent or poorly formed. Antibiotics that act intracellularly should therefore be useful, but all standard antituberculous drugs are ineffective, with the exception of ethambutol.

Prophylaxis   Prophylaxis against MAC infection can be provided by a variety of agents, including azithromycin, clarithromycin, and rifabutin, either alone or in combination.

In a double-blind trial in 667 HIV-positive patients with a CD4 count of less than 100 (i.e. $0.1 \times 10^9/l$), in which 333 patients took clarithromycin 500 mg bd and 334 took placebo, MAC infection developed in 6% of the clarithromycin group compared with 16% of the placebo group during follow-up for 10 months (6^C). Taste disturbances were reported in 11% of the patients who took clarithromycin, compared with 2% of the placebo group. Severe adverse reactions occurred at a similar rate in both groups (7 and 6%, respectively).

Primary prophylaxis with weekly azithromycin has also been shown to be effective in preventing MAC infection. In a study of 693 HIV-positive patients with a CD4 count less

than 100, 7.6% of those who took azithromycin 1200 mg weekly developed MAC infection compared with 15.3% of those who took rifabutin 300 mg daily (7^C). When rifabutin and azithromycin were combined, only 2.8% of patients developed MAC infection. However, patients taking combination therapy were more likely to discontinue it because of adverse reactions.

Treatment   Treatment of MAC infection requires combination therapy to reduce the risk of the emergence of drug resistance. A trial of triple therapy with rifabutin, ethambutol, and clarithromycin versus quadruple therapy with rifampicin, ethambutol, clofazimine, and ciprofloxacin showed that triple therapy led to faster resolution of bacteremia. Blood cultures became negative in 69% of patients taking triple therapy compared with 29% of patients taking quadruple therapy. The median survival time was 8.6 months for triple therapy and 5.2 months for quadruple therapy.

Adverse effects   In this study the most important adverse reaction was uveitis, which occurred in 24 of the 63 patients taking rifabutin 600 mg/day and three of the 53 patients taking 300 mg/day. None of the patients taking quadruple therapy developed uveitis (8^C). Initially uveitis was thought to occur only with dosages of rifabutin over 1200 mg/day. However, a recent review of 54 cases has shown that it can occur at dosages of 300–600 mg/day and is more likely to occur in patients with a low body mass (9^C). The patients studied presented with uveitis 2 weeks to 7 months after starting therapy. In all cases they were also taking fluconazole and clarithromycin, drugs that inhibit the metabolism of rifabutin and increase its serum concentrations. The uveitis in these cases responded rapidly to withdrawal of rifabutin and the administration of topical corticosteroids (10^C).

Clarithromycin appeared to cause reversible mania in two patients with AIDS being treated for disseminated MAC infection (11^c). Both had a normal premorbid mental state and developed an acute psychosis after starting clarithromycin in a dosage of 1000 mg bd. The reaction resolved on withdrawal and recurred after rechallenge. Both patients were underweight (41 and 56 kg).

REFERENCES

1. Singh J, Arora A, Garg PK, Thakur VS, Pande JN, Tandon RK. Anti-tuberculosis treatment-induced hepatotoxicity: role of predictive factors. Postgrad Med J 1995;71:359—62.
2. Sharma RP, Kathari AK, Sharma NK. Acneiform eruptions and anti-tubercular drugs. Indian J Dermatol Venereol Leprol 1995;61:26—7.
3. Woo J, Chan CH, Cheung W, Or KK, Chan K. Correlation between steady state plasma concentration of anti-tuberculosis drugs and age. Inclusion of rifampicin in the treatment regimen, adverse drug reactions and other clinical parameters. J Med 1995;26:279—94.
4. Chan CH, Or KK, Cheung W, Woo J. Adverse drug reactions and outcome of elderly patients on antituberculosis chemotherapy with and without rifampicin. J Med 1995;26:43—52.
5. Shah B, Santucci K, Sinert R, Steiner P. Acute isoniazid neurotoxicity in an urban hospital. Pediatrics 1995;95:700—4.
6. Pierce M, Crampton S, Henry D, Heifets L, LaMarca A, Montecalvo M, Wormser GP, Jablonowski H, Jemsek J, Cynamon M, Yangco BG, Notario G, Craft JC. A randomised trial of clarithromycin as prophylaxis against disseminated *Mycobacterium avium* complex infection in patients with advanced acquired immunodeficiency syndrome. New Engl J Med 1996;335:384—91.
7. Havlir DV, Dube MP, Sattler FR, Forthal DN, Kemper CA, Dunne MW, Parenti DM, Lavelle JP, White AC Jr, Witt MD, Bozzette SA, McCutchan JA. Prophylaxis against disseminated *Mycobacterium avium* complex with weekly azithromycin, daily rifabutin or both. New Engl J Med 1996;335:392—98.
8. Shafran SD, Singer J, Zarowny DP, Phillips P, Salit I, Walmsley SL, Fong IW, Gill MJ, Rachlis AR, Lalonde RG, Fanning MM, Tsoukas CM. A comparison of two regimens for treatment of *Mycobacterium avium* complex bacteraemia in AIDS: rifabutin, ethambutol, and clarithromycin versus rifampicin, ethambutol, clofazimine, and ciprofloxacin. Canadian HIV Trials Network Protocol 010 Study Group. New Engl J Med 1996;335:377—83.
9. Tseng AL, Walmsley SL. Rifabutin-associated uveitis. Ann Pharmacol 1995;29:1149—55.
10. Karbassi M, Nikou S. Acute uveitis in patients with acquired immunodeficiency syndrome receiving prophylactic rifabutin. Arch Ophthalmol 1995;113:699—700.
11. Nightingale SD, Koster FT, Mertz GJ, Loss SD. Clarithromycin-induced mania in two patients with AIDS. Clin Infect Dis 1995;20:1563—4.

31 Antihelminthic drugs

BENZIMIDAZOLES *(SED-13, 912; SEDA-17, 358; SEDA-18, 315; SEDA-19, 286)*

Albendazole and mebendazole

In a study from Italy the effect of high-dosage treatment of echinococcosis with either albendazole or mebendazole on *serum transaminase activities* has been specifically addressed in 410 patients treated with either albendazole ($n = 268$) or mebendazole ($n = 128$) (1[Cr]). Serum transaminase activities increased in 70 patients (17%), of whom 14 had concomitant liver diseases. Of the other 56 patients, 16 had taken mebendazole and 40 albendazole. The observed rise in transaminase activities was generally slight to 2—4 times normal. In one only case did the transaminase activities rise to 10 times normal. Although treatment was not withdrawn, gradual normalization of transaminase activities was usually observed. It is thought that the slight rise in serum transaminase activities is a reaction to decay of liver cysts and may therefore be indicative of the effectiveness of treatment. Although careful monitoring of liver function tests during treatment with either albendazole or mebendazole for echinococcosis is mandatory, mild increases in serum transaminase activities are no indication for withdrawal of treatment.

IVERMECTIN *(SED-13, 906; SEDA-17, 355; SEDA-18, 312; SEDA-19, 287)*

Ivermectin is a very effective microfilaricidal drug in the treatment of onchocerciasis, lymphatic filariasis, and loiasis, but not in *Mansonella perstans* infections. Adverse effects are mainly attributed to the decay of dying parasites and not to intrinsic effects of the drug itself. Several reports on the use of ivermectin in onchocerciasis and lymphatic filariasis have recently appeared.

Ivermectin and onchocerciasis Although ivermectin is an effective microfilaricidal drug and inhibits the release of intrauterine microfilariae in the uterus of the adult female worm, it does not kill the adult worm. In order to obtain a more permanent sterilizing effect on the adult female worm, ivermectin has been used in combination with albendazole in 69 patients with onchocerciasis (2[C]). The patients were given ivermectin in a single dose of 150 µg/kg, and 1 week later were randomized to receive 800 mg of albendazole ($n = 35$) or placebo ($n = 34$). The combination treatment was well tolerated but had no additional effect compared with ivermectin alone. A mild *Mazzotti-type reaction*, consisting of fever, tachycardia, and headache, occurred in 30% of patients after the initial dose of ivermectin. After ivermectin, more severe symptomatic *postural hypotension* occurred in 13 patients on the second day, and 24 patients developed fever up to 39°C within the first 72 h. There was *swelling of the limbs* on the second day in 20 patients, lasting 1—3 days. *Swelling of the face* also occurred shortly after treatment in some individuals. *Peripheral sensory phenomena*, such as soreness, burning, or pain, occurred in 14 patients within the first week. Furthermore, there were mild painful sensations without specific findings in the waist area in 27 patients, or in the chest (18), neck (14), or abdomen (eight). All of these conditions occurred shortly after treatment with ivermectin and required only mild relief of pain with paracetamol or aspirin, except for one patient who was treated with hydrocortisone because of severe lymph node pain. Additional treatment with albendazole, administered after the symptoms had subsided, did not result in new or repeated adverse effects.

Several studies on the use of ivermectin in onchocerciasis with severe skin involvement (sowda) have been published recently. In a placebo-controlled, double-blind study from Malawi (3[C]), 70 patients with onchocerciasis and heavy skin involvement received either ivermectin (150 μg/kg, 47 patients) or placebo (23 patients). Patients with edematous or lichenified skin lesions who received ivermectin had significantly more improvement then those who received placebo, although retreatment was found to be necessary more often than for onchocerciasis with ocular involvement. Common adverse effects were *itching*, initial *aggravation of skin lesions*, and *edema of the face and limbs* within the first 3 days after treatment.

In a second study from Liberia (4[C]) ivermectin was used to treat 56 patients with onchocerciasis and sowda. These patients presented before treatment with itching (98%), asymmetric chronic onchodermatitis (98%), and swelling of femoral lymph nodes (89%). Mean microfilaria densities were 1.0 microfilariae/mg in children and 0.7 microfilariae/mg in adults. After a single oral dose of 150 μg/kg of ivermectin the prevalence of carriers of microfilariae fell from 100% to 19% at 1—2 months, accompanied by significant improvement in symptoms. The adverse effects observed in 30 patients available for follow-up occurred within 72 h after treatment and consisted of *increased itching* (93%), *aggravation of dermatitis* (73%), *fever* (25%), *headache* (20%), *myalgia* (20%), and *painful swelling of lymph nodes* (13%) *or limbs* (10%). No dangerous adverse effects were noted and only symptomatic treatment was necessary. In this group of patients the symptoms tended to recur after 4—6 months, indicating the need for more frequent administration of ivermectin in patients with hyper-reactive onchodermatitis compared with patients with ocular involvement.

In a third study from Sudan, eight patients with severe asymmetric onchodermatitis (sowda) and six patients with milder onchodermatitis were treated with a single oral dose of 150 μg/kg of ivermectin (5[C]). Reactions to treatment were more common and severe in individuals with sowda, and consisted of *mus-culoskeletal pain* (seven of eight patients) and *pitting edema* (five of eight patients) starting 24—72 h after treatment. One patient developed severe swelling of a limb, with enlarged tender inguinal lymph nodes, and had to be treated with corticosteroids. *Itching* and *maculopapular rash* were also frequent.

The relation between adverse effects and serum ivermectin concentrations has been addressed in a paper from Sierra Leone (6[C]). Serum ivermectin concentrations were measured by high performance liquid chromatography in 71 patients with onchocerciasis with skin snips positive for microfilariae. After treatment, 11 patients developed severe reactions, 14 moderate reactions, 15 mild reactions, and 21 no reactions. There was no relation between serum ivermectin concentrations and the grade of adverse effects, consistent with earlier findings, again indicating that adverse effects are caused by the release of parasitic antigen, not by the drug itself. The overall mean half-life of ivermectin was 20 h.

Finally, the interaction between onchocerciasis, HIV infection, and ivermectin treatment has been investigated in an epidemiological study (7[C]). In a hyperendemic area 1910 carriers of *Onchocerca volvulus* were identified, of whom 73 (3.8%) were also infected with HIV; in addition, 276 patient without microfilariae were identified, of whom 20 (7.2%) were HIV-positive. Even in patients with both onchocerciasis and HIV infection accompanied by very low CD4 counts, there was no increase in mean microfilaria counts compared with HIV-negative patients. There was no difference in the efficacy of ivermectin in the treatment of onchocerciasis between HIV-negative and HIV-positive patients. A group of 856 microfilaria carriers, of whom 43 (5%) were HIV-positive, were treated with a single dose of 150 μg/kg of ivermectin; 356 (44%) of the HIV-negative patients and 24 (58%) of the HIV-positive patients reported adverse effects, in decreasing order of frequency: *edema of the skin*, *swelling of lymph nodes*, *fever*, *skin rash*, *conjunctivitis*, and *postural hypotension*. The prevalence of these signs was similar in HIV-negative and HIV-positive patients, but swelling of lymph nodes (25 vs. 33%) and skin rash (9 vs. 38%) were significantly more frequent in the HIV-positive group.

Ivermectin and lymphatic filariasis Ivermectin is effective in the treatment of human lymphatic filariasis, although repeated treatment is necessary. In a study from Brazil, ivermectin (single oral doses of 200 and 400 µg/kg) has been compared with diethylcarbamazine (6 mg/kg in a single oral dose) in a double-blind study in 67 patients with filariasis bancrofti (8[C]). Ivermectin reduced the number of microfilariae significantly faster than diethylcarbamazine, although the difference tended to level out after 1 month. The higher dose tended to be more effective than the lower dose, although the difference was not statistically significant. The most effective treatment consisted of the high ivermectin dose followed by diethylcarbamazine; this resulted in a reduction of microfilariae to 2.4% of pretreatment values at 2 years. Adverse effects occurred in 84% of the patients but were generally well tolerated. The nature of the adverse effects differed somewhat between ivermectin and diethylcarbamazine. Systemic symptoms were more frequent after ivermectin, while local symptoms predominated after treatment with diethylcarbamazine. *Fever* occurred in 45 vs. 4.5% of patients respectively, *malaise* in 27 vs. 9.1%, *gastrointestinal symptoms* in 18 vs. 4.5%, *respiratory symptoms* in 33 vs. 23%, *neurological symptoms* in 15 vs. 9.1%, *scrotal pain* in 9.1 vs. 50%, *inflammation in the scrotal area* in 9.1 vs. 41%, and *nodules* in 0 vs. 45%. There was no difference in the occurrence of *hematuria* (33 vs. 32%).

The treatment of bancroftian filariasis with a combination of a single oral dose of ivermectin (400 µg/kg) and a single oral dose of diethylcarbamazine (6 mg/kg) has been further studied in a large community-based study in French Polynesia (9[C]) after it had been found to be more effective than single-dose ivermectin or single-dose diethylcarbamazine alone in preventing recurrence of microfilaremia (10[C]). More than 3500 inhabitants of a Polynesian island were treated with four different regimens: a single oral dose of ivermectin 400 µg/kg, a single oral dose of diethylcarbamazine 6 mg/kg, a single oral dose of 400 µg/kg of ivermectin combined with a single oral dose of diethylcarbamazine 3 mg/kg, and a single oral dose of 400 µg/kg of ivermectin combined with a single oral dose of 6 mg/kg of diethylcarbamazine. Microfilaria counts 1 year after treatment were reduced by 80, 82, 95, and 96%, respectively. The prevalence of microfilaria carriers also fell by 11, 14, 32, and 32%, respectively. Thus, treatment of filariasis bancrofti with a combination of ivermectin 400 µg/kg and either 6 or 3 mg/kg of diethylcarbamazine is superior to treatment with either of these drugs alone. The patients were followed for 3 days after treatment. Only 3.4% of the 3711 patients treated developed adverse effects. These were mostly mild and hindered daily activities only in 29 patients (less than 1%). The intensity of adverse reactions was not related to the treatment given, but to pretreatment microfilaria counts. None of the reactions was considered serious and all disappeared after treatment with paracetamol.

Finally, in another study from Brazil the efficacy of single-dose treatment with ivermectin 400 µg/kg for filariasis bancrofti on the adult worm instead of microfilariae has been investigated in 15 men (11[C]). Longitudinal ultrasound examinations of the scrotal lymphatic vessels were performed over a period of 3—9 months. While there were important reductions in microfilaria counts, the activity of the adult worms in the scrotal lymphatics (the filaria dance sign) remained unchanged, and removal of a lymphatic vessel in one patient 8 months after treatment showed three living adult worms. It was concluded that ivermectin is not effective as a macrofilaricidal drug in filariasis bancrofti.

PRAZIQUANTEL *(SED-13, 909)*

Praziquantel is usually considered to be the most effective drug in the treatment of all types of human schistosomiasis. It is effective and usually well tolerated in single-dose treatment, although transient adverse effects, consisting of *abdominal discomfort*, *bloody diarrhea*, and *allergic reactions* (*urticaria* and *edema*), often occur, especially in the more heavily infected individuals. In a study from a hyperendemic area in Senegal there were similar, but somewhat more severe, adverse effects after treatment with a single oral dose of praziquantel 40 mg/kg for schistosomiasis mansoni in 352 stool-positive patients (12[C]). Serious but transient adverse effects occurred in a substantial number of the patients within the first 24 h and were found to be related to the pretreatment egg counts (classified as below 400, 400—1000, and over 1000). *Abdominal pain* occurred in 48% of patients (according to pretreatment egg counts 24, 31, and 22%, respectively), *diarrhea* in 22% (12, 17, and 2%), *bloody diarrhea* in 9% (3, 5, and 14%), and *vomiting* in 16% (7, 10, and 22%). Furthermore, *dizziness* occurred in 13%, *pruritus* in 4%, and *urticaria* in 4% of patients. The therapeutic results were somewhat disappointing. The parasitological cure rate at 12 weeks after treatment was only 18%, although the mean egg count of those who stayed positive was reduced by 86%. It was suggested that the low cure rates were due to intense local transmission, but reduced drug susceptibility of the parasite strain was found in one local isolate and also may play a role.

SURAMIN *(SED-13, 915; SEDA-18, 316; SEDA-19, 289)*

In a study of the use of suramin in the treatment of onchocerciasis, 20 adult men were treated with suramin to a total dose of 5 g (73—85 mg/kg) over 36 days (13[C]). The clinical effect was disappointing. At 1 year, 34% of the female worms examined after nodulectomy were still alive. The systemic adverse effects of treatment with suramin were minor—isolated cases of *nasal stuffiness, nausea, fever with chills, weakness,* or *urticaria.* There were, however, more severe *ocular reactions. Iridocyclitis* occurred in nine out of 20 patients, of whom two required treatment to prevent the formation of posterior synechiae. Strict medical surveillance of the eyes after the treatment of onchocerciasis with suramin is therefore mandatory. *Mild proteinuria* was an almost universal finding after the third dose. There was one case of *glycosuria.* In conclusion the treatment of onchocerciasis with suramin does not result in complete clearance of the infection and is liable to ocular complications. Although it also has some delayed effect on microfilaria counts, treatment with ivermectin is more effective and has fewer adverse effects.

Adverse effects of suramin in patients with prostate cancer R_x

Suramin was originally used as a macrofilaricidal drug in the treatment of onchocerciasis and African trypanosomiasis. However, its use is severely limited because of severe adverse effects. Recently there has been renewed interest in this compound because it has shown some antitumor effect, possibly through inhibition of growth factors, in the treatment of hormone-refractory prostate cancer. Its use is still highly experimental, with only a marginal effect on survival but with substantial morbidity, especially in the higher, more effective dosage schemes.

Recently, several phase I and phase II studies on the use of suramin in the treatment of hormone-refractory prostate cancer (14[C])—(21[C]) have been published, as well as a study of suramin in the treatment of metastatic colorectal cancer (22[C]), where it showed no beneficial effect, and a small review (23[R]) on its use as an antitumor drug. These studies have shown that suramin has some antitumor effect in hormone-refractory prostate cancer, but that it also causes a unique pattern of extensive adverse effects, consisting of a syndrome of general malaise, anorexia, skin rash, edema, increased serum creatinine concentrations, proteinuria, increased transaminase activities, hematological abnormalities such as leukopenia, anemia, thrombocytopenia, more rarely irreversible adrenal insufficiency, and neurological complications ranging from paresthesia to motor disturbances and a Guillain-Barré-like syndrome. The occurrence of dose-limiting toxicity increases with time and higher doses. For instance the Guillain-Barré-like polyradiculopathy is only seen with high doses and sustained plasma concentrations above 350 μg/ml; the effective serum concentration of suramin is about 250 μg/ml, whereas concentrations below 200 μg/ml are ineffective.

The adverse effects that were reported in a group of 69 patients treated for hormone-refractory prostate cancer (23[R]) were anorexia (19%), malaise and fatigue (40%), paresthesia (10%), weakness (9%), and skin rash (6%). In another group of patients (18[C]) there were higher frequencies of adverse effects: fatigue occurred in 70% and neuropathy in 16%. He-

matological abnormalities occurred frequently, but were mostly mild and consisted of neutropenia (30%), anemia (74%), thrombocytopenia (26%), and coagulopathy (30%). Other adverse effects included uremia (21%), increased serum transaminase activities (19%), nausea and vomiting (30%), constipation (9%), edema (33%), dysrhythmias (7%), mild hyperglycemia (86%), and rash (60%).

Nervous system   *The pharmacological variables associated with the development of neurological toxicity have been further studied in a phase I study in 81 patients treated with suramin, administered by continuous infusion in order to maintain a preassigned plasma concentration (175, 215, or 275 μg/ml) for a fixed duration (16[C]). Eight of 32 patients treated with the highest dosage scheme (one for 4 weeks, seven for 8 weeks) developed severe neurological motor impairment, in contrast to one patient out of 26 treated with the middle dosage scheme. A further seven patients had sensory symptoms. No serious neurological adverse effects were noted in the group of patients treated with the lowest dosage scheme. The neurological syndrome experienced by the eight patients who developed severe neuropathy was characterized by a subacute onset of asymmetric flaccid weakness and areflexia in both arms and legs, but predominantly the legs. The proximal muscle groups were more affected. These abnormalities resulted in difficulties in climbing stairs and rising from a chair. The symptoms appeared mostly at 6—8 weeks after the start of treatment, but on occasion as early as 3 weeks. In four patients the weakness progressed to total invalidity. One of these patients went on to respiratory insufficiency and had to be mechanically ventilated, later dying from pneumonia. Of the remaining seven patients, one recovered completely within 10 weeks, one recovered 70% of motor function after 6 months, one died of septicemia, and the other five died of progressive disease 3—13 months after treatment. One of*

these patients had 40% recovery of motor function, while the remaining four had no improvement. It appears that this neurological syndrome is mostly dose-related and occurs mainly with higher dosages and more prolonged treatment. When it occurs the prognosis is not good.

Skin and appendages   *The dermatological adverse effects after treatment with suramin have been especially addressed in a study of 60 patients (56 with prostatic cancer), of whom 82% had at least one cutaneous reaction after treatment with suramin (24[C]). This frequency of cutaneous reactions widely exceeds those seen with other drugs. There was a wide range of eruptions—morbilliform rashes (67%), UV recall (35%), urticaria (18%), keratotic papules (suramin keratosis) (12%), palmar erythema (10%), facial erythema (10%), generalized acute papulovesicular rashes (8%), bullous exanthems (5%), confluent erythema (5%), and reticular erythema on the dorsal aspect of the feet and legs (3%). Erythema multiforme and purpura were seen in one patient each. Most reactions occurred within 24 h after the start of treatment and were self-limiting despite continuation of treatment. Characteristic lesions associated with suramin treatment were scaling erythematous papules (suramin keratosis) and many eruptions on previously sun-exposed areas of the skin. Six patients developed severe cutaneous reactions, but no patients withdrew from treatment. Common histopathological findings were hyperkeratosis, parakeratosis, spongiosis, acanthosis, exocytosis, apoptosis, and perivascular and lymphohistiocytic infiltrates.*

In a further case of transient suramin-associated erythema multiforme, diagnosed by punch biopsy, generalized erythema started at day 1 and resolved on the following day in a 66-year-old man with prostatic cancer and metastases (25[C]). On day 15, erythematous papules appeared on the extremities and the trunk. These lesions resolved in 14 days. There were no further cutaneous reactions.

REFERENCES

Kobayashi K, Vokes KK, Vogelzang NJ, Janisch L, Soliven B, Ratain MJ. Phase I study of suramin given by intermittent infusion without adaptive control in patients with advanced cancer. J Clin Oncol 1995;13:2196−207.

2. Eisenberger MA, Sinibaldi VJ, Reyno LM, Sridhara R, Jodrell DI, Zuhowski EG, Tkaczuk KH, Lowitt MH, Hemady RK, Jacobs SC, Van Echo D, Egorin MJ. Phase I and clinical evaluation of a pharmacologically guided regimen of suramin in patients with hormone-refractory prostate cancer. J Clin Oncol 1995;13:2174−86.

3. Bitton RJ, Figg WD, Venzon DJ, Dalakos MC, Bowden C, Headlee D, Reed E, Myers CE, Cooper MR. Pharmacologic variables associated with the development of neurologic toxicity in patients treated with suramin. J Clin Oncol 1995;13:2223−9.

4. Reyno LM, Egorin MJ, Eisenberger MA, Sinibaldi VJ, Zuhowski EG, Sridhara R. Development and validation of a pharmacokinetically based fixed dosing scheme for suramin. J Clin Oncol 1995;13:2187−95.

5. Dawson NA, Cooper MR, Figg WD, Headlee DJ, Thibault A, Bergan RC, Steinberg SM, Sausville EA, Myers CE, Sartor O. Antitumor activity of suramin in hormone-refractory prostate cancer controlling for hydrocortisone treatment and flutamide withdrawal as potentially confounding variables. Cancer 1995;76:453−62.

6. Kelly WK, Curley T, Leibertz C, Dnistrian A, Schwartz M, Scher HI. Prospective evaluation of hydrocortisone and suramin in patients with androgen-independent prostate cancer. J Clin Oncol 1995;13:2208−13.

7. Kelly WK, Scher HI, Mzumdar M, Pfister D, Curley T, Leibertz C, Cohen L, Vlamis V, Dnistrian A, Schwartz M. Suramin and hydrocortisone: determining drug efficacy in androgen-independent prostate cancer. J Clin Oncol 1995;13:2214−22.

8. Kehinde EO, Terry TR, Mistry N, Horsburgh T, Sandhu DP, Bell PRF. UK studies on suramin therapy in hormone-resistant prostate cancer. Cancer Surv 1995;23:217−29.

9. Falcone A, Pfanner E, Ciancy C, Danesi R, Brunetti I, Del Tacca M, Conte PF. Suramin in patients with metastatic colorectal cancer pretreated with fluoropyrimidine-based chemotherapy. Cancer 1995;75:440−3.

10. Eisenberger MA, Sinibaldi V, Reyno L. Suramin. Cancer Pract 1995;3:187−9.

11. Lowitt MH, Eisenberger M, Sina B, Kao GF. Cutaneous eruptions from suramin. A clinical and histopathologic study of 60 patients. Arch Dermatol 1995;131:1147−53.

12. Katz SK, Medenica MM, Kobayashi K, Vogelzang NJ, Soltani K. Erythema multiforme induced by suramin. J Am Acad Dermatol 1995;32:292−3.

13. Awadzi K, Hero M, Opoku NO, Addy ET, Büttner DW, Ginger CD. The chemotherapy of onchocerciasis 18. Aspects of treatment with suramin. Trop Med Parasitol 1995;46:19−26.

14. Awadzi K, Addy ET, Opoku NO, Plenge-Bönig A, BHttner DW. The chemotherapy of onchocerciasis 20: ivermectin in combination with albendazole. Trop Med Parasitol 1995;46:213−20.

15. Burnham G. Ivermectin treatment of onchocercal skin lesions: observations from a placebo-controlled, double blind trial in Malawi. Am J Trop Med Hyg 1995;52:270−6.

16. Darge K, Büttner DW. Ivermectin treatment of hyperreactive onchodermatitis (sowda) in Liberia. Trop Med Parasitol 1995;46:206−12.

17. Baraka OZ, Mahmoud BM, Ali MMM, Ali MH, El Sheikh EA, Homeida MMA, Mackenzie CD, Williams JF. Ivermectin treatment in severe asymetric reactive onchodermatitis (sowda) in Sudan. Trans R Soc Trop Med Hyg 1995;89:312−15.

18. Njoo FL, Beek WMJ, Keukens HJ, van Wilgenburg H, Oosting J, Stilma JS, Kijlstra A. Ivermectin detection in serum of onchocerciasis patients: relationship to adverse reactions. Am J Trop Med Hyg 1995;52:94−7.

19. Fischer P, Kipp W, Kabwa P, Büttner DW. Onchocerciasis and human immunodeficiency virus in Western Uganda: prevalences and treatment with ivermectin. Am J Trop Med Hyg 1995;53:171−8.

20. Dreyer G, Coutinho A, Miranda D, Noroes J, Rizzo JA, Galdino E, Rocha A, Medeiros Z, Andrade LD, Santos A, Figueredo-Silva J, Ottesen EA. Treatment of bancroftian filariasis in Recife, Brazil: a two-year comparative study of the efficacy of single treatments with ivermectin or diethylcarbamazine. Trans R Soc Trop Med Hyg 1995;89:98−102.

21. Moulia-Pelat JP, Nguyen LN, Hascoët H, Luquiaud P, Nicolas L. Advantages of an annual single dose of ivermectin 400 µg/kg plus diethylcarbamazine for community treatment of bancroftian filariasis. Trans R Soc Trop Med Hyg 1995;89:682−5.

22. Moulia-Pelat JP, Glaziou P, Weil GJ, Nguyen LN, Gaxotte P, Nicolas L. Combination ivermectin plus diethylcarbamazine, a new effective tool for control of lymphatic filariasis. Trop Med Parasitol 1995;46:9−12.

23. Dreyer G, Noroes J, Amaral F, Nen A, Medeiros Z, Coutinho A, Addiss D. Direct assessment of the adulticidal efficacy of a single dose of ivermectin in bancroftian filariasis. Trans R Soc Trop Med Hyg 1995;89:441−3.

24. Stelma FF, Talla I, Sow S, Kongs A, Niang M, Polman K, Deelder AM, Grijseels B. Efficacy and side effects of praziquantel in an epidemic focus of *Schistosoma mansoni*. Am J Trop Med Hyg 1995;53:167−70.

25. Teggi A, Lastilla MG, Grossi G, Franchi C, De Rosa F. Increase of serum glutamic-oxaloacetic and glutamic-pyruvic transaminases in patients with hydatid cysts treated with mebendazole and albendazole. Mediterr J Infect Parasit Dis 1995;10:85−90.

32

Vaccines

Surveillance of adverse events after immunization

Surveillance systems of adverse events after immunization in the US have been variously reviewed, including critical evaluations of the limitations of the Vaccine Adverse Event Reporting System (VAERS) (described in SED-13, 919) and its predecessor, the Monitoring System for Adverse Events Following Immunization (MSAEFI) (reviewed in SEDA-13, 273; SEDA-16, 320) (1[R]), (2[R]). The authors concluded that reports to VAERS and MSAEFI are essentially non-controlled clinical case reports or case series, useful for generating hypotheses but not for testing them. The significant under-reporting of known outcomes, together with the non-specific nature of most adverse events reports, highlights the limitations of passive surveillance systems of adverse events after immunization. Other controlled studies are therefore often necessary to evaluate hypotheses raised by passive surveillance system reports: whether a given adverse event can be caused by a specific vaccine, and if so how often. However, if reporting is reasonable consistent, it may be possible to detect changes in trends of known common adverse events. In addition, passive surveillance remains a potentially cost-effective way of monitoring rare events that cannot be detected in small prelicensing trials.

Cohort studies of rare adverse events would be useful, but are generally not feasible, essentially for economic reasons. One promising alternative approach is the use of large linked databases. The databases appropriate for such studies are derived from defined populations, such as members of health maintenance organizations, universal health care systems, and Medicaid programmes. Information on both exposure (immunization records) and outcome (for example, diagnoses recording potential adverse events) is usually computerized for members of such populations. These databases can be linked for epidemiological studies assessing potential associations between immunization and outcome. Large linked databases have already been used by various groups to examine the association between DTP vaccine and sudden infant death syndrome, DTP vaccine and neurological events, and MMR vaccine and seizures. The Centers for Disease Control and Prevention (CDC) in Atlanta use large linked databases (now called Vaccine Safety Datalink) in addition to VAERS (1[R]), (3[R]). Vaccine Safety Datalink covers a defined cohort of approximately 500 000 children up to the age of 5 years.

A new epidemiological and statistical method based on linkage of routinely available computerized hospital admission records with vaccination records has been described (4[R]). This active surveillance method has been used to assess the attributable risk of convulsion after DTP and MMR immunization and to investigate the relation between MMR vaccine and idiopathic thrombocytopenic purpura in children under 2 years of age in five districts in England. The results will be found below in the sections on DTP and MMR vaccines.

Vaccine safety issues have been reviewed, with a description of the clinical problems to be addressed, standard definitions and evaluative protocols, assessment of causality, and the currently available solutions, such as clinical trials, spontaneous reporting systems, surveillance studies, ad hoc epidemiological studies, and automated databases (5[R]).

Side Effects of Drugs, Annual 20
J.K. Aronson, ed.

BACTERIAL VACCINES *(SED-13, 920; SEDA-17, 366; SEDA-18, 325; SEDA-19, 293)*

Bacille Calmette-Guérin (BCG) vaccine

Disseminated BCG infection One hundred and eight cases of disseminated BCG infection reported world-wide since 1951, including 30 cases of disseminated infection occurring during 1974 and 1994 in France, have been analysed (6[C]). Four well-defined immunodeficiency conditions predispose to disseminated BCG infection: severe combined immunodeficiency, chronic granulomatous disease, Di George syndrome, and AIDS. About half the cases of disseminated BCG infection occur without a well-defined underlying immunological defect. However, there is little doubt that children with idiopathic BCG infection are immunodeficient, and there is good evidence that their immunodeficient status is inherited: four pairs of siblings and one pair of cousins were found among 60 children with idiopathic disseminated BCG infection; in addition, among the 50 single-case families, parental consanguinity was found in seven of 24 families for whom information was available.

Osteitis Osteitis (SED-13, 922) has been reported mainly among infants immunized in the neonatal period in Sweden and Finland. The medical records of 222 children with BCG osteitis registered from 1960 to 1988 in Finland have been analysed (7[C]). The most common sites of osteitis were the metaphyses of the long bones; the lower limbs were affected more often (58%) than the upper limbs (14%). Osteitis of the sternum (15%) and ribs (11%) also occurred. With adequate treatment, the prognosis for children with BCG osteitis was good, but six children were left with sequelae, with abnormalities of the limbs in five cases and pronounced cheloid formation in the other.

The incidence of BCG osteitis correlates closely with the BCG vaccine used. Between 1960 and 1970, when the vaccine based on the Gothenburg strain was prepared in Sweden, the incidence of BCG osteitis was 7.3 per 100 000 vaccinees. There was a significant increase to 37 per 100 000 in the early 1970s when the vaccine was prepared in Copenhagen using the same Gothenburg strain. Because of the increased incidence, in 1978 the vaccine was replaced by a BCG vaccine made by Glaxo, UK. Since then, the incidence has been similar to that reported in the 1960s (6.4 per 100 000 vaccinees).

Treatment of carcinoma of the urinary bladder Intravesicular instillation of BCG is the treatment of choice for recurrent superficial transitional cell carcinoma of the bladder, and BCG instillation is described as being effective for carcinoma in situ of the bladder. However, the treatment is not free from adverse effects (SED-13, 925).

Several trials have been carried out to determine whether or not lowering the dose of BCG could reduce toxicity without comprising efficacy. In a randomized, multicenter, prospective trial in patients with superficial bladder cancer conducted by the Spanish Oncology Group in 252 patients treated with weekly instillations of 81 mg BCG and 248 patients treated with weekly instillations of 27 mg BCG, there were no significant differences in recurrence rate or progression rate, but significant differences both in local severe toxicity as well in systemic toxicity (8[C]). Somewhat different results have been reported in a study of 25 patients treated with superficial transitional cell carcinoma of the urinary bladder with weekly instillations of BCG strain Connaught 27 mg (9[C]). Efficacy was comparable to high-dose studies. However, toxicity was not reduced substantially by the low dosage of BCG. Another trial in 183 patients with papillary tumor and bladder carcinoma in situ showed no differences in progression rates between patients receiving BCG Pasteur strain 75 or 150 mg, and fewer adverse effects in patients receiving the 75-mg dose (10[C]).

Severe local and systemic side effects of BCG treatment can be treated successfully with tuberculostatic drugs, to most of which BCG is very susceptible, for up to 6 months (11[C]).

Efficacy and adverse effects of alternative treatment regimens for carcinoma in situ of the bladder have been compared with instillation of BCG in 21 patients who were treated with intravesicular instillations of Keyhole Limpet Hemocyanin (first course: 20 mg weekly for 6 weeks; second course: 20 mg monthly for 1 year or bimonthly for 2 subsequent years). Patients who did not respond to two courses were treated with regular instillations of BCG Connaught strain 120 mg. Eleven patients were free from tumor after the first or second course of Keyhole Limpet Hemocyanin. Ten patients had to have a cystectomy because of persistence or progression of carcinoma after Hemocyanin or Hemocyanin with subsequent BCG. However, instillations of BCG caused severe dysuria in 60% and fever in 40% of patients, whereas Hemocyanin treatment had only minor adverse effects (12^C). Combined therapy with mitomycin C and BCG was more effective in 28 patients with carcinoma in situ of the bladder than mitomycin alone (13^C). Compared with BCG monotherapy there were only a few adverse effects.

More adverse effects, such as *loss of bladder capacity*, have been reported in 15 patients receiving whole bladder wall photodynamic therapy for carcinoma in situ than in patients treated with instillation of BCG (14^C). The success rates were comparable.

Cholera vaccine *(SED-13, 925; SEDA-17, 366)*

Following the administration of live oral cholera vaccine (containing the attenuated strain *Vibrio cholerae* CVD 103-HgR, prepared from *V. cholerae* 01 strain 569B), there were significant rises in serum antitoxin concentrations and only few mild adverse effects (SED-13, 925). There was protective efficacy in 82–100% healthy adult volunteers and no difference in adverse effects between 25 recipients of the vaccine and 26 controls (15^C).

New vaccines are needed to prevent cholera caused by *Vibrio cholerae* 0139. When an oral single-dose cholera vaccine candidate was given to 10 volunteers there was 83% protective efficacy, and the only adverse effect, in one volunteer, was mild *diarrhea* (16^C).

Diphtheria vaccine (including diphtheria— tetanus vaccine) *(SED-13, 926)*

Booster immunization (0.5 ml) with two different diphtheria—tetanus vaccines containing 12 Lf/ml of diphtheria and tetanus toxoids was given to 313 Danish recruits (17^C). The vaccines were identical in all respects, but either aluminium hydroxide or calcium phosphate were used as adjuvant. After booster immunization, all the vaccinees had protective diphtheria and tetanus antibody titers; the median antibody content of the calcium phosphate group was higher than in the aluminium hydroxide group. Adverse reactions occurred in 57% of vaccinees, 93% being mild local reactions. Five vaccinees developed severe systemic reactions: *dizziness* or *nausea* for 1 week; *fever* of 39°C. Recruits re-immunized with the calcium phosphate-adsorbed vaccine had a significantly higher rate of adverse reactions than those re-immunized with the aluminium hydroxide-adsorbed vaccine.

Hemophilus influenzae (Hib) vaccine (including vaccines combined with the Hib component) *(SED-13, 927; SEDA-17, 367; SEDA-18, 330; SEDA-19, 293)*

Soon after birth 120 healthy infants received conjugated Hib tetanus toxoid vaccine (18^C). The vaccine was well tolerated and antibody responses showed no evidence of immunological tolerance. The most common reactions were *local redness* and *soreness or swelling at the injection site*, but the local reaction was never larger than 3 cm in diameter. *Erythema* and *fever* of 38.4°C developed in an infant 12 h after administration of vaccine. Local reactions following the second dose of the vaccine were similar to those seen after the first dose. The booster dose at 14 months caused only mild reactions.

Meningococcal vaccine *(SED-13, 938)*

The current commercially available meningococcal polysaccharide vaccines (bivalent serotypes A and C vaccine and tetravalent serotypes A, C, Y, and W135 vaccine) are not effective in children under 2 years of age. Various conjugated vaccines are therefore under development and have been evaluated in clinical trials. A serotype A and C polysaccharide-CRM197 conjugate vaccine has been compared with a commercially available non-conjugated serotype A and C vaccine in 304 Gambian infants aged 8–10 years (19^C). The new conjugate vaccine was safe and more immunogenic than the non-conjugated vaccine.

Combination meningococcal and typhoid fever vaccine A combination meningococcal and typhoid fever polysaccharide vaccine (Merieux) has been evaluated in 158 volunteers in a single-blind study (20[C]). Comparing vaccinees immunized with monocomponent vaccines or the combination vaccine, there was no significant difference in the reported frequency or duration of local and systemic reactions. However, vaccinees who received the monocomponent typhoid fever vaccine alone were less likely to complain of *swelling or pain at the injection site*.

Pertussis vaccine (including diphtheria—tetanus—pertussis vaccine, DTP or DTaP) *(SED-13, 940; SEDA-17, 370; SEDA-18, 332; SEDA-19, 297)*

Diphtheria—tetanus—pertussis vaccine is available as combinations containing either whole-cell pertussis vaccine (DTP) or acellular pertussis vaccine (DTaP). From 1991 to 1993 approximately 27 million doses of DTP vaccine and 5 million doses of DTaP vaccine have been distributed in the US. The results of a post-marketing comparison of the safety of acellular pertussis vaccines with whole-cell pertussis vaccines have been published (21[C]). The rates of reported adverse events per 100 000 immunizations were significantly lower after the administration of DTaP vaccine than after DTP vaccine for the following outcomes: all reports, 2.9 vs. 9.8; fever, 1.9 vs. 7.5; seizures, 0.5 vs. 1.7; and hospitalizations, 0.2 vs. 0.9. Brown expressed the opinion that the methods used in the post-marketing assessment—data collected through the Vaccine Adverse Event Reporting System (VAERS)—were inadequate for estimating rates of vaccine reactions (22[C]).

To facilitate future vaccine reaction data collection, an effort has been made to determine the minimum data set required to describe accurately and to compare common reactions after the administration of acellular or whole-cell pertussis vaccine with diphtheria and tetanus toxoids combined, using the results of a study including 13 acellular and two whole-cell pertussis vaccines (reviewed in SEDA-18, 332) (23[R]).

Pre-existing maternal antibodies reduced the subsequent antibody response after the administration of whole-cell pertussis vaccine but not the antibody response after acellular pertussis vaccine in infants (24[C]). There was no consistent correlation between the pre-immunization titer of pertussis antibody and the occurrence of reactions after the first immunization.

Booster pertussis immunization after primary immunization An evaluation of the results of two studies in a total of 182 children primed either with acellular or with whole cell pertussis vaccines at 2, 4 and 6 months of age and boosted with an acellular vaccine has shown that booster doses of acellular vaccine are safe and immunogenic (25[C]). Local adverse reactions after booster immunization with acellular vaccine were more common in children primed with acellular vaccine than in those primed with whole cell pertussis vaccine (68 vs. 33%). In a similar study children primed with acellular or whole cell pertussis combined with DT vaccine have been boosted with a recombinant acellular pertussis vaccine combined with DT vaccine. The vaccine was highly immunogenic and safe (26[C]).

Whole-cell pertussis vaccine Using a new method for active post-marketing surveillance of vaccine safety based on patients records (as described above in the subchapter surveillance), there was an increased relative incidence of *convulsions* occurring up to 3 days after DTP immunization (4[R]). The effect was limited to the third dose of vaccine, for which the attributable risk was one per 12 500 doses.

Acellular pertussis vaccine Various acellular pertussis vaccines have been licensed either for booster immunization or for primary as well as booster immunization in many countries (for example in the US (27[R]), Canada, and some Western European countries). A monovalent acellular pertussis vaccine developed by the National Institute of Child Health and Human Development, Bethesda, Maryland, and composed only of detoxified pertussis toxin (pertussis toxoid) has been studied in a randomized, double-blind, placebo-controlled field trial in 3450 Swedish children (28[C]), (29[R]). The children were randomized to receive either DT vaccine alone or the DT vaccine plus pertussis toxoid vaccine at 3,

5, and 12 months of age. Pertussis infection was reduced by more than 70% in the group immunized with pertussis toxoid compared with the control group. The percentages of children whose temperatures increased to more than 38°C in the first 48 h after immunization were the same. Similarly, after the third dose, *redness* occurred in 10% of the vaccinees in the pertussis toxoid group and in 8% of the controls; *swelling* occurred in 9 versus 7%.

In addition to erythromycin prevention, 630 staff members considered to be contacts during an institutional outbreak of pertussis received a half dose of DT vaccine plus acellular pertussis vaccine (30[C]). Adverse effects were reported by 344 (54%) of the immunized staff; 64 adverse effects were classified as mild local reactions and 50 as moderate systemic reactions or moderate local reactions resulting in limitation of arm movement. Three vaccinees missed one or more days of work.

Combined vaccines (DTP or DTaP vaccine combined with other antigens, such as hepatitis B or Hemophilus influenzae type b (Hib) or inactivated poliovirus (IPV))

Four-valent, five-valent, and even six-valent combination vaccines based on DTP or DTaP vaccine and including other antigens such as hepatitis B or Hib or IPV will play an important role in future immunization programs. Some such combination vaccines have already been licensed in some countries, others are expecting to be licensed soon or are under evaluation in clinical trials. In general, there are similar results when comparing seroconversion rates, mean geometric antibody titers, and adverse reactions after the administration of combination vaccines or separate injections of DTP/DTaP vaccine and other single antigen vaccines.

A DTaP plus hepatitis B virus vaccine (SmithKline Beecham Biologicals) (group 1, 20 infants) has been compared with separate DTaP and hepatitis B virus vaccines (group 2, 10 infants) and DTaP vaccine alone (group 3, 10 infants) at different injection sites (31[C]). After immunization there were no statistically significant differences between the groups for the immune responses to any of the vaccine components. *Local reactions* were observed

in only one infant (group 1) and transient slight *fever* in two vaccinees (groups 1 and 2).

Typhoid fever vaccine *(SED-13, 950; SEDA-17, 373; SEDA-18, 332)*

All published studies of a relatively new Vi capsular polysaccharide typhoid fever vaccine have been reviewed (32[R]) (see also SEDA-18, 333). In two areas in which typhoid fever is endemic protective efficacy was 55 and 75%, respectively. The vaccine was well tolerated in all trials, inducing only minor reactions in fewer than 10% of the vaccinees.

VIRAL VACCINES

Hepatitis A vaccine *(SED-13, 928; SEDA-17, 373, SEDA-18, 333)*

To increase immunogenicity, hepatitis A vaccines commercially available are coupled to adjuvant aluminium phosphate or aluminium hydroxide. However, alum precipitates provoke *inflammatory responses at the injection site*. As an alternative adjuvant, immunostimulating reconstituted influenza virosomes have been used (33[C]). In 1994, a hepatitis A vaccine including the new adjuvant was licensed in Switzerland, and registration in other countries is under way. The vaccine has been evaluated in Thailand in 79 vaccinees aged 17—35 years. A single dose of vaccine resulted in 100% seroconversion, and all vaccinees maintained protective anti-hepatitis A antibodies over the 12-month observation period. The most frequent complaints after the administration of the vaccine were *pain and swelling at the injection site* (16 and 13%, respectively), *malaise* (10%), and *headache* (7.6%). Most reactions were mild and transient, lasting for one day or less (34[C]).

Human immunodeficiency virus vaccine (including other immunization in HIV-infected persons) *(SED-13, 930; SEDA-17, 374; SEDA-18, 334; SEDA-19, 299)*

Immunization of HIV-infected persons   In addition to five other cohort studies, a study in Haiti has confirmed that the risk of complications after BCG vaccination in HIV-infected children is low and that the risk does not outweigh the benefits of BCG vaccination in populations at high risk of tuberculosis during infancy and childhood (35[C]). Mild or moderate adverse effects occurred in 19 (9.6%) of 166 infants born to HIV-seronegative mothers compared with four (31%) of 13 HIV-infected infants.

Japanese encephalitis vaccine *(SED-13, 934)*

In Japan, seven case reports of *acute disseminated encephalomyelitis* following the receipt of Japanese encephalitis vaccine occurred between 1968 and 1990 (36[R]). The rates of less than one case per million doses of vaccine are similar when comparing the vaccine based on the Nakayama-Yoken strain (used since 1954) and the vaccine based on the Beijing strain now in use.

Measles vaccine *(SED-13, 935; SEDA-19, 300)*

It has been suggested that isolation of measles virus from patients suspected of a vaccine-induced complication and subsequent characterization of such isolated virus as either wild or vaccine virus may be useful in differentiating between natural measles and vaccine-associated complications (37[C]). Using marmoset lymphoblastoid B95a cells, isolation of measles virus from throat swabs or peripheral blood leukocytes became possible at high frequency.

Measles—mumps—rubella (MMR) vaccine (including measles—mumps and measles—rubella vaccine) *(SED-13, 937; SEDA-17, 376; SEDA-19, 300)*

Reports on adverse effects received in the St Helens and Knowsley district after the UK national measles and rubella immunization campaign of November 1994 have been analysed (38[C]). As only 0.24% of vaccinees suffered from mild adverse effects, such as *nausea, dizziness, abdominal pain, headache*, and *fever*, the authors considered the vaccine safe. These results are in agreement with other studies, which have reported a rate of 0.25%

of mild adverse effects after a second dose of MMR vaccine.

Nervous system A new method for active post-marketing surveillance of vaccine safety based on patient records (see above under surveillance of adverse events following immunization) has shown risk rates of *convulsions* of one per 3000 doses of MMR vaccine administered and one per 2600 doses of MMR vaccine containing the Urabe mumps strain (4[C]).

Transverse myelitis has been reported in a 20-year-old man after MMR vaccine (39[C]). Serological tests for Epstein-Barr, mumps, measles, and rubella viruses showed a significant rise in titers of rubella antibodies only (from 30 to 240 IU for IgG and from positive to strongly positive for IgM). Post-immunization transverse myelitis is rare.

Immunological and hypersensitivity reactions In 24 of 26 children aged 1—4 years who developed anaphylactic reactions within minutes after the administration of MMR vaccine IgE antibodies against gelatin were found (40[C]).

Mumps vaccine *(SED-13, 938; SEDA-17, 377; SEDA-18, 336; SEDA-19, 301)*

Vaccine-associated mumps meningitis The Ministry of Health and Welfare in Japan withdrew the domestically produced MMR vaccine containing the Urabe mumps vaccine strain in April 1993 (SEDA-18, 336). A retrospective study has been carried out to determinate the incidence of vaccine-associated meningitis after the administration of different locally produced MMR vaccines (MHW MMR vaccine, Takeda MMR vaccine, Biken MMR vaccine, and Kitasato MMR vaccine) (41[C]). Among the three MMR vaccines (Biken vaccine excepted) the incidence of meningitis was about one in 500—900 vaccinees. The criteria for inclusion of a case of meningitis were clinical symptoms of meningitis and pleocytosis in the cerebrospinal fluid.

A somewhat different note has been sounded from France, where all mumps vaccines produced and marketed contain the Urabe vaccine strain; the incidence of vaccine-associated meningitis has been estimated using two different data sources: the national network of hospital virology laboratories and the pharmacovigilance department of the manufacturer (42[C]). The risk of vaccine-associated meningitis was assessed as one case per 28—400 doses distributed when using the laboratory network data or one case per 13 000—67 200 doses distributed when using the pharmacovigilance data. The French vaccination committee recommended that the vaccine be continued to be used whilst awaiting vaccine containing the Jeryl-Lynn strain.

Rotavirus vaccine

Animal rotaviruses, including the rhesus rotavirus and the bovine rotavirus strains, have been evaluated as live attenuated rotavirus vaccines in humans. The results of further clinical trials using a serotype 1 bovine—human rotavirus reassortant vaccine (43[C]) and both rhesus rotavirus monovalent and tetravalent reassortant vaccines (44[C]) have been published. All the vaccines were well tolerated. After the first dose of the tetravalent rotavirus reassortant vaccine there was a significant increase in *fever* (over 38°C) compared with the monovalent vaccine and controls. There was no significant increase after the first, second, or third doses in vomiting or diarrhea. The protective efficacy of the bovine—human rotavirus reassortant was 87% against severe rotavirus gastroenteritis and 64% against all symptomatic rotavirus episodes. Both rhesus rotavirus vaccines appeared to be immunogenic, inducing an immune response in 85% of the monovalent and 93% of tetravalent vaccine recipients.

Rubella vaccine

A suspected case of rubella vaccine-associated *myelitis* has been reported (see under MMR vaccine above) (39[C]).

When women were questioned by phone about joint complaints following pregnancy, there was no evidence of an association between rubella immunization and the subsequent development of arthritis in 485 women who received rubella vaccine post-partum and 493 controls matched for age, place of residence, and date of delivery (45[C]). Those who reported joint complaints were invited for detailed investigation; 19 women in the group of vaccinees (3.9%) and 16 women in the control group (3.2%) were judged to have joint symptoms compatible with the study definition of arthritis.

Retinal vasculitis has been reported after rubella immunization (46[C]). Three weeks elapsed between immunization and the onset of the first symptoms; there was high intrathecal antibody production against rubella in the cerebrospinal fluid but little or none against other viruses.

Tick-borne encephalitis vaccine *(SED-13, 949; SEDA-17, 379; SEDA-18, 337)*

The immunogenicity and safety of simultaneous administration of tick-borne encephalitis vaccine plus tick-borne encephalitis immunoglobulin has been evaluated in 60 people compared with a 61 controls given TB vaccine alone (47[C]). On day 28 median tick-borne encephalitis antibodies were twice as high in the vaccine group as in the vaccine plus immunoglobulin group. All types of adverse events (*chills, influenza-like symptoms, pain at the injection site*) were reported less often in the tick-borne encephalitis vaccine group (25 vs. 45%). After the second dose (on day 28) the rate of adverse events was 7% in both groups.

Varicella vaccine *(SED-13, 950; SEDA-17, 379; SEDA-18, 337)*

The efficacy and safety of Oka/Merck varicella vaccine have been reviewed (48[R]). The authors concluded that the vaccine is highly immunogenic and confers protection in healthy children (98%) and adolescents (50%) as well as against moderate and severe varicella in children (100%) and adolescents with leukaemia. Reported adverse effects were mild *varicelliform rashes*, occasionally accompanied by *fever* and *pain at the injection site*.

Risk factors   In children with leukemia, vaccine-associated rash was reported in up to 50% of the vaccinees. When live attenuated varicella vaccine was licensed in 1995 in the US, the Committee on Infectious Diseases reviewed its safety and efficacy and gave recommendations for its use. Because varicella virus can be cultured from vaccine recipients with skin lesions, transmission of the vaccine virus can occur. However, contacts of vaccinees with leukemia developed extremely mild illnesses, indicating that the vaccine virus remains stable. A *zoster-like illness* has been reported in eight of 9000 healthy children immunized (49[R]).

MISCELLANEOUS

Immunization in children with fibrodysplasia ossificans progressiva   A child with fibrodysplasia ossificans progressiva developed permanent *heterotopic ossification* at the injection site after intramuscular DTP immunization (50[C]). The authors considered that intramuscular injections in children with fibrodysplasia ossificans progressiva constituted a risk factor, whereas subcutaneous injections could be carried out.

REFERENCES

1. Chen RT, Rastogi SC, Mullen JR, Hayes SW, Cochi SL, Donlon JA, Wassilak SG. The Vaccine Adverse Event Reporting System (VAERS). Vaccine 1994;12:542—9.
2. Rosenthal S, Chen RT. The reporting sensitivities of two passive surveillance systems for vaccine adverse events. Am J Publ Health 1995; 85:1706—9.
3. Wassilak SG, Glasser JW, Chen RT, Hadler SC. Utility of large, linked databases in vaccine safety, particularly in distinguishing independent and synergistic effects. In: Combined vaccines and simultaneous administration. Ann NY Acad Sci 1995;754:377—82.
4. Farrington P, Pugh S, Colville A, Flower A, Nash J, Morgan-Capner P, Rush M, Miller E. A new method for active surveillance of adverse events from DTP and MMR vaccines. Lancet 1995;345:567—9.
5. Chen RT. Special methodological issues in pharmacoepidemiology studies of vaccine safety. In: Strom BL, ed. Pharmacoepidemiology, 2nd ed. Chichester 1994:581—94.
6. Casanova JL, Jouanguy E, Lamhamedi S, Blanche S, Fischer A. Immunological conditions of children with disseminated infection. Lancet 1995;346:581.
7. Kröger L, Korppi M, Brander E, Kröger H, Wasz-Höckert O, Backman A, Rapoli J, Launiala K, Katila, ML. Osteitis caused by BCG vaccination: a retrospective analysis of 222 cases. J Infect Dis 1995;172:574—6.
8. Martinez-Pineiro JA, Solsona E, Flores N, Isorna S. Improving the safety of BCG immunotherapy by dose reduction. Eur Urol 1995;27 Suppl 1:13—18.
9. Mack D, Frick J. Low-dose Bacille Calmette-Guérin (BCG) therapy in superficial high-risk bladder cancer: a phase II study with the BCG strain Connaught Canada. Br J Urol 1995; 75:185—7.
10. Pagano F, Bassi P, Piazza N, Abatangelo G, Drago-Ferrante GL, Milani C. Improving the efficacy of BCG immunotherapy by dose reduction. Eur Urol 1995;27 Suppl 1:19—22.
11. Van der Meijden APM. Practical approaches to the prevention and treatment of adverse reactions to BCG. Eur Urol 1995;27 Suppl:23—8.
12. Jurincic-Winkler C, Metz KA, Beuth J, Sippel J, Klippel KF. Effect of keyhole limpet hemocyanin and Bacillus Calmette-Guérin (BCG) instillation on carcinoma in situ of the urinary bladder. Anticancer Res 1995;15:2771—6.
13. Rintala E, Jauhiainen K, Rajala P, Ruutu M, Kaasinen E, Alfthan O, Alfthan O, Hansson E, Juusela H, Kanerva K, Korhonen H, Nurmi M, Permi J, Petays P, Tainio H, Talja M, Tuhkanen K, Viitanen J. Alternating mitomycin C and Bacillus Calmette-Guérin instillation therapy for carcinoma in situ of the bladder. J Urol 1995; 154:2050—3.
14. Hallewin MA, Baert L, Benson RC Jr. Long-term results of whole bladder wall photodynamic therapy for carcinoma in situ of the bladder. Urology 1995;45:763—7.
15. Davis R, Spencer CM. Live oral cholera vaccine. A preliminary review of its pharmacology and clinical potential in providing protective immunity against cholera. Clin Immunother 1995; 4:235—47.
16. Coster TS, Killeen KP, Waldor MK, Seattle DT, Spriggs DR, Kenner JR, Trofa A, Sadoff JC, Mekalanos JJ, Taylor DN. Safety, immunogenicity, and efficacy of live attenuated *Vibrio cholerae* O139 vaccine prototype. Lancet 1995; 345:949—52.
17. Aggerbeck H, Fenger Ch, Heron I. Booster vaccination against diphtheria and tetanus in man. Comparison of calcium phosphate and alunimium hydroxide as adjuvants—II. Vaccine 1995;13: 1366—74.
18. Kurikka S, Kayhty H, Peltola H, Saarinen L, Eskola J, Makela PH. Neonatal immunization: response to *Haemophilus influenzae* type b tetanus toxoid conjugate vaccine. Pediatrics 1995; 95:815—22.
19. Twumasi PA Jr, Kumah S, Leach A, O'Dempsey TJD, Ceesay SJ, Todd J, Broome CV, Carlone GM, Pais LB, Holder PK, Plikaytis BD, Greenwood BM. A trial of a group A plus

group C meningococcal polysaccharide-protein conjugate vaccine in African infants. J Infect Dis 1995;171:632—8.

20. Khoo SH, StClair Roberts J, Mandal BK. Safety and efficacy of combined meningococcal and typhoid vaccine. Br Med J 1995;310:908—9.

21. Rosenthal S, Chen R, Hadler S. The safety of acellular pertussis vaccine versus whole-cell pertussis vacine. A postmarketing assessment. Arch Pediatr Adolesc Med 1996;150:457—60.

22. Brown GW. Nothing to whoop about. Arch Pediatr Adolesc Med 1996;150:461—3.

23. Pichichero ME, Christy C, Decker MD, Steinhoff MC, Edwards KM, Rennels MB, Anderson EL, Englund JA. Defining the key parameters for comparing reactions among acellular and whole-cell pertussis vaccines. Pediatrics 1995;96 Suppl II:588—92.

24. Englund JA, Anderson EL, Reed GF, Decker MD, Edwards KM, Pichichero ME, Steinhoff MC, Rennels MB, Deforest A, Meade BD. The effect of maternal antibody on the serologic response and the incidence of adverse reactions after primary immunization with acellular and whole-cell pertussis vaccines combined with diphtheria and tetanus toxoids. Pediatrics 1995;96 Suppl II:580—4.

25. Halperin SA, Mills E, Barreto L, Pim C, Eastwood BJ. Acellular pertussisvaccine as a booster dose for seventeen- to nineteen-month-old children immunized with either whole cell or acellular pertussis vaccine at two, four and six months of age. Pediatr Infect Dis J 1995;14:792—7.

26. Podda A, Bona G, Canciani G, Pistilli AMC, Contu B, Furlan R, Meloni T, Stramare D, Titone L, Rappuoli R, Granoff DM, Bartalini M, Budroni M, De Luca EC, Cascio A, Cascio G, Cossu M, Orto PD, Di Leo G. Effect of priming with diphtheria and tetanus toxoids combined with whole-cell pertussis vaccine or with acellular pertussis vaccine on the safety and immunogenicity of a booster dose of an acellular pertussis vaccine containing a genetically inactivated pertussis toxin in fifteen- to twenty-one-month-old children. J Pediatr 1995;127:238—43.

27. Advisory Committee on Immunization Practices (ACIP). Pertussis vaccination: use of acellular pertussis vaccines among infants and young children. Morb Mortal Wkly Rep 1997;46:1—25.

28. Trollfors B, Taranger J, Lagergard T, Lind L, Sundh V, Zackrisson G, Lowe CU, Blackwelder W, Robbins JB. A placebo-controlled trial of a pertussis-toxoid vaccine. New Engl J Med 1995;333:1045—50.

29. Marwick C. Acellular pertussis vaccine scores high in trial. Am Med J 1995;273:1892—3.

30. Shefer A, Dales L, Nelson M, Werner B, Baron R, Jackson R. Use and safety of acellular pertussis vaccine among adult hospital staff during an outbreak of pertussis. J Infect Dis 1995;171:1053—6.

31. Kanra G, Ceyhan M, Ecevit Z, Bogaerts H, De Grave D, Hauser P, Desmons P. Primary vaccination of infants with a combined diphtheria-tetanus-acellular pertussis-hepatitis B vaccine. Pediatr Infect Dis J 1995;14:998—1000.

32. Plotkin SA, Bouveret Le Cam N. A new typhoid vaccine composed of the Vi capsular polysaccharide. Arch Intern Med 1995;155:2293—9.

33. Glück R. Liposomal hepatitis A vaccine and liposomal multiantigen combination. J Liposome Res 1995;5:467—79.

34. Poovarawan Y, Theamboonlers A, Chumdermpadetsuk S, Gluck R, Cryz J Jr. Safety, immunogenicity, and kinetics of the immune response to a single dose of virosome-formulated hepatitis A vaccine in Thais. Vaccine 1995;13:891—3.

35. O'Brien KL, Ruff AJ, Louis MA, Desormeaux J, Joseph DJ, McBrien M, Coberly J, Boulos R, Halsey NA. Bacillus Calmette-Guérin complications in children born to HIV-1-infected women with a review of the literature. Pediatrics 1995;95:414—18.

36. Ohtaki E, Matsuishi T, Hirano Y, Maekawa K. Acute disseminated encephalomyelitis after treatment with Japanese B encephalitis vaccine (Nakayama-Yoken and Beijing strains). J Neurol Neurosurg Psychiatry 1995;59:316—17.

37. Kobune F, Funatu M, Takahashi H, Fukushima M, Kawamoto A, Iizuka S, Sakata H, Yamazaki S, Arita M, Wenbo X, Li Bi Z. Characterization of measles viruses isolated after measles vaccination. Vaccine 1995;13:370—2.

38. Wiratunga EBP, O'Brien J. National measles and rubella vaccination campaign. Br Med J 1995;310:1532.

39. Joyce KA, Rees JE. Transverse myelitis after measles, mumps, and rubella vaccine. Br Med J 1995;311:422.

40. Sakaguchi M. Vaccine reaction due to gelatin. J Allergy Clin Immunol 1996;98:1058—61.

41. Ueda K, Miyazaki C, Hidaka Y, Okada K, Kusuhara K, Kadoya R. Aseptic meningitis caused by measles-mumps-rubella vaccine in Japan. Lancet 1995;346:701—2.

42. Rebiere I, Galy-Eyraud C. Estimation of the risk of aseptic meningitis associated with mumps vaccination, France, 1991-1993. Int J Epidemiol 1995;24:1223—7.

43. Treanor JJ, Clark HF, Pichichero M, Christy C, Gouvea V, Shrager D, Palazzo S, Offit P. Evaluation of the protective efficacy of a serotype 1 bovine-human rotavirus reassortant vaccine in infants. Pediatr Infect Dis J 1995;14:301—7.

44. Bernstein DI, Glass RI, Rodgers G, Davidson BL, Sack DA. Evaluation of rhesus rotavirus monovalent and tetravalent reassortant vaccines in US children. J Am Med Assoc 1995;273:1191—6.

45. Slater PE, Ben Zvi T, Fogel A, Ehrenfeld M, Ever Hadani S. Absence of an association between rubella vaccination and arthritis in underimmune postpartum women. Vaccine 1995;13:1529—32.

46. Riikonen RS. Retinal vasculitis caused by rubella. Neuropediatrics 1995;26:174—6.

47. van Hedenstrom M, Heberle U, Theobald-K.

Vaccination against tick-borne encephalitis (TBE): influence of simultaneous application of TBE immunoglobulin on seroconversion and rate of adverse events. Vaccine 1995;13:759—62.

48.   Perry CM, Bryson HM. Oka/Merck varicella vaccine: a review of its immunogenicity and protective. Clin Immunother 1995;4:396—416.

49.   Committee on Infectious Diseases. Recommendations for the use of live attenuated varicella vaccine. Pediatrics 1995;95:791—6.

50.   Lanchoney TF, Cohen RB, Rocke DM, Zasloff MA, Kaplan FS. Permanent heterotopic ossification at the injection site after diphtheria-tetanus-pertussis immunizations in children who have fibrodysplasia ossificans progressiva. J Pediatr 1995;126:762—4.

H.W. Eijkhout and W.G. van Aken

33   Blood, blood components, plasma, and plasma products

BLOOD TRANSFUSION *(SED-13, 963; SEDA-17, 387; SEDA-19, 309)*

Non-infectious adverse effects of blood transfusion Non-infectious transfusion reactions, which are diverse in nature and severity, consist of life-threatening disorders, such as *acute intravascular or extravascular hemolytic reactions, anaphylactic reactions*, transfusion-related *acute lung injury*, transfusion-associated *graft-versus-host disease*, and relatively mild conditions (such as *febrile reactions, allergies*, and *delayed hemolytic reactions*) (1[R]). Information on the pathophysiology, diagnosis, and treatment of these reactions, although derived from studies in adults, can in most instances be applied to neonates (2[R]).

Immunization and immunomodulation Transfusion of blood components can induce *alloantibodies against erythrocyte and platelet antigens and HLA antigens* (3[C]), (4[c]).

Post-transfusion *purpura* is characterized by a sudden onset of severe thrombocytopenia and hemorrhage within 5—11 days after transfusion of blood products containing platelet material (4[c]). Post-transfusion purpura occurs most frequently in women with anti-HPA-1a antibodies. It can also be induced by antibodies against other epitopes on platelet membrane GPIIb/IIIa. It is assumed that primary immunization occurs during pregnancy. The occurrence of HLA antibodies is also associated with the use of non-leukocyte-depleted transfusions (3[C]).

HLA antibodies cause immunological *platelet transfusion refractoriness* (3[C]). Primary HLA alloimmunization can be prevented by the use of leukocyte-depleted blood products.

Filtration of platelets is a more effective method than centrifugation to deplete leukocytes (3[C]). Leucocyte-reduced blood-products not only reduce the prevalence of alloimmunization, but also transmission of infectious diseases, transfusion-related acute lung injury, and immunomodulation (5[c]).

Transfusion of blood is associated with *immunosuppression* (6[R]), and in patients undergoing surgery transfusion is a risk factor for infection. Non-operative site infections are more common after blood transfusion, suggesting that the association of transfusion with infection is independent of the operative trauma. Infections can be prevented by using filtered blood components (6[R]). The association between allogeneic blood transfusions and immunosuppression in recipients undergoing curative surgery for malignant tumors has raised concern (7[R]).

In a retrospective study of 500 colorectal cancer patients blood transfusion (autologous and homologous) was associated with a significantly increased risk of *cancer recurrence* (6[R]). On the other hand, several retrospective studies have provided no definitive evidence that allogeneic blood transfusion promotes the growth of tumors. Meta-analysis was used to explain the reported disagreements across 60 clinical studies published from 1982 to 1994 (8[R]). Before adjustment for the effect of confounding, a significant deleterious transfusion effect was found for all cancer sites (except for breast), but there was large variation in the relative risks, notably for colorectal and gastric cancers. However, when the computed unadjusted transfusion effect was reduced (to adjust for the effect of confounding), the significance of the adverse transfusion effect in most cancer sites was eliminated.

It has been suggested that blood transfusion has a positive effect on the outcome of Crohn's disease, because the immunosuppressive effects of transfusion might benefit patients in the same way that steroids affect the course of the disease. In most of the studies it has been observed that non-transfused patients had higher rates of recurrence than transfused patients.

Transfusion-related *acute lung injury*, a rare, serious complication of blood transfusion, caused by immunoreactivity of leukocyte antibodies (9[c]), is characterized by respiratory distress, diffuse bilateral alveolar and interstitial infiltrates on chest X-ray, and hypoxemia. The mortality rate is 10% (10[c]). It is thought to result from concomitant transfer of HLA or granulocyte antibodies from the donor's plasma to the recipient during blood transfusion. Donor antibodies, which interact with the marginated pool of recipient granulocytes mostly in the lung and activate the complement system, cause further neutrophil sequestration and aggregation. Furthermore, complement-activated neutrophils release enzymes that are directly toxic to the pulmonary capillary endothelium.

Transfusion-associated *graft-versus-host disease* is a rare but lethal disorder, caused by engraftment and proliferation of donor lymphocytes in immunocompromised patients (10[r]). It has also been reported after massive transfusion, exchange transfusions, and multiple intrauterine transfusions, as well as in premature infants (11[c]). It is characterized by fever, a maculopapular erythematous rash, anorexia, vomiting, hepatosplenomegaly, and raised liver enzymes. In 90% of cases the course is fatal (12[R]). After filtration of blood components a small number of leukocytes remain in the units and can cause graft-versus-host disease. Irradiation (2500 cGy) is still the procedure of choice in patients at risk. It is recommended that the erythrocytes are infused within 28 days after irradiation.

Acute hemolytic transfusion reaction, the most feared reaction associated with blood component therapy, occurs approximately once for every 25 000 units of erythrocyte concentrate transfused (13[R]). Acute hemolytic transfusion reactions are caused by pre-existent erythrocyte antibodies in the recipient that bind to the transfused red blood cells. Acute hemolytic transfusion reactions induce non-specific symptoms, such as fever, nausea, dyspnea, chills, and hypotension.

Anaphylactic reactions to blood products are rare (13[R]). The most common allergen is IgA, which can cause anaphylactic reactions in patients with IgA deficiency and circulating IgA antibodies.

Febrile, non-hemolytic transfusion reaction (14[R]) is defined as a rise in temperature of at least 1°C. It occurs in approximately 1% of all transfusions and is associated with the presence of donor leukocytes in the transfusate. Reduction of the leukocyte count of donor units, which is possible by filtration, will reduce the incidence.

The short-term complications of transfusions have been studied in 219 patients with various types of cancers. During a total of 483 transfusions, 8.7% had transfusion reactions; 10% of the patients had *positive antibody screening*, requiring further work-up; 3.2% had clinically significant antibodies that required the use of antigen-negative units (15[C]).

Bacterial infections transmitted by blood transfusion   Bacterial growth in blood components, such as erythrocyte and platelet concentrates, may have serious consequences for the recipient. Although the true incidence of bacterial contamination of stored cellular blood components has not been established, it has been suggested that septic reactions after transfusions may occur as often as one per 4000 platelet transfusions (16[R]).

The effect of allogeneic blood transfusions on the incidence of bacterial infections following trauma, burns, and surgery for malignant tumors has been examined (17[R]), (18[R]). In several retrospective and non-randomized prospective studies there was a significantly higher rate of bacterial infections in allogeneic transfused patients compared with patients who received autologous blood transfusions. Properly controlled, prospective, randomized studies are needed to determine whether there is a relation between postoperative bacterial infections and allogeneic transfusions.

Septic transfusion reactions after stored erythrocyte transfusions are often due to *Yersinia enterocolitica* (19[c]). Case reports from 13 fatal and 11 non-fatal reactions due to *Yersinia enterocolitica* serotypes O2, O3, O5, O6, and O9 have shown that all but two of the reactions occurred in blood that had been stored for more than 21 days. However, the severity of the reactions was not related to storage time (20[c]), (21[R]).

Serratia marcescens has been linked to erythrocyte contamination involving a blood bag manufacturing process, while *Serratia liquifasciens* has been identified as a erythrocyte and platelet contaminant (22[R]).

Platelet transfusion may be accompanied by septicemia. The identification of the bacterial strain from blood components is traditionally done by serological typing or plaque typing. Polymerase chain reaction-based fingerprinting may be used to show growth of *Proteus mirabilis* (23[c]).

Prospective bacteriological surveillance of more than 15 000 random donor platelet concentrates for 6 months in one center indicated a bacterial contamination rate of 4.4 in 10 000 (16[R]).

In vitro studies have supported the efficacy of pre-storage leukocyte reduction in the removal of bacteria from contaminated blood components (14[R]).

Viral infections transmitted by blood transfusion Although transfusion practice has become increasingly safe over recent years, the risk of transfusion-associated infection following a unit of screened blood has not been completely eliminated. An overview of the current safety issues (24[R]) has demonstrated the magnitude of the various risks due to viral infections, bacterial contamination, protozoan disease, and clerical errors. In another review (25[R]), on viral contamination of blood components and how to reduce infectivity, it has been concluded that at present the supply of blood offers a relatively low risk of viral infection. As a result of the use of effective viral inactivation procedures, products prepared from pooled plasma are now thought to carry less risk than that associated with single-donor products. However, viral inactivation of single-donor blood cell components is expected to be developed in the near future (25[R]).

Hepatitis C continues to be the agent that is most often transmitted, while HIV and hepatitis B are least likely to be transmitted (25[R]). Transmission of hepatitis C by erythrocyte concentrate has again been described (26[c]). The implicated donation was negative with ELISA-2, but PCR positive. Post-transfusion hepatitis B by HBV-negative blood transfusion has also been described (27[c]).

Other viruses, known to be transmitted by transfusion are cytomegalovirus, parvo B19, and hepatitis A. Transmission of cytomegalovirus is of greatest concern, because it can lead to serious disease or death among premature infants and immunocompromised patients (25[R]). Parvo B19 and hepatitis A are non-enveloped viruses, which are not susceptible to many viral inactivation methods currently used.

Several surveys have reported an incidence of parvo B19 infection of 0.004—0.03% in healthy blood donors (28[c]). In 136 subjects with hemophilia the seroprevalence of parvo B19 was 82% (29[R]). Although the seroprevalence was high and indicative of past B19 infection, there was no detectable B19 viral activity or any associated long-term clinical hematological sequelae. However, a 33-year-old man with hemophilia A has been described, who acquired iatrogenic parvo B19 infection due to factor VIII concentrate (30[c]). In this patient parvo B19 infection was manifested by pancytopenia, severe septicemia, hepatic dysfunction, and neurological symptoms. The batch of factor VIII concentrate received by the patient was positive for parvo B19 DNA tested by PCR.

Parasitic infections transmitted by blood transfusion Transmission of parasitic infections, such as malaria and *Trypanosoma cruzi* (Chagas' disease) continue to be a risk.

Infection with *T. cruzi* is life-long. Current strategies for preventing transfusion-associated Chagas' disease include serological tests. However, a disadvantage of these tests is the percentage of false-positive and false-negative results (31[c]). Recent in vivo experiments have shown that leukocyte-reducing filters are able to remove significant numbers of *T. cruzi* organisms present in artificially infected blood (32[c]).

Transmission of malaria by blood transfusion is a significant problem in regions in which the disease is endemic. *Plasmodium falciparum* in particular may lead to fatalities. Studies in Vietnam have shown that PCR detects many more cases of low-level parasitemia than thick blood films (33[c]).

Other infections transmitted by blood transfusion *Creutzfeldt-Jakob disease*, a neurodegenerative disease, has been transmitted by homografts and also by pituitary tissue extracts (34[c]), (35[c]). It has been observed that the infectious agent responsible is present not only in the central nervous system, but also in a wide variety of body tissues. Despite some results from animal experiments, which suggest that transmission of the agent responsible for this disease may be transmitted by whole blood, buffy coats, and serum, epidemiological studies have not supported the contention that administration of blood transmits this disease (36[R]).

Peripheral blood stem cells

The dosage of chemotherapeutic agents in the treatment of malignancies is limited by bone-marrow suppression and various toxic effects. The use of hemopoietic progenitor cells in combination with growth factors has allowed the delivery of multiple cycles and more dose-intensive chemotherapy (37[c]), (38[c]). Peripheral blood stem cells can be mobilized by the administration of growth factors and/or chemotherapy and collected by leukapheresis. The number of peripheral blood CD34+ cells is the best predictor for the yield of the stem cells (39[c]). Peripheral blood stem cells have a number of advantages over autologous bone-marrow transplantation. Their collection does not require anesthesia, recovery after myeloablative therapy is more rapid, and the risk of contamination of residual tumor cells is possibly lower (40[c]).

Complications associated with peripheral blood stem cell transplantation can be divided into three groups.

First, complications attributable to stem cell mobilization and harvesting. Drugs, such as melphalan, that are toxic to stem cells may adversely affect the yield and performance of peripheral blood stem cells (41[c]). During mobilization and harvesting *venous catheter occlusion* may occur, the risk being increased by the use of GM-CSF (molgramostim). Chemotherapy used for cell mobilization can cause adverse effects, such as *fever* and *sepsis*, *thrombocytopenia*, *neutropenic anemia*, and *hemorrhagic cystitis*. Growth factors, used for cell mobilization, can also result in *bone pain*, *pleural effusions*, and *peripheral edema*.

The second group of complications is attributable to the high-dose conditioning regimen. *Neutropenia* can cause pneumonitis, bacteremia, and septic shock. Other complications are *hypoproliferative anemia* and *thrombocytopenia*. Abnormalities in humoral and cell-mediated immunity have also been reported. In addition, delayed engraftment, partial engraftment, or even non-engraftment have been reported.

Complications have been observed during the infusion of cryopreserved cells (42[R]). Infusion of cryopreserved peripheral blood stem cells is associated with complications such as *facial flushing*, *hemoglobinuria*, *renal insufficiency*, *cough*, and *nausea*. However, none of these complications is life-threatening.

Engraftment of peripheral blood stem cells is often associated with an *engraftment syndrome* (43[c]), which includes fever, skin rash, capillary leak, and pulmonary infiltrates. The fever during the engraftment process is non-infective. Administration of G-CSF (filgrastim) after transplantation increases the incidence of this syndrome (43[c]).

Umbilical cord blood

Human umbilical cord blood was identified as a potential source of hemopoietic progenitor cells in the 1970s (44[r]). The use of umbilical cord blood carries little risk to the donor: there is no need for general anesthesia, no blood replacement, and no discomfort. However, immediate clamping of the cord, which is necessary for the collection of cord blood, has been reported to produce cerebral hemorrhage in premature infants (45[c]), caused by the sudden increase in arterial pressure due to immediate clamping.

Umbilical cord blood contains a sufficiently large number of hemopoietic stem and progenitor cells to engraft young/small recipients (46[c]). It is indicated for the treatment of malignant and non-malignant disorders, such as juvenile chronic myelogenous leukemia and Fanconi anemia (47[R]).

An important advantage of using cord blood is the immunological naiveté of the cells, as confirmed by the low incidence and reduced severity of graft-versus-host disease. In addition, there might be a reduced risk of transmission of viral infection, for example, cytomegalovirus (44[r]), (46[c]). It is hypothesized that the rate of contamination by cytomegalovirus is significantly lower in cord blood than in donated bone-marrow.

A major disadvantage associated with the use of human umbilical cord blood is potential contamination by maternal T cells, which may precipitate life-threatening *graft-versus-host disease*. However, several groups have shown that maternal cells cannot be detected in the umbilical cord blood by cytogenic or DNA techniques (48[C]). There is also a risk of infection after vaginal delivery, when the surface of the placenta and cord come in contact with the non-sterile mucosa of the cervix and vagina and the perineal skin (44[r]). A possible disadvantage is the unwitting transmission of a genetic disease affecting hemopoietic cells (49[C]).

The following questions remain to be answered: whether the number of stem and progenitor cells in umbilical cord blood is sufficient for engraftment and repopulation of the hemopoietic system of larger recipients; whether greater HLA disparities between donor and recipient can be tolerated; whether the risk of leukemia relapse after umbilical cord blood transplantation is greater if the risk of graft-versus-host disease is lower. Another unsolved problem is whether the lower incidence of graft-versus-host disease indicates a reduction in graft-versus-leukemia activity and thus an increased risk of leukemia relapse (49[C]).

Erythrocyte substitutes

The hazards of transfusion of erythrocytes include hemolysis due to erythrocyte incompatibility, transmission of infections, and circulatory overload (50[R]). Hemoglobin solutions and perfluoro compounds are substitutes for erythrocytes. The theoretical advantages of these products are prolonged shelf-life, universal compatibility, and absence of viruses, while their oxygen delivery potential is greater than that of conventional plasma expanders (51[R]). Possible indications for erythrocyte substitutes are emergency resuscitation of trauma patients and peri-operative hemodilution.

Hemoglobin solutions are prepared from human or bovine erythrocytes. There is also a synthetic human hemoglobin prepared by recombinant DNA technology. Hemoglobin is a tetramer, which dissociates outside erythrocytes. To prevent its dissociation several techniques are used, for example polymerization, internal stabilization, encapsulation, and macromolecular linkage (50[R]).

Among the adverse effects of hemoglobin solutions *vasospasm* is one of the most prominent. Infusion of hemoglobin solution results in a *low cardiac output* with an *increase in systemic and pulmonary artery pressure*. It has been postulated that hemoglobin leaks through vascular endothelium and binds to the endothelium-derived relaxing factor, nitric oxide, causing vasospasm (50[R]), (51[R]). Polymerization or encapsulation of hemoglobin will prevent its extravasation (52[R]).

Infusion of tetrameric, stroma-free hemoglobin may cause *renal damage*. It is uncertain if impurities or α-β dimers themselves are responsible for this.

Hemoglobin is cleared by the mononuclear phagocyte system, causing blockade of this system and interfering with essential functions, such as ingestion of bacteria. Further investigation is required to investigate the possibility that free iron increases bacterial growth, leading to fulminant septicemia (51[R]). To assess safety and efficacy, clinical trials with several hemoglobin solutions have begun.

Perfluoro compounds are excreted through the lungs. There is evidence that macrophages that have ingested perfluoro compounds lose phagocytic function or are stimulated to release cytokines (50[R]). Acute adverse effects of perfluoro compounds include: *facial flushing*; *fever*, caused by the release of prostaglandins and cytokines; and 'flu-like' symptoms may occur 1—4 h after transfusion (53[R]).

Small falls in platelet count have been observed that 2—4 days after transfusion of perfluoro compounds, in one case to not lower than 80×10^9/l (53[R]) and in another to 130×10^9/l (54[c]); this is thought to be caused by interaction of platelets with the emulsion, leading to the removal of senescent platelets by the reticuloendothelial system.

Perfluorocarbons, such as perflubron, may prove to be of use as oxygen carriers in resuscitation and in intraoperative hemodilution.

Albumin *(SED-13, 973; SEDA-18, 363)*

The efficacy and safety of albumin and the colloid hetastarch have been compared in 85 patients with post-aneurysmal subarachnoid hemorrhage (55[C]). On the basis of hetastarch-associated coagulopathy (see also Chapter 34) and data that show that albumin may be the most effective agent for increasing cerebral blood flow and preventing infarction, the authors stopped using hetastarch in these patients and decided to recommend albumin exclusively.

Intravenous immunoglobulin *(SED-13, 974; SEDA-17, 390; SEDA-19, 306)*

Intravenous immunoglobulin, manufactured from pooled plasma of several thousand donors, is used in a wide variety of disorders, such as primary and secondary immune deficiencies, immune disorders (such as Kawasaki disease, dermatomyositis, and immune thrombocytopenia), and neurological diseases (such as Guillain-Barré syndrome and chronic inflammatory demyelinating polyneuropathy) (56[R]), (57[C]), (58[C]). Several mechanisms of immunomodulation by immunoglobulins have been proposed, including blockade of receptors for the Fc portion of IgG on reticuloendothelial cells, interference with activated complement, and modulation of the immune system by anti-idiotype antibodies (59[c]), (60[R]).

The rationale for the efficacy of intravenous immunoglobulin in the treatment of acute Kawasaki syndrome is poorly understood. It has been proposed that its beneficial effect could be due to the presence of antibodies that inhibit bacterial toxin (superantigen)-induced stimulation of the immune response, including cytokine-induced cell endothelial activation (61[R]).

Adverse reactions to intravenous immunoglobulin are mostly mild, and include *fever*, *headache*, *myalgia*, *nausea*, and *vomiting*. These reactions usually start 30—60 min after the onset of infusion and are effectively treated by slowing the rate of infusion (SEDA-19, 306; (59[c]), (62[c])).

Cardiovascular Hypersensitivity myocarditis has been reported in a patient with Guillain-Barré syndrome treated with intravenous immunoglobulin (63[c]).

A 43-year-old man was taking phenytoin because of partial epilepsy. He was given 0.4 g/kg of intravenous immunoglobulin on each of 2 days, and after the last dose on the second day he complained of abdominal pain, aching shoulders, and backache. He developed hypotension and subsequently died. The autopsy findings suggested cardiac failure due to hypersensitivity myocarditis. Hypersensitivity myocarditis has been associated with phenytoin, but this patient had taken phenytoin for 8 years and had never had signs of heart failure.

In this case the intravenous immunoglobulin may have triggered a hypersensitivity myocarditis, following sensitization by phenytoin.

Nervous system *Cerebral arterial vasospasm* and reversible *encephalopathy* have been observed in a 42-year-old woman with Guillain-Barré syndrome treated with intravenous immunoglobulin (64[c]). Multifocal encephalopathy developed 3 days after completion of treatment. In addition, aseptic meningitis with neutrophilic cerebrospinal fluid developed. An explanation for the encephalopathy in this patient was not found. However, aseptic meningitis has been reported several times (SEDA-19, 306), hypersensitivity through the entry of immunoglobulin molecules into the cerebrospinal fluid compartment being held responsible.

Hematological *Hemolytic anemia* and *neutropenia* may occur after infusion of intravenous immunoglobulin (SEDA-19, 307; (62[C])). Hemolysis can occur even in the presence of low titers of anti-A, anti-B, and anti-Rh (D) antibodies in intravenous immunoglobulin. Progressive neutropenia has been noted in a child with Guillain-Barré syndrome treated with intravenous immunoglobulin (59[c]). The neutropenia resolved 3 days after the end of therapy. The batches of intravenous immunoglobulin used in this patient contained a high concentration of anti-neutrophil antibodies, compared with other batches. Although the half-life of intravenous immunoglobulin is 18—23 days, the neutrophil count in this patient normalized 3 days after withdrawal. The authors proposed that when serum concentrations of immunoglobulin rise during immunoglobulin therapy, catabolism of immunoglobulin increases; this would shorten the half-life of anti-neutrophil antibodies, allowing a more rapid return of neutrophils. An alternative explanation for this phenomenon is that the anti-neutrophil antibodies in the immunoglobulin caused the neutropenia, but that the immunoglobulin itself down-regulated the immune system, resulting in normalization of serum neutrophils.

Thrombotic complications Veno-occlusive disease of the liver has been described in patients treated with intravenous immunoglobulin after bone-marrow transplantation (65^C). Intravenous immunoglobulin 0.5 g/kg was given to 45 recipients of bone-marrow from HLA-identical siblings once a week during the first 3 months after transplantation. The control group consisted of 53 previously transplanted HLA-identical siblings. The incidence of veno-occlusive disease was 16% in the immunoglobulin group compared with 6% in the control group. Although 60% of the immunoglobulin group received heparin prophylaxis, fatal veno-occlusive disease occurred in 11% of the immunoglobulin group and in none of the controls. The concentration of infused immunoglobulin correlates with the viscosity of plasma and whole blood. In veno-occlusive disease, in which sinusoidal blood flow is already reduced, the risk of microthrombosis caused by increased serum viscosity may be even higher. Necrotic hepatocytes may give rise to antigens which may react with antibodies and form immune complexes, thus enhancing thrombosis and further liver damage.

Urinary system   A potential but rare adverse effect of intravenous immunoglobulin is *deterioration in renal function* in patients with some disorders, such as systemic lupus erythematosus. The transient decline in renal function has been attributed to glomerular damage from newly formed immune complexes. Tubular damage has also been observed, resulting from an increase in blood and plasma viscosity and from the infusion of sucrose, which is included as a stabilizer of intravenous immunoglobulin (66^c).

Transmission of infectious agents Intravenous immunoglobulin is usually prepared by Cohn fractionation and finally purified by methods such as DEAE Sephadex and adsorption chromatography (SEDA-19, 307). The Cohn fractionation technique only partly reduces the risk of viral transmission, the extent of reduction varying with the type of virus. Transmission of HIV or hepatitis B in recipients of intravenous immunoglobulin has never been reported (67^R). However an association between immunoglobulin therapy (Gammagard, manufactured by Baxter) and hepatitis C infection was reported in February 1994 (68^c). In France, 233 patients exposed to Gammagard were tested for hepatitis C antibody and hepatitis C virus RNA (69^c). Nineteen patients (8.1%) were positive for hepatitis C virus RNA. The link between hepatitis C infection and the batches of Gammagard that had been used was reinforced by over-representation of the hepatitis C virus 2b genotype (58%), which contrasts with the low prevalence of this genotype in France (1%).

Among 23 patients who received Gammagard, 44% developed circulating hepatitis C virus RNA (68^c). To ensure the safety of immunoglobulin it has been suggested that all anti-hepatitis C positive donors should be excluded and all batches of immunoglobulin should be screened routinely by PCR (70^c), (71^c), (72^R). Recently manufacturers of human immunoglobulins have introduced additional chemical and physical steps, such as solvent-detergent, S-sulfonation, pasteurization, and β-propiolactone, to further improve the safety of immunoglobulins (67^R).

Clotting factors *(SED-13, 975; SEDA-17, 392; SEDA-18, 345; SEDA-19, 311)*

Clotting factors are indicated for patients with isolated or combined clotting factor deficiency. Important adverse effects are virus transmission (for example, HIV, hepatitis C), formation of inhibitors of factors VIII and IX, immunosuppression, and thrombotic complications.

Plasma-derived factor VIII concentrate and recombinant factor VIII are both used in the treatment of hemophilia A. In multicenter studies in previously untreated patients with hemophilia A treated with recombinant factor VIII mild adverse reactions occurred in 0.1—0.75%.

Continuous infusion of coagulation factor concentrates, producing steady-state plasma concentrations (73[R]), may be successful in treating hemorrhage in some patients with factor VIII inhibitors and in patients with lingual and buccal hemorrhages that have been difficult to manage by conventional approaches. In some patients continuous infusion appears to have a role in attempting to eliminate circulating alloantibodies. Continuous infusion can also be used peri-operatively (74[R]).

One of the most serious complications of replacement therapy in hemophilia A is the *development of inhibitors* (75[R]), (76[R]). Several mutations in the factor VIII gene may increase the risk of formation of inhibitors. In recently published studies of patients with severe hemophilia the frequency of inhibitors has been 15—52% in patients using intermediate pure products, 24% in patients treated with monoclonal-antibody purified products, and 19—24% in patients using recombinant factor VIII concentrate (75[R]).

Congenital factor XIII deficiency is a rare autosomal recessive disorder, for the treatment of which human placenta-derived factor XIII concentrate and plasma-derived factor XIII are available. These two products have been compared in a randomized cross-over study (77[c]). The mean half-life of factor XIII activity and antigen was almost identical for both products. The response and in vivo recovery was slightly better for plasma-derived concentrate. Five minor adverse effects were reported. The adverse effects of the plasma-derived product were mild *hematomas*, a small (0.6°C) *increase in body temperature*, and *headache*. The adverse effects of the human placenta product were slight *pressure in the throat*, mild *pruritus*, and *erythema*.

Hematological   A serious adverse effects of continuous infusion is *thrombophlebitis* at the venous access site, which can be prevented by adding heparin (74[R]). The major risk of factor IX concentrates is thrombogenicity (73[R]), attributable to small amounts of activated coagulation factors. It has been suggested that

highly purified factor IX concentrates have lower thrombogenic potential. Infection of the central venous catheter (74[R]), another complication, can be prevented by combinations of antibiotics, changes of dressing, and antimicrobial chemical solutions. Other complications may arise through problems with pump design, accuracy, and reliability (78[R]), and through air leaks in the tubing/bag before the pump unit, which may cause the pump to compress air into the patient's veins (78[R]).

Prothrombin complex, which contains clotting factors II, VII, IX, and X, is indicated for the treatment of bleeding episodes in patients with isolated or combined clotting deficiencies. Its use, however, is associated with *thrombotic complications*, including superficial/deep vein thrombosis, pulmonary embolism, cerebral embolism, arterial thrombosis, and disseminated intravascular coagulation. The thrombogenicity of prothrombin complex has been attributed to the presence of small quantities of activated factors VIIa, IXa, or Xa, or coagulant-active phospholipids (79[c]). The risk of thrombosis after the administration of prothrombin complex increases with dose, frequency of administration, and the presence of liver disease (79[c]).

Infusion of high purity factor IX concentrate results in less activation of coagulation. In 72 patients given a factor IX concentrate (Mononine), six complications have been reported (79[c]). There was only one episode of *thrombophlebitis* at the site of the infusion. None of 13 patients with a prior history of thrombosis with prothrombin complex experienced thrombotic complications. In a second study with factor IX concentrate it was concluded that factor IX concentrate in combination with an antifibrinolytic agent does not cause activation of the coagulation cascade (80[c]). Prothrombin complex contains a relatively low concentration of factor VII, compared with the concentrations of the other factors. Patients with isolated factor VII deficiency treated with prothrombin complex often suffer thrombotic complications. To prevent thrombotic complications in factor VII-deficient patients, intermediate factor VII and recombinant factor VIIa have been developed.

Immunological and hypersensitivity reactions For the production of ultrapure factor VIII concentrates (plasma-derived or recombinant), monoclonal antibodies directed against factor VIII are used. These antibodies, which are murine immunoglobulins, are present in very low concentrations in the final product. In patients given plasma-derived factor VIII concentrates, no human anti-mouse immunoglobulins were formed, while in four (6%) of 68 patients given recombinant factor VIII concentrate new human anti-mouse immunoglobulins were present; however, human anti-mouse immunoglobulins developed in 1/22 multitransfused patients during treatment with monoclonal antibody-purified plasma-derived factor VIII concentrate (81[c]).

In a 22-year-old woman with severe deficiency of von Willebrand factor, treated with factor VIII-vWF concentrate, IgG alloantibodies to von Willebrand factor occurred (82[c]). These alloantibodies resulted in *anaphylactic reactions*. No adverse effects were observed after infusion of recombinant factor VIII concentrate.

In a patient with severe hemophilia A an episode of anaphylaxis followed treatment with recombinant factor VIII (83[c]). Endotoxin contamination of the product or antibodies to recombinant product-related antigens (recombinant factor VIII, Von Willebrand factor, mouse monoclonal anti-human factor VIII, human and bovine serum albumin, polyethylene glycol 3350) were not identified. The authors suggested that pretreatment with hydrocortisone and diphenhydramine will be necessary for this patient when factor VIII concentrate is administered.

Transmission of infection The use of virucidal treatment during the production of clotting factor concentrates has improved the safety of concentrates (84[c]). In Germany 111 patients, aged 1—23 years, with hemophilia A and B and Von Willebrand disease have been tested for hepatitis C. All had used concentrates that were virus-inactivated by pasteurization for 10 h at 60°C in aqueous solution (84[c]). One of the patients was seropositive for hepatitis C; the confirmation test (recombinant immunoblot assay) was positive, while the polymerase chain reaction did not detect hepatitis C virus RNA. Although a cause-and-effect relation between concentrate infusion and infection could not be found, the authors suggested that the risk of hepatitis C transmission by pasteurized clotting concentrates is not entirely negligible. They suggested that two virus-inactivating methods should be used in the manufacture of clotting factor concentrates, in order to further increase the safety.

Risk factors In HIV-negative hemophiliacs, dysfunction of the specific immune response, such as inhibition of monocyte phagocytic function, has been observed after infusion of factor VIII concentrate (85[R]). Furthermore, a functional defect in the interaction between antigen-presenting monocytes and CD4+ cells, following exposure to bacterial antigen (85[R]), has been detected.

Proliferative responses after stimulation of lymphocytes from HIV-negative hemophiliacs are abnormal. Isolated T cells from HIV-negative hemophiliacs treated with factor VIII concentrate have reduced production of IL-2 and expression of IL-2 receptors after in vitro stimulation. There are two hypotheses to explain these abnormalities in HIV-negative hemophiliacs. One is that the abnormalities are due to chronic (re-)infection with hepatitis C. It has also been suggested that the abnormalities result from prolonged massive exposure to proteins and alloantigens present in factor VIII products. These abnormalities may cause increased susceptibility to infections and a greater risk of malignancies (85[R]).

The rate of fall in CD4 count in HIV-positive patients that was observed when intermediate pure factor VIII concentrates were used is slower when high-purity factor concentrates are used. This implies that intermediate-purity products may have some detrimental effect on the immune system (86[c]).

There is no clear relation between the quantity of clotting factors used and progression of HIV.

Erythropoietin (epoetin) *(SED-13, 978; SEDA-17, 394; SEDA-18, 348; SEDA-19, 307)*

Recombinant human erythropoietin is currently available for both intramuscular and intravenous administration. It stimulates erythropoiesis, such as in patients with renal insufficiency and renal failure, in whom anemia is due to erythropoietin deficiency. The rise in hematocrit (87[R]) that erythropoietin produces in these patients is accompanied by reduced blood transfusion requirements and improved quality of life. Patients with end-stage renal disease treated with erythropoietin require less hospitalization for cardiac, infectious, and gastrointestinal diseases, probably because of general improvement in health (88[c]). Another use of erythropoietin is in the treatment of zidovudine-induced anemia (87[R]), which may be caused by insufficient production of erythropoietin, bone-marrow unresponsiveness to erythropoietin, or infection with HIV (89[r]).

The use of erythropoietin results in lower transfusion requirements in patients with hypoproliferative anemia due to malignant diseases and chronic infections (90[C]), (91[R]), (92[c]). There is no evidence of adverse effects in patients with cancer when erythropoietin and chemotherapy are simultaneously used (91[R]), and no evidence that erythropoietin may stimulate the growth of solid tumors (90[R]). The response rate of treatment with erythropoietin in patients with anemia associated with cancer is 32–85%.

Several possible indications for erythropoietin are currently under investigation; for example, sickle cell anemia, anemia due to rheumatoid arthritis, and anemia of prematurity. It appears that in anemia of prematurity high dosages are required to obtain a response. In a study in 77 very low birth-weight preterm infants, weekly doses of erythropoietin of 300 U/kg or more reduced the use of erythrocyte transfusions (93[C]).

Erythropoietin accelerates erythrocyte recovery after allogenic bone-marrow transplantation, but has no such effect in autologous transplantation (94[R]).

Factors that may influence the response to erythropoietin include iron deficiency, underlying infections, aluminium intoxication, cyanocobalamin (vitamin B12) deficiency, and occult blood loss.

Adverse effects of erythropoietin include *hypertension, hypersensitivity encephalopathy/seizures*, a *'flu-like'* syndrome, and *thrombosis of vascular access* in dialysis patients (SEDA-19, 308).

Subcutaneous administration of erythropoietin is the preferred route, since slow release of subcutaneous depots results in a longer circulating half-life, providing more sustained plasma concentrations (87[R]), (91[R]). Subcutaneous administration can produce burning sensations at injection sites, caused by components such as citrate used in the formulation (SEDA-19, 308). It has been suggested that dilution of the vehicle with benzylalcoholic saline or reducing the injection volume to 0.1 ml can ameliorate the pain associated with injection.

Erythropoietin is contraindicated in patients in whom therapy will result in polycythemia and in patients with uncontrolled hypertension.

Cardiovascular In patients with chronic renal failure erythropoietin has been associated with *exacerbation of pre-existing hypertension* and increased *shunt thrombosis*. These adverse effects were due to excessive doses of erythropoietin and too rapid correction of anemia, rather than to direct effects of erythropoietin (87[R]).

The mechanism of hypertension is unclear, but it has been suggested that increased blood viscosity, reversal of hypoxic vasodilatation, and a direct pressor effect of erythropoietin are important (94[R]).

In a study of 20 dialysis patients treated with erythropoietin, erythrocyte mass, peripheral vascular resistance, and platelet cytosolic calcium increased, and autonomic function improved. The authors postulated that all these factors contribute to raised blood pressure during erythropoietin therapy (95[c]).

Nervous system In 4% of hemodialysis patients with anemia treated with erythropoietin seizures have been observed. However, patients with end-stage renal failure are predisposed to seizures. An incidence of 8% of seizures has been reported in dialysis patients not treated with erythropoietin.

MISCELLANEOUS

C1-esterase inhibitor concentrate

Patients with hereditary angio-edema are deficient in C1-esterase inhibitor. Hereditary angio-edema is an autosomal dominant trait and is characterized by episodic bouts of swelling of submucosal and subcutaneous tissue. C1-esterase inhibitor concentrate is a plasma-derived product that is effective in the management of acute attacks of hereditary angio-edema.

A 58-year-old woman with hereditary angio-edema and mixed connective tissue disease had cutaneous edema of her face and extremities several times a year, but infrequent attacks of laryngeal edema and abdominal pain (96^c). When she presented with laryngeal discomfort, triggered by an insect bite, she received C1-esterase inhibitor concentrate. Her dyspnea disappeared several hours later. Ten days later she had frequent attacks of cutaneous edema on her face and extremities and she also began to experience abdominal pain. No triggers or causes for these exacerbations were found.

In the absence of antibodies to C1-esterase inhibitor and other causes for this phenomenon, the authors postulated that the exacerbations were caused by the inhibitor.

REFERENCES

1. Jeter EK, Spivey MA. Noninfectious complications of blood transfusion. Hematol Oncol Clinics North Am 1995;9:187—204.
2. Holman P, Blajchman MA, Heddle N. Noninfectious adverse effects of blood transfusion in the neonate. Transfus Med Rev 1995;9:277—87.
3. Novotny VMJ, van Doorn R, Witvliet MD, Claas FHJ, Brand A. Occurrence of alleogeneic HLA and non-HLA antibodies after transfusion of prestorage filtered platelets and red blood cells: a prospective study. Blood 1995;85:1736—41.
4. Gabriel A, Lassnigg A, Kurz M, Panzer S. Post-transfusion purpura due to HPA-1a immunization in a male patient: response to subsequent multiple HPA-1a-incompatible red-cell transfusions. Transfus Med 1995;5:131—4.
5. Dzieczkowski JS, Barrett BB, Nester D, Campell M, Cook J, Sugrue M, Andersen JW, Anderson KC. Characterization of reactions after exclusive transfusion of white cell-reduced cellular blood components. Transfusion 1995;35:20—5.
6. Tartter PI. Immunologic effects of blood transfusion. Immunol Invest 1995;24:277—88.
7. Blajchman MA, Bordin JO. The tumor growth-promoting effect of allogeneic blood transfusions. Immunol Invest 1995;24:311—17.
8. Vamvakas EC. Perioperative blood transfusion and cancer recurrence: meta-analysis for explanation. Transfusion 1995;35:760—8.
9. Florell SR, Velasco S, Fine PG. Perioperative recognition, management and pathologic diagnosis of transfusion-related acute lung injury. Anesthesiology 1994;81:508—10.
10. Davey RJ. Transfusion-associated graft-versus-host disease and the irradiation of blood components. Immunol Invest 1995;24:431—4.
11. Hentschel R, Broecker EB, Kolde G, Frosch M, Friedrich W, Holzgreve W, Westphal E, Harms E. Intact survival with transfusion-associated graft-versus-host disease proved by human leukocyte antigen typing of lymphocytes in skin biopsy specimens. J Pediatr 1995:126:61—4.
12. Spector D. Transfusion-associated graft-versus-host disease: an overview and two case reports. Oncol Nurs Forum 1995;22:97—101.
13. Sloop GD, Friedberg RC. Complications of blood transfusion. Blood Transfus 1995;98:159—71.
14. Miller JP, Mintz PD. The use of leukocyte-reduced blood components. Hematol Oncol Clinics North Am 1995;9:69—90.
15. Mohandas K, Aledort L. Transfusion requirements, risks, and costs for patients with malignancy. Transfusion 1995;35:427—30.
16. Blajchman MA. Bacterial contamination of blood products and the value of pre-transfusion testing. Immunol Invest 1995;24:163—70.
17. Nielsen HJ. Detrimental effects of perioperative blood transfusion. Br J Surg 1995;82:582—7.
18. Bordin JO, Blajchman MA. Immunosuppressive effects of allogeneic blood transfusion: implications for the patient with malignancy. Hematol Oncol Clinics North Am 1995;9:205—18.
19. Kimber RJ. *Yersinia* enterocolitica and blood transfusion. Med J Aust 1995;162:277.
20. Beresford AM. Transfusion reaction due to *Yersinia enterocolitica* and review of other reported cases. Pathology 1995;27:133—5.
21. Goldman M, Delage G. The role of leukodepletion in the control of transfusion-transmitted disease. Transfus Med Rev 1995;9:9—19.
22. Krishnan LAG, Brecher ME. Transfusion-transmitted bacterial infection. Hematol Oncol Clinics North Am 1995;9:167—204.
23. Engstrand M, Engstrand L, Högman CF, Hambraeus A, Branth S. Retrograde transmission of *Proteus mirabilis* during platelet transfusion and the use of arbitrarily primed polymerase chain

reaction for bacteria typing in suspected cases of transfusion transmission of infection. Transfusion 1995;35:871—3.

24. Sloand EM, Pitt E, Klein HG. Safety of the blood supply. J Am Med Assoc 1995;274;1368—73.

25. Dodd RY. Viral contamination of blood components and approaches for reduction of infectivity. Immunol Invest 1995;24:25—48.

26. Vrielink H, van der Poel CL, Reesink HW, Zaaijer HL, Lelie PN. Transmission of hepatitis C virus by anti-HCV-negative blood transfusion. Vox Sang 1995;68:55—6.

27. Elghouzzi M-H, Couroucé A-M, Magnius LO, Lunel F, Lapierre V. Transmission of hepatitis B virus by HBV-negative blood transfusion. Lancet 1995;346:964.

28. Yoto Y, Kudoh T, Haseyama K, Suzuki N, Oda T, Katoh T. Incidence of human parvo B19 DNA detection on blood donors. Br J Haematol 1995;91:1017—18.

29. Ragni MV, Koch WC, Jordan JA. Parvo B19 infection in patients with hemophilia. Transfusion 1996;36:238—41.

30. Yee TT, Cohen BJ, Pasi KJ, Lee CA. Transmission of symptomatic parvo B19 infection by clotting factor concentrate. Br J Haematol 1996;93:457—9.

31. Grijalva MJ, Rowland EC, Powell MR, McCormick TS, Escalante L. Blood donors in vector-free zone of ecuador potentially infected with *Trypanosoma cruzi*. Am J Trop Med Hyg 1995;52:360—3.

32. Moraes-Souza H, Bordin JO, Bardossy L, MacPherson DW, Blajchman MA. Prevention of transfusion-associated Chagas' disease: efficacy of white cell-reduction filters in removing *Trypanosoma cruzi* from injected blood. Transfusion 1995;35:723—6.

33. Hang VTH, van Be T, Tran PN, Thanh LT, van Hien LV, O'Brien E, Morris GE. Screening donor blood for malaria by polymerase chain reaction. Trans Roy Soc Trop Med Hyg 1995;89:44—7.

34. Rikken B, Massa GG, Wit JM, van den Brande JL. Hypofysair groeihormoon en de ziekte van Creutzfeldt-Jakob in Nederland. Ned Tijdschr Geneeskd 1996;140:1161—5.

35. Roos RAC, Wintzen AR, Will RG, Ironside JW, van Duinen SG. Een patiënt met de ziekte van Creutzfeldt-Jakob na behandeling met humaan groeihormoon. Ned Tijdschr Geneeskd 1996;140:1190—2.

36. Brown P. Can Creutzfeldt-Jakob disease be transmitted by transfusion? Curr Opin Hematol 1995;2:472—7.

37. Long GD, Negrin RS, Hoyle CF, Kusnierz-Glaz CR, Schriber JR, Blume KG, Chao NJ. Multiple cycles of high dose chemotherapy supported by hematopoietic progenitor cells as treatment for patients with advanced malignancies. Cancer 1995;76:860—8.

38. Pettengell R, Woll PJ, Thatcher N, Dexter TM, Testa NG. Multicyclic, dose-intensive chemotherapy supported by sequential reinfusion of hematopoietic progenitors in whole blood. J Clin Oncol 1995;13:148—56.

39. Schwella N, Siegert W, Beyer J, Rick O, Zingsem J, Eckstein R, Serke S, Huhn D. Autografting with blood progenitor cells: predictive value of preapheresis blood cell counts on progenitor cell harvest and correlation of the reinfused cell dose with hematopoietic reconstitution. Ann Hematol 1995;71:227—34.

40. Legros M, Fleury J, Curé H, Condat P, Lenat A, Subtil E, Sanderson D, Communal Y, Basile M, Tavernier F, Chouffi B, Chollet P, Plagne R, Chassagne J. New methods for stem cell quantification: applications to the management of peripheral blood stem cell transplantation. Bone Marrow Transplant 1995;15:1—8.

41. Dreger P, Klöss M, Petersen B, Haferlach T, Löffler H, Loeffler M, Schmitz N. Autologous progenitor cell transplantation: prior exposure to stem cell-toxic drugs determines yield and engraftment of peripheral blood progenitor cell but not of bone marrow grafts. Blood 1995;86:3970—8.

42. Klumpp TR. Complications of peripheral blood stem cells transplantation. Semin Oncol 1995;22: 263—70.

43. Lee C-K, Gingrich RD, Hohl RJ, Ajram KA. Engraftment syndrome in autologous bone marrow and peripheral stem cell transplantation. Bone Marrow Transplantation 1995;16:175—82.

44. Jenney MEM. Umbilical cord-blood transplantation; is there a future? Lancet 1995;346:921—2.

45. Ende N. Cord blood collection: effects on newborns. Blood 1995;86:4699—708.

46. Gluckman E, Wagner J. Workshop on umbilical cord blood stem cells and transplantation. Keystone Symposia

47. Broxmeyer HE. Questions to be answered regarding umbilical cord blood hematopoietic stem and progenitor cells and their use in transplantation. Transfusion 1995;35:694—702.

48. Wagner JE, Kernan NA, Steinbuch M, Broxmeyer HE, Gluckman E. Allogeneic sibling umblical-cord-blood transplantation in children with malignant and non-malignant disease. Lancet 1995;346:214—19.

49. Kurtzberg J, Laughlin M, Graham ML, Smith C, Olson JF, Halperin EC, Ciocci G, Carrier C, Stevens CE, Rubinstein P. Placental blood as a source of hematopoietic stem cells for transplantation into unrelated recipients. New Engl J Med 1996;335:157—66.

50. Jones JA. Red blood cell substitutes: current status. Br J Anaesth 1995;74:697—703.

51. Ogden JE, Mac Donald SL. Hemoglobin-based red cell substitutes: current states. Vox Sang 1995;69:302—8.

52. Gould SA, Sehgal LR, Sehgal HL, Moss GS. The development of hemoglobin solutions as red

cell substitutes: hemoglobin solutions. Transfus Sci 1995;16:5—17.

53. Spence RK. Perfluorcarbons in the twenty-first century: clinical applications as transfusion alternatives. Artif Cells Blood Subs Immob Biotech 1995;23:367—80.

54. Keipert PE. Use of Oxygent TM, a perfluoro-chemical-based oxygen carrier as an alternative to intraoperative blood transfusion. Artif Cells Blood Subs Immob Biotech 1995;23:361—91.

55. Trumble ER, Muizelaar JP, Myseros JS, Choi SC, Warren BB. Coagulopathy with the use of hetastarch in the treatment of vasospasm. J Neurosurg 1995;82:44—7.

56. Otten A, Vermeulen M. Intravenous immuno-globulin treatment in neurological diseases. J Neurol Neurosurg Psychiatry 1995;59:359—61.

57. Bril V, Ilse WK, Pearce R, Dhanani A, Sutton D, Kong K. Pilot trial of immunoglobulin versus plasma exchange in patients with Guillain-Barr* syndrome. Neurology 1996;46:100—3.

58. Van Dijk GW, Notermans NC, Franssen H, Oey PL, Wokke JHJ. Response to intravenous immunoglobulin treatment in chronic inflamma-tory demyelinating polyneuropathy with only sen-sory symptoms. J Neurol 1996;243:318—22.

59. Tam DA, Morton LD, Stroncek DF, Leshner RT. Neutropenia in a patient receiving intraven-ous immune globulin. J Neuroimmunol 1996: 64:175—8.

60. Mouthon L, Kaveri SV, Spalter SH, Lacroix-Desmazes S, Lefranc C, Desai R, Kazatchkine MD. Mechanisms of action of intravenous im-mune globulin in immune-mediated diseases. Clin Exp Immunol 1996;104 Suppl 1:3—9.

61. Leung DYM. Kawasaki syndrome: immunom-odulatory benefit and potential toxin neutraliz-ation by intravenous immune globulin. Clin Exp Immunol 1996;104 Suppl 1:49—54.

62. Uchuya M, Graus F, Vega F, Rene R, Delat-tre J-Y. Intravenous immunoglobulin treatment in paraneoplastic neurological syndromes with antineural autoantibodies. J Neurol Neurosurg Psychiatry 1996;60:388—92.

63. Koehler PJ, Koudstaal J. Lethal hypersensitiv-ity myocarditis associated with the use of intraven-ous gammaglobulin for Guillain-Barre syndrome in combination with phenytoin. J Neurol 1996; 243:366—7.

64. Voltz R, Rosen FV, Yoursy T, Beck J, Hohlfeld R. Reversible encephalopathy with cere-bral vasospasm in a Guillain-Barré syndrome pa-tient treated with intravenous immunoglobulin. Neurology 1996;46:250—1.

65. Klaesson S, Ringdén O, Ljungman P, Aschan J, Hägglund H, Winiarski J. Does high-dose intra-venous immune globulin treatment after bone marrow transplantation increase mortality in veno-occlusive disease of the liver? Transplanta-tion 1995;60:1225—30.

66. Schroeder JO, Zeuner RA, Euler HH, Löffler H. High dose intravenous immunoglobulins in systemic lupus erythematosus: clinical and sero-logical results of a pilot study. J Rheumatol 1996;23:71—5.

67. Yap PL. The viral safety of intravenous im-mune globulin. Clin Exp Immunol 1996;104 Suppl 1:35—42.

68. Flora K, Schiele M, Benner K, Montanaro A, Johnston W, Whitham R, Press R. An outbreak of acute hepatitis C among recipients of intraven-ous immunoglobulin. Ann Allergy Asthma Immu-nol 1996;76:160—2.

69. Lefrère JJ, Loiseau P, Martinot-Peignoux M, Mariotti M, Ravera N, Thauvin M, Marcellin P, Janot C. Infection by hepatitis C virus through contaminated intravenous immune globulin: results of a prospective national inquiry in France. Transfusion 1996;36:394—7.

70. Webster ADB, Brown D, Franz A, Dusheiko G. Prevalence of hepatitis C in patients with pri-mary antibody deficiency. Clin Exp Immunol 1996;103:5—7.

71. Taliani G, Guerra E, Rosso R, Badolato MC, Luzi G, Sacco G, Lecce R, De Bac C, Aiuti F. Hepatitis C virus infection in hypogammaglobuli-nemic patients receiving long-term replacement therapy with intravenous immunoglobulin. Trans-fusion 1995;35:103—7.

72. Dodd RY. Infectious risk of plasma do-nations: relationship to safety of intravenous im-mune globulins. Clin Exp Immunol 1995;104 Suppl 1:31—4.

73. Martinowitz UP, Schulman S. Continuous in-fusion of factor concentrates: review of use on hemophilia A and demonstration of safety and efficay in hemophilia B. Acta Haematol 1995;94 Suppl 1:35—42.

74. Goldsmith JC. Rationale and indications for continuous infusion of antihemophilic factor (fac-tor VIII). Blood Coagul Fibrinolysis 1996;7 Suppl 1: S3—S6.

75. Berntorp E. Why prescribe highly purified fac-tor VIII and factor IX concentrates? Vox Sang 1996;70:61—8.

76. Strengers PFW, Zoethout R. Haemophilia: an overview of 30 years therapy. Patient Care 1996;23:3—8.

77. Brackmann HH, Egbring R, Ferster A, Fondu P, Girardel JM, Kreuz W, Masure R, Miloszweski K, Stibbe J, Zimmermann R, Krensk U, Hoos A. Pharmacokinetics and tolerability of factor XIII concentrates prepared from human placenta or plasma: a crossover randomised study. Thromb Haemostasis 1995;74:622—5.

78. Martinowitz U, Schulman S. Review of pumps for continuous infusion of coagulation factor con-centrates: what are the options? Blood Coagul Fibrinolysis 1996;7 Suppl 1:S27—S33.

79. White GC. Safety and recovery of mononine in multiple-dose, high-dose regimens. Acta Haematol 1995;94 Suppl 1:53—8.

80. Djulbegovic B, Hannan MM, Bergman GE. Concomitant treatment with factor IX concen-trates and antifibrinolytics in hemophilia B. Acta Haematol 1995;94 Suppl 1:43—8.

81. Smid WM, van der Meer J. Five-year follow-up of human anti-mouse antibody in multi-transfused HIV negative haemophilics treated

with a monoclonal purified plasma derived factor VIII concentrate. Thromb Haemostasis 1995; 74:1197—207.

82.   Bergamaschini L, Mannucci P, Federici AB, Coppola R, Guzzoni S, Agostoni A. Posttransfusion anaphylactic reactions in a patient with severe von Willebrand disease: role of complement and alloantibodies to von Willebrand factor. J Lab Clin Med 1995;125:348—55.

83.   Shopnick RI, Kazemi M, Brettler DB, Buckwalter C, Yang L, Bray G, Gomperst ED. Anaphylaxis after treatment with recombinant factor VIII. Transfusion 1996;36:358—61.

84.   Klarmann D, Kreuz W, Auerswald G, Auberger K, Rabenau H, Gürtler L, Roggendorf M. Hepatitis C and pasteurised factor VIII and IX concentrates. Thromb Haemostasis 1995;73:736—7.

85.   Allersma DP, Smid WM, Briët E. Abnormal immune parameters in HIV-seronegative haemophilic patients. Haemophilia 1996;2:65—72.

86.   Sabin CA, Pasi J, Phillips AN, Lilley P, Elford J, Lee CA. The use of intermediate-purity clotting factor concentrates and HIV disease progression in men with haemophilia. Haemophilia 1996; 2:78—81.

87.   Goodnough LT, Anderson KC. Recombinant growth factors. Transfus Sci 1995;16:45—62.

88.   Churchill DN, Muithead N, Goldstein M, Posen G, Fay W, Beecroft ML, Gorman J, Raylor DW. Effect of recombinant human erythropoietin on hospitalization of hemodialysis patients. Clin Nephrol 1995;43:184—8.

89.   Kuehl AK. Recombinant erythropoietin for zidovudine-induced anemia in AIDS. Ann Pharmacother 1995;29:7—8.

90.   Luwig H, Sundal E, Pecherstorfer M, Leitgeb C, Bauernhofer T, Beinhauer A, Samonigg H, Kappeler AW, Fritz E. Recombinant human erythropoietin for the correction of cancer associated anemia with and without concomitant cytotoxic chemotherapy. Cancer 1995;76:2319—29.

91.   Cascinu S, Catalano G, Cellerino R. Recombinant human erythropoietin in chemotherapy-associated anemia. Cancer Treat Rev 1995;21:553—64.

92.   Cascinu S, Del Ferro E, Fedeli A, Ligi M, Alessandroni P, Catalano G. Recombinant human erythropoietin treatment in elderly cancer patients with cisplatin-associated anemia. Oncology 1995;52:422—6.

93.   Shannon KM, Feith JF III, Mentzer WC, Ehrenkranz RA, Brown MS, Widness JA, Gleason CA, Bifano EM, Millard DD, Davis CB, Stevenson DK, Alverson DC, Simmons CF, Brim M, Abels RI, Phibbs RH. Recombinant human erythropoietin stimulates erythropoiesis and reduces erythrocyte transfusions in very low birth weight preterm infants. Pediatrics 1995;95:1—10.

94.   Markham A, Bryson HM. Epoetin alfa. A review of its pharmacodynamic and pharmacokinetic properties and therapeutic use in nonrenal applications. Drugs 1995;49:232—54.

95.   Liang D-Y, Chang Y-W, Ding Y-A. Effects of erythropoietin on blood pressure in patients undergoing regular hemodialysis. Acta Cardiol Sin 1995;11:139—44.

96.   Nomura S, Hashimoto J, Osawa G. Can C1 esterase inhibitor concentrate be a cause of the exacerbation of hereditary angioneurotic oedema? Vox Sang 1995;69:85.

34 Intravenous infusions: solutions and emulsions

TOTAL PARENTERAL NUTRITION *(SED-13, 994; SEDA-17, 401; SEDA-18, 358; SEDA-19, 318)*

The incidence of reported adverse effects of intravenous fluids and of total parenteral nutrition (TPN) appears to have been falling in recent years. The pathophysiological mechanisms of the complications of TPN are now well described, and individualization of treatment has become the norm. The problems of micronutrient deficiency with prolonged TPN are more successfully anticipated and prevented than in the past.

The metabolic complications of TPN are now less often reported, as they have become better understood and measures have been taken to identify and prevent them. Common problems in the past were *fat overload syndrome* (caused by phospholipid excess in the earlier formulations), *metabolic acidosis*, *hyperglycemia*, and *hypertriglyceridemia* (1[R]). These problems are now rare. Respiratory, renal, or hepatic insufficiency reduce the metabolic tolerance to calories and/or amino acids. The most common micronutrient deficiency is of *thiamine*.

INTRAVENOUS FLUIDS

Allergic and pseudoallergic reactions reported in anesthesia have been reviewed in detail (2[R]). In general, the incidence of anaphylactoid reactions is between 1:3500 and 1:20 000 anesthetic cases. The estimated mortality rate is 3—6%. Neuromuscular blocking drugs account for most of the cases of significant anaphylactoid reactions (59—70%). In this report, very low incidences were noted for allergic and pseudoallergic reactions to colloid volume expanders, dextran, hydroxyethylstarch, and gelatine formulations. In general, the risk factors for anaphylaxis are as follows: a history of IgE-mediated drug allergy, repeated anesthesia, atopy, hyperventilation tetany, and the use of neuromuscular blocking drugs in women. Risk factors for pseudoallergic reactions are emotional stress, atopic predisposition, increased sensitivity to histamine, and hyperventilation tetany; they are also more common in women. These risk factors are not specific to intravenous formulations.

Fructose

Attention has been drawn to the idiosyncratic use of fructose-based and sorbitol-based solutions for parenteral administration in Germany and German-speaking countries, where they are available for routine fluid replacement and intravenous feeding, and are widely prescribed, even after minor surgical procedures (3[r]). Elsewhere, intravenous fructose has not been used as a parenteral nutrient for about 20 years. Fructose and sorbitol (which is converted to fructose by sorbitol dehydrogenase) cause *lactic acidosis* and *hyperuricemia* (reflecting purine nucleotide breakdown in the liver). Deleterious effects have been reported after the use of parenteral fructose in critically ill patients.

The assimilation of fructose (as the free monosaccharide or derived from the oxidation of sorbitol or hydrolysis of sucrose) differs from that of sucrose. Fructose is phosphorylated rapidly in the intestine and liver by the catalytic action of ketohexosekinase (fructokinase) at the 1-carbon position. Cleavage of fructose-1-phosphate by aldolase B ensures its metabolic incorporation into the glycolytic—

Side Effects of Drugs, Annual 20
J.K. Aronson, ed.

gluconeogenic pathway. Inherited deficiency of aldolase B occurs in hereditary fructose intolerance, an autosomal recessive condition. After ingestion of fructose and related sugars in this disorder, high concentrations of fructose-1-phosphate accumulate in the liver, intestine, and proximal renal tubules, and a profound metabolic disturbance occurs. *Metabolic acidosis*, *hypophosphatemia*, *hypoglycemia*, and *hyperuricemia* result, and functional impairment and pathological injury occur in these tissues with continued administration.

Hetastarch (hydroxyethylstarch) *(SED-13, 992; SEDA-18, 361)*

The colloid hetastarch is a good alternative to albumin, because it has an extended shelf-life, carries no risk of transmitting blood-borne diseases and may be infused into patients who would refuse blood products on religious grounds. The risk of *anaphylactic reactions* to hetastarch is very small (0.0005%) (4^C).

The efficacy and safety of hetastarch and albumin have been compared in 85 patients with post-aneurysmal subarachnoid hemorrhage (4^C). Of 26 patients who developed clinical symptoms of *vasospasm*, 14 were treated with hetastarch, while the other 12 received albumin. In all patients who received hetastarch there was significant *prolongation of the partial thromboplastin time* after transfusion (pre-transfusion mean 23.9 s, post-transfusion 33.1 s), while in patients treated with albumin partial thromboplastin time was not significantly altered. The prolongation of the partial thromboplastin time resulted in *increased occult blood loss* in the hetastarch-treated patients, requiring blood transfusion in four patients. On the basis of hetastarch-associated coagulopathy and data that show that albumin may be the most effective agent for increasing cerebral blood flow and preventing infarction, the authors stopped using hetastarch in these patients and decided to recommend albumin exclusively.

REFERENCES

1. Barnoud D, Fontaine E, Leverve X. Complications métaboliques de la nutrition parenterale. Méd Nutr 1995;31:158—67.

2. Theissen JL, Zahn P, Theissen U, Brehler R. Allergische und pseudoallergische Reaktionen in der Anästhesie. Anästhesiol Intensivmed Notf Med Schmerzther 1995;30:3—12.

3. Cox TM. Therapeutic use of fructose: professional freedom, 'pharmacovigilance' and Europe. Q J Med 1995;88:225—7.

4. Trumble ER, Muizelaar JP, Myseros JS, Choi SC, Warren BB. Coagulopathy with the use of hetastarch in the treatment of vasospasm. J Neurosurg 1995;82:44—7.

35 Drugs affecting blood coagulation, fibrinolysis, and hemostasis

COUMARIN CONGENERS
(SED-13, 1033; SEDA-17, 407; SEDA-18, 366; SEDA-19, 321)

Hematological The *hemorrhagic complications* of treatment with oral anticoagulants have been reviewed (1[R]). The consensus statement concluded that bleeding rates during long-term anticoagulant therapy are substantial with high-intensity therapy and are lower with low-intensity therapy (international normalized ratio, INR, 2.0—3.0). The highest bleeding rates were seen in patients with cerebrovascular disease. In 1283 patients taking oral anticoagulant therapy for venous thromboembolism in seven trials, the median rate of major bleeding was 0.9%; there was only one fatal bleed. In trials of oral anticoagulant therapy for prosthetic heart valves, the median rate of major bleeding was 2.4% per year and the median rate of fatal bleeding was 0.7% per year. In trials of oral anticoagulant therapy for atrial fibrillation, the median rate of major bleeding was 1.7% per year and the median rate of fatal bleeding was 0.2% per year.

Bleeding during oral anticoagulant therapy may occur at unusual sites; in one case an intraneural hematoma of the median nerve reportedly caused acute *carpal tunnel syndrome* (2[c]); in another acute *vertigo* and unilateral *deafness* while on warfarin was probably due to hemorrhage in the labyrinth (3[c]).

Interactions Adverse interactions of warfarin with *non-steroidal anti-inflammatory drugs* have been systematically reviewed (4[R]). In patients taking warfarin who also require non-steroidal anti-inflammatory drugs, phenylbutazone and its analogs, high-dose aspirin, mefenamic acid, and non-steroidal anti-inflammatory drugs that are associated with a higher risk of bleeding peptic ulcer should be avoided. Patients should be closely monitored for anticoagulant control and bleeding complications if warfarin and non-steroidal anti-inflammatory drugs are used in combination.

Tenidap sodium is a novel cytokine-modulating antirheumatic agent, which is being evaluated for the treatment of rheumatoid arthritis and osteoarthritis. Tenidap sodium did not alter the pharmacodynamics and plasma protein binding of warfarin in healthy volunteers (5[C]).

The interaction of warfarin with *ticlopidine* has been carefully investigated (6[C]). Although ticlopidine caused a significant increase in mean serum R-warfarin concentration, it had no effect on S-warfarin concentration and the INR did not change significantly. The authors concluded that ticlopidine has an enantioselective kinetic interaction with warfarin, but that it is likely to be of minimal clinical significance in most patients.

Zileuton is a potent inhibitor of leukotriene biosynthesis that has been shown to be of therapeutic benefit in asthma. Zileuton had no effect on S-warfarin pharmacokinetics but significantly increased mean R-warfarin plasma concentrations, leading to prolongation of the prothrombin time by about 2 s (7[C]). The authors concluded that careful monitoring of the prothrombin time with appropriate dose titration of warfarin is recommended when zileuton and warfarin are combined.

Side Effects of Drugs, Annual 20
J.K. Aronson, ed.

HEPARINS *(SED-13, 1028; SEDA-17, 407; SEDA-18, 366; SEDA-19, 322)*

Hematological The *risk of bleeding* associated with heparin therapy has been carefully reviewed (1[R]). The consensus statement concluded that the risk of bleeding associated with intravenous heparin in patients with acute venous thrombosis is below 5%. There is some evidence to suggest that the risk of bleeding increases with the dosage of heparin. Heparin administered alone to patients with coronary artery disease is not associated with an increased risk of bleeding, but when it is given in association with thrombolytic therapy the risk of minor bleeding is increased. Recent trials have suggested that aggressive anticoagulant therapy with either intravenous heparin or hirudin used as an adjunct to thrombolytic therapy is associated with increased intracranial hemorrhage. The risk of bleeding with prophylactic low-dose subcutaneous heparin therapy is not increased in patients undergoing general surgery, but there is an increased risk of minor bleeding at the operative site in patients undergoing orthopedic surgery who receive low-dose heparin prophylaxis (1[R]).

Heparin-induced *thrombocytopenia* and *thrombosis* continue to be actively researched. As discussed in detail in SEDA-19 (p. 322), antibodies to heparin-platelet factor 4 complex bind to the platelet factor 4 receptor on platelets, and then interact with the platelet Fcγ receptor (FcγR), leading to platelet activation, thrombocytopenia, and thrombosis. There have been several recent developments.

First, improved methods have become available to detect heparin-induced platelet activation (8); an ELISA technique has been developed to demonstrate antibodies to heparin-platelet factor 4 complexes (9), (10).

Secondly, the heparin-dependent antibody is predominantly of the IgG2 subclass. A functionally important polymorphism of the Fcγ receptor has been identified; the FcγR His-131 is better activated by IgG2 binding than the FcγR Arg-131; there was a greater prevalence of FcγR His-131 in 19 patients with heparin-induced thrombocytopenia, none of whom was homozygous for FcγR Arg-131, than in 22 healthy volunteers,

allowing the conclusion that the presence of the FcγR His-131 allele is associated with a predisposition to heparin-induced thrombocytopenia and thrombosis (11[C]). This observation has been independently confirmed in a comparison of 96 patients and 100 controls (12[C]).

Thirdly, the incidence of cross-reactivity between unfractionated heparin and low molecular weight heparin in patients with heparin-induced thrombocytopenia appears to be lower than hitherto reported: seven out of nine patients with a negative cross-reactivity test were treated with dalteparin sodium without any untoward effects (13[C]). An additional report has confirmed the successful use of danaparoid in five patients with heparin-induced thrombocytopenia (14[C]). An alternative is the use of recombinant hirudin. Intravenous administration of recombinant hirudin ensured safe anticoagulation in six patients with heparin-induced thrombocytopenia and prevented rebound thromboembolism while waiting for oral anticoagulation to become effective and the platelet count to return to normal (15[C]).

Enoxaparin, a low molecular weight heparin, has been extensively reappraised (16[R]). Recent studies have reported similar incidences of hemorrhagic complications for heparin and enoxaparin.

Skin and appendages A 48-year-old woman on hemodialysis presented with a symmetrical *fixed drug eruption* above both knees, attributed to heparin sodium (17[c]). In a postmarketing surveillance study 27 (0.3%) of 9919 patients undergoing general surgery had *allergic skin reactions* during thrombosis prophylaxis with enoxaparin (18[C]).

DRUGS THAT ALTER PLATELET FUNCTION

Clopidogrel

Clopidogrel is a methyl ester of acetylticlopidine that has recently been introduced for prevention and treatment of thrombotic disorders (19[R]). Clopidogrel has been compared with aspirin in the prevention of recurrent arterial ischemic events in a large international multicenter study (20[C]). Clopidogrel proved borderline superior to aspirin. The overall safety profile of clopidogrel was at least as good as that of medium-dose aspirin. More specifically, there was no excess neutropenia in the clopidogrel group.

Ticlopidine *(SED-13, 1039; SEDA-17, 407; SEDA-18, 367; SEDA-19, 323)*

Ticlopidine, a thienopyridine derivative, is a potent inhibitor of platelet function. However, it regularly causes *neutropenia*. Another case has been reported and the literature reviewed (21[cr]).

THROMBOLYTIC AGENTS
(SED-13, 1035; SEDA-17, 407; SEDA-18, 368; SEDA-19, 323)

Hematological   An extensive review has appeared on the *hemorrhagic complications* of thrombolytic therapy in the treatment of myocardial infarction and venous thromboembolism (22[R]). The conclusions of this consensus conference were as follows. For myocardial infarction, bleeding is the only prespecified risk of thrombolytic therapy that affects the decision to treat. The risk of extracranial bleeding is virtually identical, regardless of the thrombolytic agent used within the approved dosage ranges. The risks of stroke and intracranial bleeding appear to be higher with agents other than streptokinase, although the difference is less than 0.5%. Invasive procedures are the most important predisposing factors for extracranial bleeding. The risk of major extracranial bleeding with thrombolytic therapy is related to age, size, and sex, being higher in older people, smaller people, and women. These three factors, plus prior cerebrovascular disease, are risk factors for intracranial bleeding, but they are not absolute contraindications to therapy. Aggressive adjunctive therapy with either heparin or hirudin increases the risk of intracranial bleeding associated with thrombolytic therapy. For venous thromboembolism, the consensus confer-

ence concluded that the incidence of major (clinically significant) hemorrhage in patients treated with thrombolytic drugs for acute deep venous thrombosis is 6—30%, a threefold greater incidence than with heparin alone. The incidence of hemorrhage in patients with pulmonary embolism treated with thrombolytic agents and who undergo pulmonary angiography is about 20%; these bleeds are usually catheter related.

ANTIFIBRINOLYTIC DRUGS
(SED-13, 1060; SEDA-17, 409; SEDA-19, 323)

Aprotinin

Debate continues on the justification for using aprotinin to reduce blood loss in association with primary or repeat coronary artery bypass graft surgery (23[r]). While the benefits of aprotinin on blood loss have been reconfirmed, combined data suggest that aprotinin is associated with an increased incidence of *renal failure*, and there are trends toward increases in *myocardial infarction* and *graft occlusion* and a higher mortality rate (23[r]). This outspoken view has been counterbalanced by another careful analysis, the authors of which concluded that high-dose aprotinin should be considered a valuable adjunct to aggressive blood conservation programs in patients undergoing cardiac surgery with the potential for excessive blood loss, in patients for whom transfusion is unavailable, or in patients who refuse homologous transfusions (24[R]).

Immunological and hypersensitivity reactions   The reported incidence of *anaphylactic reactions* (aprotinin is a bovine protein) in patients from recent placebo-controlled US studies was 0.3%. In two large European reviews, the incidence of *mild hypersensitivity reactions* (skin rash, hypotension, and/or *bronchospasm*) was 0.3—0.6% in patients who received mostly high-dose aprotinin. These reactions are more likely to occur in patients who have received prior aprotinin treatment (24[R]).

REFERENCES

1. Levine MN, Raskob G, Landefeld S, Hirsh J. Hemorrhagic complications of anticoagulant treatment. Chest 1995;108:276S—290S.

2. Bindiger A, Zelnick J, Kuschner S, Gellman H. Spontaneous acute carpal tunnel syndrome in an anticoagulated patient. Bull Hosp Jt Dis 1995;54:52—3.

3. Kothari M, Knopp E, Jonas S, Levine D. Presumed vestibular hemorrhage secondary to warfarin. Neuroradiology 1995;37:324—5.

4. Chan TYK. Adverse interactions between warfarin and nonsteroidal antiinflammatory drugs: mechanisms, clinical significance, and avoidance. Ann Pharmacother 1995;29:1274—83.

5. Apseloff G, Wilner KD, Gerber N. Effect of tenidap sodium on the pharmacodynamics and plasma protein binding of warfarin in healthy volunteers. Br J Clin Pharmacol 1995;39:29S—33S.

6. Gidal BE, Sorkness CA, McGill KA, Larson R, Levine RR. Evaluation of a potential enantioselective interaction between ticlopidine and warfarin in chronically anticoagulated patients. Ther Drug Monit 1995;17:33—8.

7. Awni WM, Hussein Z, Granneman GR, Patterson KJ, Dubé LM, Cavanaugh JH. Pharmacodynamic and stereoselective pharmacokinetic interactions between zileuton and warfarin in humans. Clin Pharmacokin 1995;29 Suppl 2:67—76.

8. Stewart MW, Etches WS, Boshkov LK, Gordon PA. Heparin-induced thrombocytopenia: an improved method of detection based on lumiaggregometry. Br J Haematol 1995;91:173—7.

9. Amiral J, Bridey F, Wolf M, Boyer-Neumann C, Fressinaud E, Vissac AM, Peynaud-Debayle E, Dreyfus M, Meyer D. Antibodies to macromolecular platelet factor 4-heparin complexes in heparin-induced thrombocytopenia: a study of 44 cases. Thromb Haemostasis 1995;73.21—8.

10. Arepally G, Reynolds C, Tomaski A, Amiral J, Jawad A, Poncz M, Cines DB. Comparison of PF4/heparin ELISA assay with the 14^C-serotonin release assay in the diagnosis of heparin-induced thrombocytopenia. Am J Clin Pathol 1995;104:648—54.

11. Burgess JK, Lindeman R, Chesterman CN, Chong BH. Single amino acid mutation of Fcγ receptor is associated with the development of heparin-induced thrombocytopenia. Br J Haematol 1995;91:761—6.

12. Brandt JT, Isenhart CE, Osborne JM, Ahmed A, Anderson CL. On the role of platelet FcγRIIa phenotype in heparin-induced thrombocytopenia. Thromb Haemostasis 1995;74:1564—72.

13. Ramakrishna R, Manoharan A, Kwan YL, Kyle PW. Heparin-induced thrombocytopenia: cross-reactivity between standard heparin, low molecular weight heparin, dalteparin (Fragmin) and heparinoid, danaparoid (Orgaran). Br J Haematol 1995;91:736—8.

14. Burkhard-Meier U, Söhngen D, Schultheiss HP, Greinacher A, Schwartzkopff B, Vogt M, Heyll A, Schneider W. Heparin-induced thrombocytopenia type II: successful use of Orgaran (ORG 10172) in intensive care patients. Intensive Care Med 1995;21:542—3.

15. Schiele F, Vuillemenot A, Kramarz P, Kieffer Y, Anguenot T, Bernard Y, Bassand JP. Use of recombinant hirudin as antithrombotic treatment in patients with heparin-induced thrombocytopenia. Am J Hematol 1995;50:20—5.

16. Noble S, Peters DH, Goa KL. Enoxaparin. A reappraisal of its pharmacology and clinical applications in the prevention and treatment of thromboembolic disease. Drugs 1995;49:388—410.

17. Mohammed KN. Symmetric fixed eruption to heparin. Dermatology 1995;190:91.

18. Haas S, Flosbach CW. Antithromboembolic efficacy and safety of enoxaparin in general surgery. German multicentre trial. Eur J Surg 1994;Suppl 571:37—43.

19. Feuerstein G, Nichols AJ, Ruffolo RRJr. Clopidogrel: a novel antiplatelet drug for prevention and treatment of thrombotic disorders. Exp Opin Invest Drugs 1995;4:425—30.

20. CAPRIE Steering Committee. A randomized, blinded, trial of clopidogrel versus aspirin in patients at risk of ischaemic events (CAPRIE). Lancet 1996;348:1329—39.

21. Tsatalas C, Chalkia P, Garyfallos A, Kakoulidis I, Xanthakis I. Ticlopidine-induced aplastic anaemia. Case report and review of the literature. Clin Drug Invest 1995;9:127—30.

22. Levine MN, Goldhaber SZ, Gore JM, Hirsh J, Califf RM. Hemorrhagic complications of thrombolytic therapy in the treatment of myocardial infarction and venous thromboembolism. Chest 1995;108:291S—301S.

23. Cooper BE. Aprotinin: no justification for current use. J Pharm Technol 1995;11:156—62.

24. Davis R, Whittington R. Aprotinin. A review of its pharmacology and therapeutic efficacy in reducing blood loss associated with cardiac surgery. Drugs 1995;49:954—83.

36 Gastrointestinal drugs

ANTACIDS *(SED-13, 1066; SEDA-17, 413; SEDA-18, 370; SEDA-19, 325)*

Primary-care physicians were reported in 1995 to have prescribed an antacid for 3.9% of the whole population of the North of England (1[C]), but there were no reports of significant drug interactions with antacids during the period of this review.

ANTIEMETICS

Cisapride *(SED-13, 1067; SEDA-17, 413; SEDA-18, 370; SEDA-19, 325)*

Cisapride is used mainly for the management of mild esophagitis. In a double-blind randomized comparison of cisapride 10 or 20 mg with placebo in 177 patients for 12 weeks, cisapride 20 mg qds was the most effective regimen, and there were no clinically significant changes in safety variables (2[C]). *Diarrhea* occurred more often with cisapride than placebo, and also more often in those taking the higher dose of cisapride (placebo 8.3%, cisapride 10 mg 12.5%, cisapride 20 mg 16.4%).

The combination of omeprazole 20 mg daily with cisapride 5 mg tds has been compared with omeprazole alone (3[C]). No unexpected events were observed using this combination of a prokinetic and a gastric acid antisecretory drug.

Metoclopramide *(SED-13, 1069; SEDA-17, 414)*

Metoclopramide hydrochloride is used in the treatment of gastro-esophageal reflux disease, the management of disorders of gastric emptying, and as an antiemetic after chemotherapy (4[C]). Its antidopaminergic adverse effects have long been recognised, including *extrapyramidal signs and symptoms*. There has been a large study of whether there is an increase in the use of antiparkinsonian drugs in older patients taking metoclopramide hydrochloride. Medicaid patients aged 65 years and older were enrolled into three groups: those newly prescribed a levodopa-containing medication ($n = 1253$), those prescribed an anticholinergic antiparkinsonian drug ($n = 2377$), and a control group who were not users of any antiparkinsonian therapy ($n = 16\,435$). Logistic regression was used to determine the odds ratio for the initiation for antiparkinsonian therapy in patients taking metoclopramide relative to non-users. Metoclopramide users were found to be three times more likely to start using levodopa.

A double-blind study has been performed to compare 4-day continuous infusions of either high-dose prochlorperazine ($n = 57$) or high-dose metoclopramide ($n = 56$) in patients receiving combination alkylator therapy for solid tumors (5[C]). Adverse effects that required dosage reduction or discontinuation of antiemetic drugs included *diarrhea, sedation, anxiety*, and *akathisia*. Of greater concern was a case of *second-degree heart block* in both limbs of the study, and in addition there was one patient with *bradycardia* and another with *ventricular extra beats* in the prochlorperazine group.

5-HT$_3$ RECEPTOR ANTAGONISTS *(SED-13, 1070; SEDA-17, 415; SEDA-19, 325)*

It has been concluded that it is only the expense of ondansetron, which has fewer adverse effects than the more widely used antiemetic agents, which relegates it to third-line treatment for the management and prevention

Side Effects of Drugs, Annual 20
J.K. Aronson, ed.

of post-operative emesis (6^R). Expense appears to be its worst adverse effect!

These drugs are more usually used for the control of nausea and vomiting during treatment with cytotoxic drugs. Assessment of their adverse effects is complicated because the cytotoxic drugs are usually poorly tolerated. Granisetron is the second 5-HT$_3$ receptor antagonist to become generally available, and it has been reported that in clinical trials granisetron therapy was usually well tolerated (7^R). *Headache* occurred in approximately 14% of patients receiving granisetron, constipation in 3—10%, and *diarrhea*, *weakness*, and *somnolence* in 3—5%. The reviewers noted that 5-HT$_3$ receptor antagonists have been associated with cardiovascular adverse effects, mainly *hypertension* and asymptomatic *dysrhythmias*, particularly in older patients.

Two oral dose regimens of granisetron (two doses of 1 mg separated by 12 h, or a single dose of 2 mg) have been compared. They appeared to be equally effective in controlling acute emesis during chemotherapy, but *headache* and *constipation* were frequent adverse effects (8^C). The addition of methylprednisolone to oral granisetron was reported to improve the control of delayed emesis during cisplatin treatment, without any apparent change in the adverse events profile (9^C).

Intravenous granisetron (40 µg/kg) has been assessed for the control of postoperative nausea and vomiting in a placebo-controlled study (10^C). Granisetron was more effective than placebo, and the adverse effects profile was similar in both groups ($n = 25$).

HISTAMINE H$_2$-RECEPTOR ANTAGONISTS *(SED-13, 1071; SEDA-17, 416; SEDA-18, 371; SEDA-19, 326)*

A major comparative review of the adverse effects of anti-ulcer drugs has been published (11^R).

The safety of histamine H$_2$-receptor antagonists is reflected in their recent widespread availability as over-the-counter treatments for dyspepsia. The benefit of famotidine 10 mg has been demonstrated in an innovative study of the prevention of dyspepsia in 322 patients with a history of frequent heartburn (12^C). The patients were randomized to either famotidine 10 mg or placebo 1 h before an evening meal that was likely to induce symptoms (beef stew with dumplings, an Indian curry, or chilli con carne); famotidine-treated patients had significantly less heartburn after the meal, less difficulty in getting to sleep, fewer awakenings with dyspepsia, and better control of heartburn during the night. They were also three times less likely to take an antacid during the night. In the famotidine-treated group one patient complained of each of the following symptoms: *diarrhea*, *vomiting*, *cough*, and *headache*. Only the diarrhea was considered by the attending physician to be an adverse event that had possibly been related to treatment.

An excess of tuberculosis has been reported amongst patients with a history of partial gastrectomy for the pretreatment of peptic ulcer disease, and it has therefore been questioned whether H$_2$-antagonists might be associated with an increased risk of tuberculosis (13^C). A history of daily histamine H2-antagonist use was reported in nine patients (7%) with active tuberculosis attending the Seattle-King County Tuberculosis Clinic, compared with 18 controls (5%), giving an adjusted odds rate of 0.8. The authors concluded that treatment for peptic ulcer disease has no effect on the occurrence of tuberculosis.

Famotidine

Manufacturers caution against rapid intravenous administration of ranitidine and cimetidine because of possible cardiovascular abnormalities, including bradycardia, hypotension, and dysrhythmias. Similar cautions do not appear in the product labelling for famotidine, although adverse hemodynamic effects have been reported. The effects of intravenous famotidine 20 mg have been assessed in 105 critically ill patients, 53 of whom received famotidine by rapid intravenous injection (1041 doses) and 52 by intravenous infusion (1006 doses) (14^C). Adverse effects possibly related to famotidine were observed in five patients: three in the injection group and two in the infusion group. Mild *flushing* and *tachycardia* were noted approximately 30 s after the first dose of famotidine in one patient in the injection group; these resolved within a few minutes and did not recur with subsequent famotidine injections. Another patient in the injection group had frequent *ventricular extra beats* during administration of the eleventh dose; these resolved within several minutes and did not recur with subsequent doses. *Disorientation* and *confusion* were noted in one patient in the infusion group after administration of the sixth dose; the probable cause for this change of mental status was not determined. Finally, one patient in each group developed *thrombocytopenia*, but the relation of this to treatment with famotidine was ill-defined.

Very high dosages of famotidine were given in a study in which an attempt was made to maintain intragastric pH above 6.0 in patients with a bleeding duodenal ulcer (15[C]). The mean total dose of famotidine over a 24-h period was 172 mg, but this was given without apparent adverse events.

Long-term treatment with famotidine has been assessed in patients with a history of moderate to severe erosive esophagitis. They were randomized to receive placebo ($n = 31$), famotidine 20 mg bd ($n = 69$), or famotidine 40 mg bd ($n = 72$). Famotidine was generally well tolerated, although there were sporadic increases in alanine and aspartate transaminases in a few patients (16[C]).

Roxatidine

Roxatidine 150 mg has been compared with ranitidine 300 mg in a double-blind 6-week study for the treatment of benign gastric ulceration (17[R]). Individual adverse events were experienced by at least 2% of patients in both treatment groups, *diarrhea* and *headache* being the most severe symptoms, reported by only a few patients.

PROTON PUMP INHIBITORS
(SED-13, 1075; SEDA-17, 418; SEDA-18, 373; SEDA-19, 327)

Omeprazole

A wide-ranging review of the adverse effects associated with omeprazole has been published, with particular reference to the achlorhydria-gastric carcinoid sequence (11[R]). More recently concern has shifted from concern about gastric carcinoids to the accelerated development of atrophic gastritis during profound inhibition of gastric acid secretion (18[R]). *Helicobacter pylori* is now thought to have an important role in the development of atrophic gastritis. In vivo there is little evidence that acid-suppressing drugs have any direct effect on the survival of *H. pylori* in the gastroduodenal mucosa. However, profound inhibition of gastric acid secretion quickly leads to a spreading of the bacterial infection throughout the body and fundus of the stomach, which in turn is accompanied by an increase in the associated gastritis. *H. pylori* gastritis may, in a substantial number of infected patients, ultimately lead to atrophy and intestinal metaplasia, conditions that are associated with an increased risk of gastric cancer. There is no epidemiological evidence to suggest that proton pump inhibitors are associated with accelerated development of gastric cancer, but most experts would now recommend that any patient requiring long-term treatment with a proton pump inhibitor should take treatment to eradicate *H. pylori* infection.

Gastro-esophageal reflux disease is usually a chronic problem, which will demand long-term medical treatment. The long-term management of gastro-esophageal reflux disease has been reviewed, with particular emphasis on both the efficacy and safety of gastric acid antisecretory drugs (19[R]).

Hypergastrinemia during omeprazole therapy is generally assumed to be entirely a consequence of acid suppression (20[C]). Patients with pernicious anemia have extremely high fasting plasma gastrin concentrations, due to unremitting achlorhydria. Omeprazole does not cause a further rise in plasma gastrin concentration in these patients, consistent with the hypothesis that omeprazole-induced hypergastrinemia is entirely secondary to inhibition of acid secretion.

Paradoxically, eradicating *H. pylori* infection results in a loss of some of the gastric acid antisecretory potency of omeprazole (21[C]). Intragastric pH was recorded for 24 h before and after 1 week of omeprazole 20 mg/day in 18 subjects positive for *H. pylori* before and after eradication. Eradicating *H. pylori* had no effect on intragastric acidity, but sensitivity to omeprazole was much higher before eradication (median pH 5.4) than after (median pH 3.6). The precise mechanism of this loss of antisecretory activity remains obscure, although it has been suggested that it could be a result of the production of acid-neutralizing compounds by *H. pylori* itself; for example, ammonia released by the action of urease on endogenous urea.

Urinary system Omeprazole is generally well tolerated (22[C]), (23[C]), but there have been two recent reports of *acute interstitial nephritis* (24[C]), (25[C]). One patient developed acute renal failure after the reintroduction of omeprazole, and this was due to acute interstitial nephritis, confirmed by biopsy. The second was an 83-year-old woman who developed uremia during 12 weeks of treatment with omeprazole, and a renal biopsy showed tubulo-interstitial nephritis; she recovered after treatment with dialysis, but rechallenge resulted in recurrence.

Risk factors The stomach and small intestine remain relatively sterile because of normal gastric acid secretion and normal gastrointestinal motility. Patients with scleroderma have abnormal gastrointestinal motility, and hence a tendency to overgrowth with small intestinal bacterial The abnormal motility also increases their risk of severe gastro-esophageal reflux disease, and in these patients treatment with omeprazole has often relieved misery due to severe esophageal ulceration. However, treatment with omeprazole, by removing gastric acid, increases the risk of overgrowth with small intestinal bacteria in patients with scleroderma (26[C]). Ten women with scleroderma had persistent symptoms of esophagitis uncontrolled with adequate dosages of H_2-receptor antagonists, and they were switched to omeprazole 40 mg/day for 1 month. Breath hydrogen tests were performed to assess bac-

terial overgrowth; at baseline none of the 10 patients had an abnormal hydrogen breath test, but after 1 month of omeprazole three had marked changes, indicating bacterial overgrowth. It can be anticipated that a proportion of omeprazole-treated patients with scleroderma will develop malabsorption and or malnutrition due to bacterial overgrowth of the small intestine.

Lansoprazole

Lansoprazole is usually well tolerated, and in a double-blind comparison of lansoprazole 30 mg/day and ranitidine 150 mg bd in 242 patients with erosive esophagitis the drugs were reported to be similar in terms of adverse events (27[C]). Fasting serum gastrin concentrations rose during treatment in both groups, but those taking lansoprazole had a significantly larger increase. Patients taking lansoprazole also had a significant increase in the mean number of silver-staining endocrine cells in the greater curve of the stomach, and a significant increase in the number of G-cells in the gastric antrum. These changes, similar to those seen with omeprazole, reflect drug-induced *hypergastrinemia* (11[R]).

Pantoprazole

Pantoprazole 40 mg/day has been compared with omeprazole 20 mg/day in 219 patients with benign gastric ulceration; they were treated for 1 month and both drugs were well tolerated, but there was a rise in fasting plasma gastrin concentration in both groups (28[C]). Pantoprazole 40 mg/day has also been compared with ranitidine 150 mg bd in the management of 249 patients with acute symptomatic reflux esophagitis; the frequency of adverse events was low and did not differ between the two different groups (29[C]). A similar lack of significant adverse events has been reported in further comparative trials of pantoprazole in reflux esophagitis and duodenal ulceration (30[C]), (31[C]).

OTHER ULCER-HEALING DRUGS

Bismuth compounds *(SED-13, 1077; SEDA-17, 420; SEDA 18, 374; SEDA-19, 328)*

Ranitidine bismuth citrate (GR122311X), formed from ranitidine hydrochloride and bismuth citrate (32[C]), has both the antisecretory activity of ranitidine and the mucosal protective, antipepsin and anti-*Helicobacter pylori* effects associated with bismuth salts (11[C]). It is being developed for the eradication of *H. pylori* infection, usually in combination with clarithromycin. Ranitidine bismuth citrate (200, 400, or 800 mg bd) and ranitidine hydrochloride (150 mg bd) have been compared in a multicenter, double-blind, 4-week trial in 1620 patients with duodenal ulcer. All four treatments were equally effective at healing ulcers, and ranitidine bismuth citrate alone eradicated *H. pylori* infection in about 20% of patients. Ranitidine bismuth citrate was safe and well tolerated, with an adverse events profile similar to that of ranitidine hydrochloride. Median 4-week trough bismuth concentrations were 1.3—23 ng/ml; no individual plasma bismuth concentrations were of clinical concern.

Sucralfate *(SED-13, 1078; SEDA-17, 420; SEDA-18, 374; SEDA-19, 328)*

No important new data on sucralfate have appeared since the last Annual, but its adverse effects have been reviewed (11[R]).

Helicobacter pylori **eradication regimens** *Helicobacter pylori* eradication regimens continue to increase in importance, although the best strategy remains to be established. More regimens involve the use of a gastric acid antisecretory drug together with one or two antibiotics, usually chosen from amongst amoxycillin, clarithromycin, metronidazole or tinidazole, or tetracycline (33[C])—(41[C]). A bismuth compound may also be co-prescribed. Adverse effects relate very much to the individual compounds, the most common being dysgeusia associated with clarithromy-

cin, nausea and alcohol intolerance associated with metronidazole or tinidazole, stool darkening associated with bismuth, and rashes associated with amoxycillin. Although the combinations appear to work synergistically when eradicating *H. pylori*, there appears to be no unusual pattern of adverse events associated with combinations of these drugs.

SMOOTH MUSCLE RELAXANTS *(SED-13, 1084; SEDA-19, 329)*

Mebeverine hydrochloride is used for the treatment of the irritable bowel syndrome, and its mode of action involves a reduction in the availability of calcium in colonic smooth muscle cells (42[C]). A modified-release capsule formulation of mebeverine has been compared with the standard capsule in 60 patients with irritable bowel syndrome; very few adverse events were recorded, none of which was thought to be related to mebeverine (43[R]).

Antidiarrheal drugs have been reviewed, with particular emphasis on opioids that have major effects on intestinal transit, with less well-documented pro-absorptive and anti-secretory effects (43[R]).

ANTI-INFLAMMATORY DRUGS

Salicylates *(SED-13, 1082; SEDA-17, 423; SEDA-18, 375; SEDA-19, 329)*

Sulfasalazine (salicylazosulfapyridine) occasionally causes serious blood disorders, particularly *agranulocytosis*. A general practitioner database has been used in the UK to follow up some 10 000 users of sulfasalazine and some 4000 users of mesalazine, in order to estimate the risk of blood disorders associated with these drugs (44[R]). The risk in sulfasalazine users who were being treated for arthritic disorders (6.1/1000 users) was about 10 times higher than that for users who were being treated for inflammatory bowel disease (0.6/1000 users). There was no case of blood disorders in users of mesalazine. The use of granulocyte macrophage colony-stimulating factor (GM-CSF, molgramostim) for the treatment of sulfasalazine-induced agranulocytosis has been described in a single case (45[C]).

Five weeks after starting sulfasalazine 3 g/day, a 39-year-old man was found to have no circulating neutrophils. Three days after hospital admission he was given GM-CSF 450 μg subcutaneously for 4 days. Within 3 days his white cell count had risen to 13.3×10^9/l and he remained in sustained remission.

In a survey of 45 German centres for gastroenterology it has been reported that among 1613 patients treated for acute pancreatitis in 1993, drug-induced acute *pancreatitis* was diagnosed in 22 patients (1.4%) (46[C]). Drugs held responsible were mesalazine/sulfasalazine, azathioprine, 2′,3′-dideoxyinosine (ddI), estrogens, frusemide, hydrochlorothiazide, and rifampicin. The authors suggested that in the literature, which depends upon reports of individual patients who have usually suffered severe complications, there is a suggestion that this type of drug-induced pancreatitis is highly dangerous; for example, of the 21 reported cases of azathioprine-induced pancreatitis there was a fatal outcome in 24%. This was not the finding in the German survey, in which it was concluded that drugs rarely caused acute pancreatitis, and that drug induced acute pancreatitis usually runs a benign course.

Mesalazine

Mesalazine is used for the oral and topical treatment of inflammatory bowel disease, both ulcerative colitis and more recently Crohn's disease. Mesalazine 1.5 or 3.0 g/day was given for 1 year to 169 patients with ulcerative colitis in remission (47[C]). Fewer of the group that took the larger dose relapsed, but the difference was not significant. There were no dose-related adverse events, but three patients had serious drug-related adverse events: *hepatitis*, severe *pruritus*, and *interstitial nephritis*. All recovered after withdrawal of mesalazine.

Activation of ulcerative colitis by mesalazine in two men aged 28 and 30 years was demonstrated by improvement after drug withdrawal and relapse after rechallenge with mesalazine enemas during a period of remission (48[C]).

Liver and pancreas   Of 103 patients with ulcerative colitis who took mesalazine 4 g/day for 12 months one developed *hepatitis* attributed to mesalazine (49[C]). Hepatitis was also observed in two of 44 patients who took long-term mesalazine for prevention of endoscopic recurrence after intestinal resection for Crohn's disease (50[C]).

In 163 patients who underwent surgical resection for Crohn's disease, and were randomized to treatment with either mesalazine 1.5 g bd or placebo, with follow-up for up to 72 months, mesalazine was generally well tolerated. However, one patient developed *pancreatitis* (51[C]). In a major review of drug-induced pancreatitis it was emphasized that two types of drugs used by gastroenterologists are associated with this potentially life-threatening complication: azathioprine and sulfasalazine/ mesalazine (52[R]).

Olsalazine

Olsalazine is a dimer of two molecules of 5-aminosalicylic acid (mesalazine) linked by a diazo bond. It is absorbed in the small intestine to a very small extent, but is split into its components by bacterial degradation in the colon, releasing two molecules of mesalazine. This produces a release profile that is similar to sulfalazine. Olsalazine has similar clinical activity to sulfasalazine in maintenance treatment of ulcerative colitis, but the most frequent adverse effect is *diarrhea*, which can be sufficient to halt treatment. This has been reported in five (3.1%) of 161 patients taking olsalazine 1 g/day (53[C]) and in 2.5, 5.2, and 11.7% of patients taking 0.5, 1.25, and 2.0 g/day (54[C]). Olsalazine stimulates the secretion of sodium and water along all parts of the intestine by mechanisms which are not fully understood.

Corticosteroids (*SEDA-19, 329*)

Patients with inflammatory bowel disease often develop osteoporosis, and it appears that the osteopenia is related to corticosteroid therapy rather than other disease-related variables. In a study of 49 patients with inflammatory bowel disease, only corticosteroid use was a statistically significant predictor of *reduced bone density* (55[C]). In a comparison of 152 patients with inflammatory bowel disease with 73 healthy controls, patients who had never taken corticosteroids did not have reduced bone mineral density (56[C]). Women appear to be more sensitive to this effect than men, and it is recommended that bone density measurements should be performed routinely in patients with inflammatory bowel disease (57[R]).

Budesonide has been introduced as a glucocorticoid with high topical activity, but low systemic availability, with the aim of reducing systemic effects in comparison with other glucocorticoids (58[R]). Budesonide has been tested in patients with inflammatory bowel disease when taken either by mouth as an ileal-release formulation or rectally as an enema. Generally, budesonide is more effective than placebo and similar in activity to an equivalent amount of a more conventional corticosteroid. Some mineralocorticoid adverse effects do occur during budesonide therapy, so it is not entirely devoid of systemic glucocorticoid activity. Corticosteroids are dealt with in detail in Chapter 39.

Immunosuppressive drugs

Patients who relapse during medical treatment of inflammatory bowel disease are often given azathioprine as second-line treatment, for its steroid-sparing effects. The risks of *malignancy* in inflammatory bowel disease have been reviewed (59[R]); azathioprine and its metabolite 6-mercaptopurine carry an increased risk of malignancy (60[C]). A survey of azathioprine- and cyclosporin-induced liver disease concluded that these drugs cause infrequent but sometimes significant *hepatotoxicity* (61[R]). Azathioprine causes a broad spectrum of hepatotoxic reactions, whereas cyclosporin is usually associated with cholestasis, manifested by conjugated hyperbilirubinemia. Immunosuppressive drugs are dealt with in detail in Chapter 37.

PANCREATIC ENZYME SUPPLEMENTS *(SED-13, 1086; SEDA-18, 321; SEDA-19, 330)*

Pancreatic enzyme supplements and fibrosing colonopathy ℞

Fibrosing colonopathy was first described in children with cystic fibrosis in 1994 (62[C]). A cluster of children with cystic fibrosis from one center developed fibrotic strictures in the ascending colon. A nested case-control study was performed to identify possible associations with this condition. Fourteen cases were each compared with four controls matched by date of birth from the United Kingdom Cystic Fibrosis Registry. There was a dose-related association between the occurrence of fibrosing colonopathy and the use of high-strength pancreatic enzyme formulations, particularly Nutrizym 22 and Pancrease HL, but not Creon 25 000. In another study, 99 children with cystic fibrosis were compared with 38 healthy controls; children using high-strength pancreatin were 5.2 times more likely to have a colon wall thickness of 1.5 mm or more than children using a formulation of standard strength (63[C]). A similar case from the US has been described in a 2-year-old girl with cystic fibrosis (64[C]). The Committee on Safety of Medicines has issued three recommendations (65[C]):

- *three brands of high-dose pancreatic enzyme (Pancrease HL, Nutrizym 22, and Panzytrat 25 000) should not be used in children with cystic fibrosis aged 15 years or less;*
- *the total dose of supplementary pancreatic enzymes in these patients should not exceed 10 000 lipase units/kg/day;*
- *any patient using a pancreatin formulation who complains of a new or changed abdominal symptom should be reviewed to exclude the possibility of colonic pathology.*

Creon 25 contains 25 000 units of lipase, together with increased amounts of protease and amylase. This formulation has not been associated with fibrosing colonopathy, and is usually well tolerated (66[C]).

REFERENCES

1.   Roberts SJ, Bateman DN. Prescribing of antacids and ulcer-healing drugs in primary care in the north of England. Aliment Pharmacol Ther 1995;9:137—43.

2.   Richter JE, Long JF. Cisapride for gastroesophageal reflux disease: a placebo-controlled, double-blind study. Am J Gastroenterol 1995;90: 423—30.

3.   Kimmig JM. Treatment and prevention of relapse of mild oesophagitis with omeprazole and cisapride: comparison of two strategies. Aliment Pharmacol Ther 1995;9:281—6.

4.   Avorn J, Gurwitz JH, Bohn RL, Mogun H, Monane M, Walker A. Increased incidence of levodopa therapy following metoclopramide use. J Am Med Assoc 1995;274:1780—2.

5.   Gilbert CJ, Ohly KV, Rosner G, Peters WP. Randomised, double-blind comparison of a prochlorperazine-based versus a metoclopramide-based antiemetic regimen in patients undergoing autologous bone marrow transplantation. Cancer 1995;76:2330—7.

6.   Reynolds DJM, Blogg CE. Prevention and treatment of post-operative nausea and vomiting. Presc J 1995;35:111—16.

7.   Adams VR, Valley AW. Granisetron: the second serotonin-receptor antagonist. Ann Pharmacother 1995;29:1240—51.

8.   Maisano R, Adamo V, Settineri N, Pergolizzi S, Scimone A, Altavilla G. Efficacy of two oral dose regimens of granisetron. Anticancer Res 1995;15:2287—90.

9.   Gebbia V, Testa A, Valenza R, Cannata G, Tirrito ML, Gebbia N. Oral granisetron with or without methylprednisolone versus metoclopramide plus methylprednisolone in the management of delayed nausea and vomiting induced by cisplatin-based chemotherapy. Cancer 1995;76: 1821—8.

10.   Fujii Y, Tanaka H, Toyooka H. Prevention of post operative nausea and vomiting with granisetron: a randomised, double-blind comparison with droperidol. Can J Anaesth 1995;42:852—6.

11.   Piper DW. A comparative overview of the adverse effects of antiulcer drugs. Drug Saf 1995;12:120—38.

12.   Mann SG, Murakami A, McCarroll K, Rao AN, Cottrell J, Mehentee J, Morton R. Low dose famotidine in the prevention of sleep disturbance caused by heartburn after an evening meal. Aliment Pharmacol Ther 1995;9:395—401.

13.   Buskin SE, Weiss NS, Gale JL, Nolan CM. Tuberculosis in relation to a history of peptic ulcer disease and treatment of gastric hyperacidity. Am J Epidemiol 1995;141:218—24.

14.   Fish DN. Safety and cost of rapid iv injection of famotidine in critically ill patients. Am J Health-Syst Pharm 1995;52:1889—94.

15.   Delchier J-C, El Amine I, Roudot-Thoraval F, Elouaer-Blanc L, Lamarque D, Stanescu L. Maintenance of gastric pH above 6 with intravenous famotidine in patients with a bleeding duodenal ulcer. Aliment Pharmacol Ther 1995; 9:191—6.

16.   Simon TJ, Roberts WG, Berlin RG, Hayden LJ, Berman RS, Reagan JE. Acid suppression by famotidine 20 mg daily or 40 mg twice daily in preventing relapse of endoscopic recurrence of erosive esophagitis. Clin Ther 1995;17:1147—56.

17.   Brandstatter G, Marks IN, Lanza F, Kogut D, Cobert B, Savitsky JP, Bender W, Labs R, Wurzer H, on behalf of the Multicenter Roxatidine Cooperative Study Group. A multicentre, randomized, double-blind comparison of roxatidine with ranitidine in the treatment of patients with uncomplicated benign gastric ulcer disease. Clin Ther 1995;17:467—78.

18.   Kuipers EJ, Lee A, Klinkenberg-Knol EC, Meuwissen SGM. The development of atrophic gastritis—*Helicobacter pylori* and the effects of acid suppressive therapy. Aliment Pharmacol Ther 1995;9:331—40.

19.   Klinkenberg-Knol EC, Festen HPM, Meuwissen SGM. Pharmacological management of gastro-oesophageal reflux disease. Drugs 1995; 49:695—710.

20.   Banerjee S, Ardill JES, Beattie AD, McColl KEL. Effect of omeprazole and feeding on plasma gastrin in patients with achlorhydria. Aliment Pharmacol Ther 1995;9:507—12.

21.   Verdu EF, Armstrong D, Idstrom J-P, Labenz J, Stolte M, Dorta G, Borsch G, Blum AL. Effect of curing *Helicobacter pylori* infection on intragastric pH during treatment with omeprazole. Gut 1995;37:743—8.

22.   Interdisciplinary Group for Ulcer Study. Six months of omeprazole 20 mg daily, 20 mg every other day or 40 mg at weekends in duodenal ulcer patients: a multicenter, prospective, comparative study. Digestion 1995;56:181—6.

23.   Bate CM, Booth SN, Crowe JP, Mountford RA, Keeling PWN, Hepworth-Jones B, Taylor MD, RichardsonPDI, and the Solo Investigator Group. Omeprazole 10 mg or 20 mg once daily in the prevention of recurrence of reflux oesophagitis. Gut 1995;36:492—8.

24.   Fleury D, Storkebaum H, Mougenot B, Bridoux F, Gobert P, Lemaitre V, Vanhille Ph. Acute interstitial nephritis due to omeprazole. Clin Nephrol 1995;44:129.

25.   Laursen LS, Havelund T, Bondesen S, Hansen J, Sanchez G, Sebelin E, Fenger C, Lauritsen K. Omeprazole in the long-term treatment of gastro-oesophageal reflux disease. Scand J Gastroenterol 1995;30:839—46.

26.   Gough A, Andrews D, Bacon PA, Emery P. Evidence of omeprazole-induced small bowel bacterial overgrowth in patients with scleroderma. Br J Rheum 1995;34:976—7.

27.   Robinson M, Sahba B, Avner D, Jhalas N, Greski-Rose PA, Jennings DE. A comparison of lansoprazole and ranitidine in the treatment of erosive oesophagitis. Aliment Pharmacol Ther 1995;9:25—31.

28.   Witzel L, Gutz H, Huttemann W, Schepps W.

Pantoprazole versus omeprazole in the treatment of acute gastric ulcers. Aliment Pharmacol Ther 1995;9:19—24.

29. Koop H, Schepp W, Dammann HG, Schneider A, Luhmann R, Classen M. Comparative trial of pantoprazole and ranitidine in the treatment of reflux esophagitis. J Clin Gastroenterol 1995;20:192—5.

30. Corinaldesi R, Valentini M, Belaiche J, Colin R, Geldof H, Maier C, and the European Pantoprazole Study Group. Pantoprazole and omeprazole in the treatment of reflux oesophagitis: a European multicentre study. Aliment Pharmacol Ther 1995;9:667—71.

31. Beker JA, Bianchi Porro G, Bigard M-A, Delle Fave G, Devis G, Gouerou H, Maier C. Double-blind comparison of pantoprazole and omeprazole for the treatment of acute duodenal ulcer. Eur J Gastroenterol Hepatol 1995;7:407—10.

32. Bardhan KD, Hawkey CJ, Long RG, Morgan AG, Wormsley KG, Moules IK, Brocklebank D, on behalf of the UK Lansoprazole Clinical Research Group. GR112311X (ranitidine bismuth citrate), a new drug for the treatment of duodenal ulcer. Aliment Pharmacol Ther 1995;9:145—51.

33. Reilly TG, Ayres RCS, Poxon V, Walt RP. Helicobacter pylori eradication in a clinical setting: success rates and the effect on the quality of life in peptic ulcer. Aliment Pharmacol Ther 1995;9:483—90.

34. Bayerdorffer E, Miehlke S, Mannes GA, Sommer A, Hochter W, Weingart J, Heldwein W, Klann H, Simon T, Schmitt W, Bastlein E, Eimiller A, Hatz R, Lehn N, Dirschedl P, Stolte M. Double-blind trial of omeprazole and amoxicillin to cure Helicobacter pylori infection in patients with duodenal ulcers. Gastroenterology 1995;108:1412—17.

35. Labenz J, Stolte M, Ruhl GH, Becker T, Tillenburg B, Sollbohmer M, Borsch G. One-week low-dose triple therapy for the eradication of Helicobacter pylori infection. Eur J Gastroenterol Hepatol 1995;7:9—11.

36. Moayyedi P, Sahay P, Tompkins DS, Axon ATR. Efficacy and optimum dose of omeprazole in a new 1-week triple therapy regimen to eradicate Helicobacter pylori. Eur J Gastroenterol Hepatol 1995;7:835—40.

37. Gotz JM, Veenendaal RA, Veselic M, Bernards S, Lamers CBHW. Triple therapy with ranitidine, clarithromycin, and metronidazole in the treatment of Helicobacter pylori. Scand J Gastroenterol 1995;30:34—7.

38. Yousfi MM, El-Zimaity HMT, Al-Assi MT, Cole RA, Genta RM, Graham DY. Metronidazole, omeprazole and clarithromycin: an effective combination therapy for Helicobacter pylori infection. Aliment Pharmacol Ther 1995;9:209—12.

39. Bell GD, Bate CM, Axon ATR, Tildesley G, Kerr GD, Green JRB, Emmas CE, Taylor MD. Addition of metronidazole to omeprazole/amoxycillin dual therapy increases the rate of Helicobacter pylori eradication: a double-blind, randomised trial. Aliment Pharmacol Ther 1995;9:513—20.

40. Logan RPH, Bardhan KD, Celestin LR, Theodossi A, Palmer KR, Reed PI, Baron JH, Misiewicz JJ. Eradication of Helicobacter pylori and prevention of recurrence of duodenal ulcer: a randomised, double-blind, multi-centre trial of omeprazole with or without clarithromycin. Aliment Pharmacol Ther 1995;9:417—23.

41. Bell GD, Powell KW, Burridge SM, Bowden AF, Atoyebi W, Bolton GH, Jones PH, Brown C. Rapid eradication of Helicobacter pylori infection. Aliment Pharmacol Ther 1995;9:41—6.

42. Van Outryve M, Mayeur S, Meeus MA, Rosillon D, Hendrickx B, Ceuppens M. A double-blind crossover comparison study of the safety and efficacy of mebeverine sustained release in the treatment of irritable bowel syndrome. J Clin Pharmacol Ther 1995;20:277—82.

43. Schiller LR. Anti-diarrhoeal pharmacology and therapeutics. Aliment Pharmacol Ther 1995;9:87—106.

44. Jick H, Myers MW, Dean AD. The risk of sulfasalazine- and mesalazine-associated blood disorders. Pharmacotherapy 1995;15:176—81.

45. Roddie P, Dorrance H, Cook MK, Rainey JB. Treatment of sulphasalazine-induced agranulocytosis with granulocyte macrophage-colony stimulating factor. Aliment Pharmacol Ther 1995;9:711—12.

46. Lankisch PG, Droge M, Gottesleben F. Drug induced acute pancreatitis: incidence and severity. Gut 1995;37:565—7.

47. Fockens P, Mulder CJJ, Tytgat GNJ, Blok P, Ferwerda J, and the Dutch Pentasa Study Group. Comparison of the efficacy and safety of 1.5 compared with 3.0 g oral slow-release mesalazine (Pentasa) in the maintenance treatment of ulcerative colitis. Eur J Gastroenterol Hepatol 1995;7:1025—30.

48. Sturgeon JB, Bhatia P, Hermens D, Miner PB. Exacerbation of chronic ulcerative colitis with mesalazine. Gastroenterology 1995;108:1889—93.

49. Miner P, Hanauer S, Robinson M, Schwartz J, Arora S, and Pentasa UC Maintenance Study Group. Safety and efficacy of controlled-release mesalazine for maintenance of remission in ulcerative colitis. Dig Dis Sci 1995;40:296—304.

50. Brignola C, Cottone M, Pera A, Ardizzone S, Scribano ML, de Franchis R, D'Arienzo A, D'Albasio G, Pennestri D, and the Italian Cooperative Study Group. Mesalazine in the prevention of endoscopic recurrence after intestinal resection for Crohn's disease. Gastroenterology 1995;108:345—9.

51. McLeod RS, Wolff BG, Steinhart AH, Carryer PW, O'Rourke K, Andrews DF, Blair JE, Cangemi JR, Cohen Z, Cullen JB, Chaytor RG, Greenberg GR, Jaffer NM, Jeejeebhoy KN, MacCarty RL, Ready RL, Weiland LH. Prophylactic mesalazine treatment decreases postoperative recurrence of Crohn's disease. Gastroenterology 1995;109:404—13.

52. McArthur KE. Drug-induced pancreatitis. Aliment Pharmacol Ther 1996;10:23—8.

53. Kruis W, Judmaier G, Kayasseh L, Stolte M, Theuer D, Scheurlen C, Hentschel E, Kratochvil P. Double-blind dose-finding study of olsalazine versus sulphasalazine as maintenance therapy for ulcerative colitis. Eur J Gastroenterol Hepatol 1995;7:391—6.

54. Nilsson A, Danielsson A, Lofberg R, Benno P, Bergman L, Fausa O, Florholmen J, Karvonen A-L, Kildebo S, Kollberg B, Lindberg G, Loof L, Stig R, Tanghoj H. Olsalazine versus sulphasalazine for relapse prevention in ulcerative colitis: a multicenter study. Am J Gastroenterol 1995; 90:381—7.

55. Bernstein CN, Seeger LL, Sayre JW, Anton PA, Artinian L, Shanahan F. Decreased bone density in inflammatory bowel disease is related to corticosteroid use and not disease diagnosis. J Bone Mineral Res 1995;10:250—6.

56. Silvennoinen JA, Karttunen TJ, Niemela SE, Manelius JJ, Lehtola JK. A controlled study of bone mineral density in patients with inflammatory bowel disease. Gut 1995;37:71—6.

57. Compston JE. Osteoporosis, corticosteroids and inflammatory bowel disease. Aliment Pharmacol Ther 1995;9:237—50.

58. Spencer CM, McTavish D. Budesonide. A review of its pharmacological properties and therapeutic efficacy in inflammatory bowel disease. Drugs 1995;50:854—72.

59. Forbes A, Reading NG. The risks of malignancy from either immunosuppression or diagnostic radiation in inflammatory bowel disease. Aliment Pharmacol Ther 1995;9:465—70.

60. Bouhnik Y, Lémann M, Mary J-Y, Scemama G, Ta6 R, Matuchansky C, Modigliani R, Rambaud J-C. Long-term follow-up of patients with Crohn's disease treated with azathioprine or 6-mercaptopurine. Lancet 1996;347:215—9.

61. Kowdley KV, Keeffe EB. Hepatotoxicity of transplant immunosuppressive agents. Gastroenterol Clin North Am 1995;24:991—1001.

62. Smyth RL, Ashby D, O'Hea U, Burrows E, Lewis P, van Velzen D, Fofhr JA. Fibrosing colonopathy in cystic fibrosis: results of a case-control study. Lancet 1995;346:1247—51.

63. MacSweeney EJ, Oades PJ, Buchdahl R, Rosenthal M, Bush A. Relation of thickening of colon wall to pancreatic-enzyme treatment in cystic fibrosis. Lancet 1995;345:752—6.

64. Ablin DS, Ziegler M. Ulcerative type of colitis associated with the use of high strength pancreatic enzyme supplements in cystic fibrosis. Pediatr Radiol 1995;25:113—16.

65. Pancreatic enzyme supplements and fibrosing colonopathy. WHO Drug Information 1996; 10:43—4.

66. Friesen C, Prestidge C. Comparison of a high-strength pancreatic enzyme preparation and a standard-strength preparation in cystic fibrosis. Adv Ther 1995;12:236-44.

37 Drugs acting on the immune system

THERAPEUTIC CYTOKINES

INTERFERONS *(SED-13, 1090; SEDA-18, 351; SEDA-19, 334)*

Interferon-α

Recent literature has focused on treatment strategies and the safety of interferon-α in chronic viral hepatitis (1[R]), (2[R]), (3[r]), the only effective and approved therapy in this setting. Depending on criteria for defining adverse effects, two independent Italian reports have shown that the incidence of major or important adverse effects during treatment for chronic hepatitis is variable, with an incidence of 1.3% in 11 241 patients (4[C]) and 25% in 659 patients (5[C]). Non-response to treatment, cirrhosis, age over 50—60 years, female sex, medium/high total dose, and duration of treatment were significant risk factors. In another study with high-dose interferon-α (18—70 million units weekly), dosage reduction or withdrawal was necessary in 31% of 987 patients, mostly because of *flu-like symptoms*, *leukopenia*, or *thrombocytopenia* (6[C]). In addition, significant but reversible adverse effects occurred in 12% of the other 677 patients, symptoms of *depression* and *thyroid disorders* being the most frequent. Interferon-α is sometimes used in acute hepatitis C in which it has produced only mild adverse effects (7[c]).

Cardiovascular Severe or life-threatening cardiotoxicity has mostly been reported in cancer patients or in those receiving high-dose interferon-α, but it has also occurred during the treatment of chronic viral hepatitis C in patients without evidence of previous cardiac disease and receiving low-dose interferon-α. Recent case reports have included reversible *cardiogenic shock* (8[c]), *acute cardiorespiratory arrest* without evidence of myocardial necrosis (9[c]) and severe *left ventricular dysfunction* (10[c]). Such events are very rarely reported, as only seven patients had cardiovascular toxicity (three *myocardial infarction*, one *angina*, and three *dysrhythmias*) among 11 241 patients treated for chronic viral hepatitis (4[C]). Based on a single case report, interferon-α-associated recurrent pericarditis was not considered an absolute contraindication to subsequent treatment (11[c]).

Interferon-α was confirmed to have caused severe *Raynaud's phenomenon* in four patients (12[c])—(14[c]). Continuation of treatment was complicated by digital necrosis requiring surgical excision in two patients, and arteriography disclosed distal artery occlusions or narrowing. Raynaud's phenomenon affecting both hands and feet was experienced within 1—60 months of treatment (median dose: 30 MU/week) in 13 of 25 patients with chronic myelogenous leukemia (15[c]). Vasospasm is presumably the underlying mechanism. Repetitive episodes of *chest pain* at rest, only on days of administration of interferon-α and within 10 min to 10 h after each injection, have been reported in a 54-year-old woman with a predisposition to coronary vasospasm (16[c]).

Respiratory Interferon-α-induced *interstitial pneumonitis* has previously been reported from Japan, and the role of concomitant herbal medicines cannot be ruled out in several patients. Other cases have involved Western patients with multiple myeloma (17[c]) or cutaneous T-cell lymphoma (18[c]).

Nervous system Interferon-α can induce or

unmask *myasthenia gravis*. Four additional cases associated with serum antiacetylcholine receptor antibodies have been described in patients with chronic hepatitis C (19[c]), (20[c]), chronic myelogenous leukemia (21[c]), or renal cell carcinoma (22[c]). In the last case, both interferon-α and IL-2 were used. A familial genetic predisposition was found once (19[c]) and myasthenia gravis was restricted to oculo-bulbar symptoms in two patients (20[c]), (22[c]).

Evidence of *seizures* induced by interferon-α has emerged from a retrospective investigation in 311 chronic hepatitis patients, four (1.3%) of whom experienced generalized tonic-clonic seizures after 2—14 months of treatment, a rate far higher than the 0.03—0.05% annual rate of new seizure onset in the general population (23[C]). All four patients were being treated for hepatitis B or D and two also had glomerulonephritis.

Reversible *chorea* with antinuclear and anti-DNA antibodies and progressive coagulation disorders associated with an anti-prothrombinase type of lupus anticoagulant has been reported in a 15-year-old girl after treatment with interferon-α for chronic myelogenous leukemia for 5 years (24[c]).

Neuropathy has been described in cancer patients and more recently in patients with chronic active hepatitis. One patient experienced an acute exacerbation of peripheral neuropathy shortly after interferon-α was started (25[c]). Another patient developed a severe but spontaneously reversible mononeuropathy of the lower limb on withdrawal of interferon-α (26[c]). Diffuse loss of tactile and thermal sensitivity suggesting a neuropathy of circumscribed areas has also been reported (27[c]).

Psychiatric In patients with chronic myelogenous leukemia, *mood disturbances*, *neurocognitive slowing*, and *memory difficulty*, consistent with a mild fronto-subcortical dysfunction, were more frequent in 25 patients treated with interferon-α compared with 16 patients who had not receive interferon, but the study was poorly controlled (28[C]). The mechanism is still largely unknown. Naltrexone improves interferon-α-induced cognitive dysfunction, and an excitatory effect on opioid receptors is therefore possible (29[c]). Although co-infection with HIV was previously thought to be a risk factor, there were few neuropsychological changes in 18 asymptomatic HIV-1 positive patients treated with natural interferon-αN3 for 12—24 weeks (30[C]).

Severe *depression* and *attempted suicide* are the most severe psychiatric consequences. In 11 241 patients treated for chronic viral hepatitis, reversible *acute psychosis* was found in 10 and attempted suicide was reported in two (4[C]). However, in preliminary results of a French prospective study of 219 patients with chronic viral hepatitis, four attempted suicide, of whom two died from hanging 5 months after interferon-α withdrawal, suggesting an incidence higher than expected (31[c]). In Japan a 3.4% incidence of depressive disorders has been reported in 677 patients receiving high-dose interferon-α, including two patients who attempted suicide (6[C]). Risk factors, such as depressive disorders or addictive behavior, have been found in two patients who attempted suicide within 2 months after starting interferon-α (32[c]).

Endocrine, metabolic A large amount of data has accumulated on *thyroid abnormalities*. In recent studies the rate of clinical thyroid disorders in patients with chronic hepatitis C receiving interferon-α for 12 months ranged from 7—8% (33(34[C]) to 16% (35[C]) and up to 31% (36[C]). The results of the largest prospective study, involving 207 patients, showed that 7.7% of patients (all of whom were women) had thyroid disorders before any treatment, with thyroid antibodies in 6.7% and hypothyroidism in 4.8% (37[C]). This incidence was suggested to be similar to that of the general population of similar sex and age. Among 144 patients without any thyroid dysfunction who subsequently received interferon-α for 12 months, eight (5.6%) developed antithyroid antibodies (4.9%) and/or hypothyroidism (2.8%). Antithyroid antibodies were found in all but one patient with hypothyroidism, and women (15%) were affected significantly more often than men (1%). The mean age of patients with thyroid disorders was also significantly higher than those with no anomalies, but transient hypothyroidism has also been described in children (38[c]). Other autoantibodies, for example antinuclear and anti-dsDNA, and clinical signs of autoimmune disorders (hepatitis and Sjögren's syndrome) were significantly more frequent in patients with thyroid disorders (37[C]). Patients with previous autoimmune thyroid abnormalities are clearly predisposed to develop a potentially severe form of hypothyroidism with TSH receptor antibodies (39[C]) or biphasic thyroiditis (40[C]). Thyroid dysfunction (especially hypothyroidism) is usually mild and/or transient upon interferon-α discontinuation with most cases resolving within 24 weeks (33[C]), (37[C]). Even severe interferon-α-induced hypothyroidism completely reversed spontaneously (40[c]) or after subsequent withdrawal of L-thyroxine (41[c]). However, other investigators have found long-lasting hypothyroidism (36[C]) and severe hyperthyroidism sometimes required radical radioiodine therapy with subsequent need for thyroxine replacement (42[c]). Finally, surveillance of thyroid disorders should probably be extended after withdrawal, as clinical thyroid dysfunction sometimes appears several months later (33[C]), (36[C]).

Apart from thyroid function, concentrations of other serum hormone (i.e. calcitonin, TSH, LH, FSH, prolactin, growth hormone, cortisol, testosterone, estradiol) were not altered by 6 months of interferon-α treatment in 31 patients (43[C]), but concentrations of insulin-like growth factor I were increased and negatively correlated with aminotransferase activities.

Exacerbation or de novo diabetes mellitus by interferon-α has been confirmed in eight additional patients treated for chronic hepatitis C or cancer. Risk factors, such as obesity and a family or previous history of glucose intolerance, were sometimes identified in the development of insulin-dependent (44[c]), (45[c]) or non-insulin-dependent diabetes mellitus (46[c]), but have been inconsistently found (47[c]). Islet cell antibodies were positive (44[c]) or negative (46[c]), (47[c]), so that impaired glucose tolerance or the triggering of an autoimmune phenomenon were both possible. A progressive increase in insulin requirements within 3 months of interferon-α was also noticed in a previously well-controlled 66-year-old man (48[c]). Acute worsening of diabetes mellitus has also been reported in three patients treated with both interferon-α and IL-2 for advanced malignancy (49[c]). One patient

was found dead from possible hyperglycemic coma. Although an increased expression of interferon-α in the pancreases of patients with type I diabetic argues for a causal role of this cytokine in the development of diabetes (50[C]), such an event is probably very rare and diabetes mellitus was reported in only 10 of 11 241 patients treated for chronic hepatitis C (4[C]). In addition, a retrospective study has shown that the prevalence of diabetes mellitus is spontaneously higher than expected in patients with chronic hepatitis C, but not chronic hepatitis B, compared with the general population (51[C]).

The possible development of insulin autoantibodies has been confirmed, as they were found in six of 58 patients with chronic viral hepatitis B or C after 6 months of interferon-α treatment compared with two of 60 patients before treatment (52[C]).

The effect of interferon-α on *blood lipids* has been extensively investigated. Serum concentrations of apoprotein B100, lipoprotein(a), and apoprotein B100/apoprotein A1 ratio were significantly lower in 25 untreated patients with chronic active hepatitis C compared with 25 healthy controls (53[C]). Treatment with interferon-α for 6 months caused a significant rise in serum triglyceride and lipoprotein(a) concentrations and a fall in total cholesterol, HDL-cholesterol, LDL-cholesterol, and apoprotein A1, suggesting a possible increased cardiovascular risk. The clinical relevance of interferon-induced changes in lipid profile awaits further investigation, as no pancreatic or cardiovascular complications were noted in patients who developed very high serum triglyceride concentrations (54[c]), (55[C]).

Hematological Significant *thrombocytopenia* and *neutropenia* are the most frequent hematological adverse effects of interferon-α. Although autoimmune thrombocytopenia and hepatitis C virus infection may be associated (56[R]), (57[R]), interferon-α is a possible cause in the induction (58[c]) or exacerbation (59[c]), (60[c]) of life-threatening idiopathic thrombocytopenic purpura. Based on a single case report in a 28-year-old woman with natural interferon-α-induced antinuclear antibody-associated purpuric thrombocytopenia, interferon-β has been proposed as a safe and effective alternative (61^c), (62^c).

The development or acute exacerbation of *autoimmune hemolytic anemia* has been reported in nine patients treated with interferon-α for various hematological malignancies (63^C). Exacerbation occurred within 1—21 days of treatment, whereas de novo appearance was diagnosed after 3—38 months. In chronic myelogenous leukemia, immune-mediated hemolysis was reported to occur in seven (1%) of 581 patients receiving interferon-α alone or as part of a chemotherapeutic regimen (64^C). By contrast, a severe form of Coombs' negative hemolytic anemia with mild bone-marrow erythroid hypoplasia has been reported in a 30-year-old woman with chronic hepatitis C (65^c).

Neutropenia is frequent and sometimes treatment-limiting, but complete agranulocytosis completely resolving after treatment with G-CSF has been observed (66^c).

In contrast to previous findings (SEDA-19, 335), Dutch authors have been unable to detect an increase in anti-factor VIII antibodies in patients with hemophilia A receiving interferon-α for chronic hepatitis C: two out of 21 interferon-treated patients had anti-factor VIII antibodies compared with three of 14 untreated patients with hemophilia A (67^C). A high prevalence of *anti-phospholipid antibodies* has also been found in patients infected with hepatitis C, but the causative role of interferon-α and the clinical relevance of these findings remains to be more clearly established (68^c). However, lower limb venous thrombosis was observed after 4 months of interferon-α for chronic hepatitis C in a 49-year-old man with familial asymptomatic antithrombin III deficiency and anticardiolipid antibodies (69^c).

Liver   Rare cases of fatal *liver failure* have been described in patients with decompensated cirrhosis caused by chronic hepatitis B, but also in patients with severe chronic hepatitis C. Among 11 241 patients, four patients (0.035%), two of whom had initial evidence of poor hepatic reserve, died of fulminant liver failure after 8—33 weeks of interferon-α (4^C).

Although an unexplained 5% incidence of *autoimmune hepatitis* has been found in pa-

tients with chronic hepatitis C (70^C), interferon-α-induced de novo hepatitis without pre-existing autoimmune disorders is supposedly a rare and usually self-limited complication (6^c), (71^c). However, *primary biliary cirrhosis* has been reported once (72^c). On the other hand, the co-existence of serological markers for autoimmune hepatitis and hepatitis C virus infection poses a dilemma, because of possible exacerbation of liver necrosis by interferon-α. In sharp contrast to previous results (SED-13, 1094), interferon-α was considered effective and safer than prednisone in two studies of patients (12 in each study) with antibodies to liver and kidney microsomes or nuclear antigens (73^C), (74^C). Similar safety of interferon-α was found in seven patients with chronic hepatitis C positive for antimitochondrial antibodies (75^C). Close monitoring of liver function is still strongly recommended to detect any acute exacerbation of liver disease in these patients. Indeed, interferon-α-induced reversible fulminant hepatitis has been reported in a patient with antiliver cytosol antibody autoimmune type 2 hepatitis, misdiagnosed as chronic hepatitis C (76^c). Finally, interferon-α has also been considered as a probable cause of *granulomatous hepatitis* in two cases (77^c).

Gastrointestinal   *Ischemic colitis*, a previously unreported adverse effect of interferon-α, has been described in two of 280 patients treated for chronic hepatitis C (78^C).

Urinary system   Renal disorders with interferon-α have mostly been reported in patients being treated for malignancies. Minimal-change *glomerulonephritis* with recurrent gross proteinuria on readministration of interferon-α in a 32-year-old man treated for chronic myeloid leukemia was in keeping with rare instances of renal toxicity (79^c). The combination of interferon-α and IL-2 has also been implicated in one case of pauci-immune glomerulonephritis with rapidly progressive and fatal renal failure (80^{cr}).

Skin and appendages   There is a relation between several skin disorders (cryoglobulin-associated vasculitis, lichen planus, sporadic porphyria cutanea tarda) and a high prevalence of hepatitis C infection (81[R]). A detrimental role of interferon-α should therefore be regarded cautiously, particularly with respect to lichen planus. Indeed, reports have suggested both the development and/or exacerbation of *lichen planus* (82[c]), (83[c]) or its disappearance (83[c]), (84[c]) following treatment with interferon-α. Although an association between polyarteritis nodosa and hepatitis C has also been suggested (81[R]), interferon-α was regarded as a possible cause of a severe *systemic vasculitis* similar to polyarteritis nodosa which occurred after only 10 days of treatment (85[c]).

Severe *cutaneous necrosis* at subcutaneous injections sites of interferon-α has mostly been described in patients with cancer (86[c]), but it can also occur in patients receiving lower dosages for the treatment of chronic viral hepatitis (87[c]).

Vitiligo, previously reported with interferon-α during cancer chemotherapy, has also been seen in two patients treated for chronic hepatitis C (88[c]), (89[c]).

Special senses *Retinopathy* and *visual* loss continue to be reported (90[C]), (91[c]), and retinal abnormalities should be regularly monitored to prevent severe retinal damage during treatment with interferon-α. In two prospective analyses of 50 and 63 patients with chronic hepatitis C, mild retinopathy with asymptomatic soft exudates or hemorrhages was found in 57—86% (92[C]), (93[C]). In most patients, the onset of retinopathy was noted within 8 weeks of treatment with natural or recombinant interferon-α. However, visual symptoms occurred in only a minority of patients and resolved spontaneously despite continuation of treatment. Diabetes mellitus and hypertension were again found to be significant risk factors in both studies. Experimental data have suggested that interferon-α-induced increased leukocyte adherence to vascular endothelium is a possible cause of retinal microinfarction (94). Retinopathy was not found in patients treated with topical or subconjunctival interferon-α (95[r]).

Musculoskeletal *Myositis* has been reported after 6 months of interferon-α, with further exacerbation after each subsequent infusion of IL-2 for metastatic renal cell carcinoma

(96[c]). Another case of polymyositis, reversible with corticosteroid treatment, has been reported in a 47-year-old man treated for chronic hepatitis C (97[c]), but hepatitis C infection per se is also a possible cause of an inflammatory myopathy (98[c]). Acute rhabdomyolysis and multiorgan failure occurred after the first course of interferon-α for metastatic melanoma, but the contribution of other drugs (e.g. IL-2) cannot be ruled out (99[c]).

Immunological and hypersensitivity reactions The effects of interferon-α on the prevalence and significance of autoantibodies have been further investigated in patients with chronic hepatitis B (100[C]) or C (101[C]), (102[C]). Interferon-α is often associated with various autoantibodies, but their clinical relevance seems to be limited. Except in patients with pre-existing thyroid antibodies, they are not a contraindication to treatment. The description of non-organ-specific autoimmune disorders is limited to case reports of the occurrence or exacerbation of *lupus-like syndrome* (103[c]), (104[c]) or *polyarthritis* (105[c]), (106[c]), which were respectively found in one and two patients among 677 treated with interferon-α (6[C]).

The first reported case of *Sjögren's syndrome* attributed to interferon-α treatment for chronic hepatitis C (107[c]) should be regarded with caution, because a possible association between Sjögren's syndrome and hepatitis C virus infection has been suggested (81[R]).

Miscellaneous In two patients treated for chronic hepatitis C, interferon-α induced the appearance (108[c]) or the recurrence (109[c]) of pulmonary or generalized *sarcoidosis*, suggesting that interferon-α is involved with or trigger the sarcoid reaction.

Interferon-α-associated histologically-proen *histiocytic cytophagic panniculitis*, not previously reported, has been described in a 59-year-old woman treated for chronic hepatitis C (110[c]). She developed edema after 2 months of treatment, then exophthalmos, markedly increased transaminase activities, pancytopenia, and disseminated intravascular coagulation, despite withdrawal of interferon-α. She died 2 months later from hemorrhagic shock due to massive abdominal wall bleeding.

The clinical relevance of *anti-interferon antibodies* has been more extensively investigated. Neutralizing antibodies were detected within 2—4 months of treatment in most initial responders (275 patients in three studies) with secondary disease reactivation while on interferon-α2a therapy for chronic hepatitis C (111[C])—(113[C]). Biochemical reactivation has been observed simultaneously or soon after the development of neutralizing antibodies; replacement by natural lymphoblastoid human interferon-α restored a complete response without the reappearance of anti-interferon antibodies in six out of nine non-responders with anti-interferon neutralizing antibodies (114[C]). Hepatitis C virus genotype 3a has been suggested to be more often associated with the development of antibodies (112[C]). Failure to respond to treatment because of interferon-α2a antibody-mediated resistance has also been observed in patients with cutaneous T-cell lymphoma (115[C]), chronic granulocytic leukemia (116[c]), or chronic myelogenous leukemia (117[c]), who had an initial response and secondary loss of efficacy. Again, a restored response is possible by the use of natural interferon-α (116[c]), (117[c]).

Risk factors *Interferon and transplantation* Based on the results of recent studies suggesting the deleterious influence of interferon-α on renal allograft function (118[C]), this treatment has been strongly questioned, at least in transplant patients with hepatitis C infection (119[r]). Chronic liver allograft rejection was also observed in five of 14 patients treated with interferon-α (of whom three required re-transplantation) compared with one of 32 untreated patients (120[C]). As there is no definitive evidence of increased liver graft rejection by interferon-α from other studies (121[r]), the safety and efficacy of interferon-α in organ-transplant patients warrants further studies. Interferon-α has been also associated with a dose-dependent increased incidence of graft-versus-host disease in seven patients, including one fatal case, when given early (at a median of 3 months) after allogeneic bone-marrow transplantation (122[C]).

Interferon and HIV disease Interferon-α has

been investigated in nine patients (123[C]) and 79 patients (124[C]) infected with HIV. No serious unexpected adverse effects or opportunistic infections were detected, although there was an unexplained sudden fall in CD4+ cell count in 5% of the 57 patients in another study (125[C]).

Tumor-inducing effects Concern related to second malignancies or chromosomal abnormalities in cancer patients (mostly myeloid leukemia) treated with interferon-α has again been stressed in several case reports (126[c]), (127[c]) and clinical studies (128[Cr]), but recently no evidence has been found of an increased relative risk of a second cancer, at least in patients treated for hairy cell leukemia (129[C]), (130[c]).

Second-generation effects Uncomplicated and successful outcome of pregnancy has been reported in five patients with thrombocythemia (one), chronic myelogenous leukemia (two), Hodgkin's disease (one), and chronic hepatitis C (one), including exposure during (131[c]), (132[c]) or after (133[c]), (134[c]) the period of embryogenesis (i.e. the first 10 weeks after the last menstrual period). Very low concentrations of interferon-α were found immediately post-partum in the serum of two newborns (less than 1 U/ml) or in breast milk (1.4—6 U/ml), compared with maternal serum concentrations (21 and 58 U/ml, respectively) (134[c]). Unfortunately, long-term follow-up is not yet available for these newborns, except normal development at 2 years of age in one case (131[c]).

Interactions The simultaneous use of interferon-α and *angiotensin-converting enzyme inhibitors* (enalapril or captopril) caused additive and early-occurring hematological toxicity (severe but reversible neutropenia) in three patients treated for type II mixed cryoglobulinemia (135[C]). Recurrence of neutropenia after retreatment with both drugs was reported in one patient, whereas neutropenia was not observed in the other 35 patients who received interferon-α alone.

Interferon-β

Interferon-β has been approved for the treatment of multiple sclerosis, and the results of a consensus conference on its use have been published (136[R]). However, a large debate has emerged about the unclear evidence for its efficacy and the cost of treatment (137), (138).

Adverse effects of interferon-β1b have been analysed in 72 patients (139[C]). *Influenza-like symptoms, fatigue, skin reactions, leukopenia, headache*, and *depression* were the most frequent. Discontinuation of treatment was reported in 18% of patients and was more frequent in patients with chronic progressive disease (63%). In contrast to earlier suggestions, there was a significant correlation between chronic progressive disease, fatigue, and depression in patients who decided to discontinue treatment. Results from a multicenter phase III trial in 301 patients with multiple sclerosis (140[C]) and a study of 12 healthy volunteers (141[C]) have shown a very similar profile of adverse effects for interferon β1a, i.e. mainly constitutional symptoms. Similar findings have been noted in 25 patients treated with intralesional interferon-β1a for condyloma acuminatum (142[c]).

Psychiatric   Although the reference study in multiple sclerosis concluded that depressive symptoms and suicide attempts were more probably related to the disease than to interferon-α treatment (143[C]), concern arose about *suicide and attempted suicide*. A history of depression was not considered an absolute contraindication to treatment, but previous suicide attempts and current depression should be carefully evaluated before treatment (136[r]). Analysis with single photon emission computed tomography in one patient treated for acute hepatitis C showed that symptoms of depression were associated with a marked decrease in inferior frontal cortex cerebral blood flow (144[c]).

Endocrine, metabolic   One previous study in patients with hematological malignancies failed to identify thyroid dysfunction. Another study in 11 patients without pre-existing thyroid disease and treated with daily injections for 8 weeks for chronic hepatitis C showed a slight fall in triiodothyronine and an increase in thyroid-stimulating hormone, both significant and reversible within 4—8 weeks after withdrawal (145[C]). Antithyroid antibodies were not found.

Hematological   Interferon-β has been reported to cause a reversible *autoimmune hemolytic anemia* during treatment for chronic hepatitis C (146[c]).

Skin and appendages   Whilst reactions at injection sites are common, rare but severe *skin necrosis* have been reported following high-dose and even low-dose interferon-β (147[c]). *Local reactions* to subcutaneous injections (32 million units daily) for multiple sclerosis have been described (148[C]). Among 400 patients, eight (2%) experienced a reversible local reaction within 6—19 weeks, consisting of sharply delimited *cutaneous ulcers* or *painful nodules* in seven and *pustular exacerbation of quiescent psoriasis* in one. Overall, interferon-β seems to be more often associated with cutaneous ulceration than other interferons.

Immunological and hypersensitivity reactions   The first case of a hypersensitivity reaction has been reported in a 41-year-old woman who experienced *facial and laryngeal edema* with subsequent *chronic urticaria*, reversible on withdrawal (149[c]). Hives and angio-edema occurred after rechallenge, but skin tests to interferon-β were negative. Successful desensitization by progressively increasing the dose of interferon-β was later achieved.

After 3 years of treatment, *neutralizing antibodies* to interferon β-1b are detected in 38% of patients receiving eight million units and are significantly associated with a reduction in therapeutic efficacy (143[C]). Further analysis has confirmed that relapse rates are similar in patients with neutralizing antibodies compared with placebo-treated patients, and these authors concluded that the decision to discontinue treatment should be made individually based on clinical response and a positive titer of neutralizing antibodies with the use of a reliable assay (150[C]). Neutralizing antibodies to interferon β-1a have been observed in 22% of patients after 2 years (140[C]).

Miscellaneous One additional case of interferon-β-associated *sarcoidosis* has been reported (151[c]). The patient's sister had had sarcoidosis, suggesting a predisposing genetic background and possible exacerbation of silent sarcoidosis.

Interferon-γ

After a mean follow-up period of 2.5 years in 58 children treated for chronic granulomatous disease, there were no severe adverse effects or consequences on growth and development (152[C]), (153[C]). Interferon-γ also improved the cutaneous symptoms of systemic sclerosis, but 10 of 20 patients had to discontinue interferon-γ in one study because of exacerbation of *Raynaud's syndrome* in five, *constitutional symptoms* in two, *renal crises* in two, and moderate *pancytopenia* in one (154[C]). In contrast, others using a thrice-weekly regimen found a reasonable safety profile in this setting in 16 patients, with severe *flu-like symptoms* as the most frequent adverse effect (155[C]).

Cardiovascular *Ventricular tachycardia* after injection of interferon-γ has been reported in a 34-year-old woman with underlying ventricular extra beats (155[c]).

Gastrointestinal Severe *aphthous stomatitis* associated with increased antinuclear antibody titers in a 19-year-old man treated for systemic sclerosis has been definitely related to treatment, as demonstrated by rechallenge with another injection of interferon-γ (155[c]).

Urinary system Acute renal failure is extremely rare with interferon-γ. Interferon-γ was implicated in a case of minimal-change *nephrotic syndrome* and *acute interstitial nephritis* in a 70-year-old man treated for 1 year for metastatic renal cell carcinoma (156[c]).

Skin and appendages Severe *erythroderma* has been reported in five of 10 patients after interferon-γ was added to cyclosporin after autologous bone-marrow transplantation (157[C]).

Miscellaneous *Antibodies* to recombinant interferon-γ have not been previously reported, but they did occur in a patient with systemic macrocytosis who had an initial response to subcutaneous treatment and secondary failure after 4 months (158[c]).

INTERLEUKINS *(SED-13, 1101; SEDA-17, 432; SEDA-19, 338)*

Interleukin-1 (IL-1)

IL-1 has a wide spectrum of adverse effects, most of which are dose-dependent and usually easily manageable. The main limitation of IL-1 is rather due to its modest antitumor activity and limited hemopoietic effects, so that combination with other cytokines has been proposed (159[R]).

Cardiovascular A possible association between IL-1-induced severe *hypotension* requiring phenylephrine and its antitumor activity has been suggested in patients with nonvisceral metastases (160[C]).

Endocrine, metabolic Treatment for 1 week with IL-1α and IL-1β produces various transient or reversible endocrine effects, including *increases in cortisol, growth hormone, prolactin, and thyroid-stimulating hormone*, and *reductions in testosterone, FSH, and LH*, but without apparent clinical endocrinopathies (161[C]).

Interleukin-2 (IL-2)

The lack of effect of lymphokine-activated killer (LAK) cells to improve the antitumor activity of IL-2 has been confirmed in a comparison of IL-2 alone ($n = 36$) and IL-2 plus LAK cells ($n = 35$) (162[C]). In addition, more patients experienced *pulmonary toxicity* and *hypotension* than those who received IL-2 alone for advanced renal cell carcinoma. Conjugation of polyethylene glycol to IL-2 (PEG-IL-2) did not increase antitumor activity in 64 patients compared with IL-2 alone ($n = 60$), but produced significantly less hypotension requiring vasopressors and need for intensive care support (163[C]).

The optimal safe and effective dose and schedule of administration of IL-2 has still not been defined. Evidence is accumulating that lower doses of IL-2 or its use in combination with interferon-α are as effective as higher doses in the treatment of renal cell carcinoma with substantially less toxicity (164[R]).

Low-dose IL-2 has recently emerged as a possible safe treatment of HIV infection (165[r]). Adverse effects in HIV infection fall within the usual scope of low-dose IL-2 toxicity, fever, malaise, fatigue, and asymptomatic hyperbilirubinemia being the most frequent, and treatment withdrawal for adverse effects is required in 17% of 31 patients (166[C]).

A wide range of IL-2-induced adverse effects is associated with the *vascular leak syndrome*. Using an experimental rat model, dose-dependent colonization of mesenteric lymph nodes with *Escherichia coli* was observed in IL-2-treated animals, showing that IL-2 produces bacterial translocation in the gut (167). This, together with histological evidence of dilated lymphatics and mucosal disruption, was suggested to account for increased membrane permeability and subsequent loss of fluid into visceral and soft tissues.

Cardiovascular   Adverse cardiovascular effects remain a major limitation for high-dose IL-2, and atypical manifestations can be observed, as illustrated in two patients without a history of cardiopulmonary disease (168[c]). The first patient, a 63-year-old woman, experienced unusually severe but reversible *biventricular myocardial hypocontractility* and the second, a 61-year-old woman, developed *regional aneurysmal dilatation of the left ventricle* associated with profound dyskinetic changes which subsequently resolved. Using two-dimensional and Doppler echocardiography in 19 patients, a ratio of maximal flow velocity in early diastole to maximal flow velocity in late diastole lower than 1.0 before treatment has been suggested to be helpful to anticipate severe cardiovascular toxicity, which occurred in six patients (169[C]). The same group of investigators also found a dose-dependent and progressive increase in plasma nitrate and nitrite concentrations in 10 patients who underwent multiple IL-2 cycles, positively correlated with the severity of hypotension but not with the occurrence of cardiac toxicity (170[C]).

Nervous system   IL-2-associated central neuropsychiatric adverse effects are usually considered to result from increased brain water content. Autoimmunity associated wtih *cerebral vasculitis* is another possibility (171[c]).

A 34-year-old woman developed reversible somnolence and hallucinations during her first course of IL-2, and experienced progressive paralysis of the right upper limb and bilateral cerebellar syndrome the day after the end of a second 5-day course. Multiple cerebral and cerebellar ischemic lesions were seen on magnetic resonance imaging, as well as antinuclear antibodies, hypothyroidism with antimicrosomal antibodies, and histological features of leukocytoclastic vasculitis, suggesting immunologically mediated cerebral vasculitis.

The peripheral nervous system can also be involved, with reports of *nerve entrapment syndrome* (172[C]), (173[c]). Typical symptoms of unilateral or bilateral carpal tunnel syndrome during or soon after infusion of IL-2 for renal cell carcinoma were found retrospectively in seven men and one woman, three of whom had recurrent symptoms after a subsequent course (172[c]). In five patients, electrophysiological studies showed sensorimotor median neuropathy with possible axonal dysfunction and demyelination at the wrist. Interstitial edema and local fluid accumulation as a result of increased vascular permeability (vascular leak syndrome) is a likely mechanism of this adverse effect.

Endocrine, metabolic   Interleukin-2 commonly causes *thyroid disorders*. In a study of 281 cancer patients undergoing their first treatment with IL-2 in a low dose (72 000 IU/kg) or a high dose (720 000 IU/kg), 41% of previously euthyroid patients developed thyroid dysfunction (174[C]). Hypothyroidism was the most common finding (35% of patients), but required thyroxine replacement in only 9%. In contrast, subclinical or overt hyperthyroidism was found in only 7% of initially euthyroid patients. As previously reported, the incidence of thyroid abnormalities increased with treatment duration. There was no significant difference in the incidence of thyroid disorders between high-dose and low-dose regimens, and no association with the underlying disease, namely melanoma or renal cancer.

Insulin-dependent diabetes mellitus has been described in a 45-year-old woman with colorectal cancer and a family history of type II diabetes (175[c]). She developed hyperglycemia requiring glibenclamide after 2 weeks of low-dose IL-2 and a recurrence with the need for insulin after rechallenge. Convincing evidence was also given by the finding of islet cell antibodies during therapy, but not before or after, and a fall in insulin requirements after the completion of treatment.

Liver   The possible mechanism of IL-2 *hepatotoxicity* has been investigated in an animal model (176). Activation of Kupfer cells resulted in the release of cytokines, such as tumor necrosis factor, which in turn activated leukocytes and hepatic sinusoidal endothelial cells, and induced the expression of adhesion molecules, with consequent impairment of sinusoidal blood flow and microscopic areas of hepatic ischemia.

Skin and appendages   A wide spectrum of cutaneous disorders has been described, diffuse and usually benign *erythematous macular eruptions* being the most frequent (177[R]). A high-incidence of diffuse rash has been observed after IL-2 as consolidative immunotherapy early after autologous bone-marrow transplantation in 19 patients, of whom 70% experienced skin erythema after high-dose IL-2; further histological examination in nine of these patients showed evidence of a *graft-versus host disease* (GVHD)-like reaction in seven cases (178[c]). Similar features with grade II histological cutaneous GVHD and/or T cell epidermal infiltrate were observed among 14 patients, of whom 85% developed a generalized rash that resolved spontaneously (179[c]). However, such cutaneous toxicity has not been confirmed by others in 26 patients receiving low-dose IL-2, and only nodular lesions at the injection sites were observed (180[c]).

Long-term and intermittent treatment with low-dose IL-2 after remission of secondary acute myeloid leukemia was involved in a typical case of *leukocytoclastic vasculitis*, not previously described (181[c]). The first symptoms developed after 14 months of treatment, resolved within 4—5 days, but reappeared with the subsequent requirement of continuous oral corticosteroid. Serum complement concentrations were reduced and IgG-containing immunocomplexes present.

Musculoskeletal   Muscular toxicity has not been previously reported. Biopsy-proven severe *necrotizing myositis* developed after the sixth dose of IL-2 in a 50-year-old man with metastatic renal cancer (182[c]). Histological examination showed features similar to those of dermatomyositis, which, together with the presence of antinuclear antibodies, suggested an autoimmune mechanism. Complete recovery occurred within 3 weeks.

Interleukin-3 (IL-3)

When given alone, IL-3 has limited clinical effects. However, an enhanced hemopoietic response has been obtained with PIXY321, a genetically engineered GM-CSF/IL-3 fusion protein (183[R]). As expected from the known adverse effects of both of these cytokines, PIXY321 caused only mild-to-moderate adverse effects, *erythema*, *reactions at the site of injection*, *constitutional symptoms*, and *gastrointestinal symptoms* being the most frequent.

Skin and appendages   Mild cutaneous reactions at the injection site are frequent with IL-3. In a 50-year-old woman with IL-3-induced *pruritic and erythematous indurated lesions at the injection site*, the histological features closely resembled those observed with GM-CSF and consisted of superficial and deep perivascular infiltrate with no evidence of vasculitis (184[c]). In contrast, histological evidence of hypersensitivity vasculitis was noted at the injection site in a man infected with HIV-1 (185[c]).

Miscellaneous   The first case of *capillary vascular syndrome* has been described (186[c]).

During the first 11 days of treatment for aplastic anemia, a 39-year-old woman successively developed conjunctivitis, fever and headache, antibacterial-responsive catheter-related septicemia, a generalized papular hemorrhagic skin eruption, and symptoms of peripheral neuropathy. Complete paralysis and increased bleeding tendency later developed despite IL-3 withdrawal, and high-dose steroids and immunoglobulin treatment. She died on day 25 with profuse bleeding and features suggestive of disseminated intravascular coagulation. Diffuse hemorrhages involving peripheral nerves, histological signs suggesting increased vascular permeability, and massive reactive erythrophagocytosis were found at autopsy.

In this case, excessive stimulation of macrophages and secondary cytokines secretion was thought to be involved.

Interleukin-4 (IL-4)

The combination of IL-2 and IL-4 in refractory malignancies in 39 patients has been evaluated and deemed to produce no additional adverse effects to those noted with IL-2 alone (187[C]).

IL-4 administration to 31 patients for 1–13 weeks had no significant effect on serum concentrations of hormones (adrenocorticotropin, cortisol, thyrotropin, thyroxine, prolactin) or lipids (188[C]).

Vitiligo occurred 1 month after IL-4 had been started in a 30-year-old woman with metastatic malignant melanoma (189[c]). She also developed permanent *hyperthyroidism* 14 months after the last course of IL-4, and Grave's disease was diagnosed. Both adverse effects and the further complete remission of melanoma suggested a common immune cause.

Interleukin-6 (IL-6)

Clinical trials of IL-6 as thrombopoietic or antitumor agent are still being carried out (190[R]). Recent trials in patients treated for metastatic renal carcinoma ($n = 40$) (191[C]) or myelodysplastic syndrome ($n = 22$) (192[C]) have shown that IL-6 causes moderate and reversible adverse effects, *fever*, *flu-like symptoms*, *nausea*, and *weight loss* being the most frequent.

Endocrine, metabolic The endocrine effects of IL-6 have been investigated in five men (193[C]). Serum thyrotropin and total serum concentrations of T_3 and T_4 fell after 3 weeks, while serum luteinizing hormone concentrations increased. Concentrations of other hormones, such as testosterone, follicle-stimulating hormone, growth hormone, and prolactin were not significantly affected.

Hematological IL-6-induced *normochromic*

normocytic anemia rarely requires blood transfusion. In 15 cancer patients there was a mean 19% reduction in hemoglobin concentration over a period of 3 days during week 4 of a 6-week course of subcutaneous IL-6 (150 μg/day) (194[C]). Serum iron concentrations fell significantly and plasma volume increased by 18%, but erythrocyte volume was unchanged, indicating hemodilution as the primary mechanism.

Miscellaneous The administration of subcutaneous recombinant IL-6 induced *anti-IL-6 antibodies* in 15% of 49 patients treated for metastatic renal cell cancer, but only one had neutralizing antibodies (191[C]).

Other interleukins

Several other cytokines are currently under investigation and their adverse effects profiles seem to be similar to those of other cytokines.

In 54 healthy volunteers receiving single doses of IL-10 (0.1–100 μg/kg), only mild to moderate *flu-like symptoms*, with fever, chills, headache, and myalgia, were observed at the highest dose (195[C]). In another study in 22 healthy volunteers receiving single doses (1–25 μg/kg), no adverse effects were noted, but two patients had new occurrence or transient exacerbation of mild reversible *first-degree atrioventricular block* 2 h after intravenous administration (196[c]).

Dose-related adverse effects of subcutaneous IL-11 administered for its thrombopoietic activity, consisted of moderate constitutional symptoms (*myalgia/arthralgia*, *fatigue*, and *headache*, but without fever), with a maximum tolerated dose of 75 μg/kg. Moderate weight gain with *edema* and *anemia* due to plasma volume expansion have also been observed (197[c]), as well as transient but symptomatic *atrial dysrhythmias* (198[c]).

IL-12 is regarded as a potential immunotherapeutic agent (199[R]). Multiple organ adverse effects of IL-12 resulted in two deaths among 13 renal cancer patients, and were attributed to the schedule of IL-12 administration, multiple high-doses having been given without an initial single dose (200[r]).

COLONY-STIMULATING FACTORS *(SED-13, 1111; SEDA-17, 395; SEDA-18, 349; SEDA-19, 342)*

Guidelines for the use of hemopoietic growth factors have been proposed (201[R]). Very few comparisons of recombinant growth factors are available, but it has been suggested that intravenous G-CSF is better tolerated, mild to moderate adverse effects requiring dosage adjustment or temporary treatment withdrawal being more common in treated patients with GM-CSF (202[C]). In addition, *weight gain, hypotension, dyspnea,* or *deep venous thrombosis*, suggesting a moderate *capillary leak syndrome*, occurred only in patients treated with GM-CSF.

Treatment with G-CSF in children was considered as reasonably safe (201[R]). Follow-up of 21 infants (median age 25 months) who had received a 3-day course of G-CSF at birth for presumed bacterial sepsis showed no abnormalities in hematological or immunological profile or developmental status (203[C]).

Granulocyte colony-stimulating factor (G-CSF; filgrastim and lenograstim)

Cardiovascular   A new case of acute arterial thrombosis has been described in a 44-year-old man without cardiovascular risk factors who received filgrastrim after chemotherapy (204[c]). Arterial thrombosis in the distal aorta occurred after 7 days of treatment and required balloon angioplasty and subsequent thrombectomy. Thrombosis was suggested to be secondary to filgrastrim-induced increase in platelet count and aggregation. In addition, increased platelet count and abnormalities of platelet aggregation recurred after rechallenge. Similarly, G-CSF administration in healthy volunteers induced increased platelet aggregation, indicating possible hypercoagulability (205[C]).

Endocrine, metabolic   Acute administration of G-CSF did not produce significant changes in serum concentrations of hormones (cortisol, GH, PRL, FSH, LH, TSH, or melatonin) in eight patients with cancers (206[C]).

Hypothyroidism with thyroid microsomal and thyroglobulin antibodies has been reported in a 40-year-old woman who received filgrastrim (in a 10-day course, three times) after each cycle of chemotherapy for breast cancer (207[c]).

Exacerbation of *pseudogout* after G-CSF administration and rechallenge has been reported in a 70-year-old woman (208[c]).

Hematological   Unexpectedly more frequent and severe *thrombocytopenia* occurred after chemotherapy in 18 patients given G-CSF until 2 days before than in 18 controls who received G-CSF only after chemotherapy (209[C]). The administration of G-CSF for mobilization before allogeneic transplantation has also been suggested to account for prolonged but asymptomatic thrombocytopenia in a 44-year-old healthy donor (210[c]).

Liver   In contrast to concern that growth factors might stimulate allograft rejection, G-CSF in the early phase of liver transplantation significantly reduced the incidence of rejection in 37 treated patients compared with 49 untreated (211[C]).

Urinary system   A transient *increase in serum creatinine concentration* has been reported in a 18-year-old man with non-Hodgkin's lymphoma (212[c]), whereas G-CSF therapy for ganciclovir-induced neutropenia has been suggested to contribute to reduced diuresis and a further acute rejection episode in a 38-year old man with a renal transplant (213[c]). However, no apparent increase in the risk of renal allograft rejection has so far been observed (214[C]).

Skin and appendages   Although rare, a wide spectrum of cutaneous disorders has been reported (177[R]). In two patients who experienced *localized skin lesions*, histological examination erroneously diagnosed the presence of malignant cells, which were subsequently recognized as inflammatory macrophages (215[c]).

Progressively generalized, but well-delimited *erythematous papules or plaques*, sometimes markedly indurated, were noted and subsequently disappeared after G-CSF discontinuation or dosage reduction in three patients (216[cr]). Skin histology showed mild spongiosis with exocytosis of lymphocytes, a perivascular infiltrate with neutrophils or mononuclear cells, and accumulation of large plump dermal macrophages. Several adhesion molecules were also expressed in the skin.

G-CSF induces or facilitate the occurrence of several types of neutrophilic dermatitis. Sweet's syndrome has been reported for the first time in a 5-year-old girl with glycogen storage disease type Ib, associated with chronic neutropenia (217[c]). Cutaneous lesions, fever, and the histological features of Sweet's syndrome were noted after 2 years of treatment with filgrastrim. Symptoms disappeared after dosage reduction from 60 to 50 µg/day, so that a spontaneously reversible case of Sweet's syndrome cannot be ruled out. An unusual case of Sweet's syndrome localized to an arm affected by lymphedema and reversible on withdrawal of G-CSF has also been reported in a 45-year-old woman (218[c]).

Short-term treatment with G-CSF for Felty's syndrome in a 59-year-old man was also associated with *leukocytoclastic vasculitis* (219[c]). Concern about the safety of G-CSF in patients with Felty's syndrome was raised in this report and others (220[c]). G-CSF has been implicated in a severe exacerbation of *acne* in a 17-year-old boy, with severe inflammatory cystic lesions after rechallenge (221[c]).

Special senses   Reversible bilateral acute *iritis* in a 44-year-old donor of peripheral blood progenitor cells was attributed to a 4-day course of G-CSF (222[c]), and the triggering of an autoimmune phenomenon was suggested.

Musculoskeletal system   Exacerbation of symptoms of rheumatoid arthritis have been reported in a patient with definite rheumatoid arthritis (223[c]) and in one with Felty's syndrome (220[c]), and an excessive rise in neutrophil count was suggested to account for the flare-up.

Immunological and hypersensitivity reactions   Although IgE-specific antibodies have not yet been detected, filgrastrim is undoubtedly associated with type I hypersensitivity, as shown by another report of a *generalized urticarial reaction* with *angio-edema*, and positive skin-prick and intradermal tests in a

19-year-old woman (224[c]) or the recurrence of angio-edema after rechallenge in a 44-year-old man (225[c]).

Tumor-inducing effects   In reviewing clinical trials with GM-CSF or G-CSF for acute leukemias, the risk of stimulating a leukemic clone has been considered to be probably very low (226[R]). In addition, in vivo leukemic resurgence during G-CSF administration was not correlated with in vitro blast response to this cytokine and occurred in patients who had fewer blast G-CSF receptors with a higher affinity, whether they had received G-CSF or not (227[R]).

The role of G-CSF in the occurrence of *myelodysplastic syndrome* or *acute myelogenous leukemia* with an abnormal karyotype (e.g. monosomy 7) has again been stressed in the context of four patients treated for severe congenital neutropenia or aplastic anemia (228[c])−(231[c]). In vitro proliferation of leukemic blasts showed sensitivity to G-CSF, but not to erythropoietin or IL-6, in a 20-year-old man who was also receiving erythropoietin, cyclosporin, anti-thymocyte globulin, and IL-6 (229[c]). In spite of unresolved problems, it was even stated that the clinical benefits of G-CSF outweigh the hazard of leukemogenesis, but careful monitoring of morphological bone-marrow changes and cytogenetic studies have also been recommended (232[r]).

High-dosage G-CSF in healthy donors to mobilize peripheral blood progenitors before allogeneic transplantation has been considered reasonably safe, with only mild to moderate *bone pain* and *headaches* (233[C]). Analysis of peripheral blood, bone-marrow, and karyotype showed no abnormalities in three volunteers who had received G-CSF 5 years before, to mobilize peripheral stem cells for allogeneic transplantation (234[C]).

Transient *leukoerythroblastosis* after G-CSF has been reported in a 48-year old man with acute myelomonocytic leukemia (235[c]).

Interactions   There was a 30% increase in *theophylline* clearance after G-CSF or GM-CSF in 22 patients undergoing bone-marrow transplantation (236[C]).

Interference with diagnostic routines   When blood glucose was analysed on the Ektachem

700 analyser in asymptomatic patients treated with G-CSF, artifactual *hypoglycemia* was observed and suggested to be the result of a high rate of glucose depletion by granulocytes in vitro, because of a lag time of 2.5 h between sampling and assay in the absence of an inhibitor of glycolysis (237[C]).

Granulocyte-macrophage colony-stimulating factor (GM-CSF; molgramostim, sargramostim)

Psychiatric   *Manic disorders* requiring antipsychotic drugs were attributed to a 1-month course of GM-CSF (molgramostim) for chronic neutropenia in a 41-year-old woman who had previously tolerated G-CSF therapy for 2 years (238[c]).

Endocrine, metabolic   A transient *rise in serum lactate dehydrogenase* (LDH) activity sometimes occurs in cancer patients receiving supportive treatment with GM-CSF or G-CSF. In a retrospective analysis of 52 courses of therapy in responding patients, serum LDH increased from 37 to 85% for leukocyte counts ranging from 5 to 15×10^9/l (239[C]). There was a linear relation between the leukocyte count during hematological recovery and increased serum LDH. The LDH became normal and the leukocyte count fell when the growth factors were withdrawn.

Skin and appendages   Severe cutaneous reactions localized to the injection site occurred in 11 patients with breast cancer and one patient with a malignant teratoma after three to four injections of GM-CSF (240[C]). Whereas lesions gradually improved within 2—3 weeks, subsequent rechallenge produced similar eruptions.

Miscellaneous   A possible GM-CSF-induced increase in relapse rate of autologous bone-marrow transplantation was retrospectively noted in a few children treated for acute myelogenous leukemia (241[C]).

Tumor-inducing effects   One concern raised by the use of GM-CSF in patients with myelodysplastic syndrome or related hematological disorders is the possibility of growth stimulation of blasts cells or accelerated occurrence of acute leukemia (242[R])(243[C]). In addition, experiments in human cells have shown expression of GM-CSF receptors by Langerhans' histiocytosis cells, suggesting that GM-CSF should not be used in this setting (244.

Interactions   A significant association between GM-CSF or G-CSF administration and the development of reversible, but severe atypical neuropathy has been found in patients undergoing *vincristine*-containing chemotherapy regimens (245[C]). Indeed, 11 of 28 patients with severe atypical neuropathy had received hemopoietic growth factors compared with only one of 26 patients who had not. There was evidence of a synergistic effect of both hemopoietic growth factors and cumulative vincristine dose.

In a phase III trial of *chemotherapy* plus *radiotherapy* for limited small-cell lung cancer, 107 patients randomized to receive GM-CSF had significantly more adverse effects, more deaths (due to pulmonary complications, sepsis, arterial thrombosis) and more non-hematological adverse effects (246[C]).

Macrophage colony-stimulating factor (M-CSF)

Exacerbation of *glomerular injury* has been reported in a 59-year-old man with acute myeloblastic leukemia and a previous history of mild proteinuria (247[c]). He experienced recurrent nephrotic syndrome with reversible glomerular hypercellularity and marked glomerular macrophage infiltration after the fourth and fifth courses of M-CSF, without further anomalies after chemotherapy alone.

MONOCLONAL ANTIBODIES
(SED-13, 1131; SEDA-17, 391, 433; SEDA-18, 342; SEDA-19, 353)

Orthoclone OKT3

The pharmacological properties and therapeutic use of OKT3 in prophylaxis of allograft rejection have recently been reviewed (248[r]). OKT3 prophylaxis was more effective than standard triple therapy in patients with renal and hepatic, but not cardiac, transplants. Efforts have also been made to reduce the risk of renal dysfunction (referred to as '*cytokine nephropathy*') and *intragraft thromboses*. In a retrospective comparison of 345 renal transplant patients, increased hydration, the use of diltiazem, and reduction of methylprednisolone dosage reduced the nephrotoxic effects of OKT 3 and decreased both delayed graft function and post-operative intragraft thrombosis (249[C]). Although pentoxifylline was proposed to prevent OKT3-induced *cytokine release syndrome*, this view was not supported by a double-blind placebo-controlled trial in 46 patients (250[C]). On the other hand, meperidine (pethidine) has been proposed as a valuable drug to mitigate symptoms of the cytokine release syndrome, but based on only three patients (251[c]).

Special senses   *Visual loss* is very rarely reported with OKT3. In one case, severe progressive visual disturbances occurred shortly after OKT3 administration in a 30-year-old woman with fully corrected myopia (252[c]). Fundoscopic examination and fluorescein angiography suggested an immune complex vasculitis and thrombosis, and there was no improvement in visual acuity after 2 months.

Miscellaneous   Although *influenza A pneumonitis* has rarely been reported and usually has a benign course in organ-transplant patients, a very severe case requiring mechanical ventilation has been described in a 51-year-old man after a 10-day course of OKT3 for heart transplant rejection (253[c]).

Immunological and hypersensitivity reactions   Very few cases of *anaphylactic reactions* with specific IgE antibodies have been reported after OKT3. Anti-OKT3 IgE antibodies were identified after 10—25 days of treatment in only six of 181 tested patients, and were undetectable within 3 months (254[C]). These antibodies were detected only in patients with high titers of anti-OKT3 IgG antibodies, particularly blocking antibodies, thus delineating a possibly predisposed population.

Tumor-inducing effects   Whether the increased risk of neoplasia associated with OKT3-based immunosuppression is due to the drug itself or to the overall degree of immunosuppression is still debated. The degree of immunosuppression undoubtedly plays a critical role, and it has been suggested that high-dose OKT3, increased treatment duration, multiple courses of treatment and early retreatment increases the risk of neoplasia (248[r]). Using data from postmarketing surveillance and the literature, the reporting rate of malignancies in OKT3-treated patients was 0.57%, but the method of analysis was subject to many biases, such as under-reporting (255[R]).

Other monoclonal antibodies

A large number of monoclonal antibodies directed against cytokine or cellular targets are being developed in an attempt to attack specific mechanisms involved in the pathophysiology of transplant rejection, sepsis, and inflammatory diseases. In 1995, at least 69 monoclonal antibodies were investigated in clinical trials (256[r]), and it is beyond the scope of this chapter to review all available studies, which usually included very few patients. The reader can refer to recent general reviews (257[R])—(259[R]).

For the prevention of acute rejection in renal or heart transplantation, promising results have been obtained with BT563, a monoclonal anti-interleukin-2 receptor antibody, without severe adverse effects ($n = 30$) (260[C]). In particular, the typical *cytokine release syndrome* was not reported in 31 patients treated with BT563, whereas the majority of 29 patients treated with OKT3 had symptoms of the syndrome (261[C]).

Among the anti-T cell therapy used in rheumatoid arthritis, a chimeric murine/human CD4 monoclonal antibody (cM-T412) produced only limited adverse effects, namely *flu-like symptoms* (fever, chills, nausea, headache) and transient *hypotension*, presumably related to increased serum IL-6 concentrations (262[R]) and dose-dependent in nature (263[C]).

Although the adverse effects of most monoclonal antibodies were very few or benign, the possibility of more severe or unusual complications should be carefully considered. For example, severe *migratory polyarthritis* with *fever*, an *urticarial rash*, and *renal involvement* (hematuria and proteinuria), responding to high-dose corticosteroids only, has been reported 6 days after the first dose of CAMPATH-1G, a rat antihuman monoclonal antibody reactive against CDw52 antigens, before marrow transplantation in a 25-year-old patient (264[c]). As this patient was a zoo ranger with previous exposure to rat proteins through frequent bites, an immunologically-mediated reaction was deemed possible. In addition, several patients developed *auto-antibodies*, such as antinuclear antibodies, anti-DNA, or anticardiolipin antibodies, in trials performed with cA2, a chimeric monoclonal anti-TNF-α antibody, or CDP-571, an engineered human anti-TNF-α antibody (258[r]). The significance of these findings is still unknown, as no patients developed clinical symptoms of systemic lupus erythematosus.

IMMUNOSUPPRESSIVE DRUGS
(SED-13, 1118; SEDA-19, 345)

Experience with immunosuppressive agents has been mostly acquired in the field of transplantation, but several agents are also used for autoimmune diseases. The ideal, safe, target-specific immunosuppressive agent has not yet been found (265[r]), and several new agents are under investigation (266[R]), (267[R]).

Malignancies and infectious diseases   Data on cancer incidence in immunosuppressed transplant patients are accumulating. Recent follow-up studies have confirmed that immunosuppression per se rather than a single agent is responsible for the increased risk of cancer (268[C]) – (272[C]); in these studies 2366 cancers occurred in 9917 patients.

Infection is the major complication in immunosuppressed patients. Involved pathogens and risk factors are numerous, as has been discussed in several recent reviews (273[R]) – (275[R]). Based on an analysis of medical and autopsy reports, the main causes of death in 102 renal transplant patients were infection (70%) and cardiovascular complications (276[C]). Infectious agents were bacteria (50%) and fungi (29%), of which candida and cryptococcus were the most frequent. Sites of infections were disseminated in 39% of cases or involved a single organ, such as the lung (24%) and the kidney (14%).

Azathioprine *(SED-13, 1120; SEDA-17, 525; SEDA-19, 346)*

Hematological   A follow-up study of 157 patients treated for Crohn's disease showed that the potential long-term risks (mainly hematological adverse effects and malignancies) of azathioprine or 6-mercaptopurine over 4 years outweighed the therapeutic benefit (277[C]).

Pure *erythroid aplasia* has been rarely described and exclusively as case reports in renal transplant patients (278[cr]).

Liver and pancreas   The spectrum of azathioprine-induced hepatotoxicity has been reviewed (279[R]). *Hepatitis* was found retrospectively in 21 (2%) of 1035 renal transplant patients and hepatitis B or C infections were suggested to increase the risk of azathioprine hepatotoxicity (280[C]). Complete histological reversal of azathioprine-induced veno-occlusive hepatitis was reported on a post-mortem examination performed on a 50-year-old man 11 months after azathioprine withdrawal (281[c]).

Pancreatitis has mostly been observed in patients with inflammatory bowel disease, as illustrated by three further cases (282[c]), (283[c]). In a 33-year-old man recurrence was observed within hours after 6-mercaptopurine administration and 2 h after an extremely low dose of azathioprine (282[c]). Acute lethal hemorrhagic pancreatitis has also been reported in a 16-year-old girl taking a multidrug regimen for systemic lupus erythematosus (284[c]).

Musculoskeletal system   *Rhabdomyolysis* as a feature of azathioprine hypersensitivity syndrome has been reported for the first time in a 76-year-old man with pemphigus foliaceus after 16 days of treatment (285[c]).

Hypersensitivity reactions   Multiorgan involvement is common in azathioprine hypersensitivity, but isolated *fever* and *rigors* are sometimes observed (286[c]). *Leukocytoclastic cutaneous vasculitis* is not a classical feature, but should also be considered as part of the diagnosis (287[c]), and it was found in four of

43 patients with rheumatoid arthritis who also developed fever and leukocytosis during treatment with azathioprine (288[C]). Azathioprine hypersensitivity associated with reversible *interstitial nephritis* has also been documented in four patients, including two renal transplant patients; excluding rejection might be difficult in such cases (289[c]).

Interactions Life-threatening hematological toxicity due to an interaction of azathioprine with *allopurinol* is still a problem leading to substantial costs (290[c]). Reduction in azathioprine dosage by at least two-thirds is recommended in patients taking allopurinol, but compliance with these guidelines was observed in only 58% of 24 patients with heart or lung transplants (291[C]). In addition, although adequate azathioprine dosage reduction reduces the incidence of cytopenias, the risk exists even after the first month of the combination. Close and prolonged hematological monitoring is therefore necessary whatever the dosage of azathioprine.

A possible synergistic effect of azathioprine and *isotretinoin* on the occurrence of curly hair has been suggested in three transplant patients treated for cyclosporin-induced acne (292[c]).

The addition of azathioprine to long-term well-tolerated *methotrexate* treatment in 43 patients with refractory rheumatoid arthritis resulted in hypersensitivity reactions in four patients (288[c]), and methotrexate was thought to have increased the risk of azathioprine toxicity.

Tumor-inducing effects The long-term risk of cancer in azathioprine-treated patients has been investigated in a case-control study of 1191 patients with multiple sclerosis (293[C]). The adjusted odds ratio was 1.3 for 1 month to 5 years of treatment, 2.0 for 5–10 years, and 4.0 for more than 10 years of treatment; however, none of these changes was significant. Nevertheless, a significant association was found for cumulative dosage higher than 600 g. Taken together, these results suggest a low risk of cancer in the population but a dose-dependent increase during long-term treatment. Soft-tissue carcinoma after treatment for 6 years for rheumatoid arthritis has been reported in an 85-year-old woman

(294[c]). Spontaneous regression was noted within 1 year after azathioprine withdrawal and no recurrence during 5 years of follow-up.

Azathioprine and 6-mercaptopurine may carry a slightly increased risk of malignancy in inflammatory bowel disease (295[R]), and a follow-up study of 157 patients treated for Crohn's disease has shown that the potential long-term risks (mainly hematological adverse effects and malignancies) of azathioprine or 6-mercaptopurine over 4 years outweighed the therapeutic benefit (277[C]).

Cyclophosphamide *(SED-13, 1122; SEDA-17, 518, 522, 524, 526; SEDA-19, 347)*

Endocrine, metabolic *Menstrual disorders* and *ovarian failure* after oral or intravenous pulses of cyclophosphamide for systemic lupus erythematosus have been analysed in two retrospective studies (296[C]), (297[C]). The first study in 30 prepubertal and peripubertal girls found oligomenorrhea in 20% of patients and sustained amenorrhea in 5%, but the underlying disease or corticosteroids may have also played a role (296[C]). The second study was a comparison of the rate of ovarian failure in 35 adult women treated with pulse cyclophosphamide with 20 women treated with azathioprine or 35 healthy age-matched controls (297[C]). Ovarian failure was reported in 54, 5.5, and 3.0% of premenopausal patients, whereas menopause occurred at mean ages of 38, 44, and 45 years, respectively. Of the women treated before the age of 40 years, 41% developed premature ovarian failure. Older age at the start of treatment, treatment duration, and the degree of bone-marrow suppression were significant risk factors for ovarian failure.

Liver *Hepatitis* is infrequently reported in children receiving cyclophosphamide. Completely reversible acute icteric hepatitis has been reported in a 5-year-old girl within 9 weeks of treatment for minimal change nephrotic syndrome (298[c]).

Skin and appendages Severe *Stevens-Johnson syndrome* has been reported in two patients, including one with positive rechallenge

(299[c]). A 55-year-old woman with Wegener's granulomatosis experienced cutaneous lesions after 48 days of cyclophosphamide. Estimated epidermal loss was 20% of body surface area. A widespread eruption and atypical target lesions reappeared 8 days after rechallenge 2 years later.

Miscellaneous   An increased risk of *infectious diseases* is a well-known complication of cyclophosphamide, but it is sometimes difficult to determine the relative contributions of the disease and the treatment. Disseminated cryptococcosis in a 33-year-old woman treated for lupus nephritis probably involved prolonged immunosuppression with high-dosage corticosteroids and cyclophosphamide (300[c]).

The additional role of cyclophosphamide in infections has been exemplified in a retrospective study of 100 patients with systemic lupus erythematosus, 45% of whom developed serious bacterial infections (58%), opportunistic infections (24%), or herpes zoster (18%), compared with 12% in those taking high-dosage steroids alone (301[c]). In addition, infections were more frequent in patients treated with sequential intravenous and oral cyclophosphamide (68%) than in those on intravenous (39%) or oral (40%) cyclophosphamide, leukopenia being an additional risk factor.

Tumor-inducing effects   A retrospective analysis of *bladder toxicity* in 145 patients followed for a mean 8.5 years, who had taken long-term oral cyclophosphamide for Wegener's granulomatosis showed that half of the patients had microscopic or gross non-glomerular hematuria, among whom 70% had macroscopic features compatible with cyclophosphamide-induced bladder injury on cystoscopy (302[c]). Overall, seven patients (5%) developed bladder cancer at 7 months to 15 years after the start of treatment, a 31-fold higher incidence than in the general population. Six patients had received a total cumulative dose higher than 100 g for a cumulative duration of treatment of more than 2.7 years. All had previously experienced at least one episode of non-glomerular hematuria, whereas none of the patients who did not experience hematuria during or after treatment developed bladder cancer. Hematuria was the only significant risk factor for bladder cancer, suggesting the need for regular monitoring with cystoscopy in cyclophosphamide-treated patients.

Cyclosporin *(SED-13, 1123; SEDA-17, 520, 522, 523; SEDA-19, 348)*

Cyclosporin is being increasingly used in non-transplant patients. In early active rheumatoid arthritis, low-dosage cyclosporin (3 mg/kg/day; $n = 167$) was more effective than conventional antirheumatic drugs ($n = 173$) and associated with less premature withdrawal because of adverse effects (303[c]). *Hypertension* and *worsening of renal function* were the most frequent, but were easily manageable with dosage reduction and antihypertensive therapy. In contrast, the increased incidence of adverse effects during long-term cyclosporin treatment in 122 patients with severe psoriasis treated for 3—76 months was deemed to be unacceptable, since 14 and 41% had to discontinue treatment after 1 and 4 years because of adverse effects (304[c]). However, in another study of 217 patients treated for 6—30 months conflicting views were expressed (305[c]).

Cardiovascular   Cardiovascular disease is a major cause of morbidity and mortality after renal transplantation, and risk factors are numerous (306[c]). Higher whole blood cyclosporin concentrations were found during the preceding months in patients who experienced *thromboembolic complications*, compared with patients who had no cardiovascular complications; thromboembolic complications were also more common in patients who received triple therapy (8% of 126) compared with those who received cyclosporin plus prednisone (20% of 118) (307[c]).

Nervous system   Based on a re-analysis of 138 reported cases, cyclosporin-associated neurotoxicity has been comprehensively reviewed (308[R]). The brain, cerebellum, spinal cord, and peripheral nerves can be affected. The main risk factors include supratherapeutic whole-blood concentrations, drug interactions, and hypocholesterolemia. Cyclosporin-induced vasculopathy, with endothelial injury and disturbance of the blood—brain barrier, is the postulated mechanism. In liver transplantation, neurotoxicity has been reported to occur in 46 (12%) of 386 cyclosporin-treated patients, within 2 weeks in 85% (309[C]). All the patients had *tremors* and *restlessness*, 20 had *acute psychotic episodes* associated with inappropriate crying and laughing, paranoid behavior, or visual hallucinations, and eight had generalized *tonic-clonic seizures*; *speech abnormalities* and *cortical blindness* were found in only three and two patients, respectively. Symptoms usually reversed within 1—3 days after temporary withdrawal and dosage reduction, whereas whole blood cyclosporin concentrations were in the target range in 40% of the patients. Three patients later tolerated tacrolimus. In contrast to other reports, white matter abnormalities were not found on magnetic resonance imaging, and this was attributed to the early recognition and management of neurotoxicity.

Reports of other forms of cyclosporin neurotoxicity continue to appear, including cases of *leukoencephalopathy* with cerebellar hemorrhage and progressive multifocal leukoencephalopathy at the time of autopsy (310[c]), isolated *cerebellar syndrome* (311[c]), *acute cerebellar edema* with progressive brain-stem compression requiring craniectomy (312[c]), *cortical blindness* (313[cr]), (314[c]) with sudden and early occurrence of permanent blindness (not previously described) (315[c]), slowly reversible *speech disorders* associated with mutism (316[C]), and features of *parkinsonism* (317[c]). The identification of transient cerebral perfusion abnormalities on single-photon emission computed tomography of the brain has been suggested to be a reliable indicator of cyclosporin neurotoxicity (318[c]).

Endocrine, metabolic   The role of cyclosporin in *hyperlipidemia* is controversial. Two independent groups have been unable to find an association between hyperlipidemia and cyclosporin in a total of 647 renal transplant patients (319[C]), (320[C]); hyperlipidemia was influenced by impaired renal function, diuretics and β-blockers, increased age, and female sex.

The contributory role of cyclosporin in homocysteinemia, another recognized risk factor for the development of atherosclerosis, has also been studied in renal transplant patients (321[C]). Cyclosporin-treated patients ($n = 67$) had significantly higher plasma homocysteine concentrations than both transplant patients not treated with cyclosporin ($n = 17$) and non-transplant patients with renal insufficiency ($n = 53$). Plasma homocysteine concentrations were also higher in renal transplant patients with a history of atherosclerotic disease.

Mineral and fluid balance   *Hyperkalemia* has been thoroughly investigated in 11 of 24 children with renal transplants taking cyclosporin (322[C]). Possible mechanisms included inhibition of distal nephron potassium secretion, a reduction in distal tubular flow rate, and cellular potassium leak into the extracellular fluid.

Hematological   Cyclosporin-induced *hypercoagulability* with increased plasma fibrinogen, prothrombin fragment 1 + 2, and von Willebrand factor antigen has been suggested in 10 patients with aplastic anemia who were receiving cyclosporin compared with 11 who were not and 38 healthy controls (323[C]).

Liver   Cyclosporin-related hepatotoxicity in transplant patients, namely *cholestasis* with conjugated hyperbilirubinemia, has been extensively reviewed (279[R]).

It has recently been found that the presence of underlying chronic viral hepatitis increased the severity of cyclosporin-induced cholestasis (324[C]). There are very few data in the non-transplant setting, but a synergistic effect of total parenteral nutrition and cyclosporin in the incidence of hepatotoxicity in patients treated for acute ulcerative colitis has been suggested (325[C]).

Urinary system   Very comprehensive reviews have recently been published on chronic cyclosporin nephrotoxicity (326[R])—(328[R]). New data have largely confirmed or have not added significantly to what was already known. It is as yet unclear to what extent long-term cyclosporin contributes to *progressive renal failure*, and what is the effective dosage that does not lead to *renal fibrosis*. In renal transplant patients, prospective large-scale studies of renal structure and function, to exclude chronic graft rejection, are still lacking. In one study there was no clear correlation between histological renal findings and various measures of renal function in 19 patients (329[C]). The results of a randomized controlled study in 128 patients (330[C]), suggesting that conversion from cyclosporin to azathioprine 3 months after transplantation led to better renal function, have been strongly debated.

There were histological features of cyclosporin nephrotoxicity in 8% of patients with rheumatoid arthritis treated for a mean duration of 19 months, and no significant progression of lesions was noted in the 14 patients who underwent a second biopsy after a mean of 39 months of cyclosporin therapy (331[C]). Nephropathy was not observed in the 22 rheumatoid patients treated with the currently recommended starting dose and maximum daily dose. Similar reassuring results have been obtained by others (332[C]).

Thrombotic microangiopathy/hemolytic-uremic syndrome, attributed to cyclosporin injury to the vascular endothelium, is a possible cause of acute graft loss in renal transplant patients. In a case-controlled retrospective series of 13 kidney or kidney/pancreas transplant patients who developed thrombotic microangiopathy after cyclosporin (12 patients) or tacrolimus (one patient), reintroduction of cyclosporin or conversion to tacrolimus was successfully used in 92% of patients after the addition of isradipine, aspirin, and pentoxifylline (333[C]). In addition, creatinine clearance during a 2-year follow-up period was similar to that of a control group.

Skin and appendages   *Distichiasis* (the presence of accessory eyelashes), resulting in ocular irritation, has been reported in a 54-year-old man with cyclosporin-associated trichomegaly (334[c]).

Most cases of acne in transplant patients are attributed to steroid treatment, and cyclosporin is very rarely involved. However, resolution of severe isotretinoin-resistant *nodulocystic lesions of acne conglobata* was obtained only after cyclosporin withdrawal in a 22-year-old man (335[c]).

Teeth and gums   The clinical, ultrastructural and histochemical features of *gingival overgrowth*, a frequent adverse effect of cyclo-

sporin, continue to be investigated (336[C]), (337[C]). Cyclosporin-induced inhibition of prostaglandin I_2 synthesis has been suggested as the possible mechanism (338[C]).

Musculoskeletal system   *Bone pain*, affecting mostly the lower limbs, and without evidence of avascular necrosis, is increasingly reported in transplant patients, but only in those taking cyclosporin (339[C]). In addition, acute osteo-articular pains, reversible on cyclosporin withdrawal, have also been described in a 32-year-old woman with acute ulcerative colitis (340[c]).

The possible contribution of cyclosporin to bone loss and subsequent *osteoporosis* in transplant patients is still debated. In addition to experimental findings, the results of a prospective assessment of bone mineral density and biochemical parameters in 24 heart transplant patients, suggested that cyclosporin increases bone turnover as well (341[C]).

Overdosage   An unexpectedly high cyclosporin serum concentration (6640 ng/ml) and half-life (55 h) have been reported in a 31-year-old man after an intravenous infusion of high-dose cyclosporin (21 mg/kg for 60 h) for stage 4B Hodgkin's lymphoma (342[c]). He subsequently developed acute renal tubular necrosis and died.

Interactions   Many studies or case reports accumulate each year on cyclosporin drug interactions and have been recently comprehensively reviewed (343[R]).

Although one previous study suggested that *amlodipine* did not interact with cyclosporin, a longer duration of treatment (5 mg/day for 7 weeks in 11 patients) produced an average 40% increase in cyclosporin blood concentrations (344[C]).

An increase in cyclosporin concentration requiring a 20% reduction in dosage has been already reported in two patients taking *glipizide*, and a 57% increase in steady-state plasma cyclosporin concentrations has now been reported in six patients taking *glibenclamide* (345[CR]).

Increased blood cyclosporin concentrations have been reported once during treatment with *nefazodone* (346[c]) or *fluoxetine* (347[c]). However, results in 13 transplant patients suggested that fluoxetine does not affect cyclosporin concentrations or renal function (348[C]).

In contrast to a previous case report, there were no changes in cyclosporin concentrations in six patients who took *azithromycin* (349[c]). Several investigators have even proposed azithromycin to improve cyclosporin-induced gingival hyperplasia (350[C]). Norfloxacin with cyclosporin has been proposed to be a safe combination (344[R]), but other clinical and experimental data have recently suggested that norfloxacin inhibited cyclosporin metabolism (351[C]).

Co-administration of Liqui-E, a water-soluble *vitamin E* formulation, increased oral cyclosporin absorption and produced significant lowering in cyclosporin dosage requirements, with a 26% reduction in drug costs in 26 transplant patients (352[C]).

Acute myopathy could well have resulted from enhanced muscular toxicity when a combination of cyclosporin with *pyrazinamide* was given to a 39-year-old woman with a renal transplant (353[c]).

Mizoribine

Mizoribine is considered a valuable and safe alternative to azathioprine, with a reduced incidence of leukopenia (354[c]).

Mycophenolate mofetil *(SED-13, 1130; SEDA-19, 351)*

The pharmacology and plasma concentration monitoring of mycophenolate mofetil have been reviewed (355[R]), (356[R]). The final results from the third pivotal trial of mycophenolate mofetil (2 or 3 g, $n = 173$ and 164, respectively) versus azathioprine ($n = 166$) to prevent rejection in renal transplant patients showed a partially dose-dependent increase in the incidence of *gastrointestinal disorders*, *leukopenia*, and tissue invasive *cytomegalovirus infection*, compared with azathioprine (357[C]). Whether mycophenolate mofetil is associated with a slightly increased incidence of *lymphoproliferative disorders* is as yet unresolved. Mycophenolate was putatively involved in the occurrence of *fever, exudative pharyngitis, adynamic ileus,* and *myocardial dysfunction* in a 14-year old renal transplant

patient; all symptoms resolved on withdrawal (358[c]).

Rapamycin (sirolimus)

Rapamycin is an immunosuppressant structurally related to tacrolimus, but with a different mechanism of action. No serious adverse effects have been noted in preliminary trials, with only one case of *thrombocytopenia* probably related to the drug (359[c]) and significant reversible reductions in platelet and white blood cell counts (360[c]).

Tacrolimus *(SED-13, 1130; SEDA-19, 351)*

Despite structural differences, cyclosporin and tacrolimus share a very similar spectrum of adverse effects. Based on a consensus conference, recommendations on tacrolimus monitoring have been proposed (361[R]). Although the steroid-sparing effect of tacrolimus is deemed to be greater than that of cyclosporin, evidence for an improved toxicity profile is puzzling.

In a retrospective and uncontrolled review of 49 children with heart transplants who received tacrolimus as the primary agent, the most common long-term adverse effects (mean duration of follow-up 29 months) were *anemia* (61%), *renal toxicity* (37%), *hyperkalemia* (53%), *eosinophilia and allergic symptoms* (32%), and *gastrointestinal disorders* (24%) (362[C]). In sharp contrast to cyclosporin, gingival hyperplasia, hirsutism, and coarsening of facial features have not been observed (362[C]), (363[C]).

Cardiovascular Whilst no significant differences on mean arterial blood pressure were found between tacrolimus and cyclosporin-treated renal transplant patients (15 of each), antihypertensive drugs were less frequently used in tacrolimus-treated patients (364[C]). Other investigators have suggested that the prevalence of hypertension is lower in tacrolimus-treated heart transplant patients (363[C]). Severe *anasarca* and *symmetrical cardiomyopathy* with successful replacement with cyclosporin have been described (365[c]).

Nervous system A possibly higher incidence

of neurotoxic effects has been reported in 92 patients treated with tacrolimus (366[C]).

Leukoencephalopathy within 3—12 months of treatment has been described in three liver transplant patients, aged 34—51 years (367[C]). All had severe headaches, vomiting, and generalized seizures, and neuroimaging showed abnormalities in the white matter, predominantly in the parietal and occipital lobes. Cerebral biopsy showed non-specific demyelination in one patient. The clinical, radiological, and neuropathological examinations were thus similar to those reported with cyclosporin. Very similar acute symptoms together with cortical blindness and diffuse magnetic resonance imaging abnormalities have been reported in three other patients out of 50 taking tacrolimus for the prevention of graft-versus-host disease after bone-marrow transplantation (368[C]). Hemorrhage on neuroimaging were also found. Further cyclosporin administration is sometimes well-tolerated.

Although neurological symptoms are usually reversible, persistent *dysarthria* and *speech apraxia* have been described in a 46-year-old woman 8 months after their occurrence and despite tacrolimus withdrawal (369[c]).

Endocrine, metabolic Tacrolimus has been associated with a higher prevalence of *hyperglycemia* and *insulin-dependent diabetes mellitus* (10—20% in adults and only 2% in children) (362[e]), (366[C]), (370[e]), (371[e]). However, diabetes mellitus was observed in three of 19 patients aged 11—16 years, although only one required prolonged insulin maintenance (370[C]). Detection of at-risk patients has been considered by using the 75 g oral glucose tolerance test in 18 renal transplant patients (372[C]). There was a possible correlation between impaired glucose tolerance or a diabetic pattern before transplantation and the later development of post-transplant diabetes mellitus. In contrast, only one of 154 pancreas transplant patients required long-term insulin maintenance (373[C]), and complete reversal of severe tacrolimus-induced diabetes was usually observed after conversion to cyclosporin (371[C]), (373[C]).

Hematogical *Hemolytic-uremic syndrome* and *thrombotic thrombocytopenic purpura* have occasionally been described, and the possible contribution of tacrolimus in the early development of thrombotic thrombocytopenic purpura during prophylaxis for graft-versus-host disease after bone-marrow transplantation (374[c]) or in the occurrence of hemolytic-uremic syndrome in the post solid-organ transplantation period (375[c]) has been substantiated in four additional patients. The first two improved after tacrolimus withdrawal and repetitive plasma exchanges, but one died from acute graft-versus-host disease (374[c]). Another patient had recurrence of hemolytic anemia after tacrolimus rechallenge, whereas the fourth patient was later successfully treated with cyclosporin (375[c]), confirming that cross-reactions between the two drugs are not obligatory.

Regressive pure *erythroid aplasia* has been reported in a 34-year-old man during treatment for renal transplantation, with no further recurrence after cyclosporin administration (376[c]).

Urinary system Very similar clinical and morphological patterns of *nephrotoxicity* are observed with tacrolimus and cyclosporin. However, 11 kidney/pancreas transplant patients who had severe cyclosporin nephrotoxicity or persistent rejection with documented arteriolopathy on renal histology were all successfully switched to tacrolimus with resulting improvement or stabilization of renal function and no deleterious effect on glucose metabolism (377[C]).

Miscellaneous In additional studies there have been no significant differences in the incidences of *major infections* between tacrolimus and cyclosporin (363[C]), (366[C]). However, an unexplained changing pattern of microbial causes of pneumonia has been noted in liver transplant patients taking tacrolimus, with *Legionella* and fungal pneumonia (*Aspergillus fumigatus* and *Cryptococcus neoformans*) as the cause in 16 and 37% of episodes of pneumonia respectively, and all direct deaths due to pneumonia involved fungal infection (378[C]).

Tumor-inducing effects The incidence of post-transplant *lymphomas* appeared to be equal between cyclosporin and tacrolimus, but a possible increased risk of post-transplant lymphomas, all originating in the large or small bowel, has been suggested in pancreas transplant patients (373[C]).

Interactions Most of the suspected tacrolimus interactions are derived from in vitro studies or extrapolated from cyclosporin. Currently known interactions have been reviewed (SED-13, 1131). In contrast to the oral route of administration, intravenous *fluconazole* caused a non-significant increase in steady-state concentrations of intravenous tacrolimus in 15 patients (379[C]).

IMMUNOENHANCING DRUGS

Levamisole *(SED-13, 1135; SEDA-17, 434; SEDA-18, 316; SEDA-19, 354)*

In a group of 929 patients with colorectal cancer, followed for 5 years, the effect of combination treatment with levamisole and fluorouracil (304 patients) was compared with levamisole alone (315 patients) or observation only (310 patients) (380[C]). The combination treatment consisted of fluorouracil (450 µg/m^2 i.v.) weekly for 48 weeks and levamisole (50 mg orally tds) for 3 days repeated every 2 weeks for 1 year. The combination treatment reduced the recurrence rate of Dukes C colorectal cancer by 40% and mortality by 33% at 5 years compared with observation only or levamisole alone. Reactions to levamisole alone were generally mild and infrequent, and

included *nausea, dermatitis, fatigue, arthralgia,* and *taste change.* Mild fully reversible *bone-marrow depression* occurred in 90% of patients. These adverse effects were more fully described in an earlier report by the same authors (381[C]). Toxicity in the patients treated with the combination of levamisole and fluorouracil resembled the toxicity caused by fluorouracil alone and consisted of *nausea,* infrequent *vomiting, stomatitis, diarrhea, dermatitis, fatigue,* and mild *alopecia.* There was a mild *disturbance in liver function tests* in 40% of patients. Half of the patients had mild *bone-marrow depression,* usually limited to mild leukopenia. There was one death due to profound leukopenia and sepsis.

In a further study of the use of levamisole and fluorouracil in Dukes C colorectal cancer levamisole added substantial granulocyte toxicity to treatment with fluorouracil or levamisole alone; 41 patients were treated with fluorouracil alone and 50 with levamisole and fluorouracil in combination (382[C]). There was *severe granulocyte toxicity* in 3.4 and 17% of patients, respectively. Although leukopenia is by far the most frequent hematological adverse effect after treatment with levamisole, other hematological toxic effects can occur, even several years after the start of treatment (383[C]). *Thrombocytopenia* occurred two years after continuous treatment with levamisole in a dose of 2.5 mg/kg on two consecutive days per week for melanoma. The thrombocyte count normalized after the discontinuation of levamisole but reappeared on rechallenge. There was a rapid permanent normalization after the withdrawal of levamisole.

REFERENCES

1. Niederau C, Heintges T, Lange S, H ussinger D. Treatment of chronic hepatitis C with α-interferon: an analysis of the literature. Hepato-Gastroenterology 1996;43:1544—6.
2. Saracco G, Rizzetto M. A practical guide to the use of interferons in the management of hepatitis virus infections. Drugs 1997;53:74—85.
3. Terrault N, Wright T. Interferon and hepatitis C. New Engl J Med 1995;332:1509—11.
4. Fattovich G, Giustina G, Favarato S, Ruol A. A survey of adverse events in 11,241 patients with chronic viral hepatitis treated with α interferon. J Hepatol 1996;24:38—47.
5. De Sanctis GM, D'Errico DAF, Leonetti G,

Di Giulio A, Bianchi P, Goldoni E, Barbacini IG, Errera G, Chircu LV. Occurrence of major side effects in patients with chronic viral liver disease treated with interferons. Mediter J Infect Parasit Dis 1995;10:225—30.
6. Okanoue T, Sakamoto S, Itoh Y, Minami M, Yasui K, Sakamoto M, Nishioji K, Katagishi T, Nakagawa Y, Tada H, Sawa Y, Mizuno M, Kagawa K, Kashila K. Side effects of high-dose interferon therapy for chronic hepatitis C. J Hepatol 1996;25:283—91.
7. Camma C, Almasio P, Craxi A. Interferon as treatment for acute hepatitis C. A meta-analysis. Dig Dis Sciences 1996;41:1248—55.

8. Teragawa H, Hondo T, Amano H, Watanabe Y, Ohe H, Hattori N, Watanabe Y, Hino F, Ohbayashi M. Cardiogenic shock following recombinant α-2b interferon therapy for chronic hepatitis C: a case report. Jpn Heart J 1996;37:137—42.

9. Giraud O, Thomas F, Jupas JJ, Ravaud Y. Arrêt cardio-respiratoire et traitement par interféron α-2a. Réanim Urgences 1995;4:645.

10. Mateo R, Jethmalani S, Angus DC, Gorcsan J III, Uretsky B, Fung J. Interferon-associated left ventricular dysfunction in a liver transplant recipient. Dig Dis Sci 1996;41:1500—3.

11. Fava S, Luoni M, Stioui S. Pericarditis during interferon-α therapy in chronic myelogenous leukemia. Haematologica 1996;81:484.

12. Bachmeyer C, Farge D, Gluckman E, Miclea JM, Aractingi S. Raynaud's phenomenon and digital necrosis induced by interferon-α. Br J Dermatol 1996;135:481—3.

13. Creutzig A, Freund M. Severe Raynaud's syndrome associated with interferon therapy: a case history. Angiology 1996;47:185—7.

14. Mineur P. Digital necrosis associated with chronic myeloid leukaemia: a rare paraneoplastic phenomenon or toxicity or recombinant interferon? Acta Clin Belg 1996;51:61—2.

15. Creutzig A, Caspary L, Freund M. The Raynaud phenomenon and interferon therapy. Ann Intern Med 1996;125:423.

16. Tanaka H, Yamakado T, Emi Y, Nabeshima K, Itoh S, Nakano T. Interferon-induced coronary-vasospasm: a case history. Angiology 1995; 46:1139—43.

17. Lustman F, Salhadin A, Nouwynck C, Hanson B. Pneumonie interstitielle à la suite d'un traitement par interféron-α. Presse Med 1995;24:1910.

18. Nouri K, Valor R, Rodriguez M, Kerdel FA. Interferon α-induced interstitial pneumonitis in a patient with cutaneous T-cell lymphoma. J Am Acad Dermatol 1996;35.269—70.

19. Mase G, Zorzon M, Biasutti E, Vitrani B, Cazzato G, Urban F, Frezza M. Development of myasthenia gravis during interferon-α treatment for anti-HCV positive chronic hepatitis. J Neurol Neurosurg Psychiatry 1996;60:348—9.

20. Piccolo G, Franciotta D, Versino M, Alfonsi E, Lombardi M, Poma G. Myasthenia gravis in a patient with chronic active hepatitis C during interferon-α treatment. J Neurol Neurosurg Psychiatry 1996;60:348.

21. Lensch E, Faust J, Nix WA, Wandel E. Myasthenia gravis after interferon-α treatment. Muscle Nerve 1996;July:927—8.

22. Rohde D, Sliwka U, Schweizer K, Jakse G. Oculo-bulbar myasthenia gravis induced by cytokine treatment of a patient with metastasized renal cell carcinoma. Eur J Clin Pharmacol 1996;50:471—3.

23. Shakil AO, Di Bisceglie AM, Hoofnagle JH. Seizures during α interferon therapy. J Hepatol 1996;24:48—51.

24. Neau JP, Guilhot F, Boinot C, Dumas P, Tantot AM, Gil R. Development of chorea with lupus anticoagulant after interferon therapy. Eur Neurol 1996;36:235—6.

25. La Civita L, Zignego AL, Lombardini F, Monti M, Longombardo G, Pasero G, Ferri C. Exacerbation of peripheral neuropathy during α-interferon therapy in a patient with mixed cryoglobulinemia and hepatitis B virus infection. J Rheumatol 1996;23:1641—3.

26. Maeda M, Ohkoshi N, Hisahara S, Mizusawa H, Shoji S. Mononeuropathy multiplex in a patient receiving interferon α therapy for chronic hepatitis C. Rinsho Shinkeigaku 1995;35:1048—50.

27. Malaguarnera M, Pistone G, Trovato BA, Panebianco P, Rampello L. Impaired thermal and tactile sensitivity during interferon-α treatment. Clin Drug Invest 1996;12:271—3.

28. Pavol MA, Meyers CA, Rexer JL, Valentine AD, Mattis PJ, Talpaz M. Pattern of neurobehavorial deficits associated with interferon α therapy for leukemia. Neurology 1995;45:947—50.

29. Valentine AD, Meyers CA, Talpaz M. Treatment of neurotoxic side effects of interferon-α with naltrexone. Cancer Invest 1995;13:561—6.

30. Mapou RL, Law WA, Wagner K, Malone JL, Skillman DR. Neuropsychological effects of interferon α-N3 treatment in asymptomatic human immunodeficiency virus-1-infected individuals. J Neuropsychiatry Clin Neurosci 1996;8:74—81.

31. Rifflet H, Vuillemin E, Oberti F, Laine P, Calès P. Interferon et suicide au cours des hépatites virales chroniques. Gastroenterol Clin Biol 1996;20:68.

32. Bourat L, Larrey D, Michel H. Tentative de suicide lors du traitement d'une hépatite chronique virale C par interféron. A propos de deux cas. Gastroenterol Clin Biol 1995;19:1063.

33. Carella C, Amato G, Biondi B, Rotondi M, Morisco F, Tuccillo C, Chiuchiolo N, Signoriello G, Caporaso N, Lombardi G. Longitudinal study of antibodies against thyroid in patients undergoing interferon-α therapy for HCV chronic hepatitis. Horm Res 1995;44:110—4.

34. Murakami T, Masumoto T, Michitaka K, Horiike N, Hino H, Okada S, Kitai K, Onji M. Prediction of interferon-α-induced thyroid dysfunction in patients with chronic hepatitis C. J Gastroenterol Hepatol 1995;10:528—31.

35. Minelli R, Girasole G, Pedrazzoni M, Giuliani N, Schianchi C, Giuberti T, Braverman LE, Salvi M, Roti E. Lack of increased serum interleukin-6 and soluble IL-6 receptor concentrations in patients with thyroid diseases following recombinant human interferon α therapy. J Invest Med 1996;44:370—4.

36. Preziati D, La Rosa L, Covini G, Marcelli R, Rescalli S, Persani L, Del Ninno E, Meroni PL, Colombo M, Beck-Peccoz P. Autoimmunity and thyroid function in patients with chronic active hepatitis treated with recombinant interferon α-2a. Eur J Endocrinol 1995;132:587—93.

37. Marazuela M, Garcia-Buey L, Gonzalez-

Fernandez B, Garcia-Monzon C, Arranz A, Borque MJ, Moreno-Otero R. Thyroid autoimmune disorders in patients with chronic hepatitis C before and during interferon-α therapy. Clin Endocrinol 1996;44:635—42.

38. Abdul-Jabbar MA, Ehrlich RM, Mann N, Roberts EA. Transient hypothyroidism in a child treated with α-interferon for chronic hepatitis B infection. Clin Pediatr 1995;34:663—5.

39. Chen FQ, Okamura K, Sato K, Kuroda T, Mizokami T, Fujikawa M, Tsuji H, Okamura S, Fujishima M. Reversible primary hypothyroidism with blocking or stimulating type TSH binding inhibitor immunoglobulin following recombinant interferon-α therapy in patients with pre-existing thyroid disorders. Clin Endocrinol 1996;45:207—14.

40. Uchida K, Matsui A, Nakano S, Kigoshi T, Morimoto S. Painless thyroiditis occuring during long-term treatment with interferon-α in a patient with chronic active hepatitis C. South Med J 1996;89:81—3.

41. Sato K, Miyakawa M, Demura H. Reversible, extremely severe hypothyroidism in a patient with chronic hepatitis C treated with interferon-α. Thyroid 1996;6:249—52.

42. Wada M, Hiraizumi W, Fujimoto M, Kinugasa A, Shintani S, Sawada K, Shimoyama T, Suehiro M, Fukuchi M. Occurence of Graves' disease during retreatment with interferon-α2a for chronic hepatitis C. Intern Med 1995;34:1097—100.

43. Del Monte P, Bernasconi D, De Conca V, Randazzo M, Meozzi M, Badaracco B, Mesiti S, Marugo M. Endocrine evaluation in patients treated with interferon-α for chronic hepatitis C. Horm Res 1995;44:105—9.

44. Mathieu E, Fain O, Sitbon M, Thomas M. Diabète auto-immun après traitement par interféron —. Presse Med 1995;24:238.

45. Shiba T, Morino Y, Tagawa K, Fujino H, Unuma T. Onset of diabetes with high titer anti-GAD antibody after IFN therapy for chronic hepatitis. Diabetes Res Clin Pract 1995;30:237—41.

46. Chédin P, Cahen-Varsaux J, Boyer N. Non-insulin-dependant diabetes mellitus developing during interferon-α therapy for chronic hepatitis C. Ann Intern Med 1996;125:521.

47. Murakami M, Iriuchijima T, Mori M. Diabetes mellitus and interferon-α therapy. Ann Intern Med 1995;123:318.

48. Campbell S, McLaren EH, Danesh BJ. Rapidly reversible increase in insulin requirement with interferon. Br Med J 1996;313:92.

49. Whitehead RP, Hauschild A, Christophers E, Figlin R. Diabetes mellitus in cancer patients treated with combination interleukin 2 and α-interferon. Cancer Biother 1995;10:45—51.

50. Huang X, Yuan J, Goddard A, Foulis A, James RFL, Lernmark A, Pujol-Borrell R, Rabinovitch A, Somoza N, Stewart TA. Interferon expression in the pancreases of patients with type II diabetes. Diabetes 1995;44:658—64.

51. Fraser GM, Harman I, Meller N, Niv Y, Porath A. Diabetes mellitus is associated with chronic hepatitis C but not chronic hepatitis B infection. Isr J Med Sci 1996;32:526—30.

52. Di Cesare E, Previti M, Russo F, Brancatelli S, Ingemi MC, Scoglio R, Mazzu N, Cucinotta D, Raimondo G. Interferon-α therapy may induce insulin autoantibody development in patients with chronic viral hepatitis. Dig Dis Sci 1996;41:1672—7.

53. Malaguarnera M, Giugno I, Ruello P, Pistone G, Restuccia S, Trovato BA. Effect of interferon on blood lipids. Clin Drug Invest 1996;11:43—8.

54. Jaubert D, Hadjali Y, De Jaureguiberry JP. Hypertriglycéridémies sous interféron α. Presse Med 1996;25:820.

55. Penarrubia MJ, Steegmann JL, Lavilla E, Casado F, Requena MJ, Pico M, Arranz R, Fernandez-Ranada JM. Hypertriglyceridemia may be severe in CML patients treated with interferon-α. Am J Hematol 1995;49:240—1.

56. Nagamine T, Ohtuka T, Takehara K, Arai T, Takagi H, Mori M. Thrombocytopenia associated with hepatitis C viral infection. J Hepatol 1996;24:135—40.

57. Pawlotsky JM, Bouvier M, Fromont P, Deforges L, Duval J, Dhumeaux D, Bierling P. Hepatitis C virus infection and autoimmune thrombocytopenic purpura. J Hepatol 1995;23:635—9.

58. Khan HA, Khawaja FI, Mahrous ARS. Life-threatening severe immune thrombocytopenia after α-interferon therapy for chronic hepatitis C infection. Am J Gastroenterol 1996;91:821—2.

59. Bacq Y, Sapey T, Gruel Y, Fimbel B, Degenne D, Barin F, Metman EH. Exacerbation d'un purpura thrombopénique auto-immun au cours du traitement par l'interféron chez une femme atteinte d'une hépatite chronique virale C. Gastroenterol Clin Biol 1996;20:303—6.

60. Maïga MY, Oberti F, Foussard C, Calès P. Purpura thrombopénique auto-immun après traitement d'une hépatite chronique virale C par l'interféron. Gastroenterol Clin Biol 1995;19:739—40.

61. Tappero G, Guerrasio A, Gallo M, Negro F, Hadengue A, Angeli A. Interferon-induced 'lupoid' thrombocytopenia in chronic hepatitis C. J Hepatol 1996;24:124.

62. Tappero G, Negro F, Farina M, Gallo M, Angelo A, Hadengue A. Safe switch to β-interferon treatment of chronic hepatitis C after α-interferon-induced autoimmune thrombocytopenia. J Hepatol 1996;24.

63. Andriani A, Bibas M, Callea V, Derenzo A, Chiurazzi F, Marceno R, Musto P. Autoimmune hemolytic anemia during α interferon treatment in nine patients with hematological diseases. Haematologica 1996;81:258—60.

64. Sacchi S, Kantarjian H, O'Brien S, Cohen PR, Pierce S, Talpaz M. Immune-mediated and unusual complications during interferon α therapy in chronic myelogenous leukemia. J Clin Oncol 1995;13:2401—7.

65. Takase K, Nakano T, Hamada M, Shiraki K,

Oohashi Y, Kihira T, Tameda Y. Hemolytic anemia provoked by recombinant α-interferon. J Gastroenterol 1995;30:795—7.

66. Higashi Y, Sakai K, Tada S, Miyase S, Nakamura T. Agranulocytosis induced by interferon-α therapy for chronic hepatitis C. J Gastroenterol Hepatol 1996;11:1012—5.

67. Mauserbunschoten EP, Damen M, Reesink HW, Roosendaal G, Chamuleau RAFM, van den Berg HM. Formation of antibodies to factor VII in patients with hemophilia A who are treated with interferon for chronic hepatitis C. Ann Intern Med 1996;125:297—9.

68. Matsuda J, Saitoh N, Gotoh M, Gohchi K, Tsukamoto M, Syoji S, Miyake K, Yamanaka M. High prevalence of anti-phospholipid antibodies and anti-thyroglobulin antibody in patients with hepatitis C virus infection treated with interferon-α. Am J Gastroenterol 1995;90:1138—41.

69. Durand JM, Cretel E, Kaplanski G, Juhan-Vague I, Soubeyrand J. Thrombose et traitement par interféron. Rev Med Int 1995;16 Suppl 1:161s.

70. Garcia-Buey L, Garcia-Monzon C, Rodriguez S, Borque MJ, Garcia-Sanchez A, Iglesias R, De-Castro M, Mateos FG, Vicario JL, Balas A, Moreno-Otero R. Latent autoimmune hepatitis triggered during interferon therapy in patients with chronic hepatitis C. Gastroenterology 1995; 108:1770—7.

71. Cianciara J, Laskus T. Development of transient autoimmune hepatitis during interferon treatment of chronic hepatitis B. Dig Dis Sci 1995;8:1842—4.

72. D'Amico E, Paroli M, Fratelli V, Palazzi C, Barnaba V, Callea F, Consoli G. Primary biliary cirrhosis induced by interferon-α therapy for hepatitis C virus infection. Dig Dis Sci 1995;40:2113—6.

73. Calleja JL, Albillos A, Cacho G, Iborra J, Abreu L, Escartin P. Interferon and prednisone therapy in chronic hepatitis C with non-organ-specific antibodies. J Hepatol 1996;24:308—12.

74. Todros L, Saracco G, Durazzo M, Abate ML, Touscoz G, Scaglione L, Verme G, Rizzetto M. Efficacy and safety of interferon α therapy in chronic hepatitis C with autoantibodies to liver-kidney microsomes. Hepatology 1995;22:1374—8.

75. Grimbert S, Johanet C, Bendjaballah F, Homberg JC, Poupon R, Beaugrand M. Antimitochondrial antibodies in patients with chronic hepatitis C. Liver 1996;16:161—5.

76. Gschwantler M, Schrutka-Kölbl C, Weiss W. Acute exacerbation of antiliver cytosol antibody-positive autoimmune chronic hepatitis by α-interferon. Am J Gastroenterol 1995;90:2239—340.

77. Propst A, Propst T, Dietze O, Kathrein H, Judmeier G, Vogel W. Development of granulomatous hepatitis during treatment with interferon-α2b. Dig Dis Sci 1995;40:2117—8.

78. Tada H, Saitoh S, Nakagawa Y, Hirana H, Morimoto L, Shima T, Shimamoto K, Okanoue T, Kashima K. Ischemic colitis during interferon-α treatment for chronic active hepatitis C. J Gastroenterol 1996;31:582—4.

79. Rettmar K, Kienast J, van de Loo J. Minimal change glomerulonephritis with reversible proteinuria during interferon α-2a therapy for chronic myeloid leukemia. Am J Hematol 1995;49:355—6.

80. Parker MG, Atkins MB, Ucci AA, Levey AS. Rapidly progressive glomerulonephritis after immunotherapy for cancer. J Am Soc Nephrol 1995;5:1740—4.

81. Pawlotsky JM, Dhumeaux D, Bagot M. Hepatitis C virus in dermatology. Arch Dermatol 1995;131:1185—93.

82. Areias J, Velho GC, Cerquiera R, Barbedo C, Amaral B, Sanches M, Massa A, Saraiva AM. Lichen planus and chronic hepatitis C: exacerbation of the lichen under interferon-α-2a therapy. Eur J Gastroenterol Hepatol 1996;8:825—8.

83. Doutre MS, Couzigou P, Beylot-Barry M, Beylot C, Quinton A. Lichen plan et hépatite C. Hétérogénéité évolutive de 6 cas traités par l'interféron α. Gastroenterol Clin Biol 1996; 20:709—10.

84. Hildebrand A, Kolde G, Luger TA, Schwarz T. Successful treatment of generalized lichen planus with recombinant interferon α-2b. J Am Acad Dermatol 1995;33:880—3.

85. Pateron D, Fain O, Sehonnou J, Trinchet JC, Beaugrand M. Severe necrotizing vasculitis in a patient with hepatitis C virus infection treated by interferon. Clin Exp Rheumatol 1996;14:79—81.

86. Azagury M, Pauwels C, Kornfeld S, Bataille N, Perie G. Severe cutaneous reactions following interferon injections. Eur J Cancer 1996; 32A:1821.

87. Kontochristopoulos G, Stavrinos C, Aroni K, Tassopoulos NC. Cutaneous necrosis by subcutaneous injection of α-interferon in a patient with chronic type B hepatitis. J Hepatol 1996;25:271.

88. Bernstein D, Reddy KR, Jeffers L, Schiff E. Canities and vitiligo complicating interferon therapy for hepatitis C. Am J Gastroenterol 1995;90:1176—7.

89. Simsek H, Savas C, Akkiz H, Telatar H. Interferon-induced vitiligo in a patient with chronic viral hepatitis C infection. Dermatology 1996;193:65—6.

90. Mori T, Asakura A, Nakajima S, Ono M, Kano A. Visual function in patients with chronic C hepatitis treated with interferon. Folia Ophthalmol Jpn 1995;46:482—5.

91. Shahidullah AB, Cerulli MA, Berman DH. Interferon may cause retinopathy during hepatitis therapy. Am J Gastroenterol 1995;90:1543.

92. Kawano T, Shigehira M, Uto H, Kato J, Hayashi K, Maruyama T, Kuribayashi T, Chuman T, Futami T, Tsubouchi H. Retinal complications during interferon therapy for chronic hepatitis C. Am J Gastroenterol 1996;91:309—13.

93. Soushi S, Kobayashi F, Obazawa H, Kigasawa K, Shiraishi K, Itakura M, Matsuzaki S. Evaluation of risk factors of interferon-associated retinopathy in patients with type C chronic active hepatitis. Nippon Ganka Gakkai Zasshi 1996;100:69—76.

94.   Nishiwaki H, Ogura Y, Miyamoto K, Matsuda N, Honda Y. Interferon α induces leukocyte capillary trapping in rat retinal microcirculation. Arch Ophthalmol 1996;114:726—30.

95.   Gillies MC. Potential use of interferon-α in ophthalmological disorders. Clin Immunother 1996;6:383—94.

96.   Finger DR, Plotz PH, Heywood G. Myosotis following treatment with high dose interleukin-2 for malignancy. J Rheumatol 1995;22:2188.

97.   Solis RA, Pomales SY, Torres EA. Polymyositis induced by interferon α-2b in a patient with chronic hepatitis C. Am J Gastroenterol 1996;91:2041.

98.   Harada M, Sata M, Yoshida H, Noguchi S, Yamakawa Y, Mimura Y, Ohishi M, Ayabe M, Tanikawa K. Inflammatory myopathy associated with hepatitis C virus infection: a report of four cases. Int Hepatol Commun 1995;4:195—200.

99.   Anderlini P, Buzaid AC, Legha SS. Acute rhabdomyolysis after concurrent administration in interleukin-2, interferon-α and chemotherapy for metastatic melanoma. Cancer 1995;76:678—9.

100.   Gregorio GV, Jones H, Choudhuri K, Vegnente A, Bortolotti F, Miel-Vergani G, Vergani D. Autoantibody prevalence in chronic hepatitis B virus infection: effect of interferon α. Hepatology 1996;24:520—3.

101.   Heller J, Musiolik J, Homrighausen A, Sauerbruch T, Spengler U. Vorkommen und Bedeutung von Autoantikörpen im Rahmen der Interferontherapie der chronischen Hepatitis C. Dtsch Med Wochenschr 1996;121:1179—83.

102.   Noda K, Enomoto N, Arai K, Masuda E, Yamada Y, Suzuki K, Tanaka M, Yoshiara H. Induction of antinuclear antibody after interferon therapy in patients with type-C chronic hepatitis: its relation to the efficacy of therapy. Scand J Gastroenterol 1996;31:716—22.

103.   Morris LF, Lemak NA, Arnett FC Jr, Jordon RE, Duvic M. Systemic lupus erythematosus diagnosed during interferon α therapy. South Med J 1996;89:810—4.

104.   Yoshida A, Morozumi K, Takeda A, Koyama K, Oikawa T. Systemic lupus erythematosus-like serological disorders and nephropathy after interferon-α therapy of chronic hepatitis C. Jpn J Rheumatol 1995;6:47—52.

105.   Carli P, De Jauréguiberry JP, Paris JF, Marlier S, Galzin M, Chagnon A. Polyarthrite au cours d'un traitement par interféron α. Deux observations. Presse Med 1995;24:1709.

106.   Jumbou O, Berthelot JM, French N, Bureau B, Litoux P, Dréno B. Polyarthritis during interferon α therapy: 3 cases and a review of the literature. Eur J Dermatol 1995;5:581—4.

107.   Unoki H, Moriyama A, Tabaru A, Masumoto A, Otsuki M. Development of Sjögren's syndrome during treatment with recombinant human interferon-α-2b for chronic hepatitis C. J Gastroenterol 1996;31:723—7.

108.   Teragawa H, Hondo T, Takahashi K, Watanabe H, Ohe H, Hattori N, Watanabe Y, Amano H, Hino F, Ohbayashi M, Urushihara T, Yone-hara S. Sarcoidosis after interferon therapy for chronic active hepatitis C. Intern Med 1996;35:19—23.

109.   Nakajima M, Kubota Y, Miyashita N, Niki Y, Matsushima T, Manabe T. Recurrence of sarcoidosis following interferon α therapy for chronic hepatitis C. Intern Med 1996;35:376—9.

110.   Kuno M, Mimori A, Fujii T, Takeda A, Masuyama J, Yoshio T, Minota S, Kano S. Histiocytic cytophagic panniculitis which developed during interferon-α therapy. Intern Med 1996;35:115—8.

111.   Antonelli G, Giannelli G, Currenti M, Simeoni E, Del Vecchio S, Maggi F, Pistello M, Roffi L, Pastores G, Chemello L, Dianzani F. Antibodies to interferon (IFN) in hepatitis C patients relapsing while continuing recombinant IFN-α 2 therapy. Clin Exp Immunol 1996; 104:384—7.

112.   Hanley JP, Jarvis LM, Simmonds P, Ludlam CA. Development of anti-interferon antibodies and breakthrough hepatitis during treatment for HCV infection in haemophiliacs. Br J Haematol 1996;94:551—6.

113.   Roffi L, Colloredo Mels G, Antonelli G, Bellati G, Panizzuti F, Piperino A, Pozzi M, Ravizza D, Angeli G, Dianzani F, Mancia G. Breakthrough during recombinant interferon α therapy in patients with chronic hepatitis C virus infection: prevalence, etiology and management. Hepatology 1995;21:645—9.

114.   Milella M, Antonelli G, Santantonio T, Giannelli G, Currenti M, Monno L, Turriziani O, Pastore G, Dianzani F. Treatment with natural IFN of hepatitis C patients with or without antibodies to recombinant IFN. Hepato-Gastroenterology 1995;42:201—4.

115.   Rajan GP, Seifert B, PrHmmer O, Joller-Jemelka HI, Burg G, Dummer R. Incidence and in-vivo relevance of anti-interferon-antibodies during treatment of low-grade cutaneous T-cell lymphomas with interferon α-2a combined with acitretin or PUVA. Arch Dermatol Res 1996;288:543—8.

116.   Tefferi A, Grendahl DC. Natural leucocyte interferon-α therapy in patients with chronic granulocytic leukemia who have antibody-mediated resistance to treatment with recombinant interferon-α. Am J Hematol 1996;52:231—3.

117.   Russo D, Candoni A, Zuffa E, Minisini R, Silvestri F, Fanin R, Zaja F, Martinelli G, Tura S, Botta G, Baccarani M. Neutralizing anti-interferon-α antibodies and response to treatment in patients with Ph(+) chronic myeloid leukaemia sequentially treated with recombinant (α 2a) and lymphoblastoid interferon-α. Br J Haematol 1996;94:300—5.

118.   Rostaing L, Izopet J, Baron E, Duffaut M, Puel M, Durand D. Treatment of chronic hepatitis C with recombinant interferon-α in kidney transplant recipients. Transplantation 1995;59:1426—31 (also in Nephron 1996;74:512—6).

119.   Pohanka E, Kovarik J. Is treatment with interferon-α in renal transplant recipients still justified? Nephrol Dial Transplant 1996;11:1192—3.

120. Féray C, Samuel D, Gigou M, Paradis V, David MF, Lemonnier C, Reynès M, Bismuth H. An open trial of interferon α recombinant for hepatitis C after liver transplantation: antiviral effects and risk of rejection. Hepatology 1995;22:1084—9.

121. Min AD, Bodenheimer HC. Does interferon precipitate rejection of liver allografts? Hepatology 1995;22:1333—5.

122. Samson D, Volin L, Schanz U, Bosi A, Gahrton G. Feasibility and toxicity of interferon maintenance therapy after allogeneic BMT for multiple myeloma: a pilot study of the EBMT. Bone Marrow Transplant 1996;17:759—62.

123. Mauss S, Heintges T, Adams O, Albrecht H, Niederau C, Jablonowski H. Treatment of chronic hepatitis C with interferon-α in patients infected with the human immunodeficiency virus. Hepato-Gastroenterology 1995;42:528—34.

124. Rivero J, Limonta M, Aguilera A, Fraga M, Lopez-Saura P. Use of recombinant interferon-α in human immunodeficiency virus (HIV)-infected individuals. Biotherapy 1995;8:23—31.

125. Soriano V, Garcia-Samaniego J, Bravo R, Castro A, Odriozola PM, Gonzalez J, Colmenero M, Carballo E, Suarez D, Libre JM, Alberdi JC, Pedreira J, Gonzales-Lahoz J. Efficacity and safety of α-interferon treatment for chronic hepatitis C in HIV-infected patients. J Infect 1995;31:9—13.

126. Izumi T, Imagawa S, Hatake K, Miura Y, Ariyama T, Inazawa J, Abe T. Philadelphia chromosome-negative cells with trisomy 8 after busulfan and interferon treatment of Ph1-positive chronic myelogenous leukemia. Int J Hematol 1996;64:73—7.

127. Mahé B, Gaillard F, Labadie F, Papin S, Letortorec S, Moreau P, Harousseau JL, Milpied N. Occurrence of a T cell lymphoma in a patient with chronic myeloid leukemia treated with α interferon. Leuk Lymphoma 1995;19:515—7

128. Johansson B, Fioretos T, Billström R, Mitelman F. Aberrant cytogenetic evolution pattern of Philadelphia-positive chronic myeloid leukemia treated with interferon-α. Leukemia 1996;10:1134—8.

129. Pawson R, A'Hern R, Catovsky D. Second malignancy in hairy cell leukaemia: no evidence of increased incidence after treatment with interferon α. Leuk Lymphoma 1996;22:103—6.

130. Troussard X, Henry-Amar M, Flandrin G. Second cancer risk after interferon therapy. Blood 1994;84:3242—4.

131. Ferrari VD, Jirillo A, Lonardi F, Pavanato G, Bonciarelli G. Pregnancy during α-interferon therapy in patients with advanced Hodgkin's disease. Eur J Cancer 1995;31A:2121—2.

132. Masbou J, Larrey D, Michel H. Traitement par interféron α-2a recombinant et grossesse chez une malade atteinte d'hépatite chronique virale C. Gastroenterol Clin Biol 1995;19:961—2.

133. Delage R, Demers C, Cantin G, Roy J. Treatment of essential thrombocythemia during pregnancy with interferon-α. Obst Gynecol 1996;87:814—7.

134. Haggstrom J, Adriansson M, Hybbinette T, Harnby E, Thorbert G. Two cases of CML treated with α-interferon during second and third trimester of pregnancy with analysis of the drug in the new-born immediately postpartum. Eur J Haematol 1996;57:101—2.

135. Casato M, Pucillo LP, Leoni M, di Lullo L, Gabrielli A, Sansonno D, Dammacco F, Danieli G, Bonomo L. Granulocytopenia after combined therapy with interferon and angiotensin-converting enzyme inhibitors: evidence for a synergistic hematologic toxicity. Am J Med 1995;99:386—91.

136. Lublin FD, Whitaker JN, Eidelman BH, Miller AE, Arnason BGW, Burks JS. Management of patients receiving interferon β-1b for multiple sclerosis: report of a consensus conference. Neurology 1996;46:12—8.

137. Anonymous. Euromedicines evaluation: the striptease begins. Lancet 1996;347:483 (see also Harvey P. Why interferon β 1b was licensed is a mystery. Br Med J 1996;313:297—8 and Napier JC. Reputation of interferon β-1b. Lancet 1996;347:968).

138. Richards RG. Interferon β in multiple sclerosis. Clinical cost effectiveness falls at the first hurdle. Br Med J 1996;313:1159.

139. Neilley LK, Goodin DS, Goodkin DE, Hauser SL. Side effect profile of interferon β-1b in MS: results of an open label trial. Neurology 1996;46:552—4.

140. Jacobs LD, Cookfair DL, Rudick RA, Herndon RM, Richert JR, Salazar AM, Fischer JS, et al. Intramuscular interferon β-1a for disease progression in relapsing multiple sclerosis. Ann Neurol 1996;39:285—94.

141. Salmon P, Le Cotonnec JY, Galazka A, Abdul-Ahad A, Darragh A. Pharmacokinetics and pharmacodynamics of recombinant human interferon-β in healthy male volunteers. J Interferon Cytokine Res 1996;16:759—64.

142. Monsonego J, Cossot G, Ince SE, Galazka AR, Abdul-Ahad AK. Randomised double-blind trial of recombinant interferon-β for condyloma acuminatum. Genitourin Med 1996;72:111—4.

143. The IFNB Multiple Sclerosis Study Group and the University of British Columbia MS/MRI Analysis Group. Interferon β-1b in the treatment of multiple sclerosis: final outcome of the randomized controlled trial. Neurology 1995;45:1277—85.

144. Sasaki M, Sata M, Suzuki H, Uchimura Y, Murashima S, Tanaka K, Uchimura N, Nakamura J, Ishibashi M, Tanikawa K. Change in cerebral blood flow in an acute hepatitis C patient with depressive state while receiving interferon. Int Hepatol Commun 1996;5:354—60.

145. Nagai Y, Ohsawa K, Ieki Y, Kobayashi KI. Effect of interferon-β on thyroid function in patients of chronic hepatitis C without preexisting autoimmune thyroid disease. Endocr J 1996;43:545—9.

146. Kazuta Y, Watanabe N, Sagawa K, Kobayashi H, Kojima T, Funabashi H, Moritoh T, Kasukawa R. A case of autoimmune hemolytic anemia

induced by IFN-β therapy for type-C chronic hepatitis. Fukushima J Med Sci 1995;41:43—9.

147. Benincasa P, Bielory L. Necrotizing cutaneous lesions as a complication of subcutaneous interferon β-1b. J Allergy Clin Immunol 1996; 97:343.

148. Webster GF, Knobler RL, Lublin FD, Kramer EM, Hochman LR. Cutaneous ulcerations and pustular psoriasis flare caused by recombinant interferon β injections in patients with multiple sclerosis. J Am Acad Dermatol 1996;34:365—7.

149. Young MC, Otis J. Interferon β-1b hypersensitivy and desensitization. J Allergy Clin Immunol 1996;97:345.

150. The IFNB Multiple Sclerosis Study Group and the University of British Columbia MS/MRI Analysis Group. Neutralizing antibodies during treatment of multiple slcerosis with interferon β-1b: experience during the first three years. Neurology 1996;47:889—94.

151. Bobbio-Pallavicini E, Valsecchi C, Tacconi F, Moroni M, Porta C. Sarcoidosis following β-interferon therapy for multiple myeloma. Sarcoidosis 1995;12:140—2.

152. Bemiller LS, Roberts DH, Starko KM, Curnutte JT. Safety and effectiveness of long-term interferon γ therapy in patients with chronic granulomatous disease. Blood Cells Mol Dis 1995;21:239—47.

153. Weening RS, Leitz GJ, Seger RA. Recombinant human interferon-γ in patients with chronic granulomatous disease. European follow up study. Eur J Pediatr 1995;154:295—8.

154. Polisson RP, Gilkeson GS, Pyun EH, Pisetsky DS, Smith EA, Simon LS. A muticenter trial of recombinant human interferon γ in patients with systemic sclerosis: effects on cutaneous fibrosis and interleukin-2 receptor levels. J Rheumatol 1996;23:654—8.

155. Vlachoyianniopoulos PG, Tsifetaki N, Dimitriou I, Galaris D, Papiris SA, Moutsopoulos HM. Safety and efficacy of recombinant γ interferon in the treatment of systemic sclerosis. Ann Rheum Dis 1996;55:761—8.

156. Tashiro M, Yokoyama K, Nakayama M, Yamada A, Ogura Y, Kawaguchi Y, Sakai O. A case of nephrotic syndrome developing during postoperative γ interferon therapy for renal cell carcinoma. Nephron 1996;73:685—8.

157. Horn TD, Altomonte V, Vogelsang G, Kennedy MJ. Erythroderma after autologous bone marrow transplantation modified by administration of cyclosporine and interferon γ for breast cancer. J Am Acad Dermatol 1996;34:413—7.

158. Fiehn C, PrHmmer O, Gallati H, Heilig B, Hunstein W. Treatment of systemic mastocytosis with interferon-γ: failure after appearance of anti-IFN-γ antibodies. Eur J Clin Invest 1995;25:615—8.

159. Veltri S, Smith JW II. Interleukin 1 trials in cancer patients: a review of the toxicity, antitumor and hematopoietic effects. Stem Cells 1996; 14:164—76.

160. Janik JE, Miller LL, Longo DL, Powers GC, Urba WJ, Kopp WC, Gause BL, Curti BD, Fenton RG, et al. Phase II trial of interleukin-1α and indomethacin in treatment of metastatic melanoma. J Natl Cancer Inst 1996;88:44—9.

161. Curti BD, Urba WJ, Longo DL, Janik JE, Sharfman WH, Miller LL, Cizza G, Shimizu M, Openheim JJ, Alvord WG, Smith JW II. Endocrine effects of IL-1α and β administered in a phase I trial to patients with advanced cancer. J Immunother 1996;19:142—8.

162. Law TM, Motzer RJ, Mazumdar M, Sell KW, Walther PJ, O'Connel M, Khan A, Vlamis V, Vogelzang NJ, Bajorin DF. Phase III randomized trial of interleukin-2 with or without lymphokine-activated killer cells in the treatment of patients with advanced renal cell carcinoma. Cancer 1995;76:824—32.

163. Yang JC, Topalian SL, Schwartzentruber DJ, Parkinson DR, Marincola FM, Weber JS, Seipp CA, White DE, Rosenberg SA. The use of polyethylene glycol-modified interleukin-2 (PEG-IL-2) in the treatment of patients with metastatic renal cell carcinoma and melanoma. A phase I study and a randomized prospective study comparing IL-2 alone versus IL-2 combined with PEG-IL-2. Cancer 1995;76:687—94.

164. Stadler WM, Vogelzang NJ. Low-dose interleukin-2 in the treatment of metastatic renal-cell carcinoma. Semin Oncol 1995;22:67—73.

165. Piscitelli SC, Minor JR. Role of interleukin-2 in managing infection with the human immunodeficiency virus. Am J Health-Syst Pharm 1995;52:541—2.

166. Kovacs JA, Vogel S, Albert JM, Falloon J, Davey RT, Walker RE, Polis MA, Spooner K, Metclaf JA, Baseler M, Fyfe G, Lane HC. Controlled trial of interleukin-2 infusions in patients infected with the human immunodeficiency virus. New Engl J Med 1996;335:1350—6.

167. Reynolds JV, Murchan P, Leonard N, Gough DB, Clarke P, Keane FBV, Tanner WA. High-dose interleukin 2 promotes bacterial translocation from the gut. Br J Cancer 1995;72:634—6.

168. Du Bois IS, Udelson JE, Atkins MB. Severe reversible global and regional ventricular dysfunction associated with high-dose interleukin-2 immunotherapy. J Immunother 1995;18:119—23.

169. Citterio G, Fragasso G, Rossetti E, Di Lucca G, Bucci E, Foppoli M, Guerrieri R, Matteucci P, Polastri D, Scaglietti U, Tresoldi M, Chierchia SL, Rugarli C. Isolated left ventricular filling abnormalities may predict interleukin-2-induced cardiovascular toxicity. J Immunother 1996;19:134—41.

170. Citterio G, Pellegatta F, Di Lucca G, Fragasso G, Scaglietti U, Pini D, Fortis C, Tresoldi M, Rugarli C. Plasma nitrate plus nitrite changes during continuous intravenous infusion interleukin-2. Br J Cancer 1996;74:1297—301.

171. Michel M, Vincent F, Sigal R, Damaj G, Bensoussan TA, Leclercq B, Escudier B. Cerebral vasculitis after interleukin-2 therapy for renal cell carcinoma. J Immunother 1995;18:124—6.

172. Puduvalli VK, Sella A, Austin SG, Forman AD. Carpal tunnel syndrome associated with interleukin-2 therapy. Cancer 1996;77:1189—92.

173. Sikora SS, Samsonov ME, Dookeran KA, Edington H, Lotze MT. Peripheral nerve entrapment: an unusual adverse event with high-dose interleukin-2 therapy. Ann Oncol 1996;7:535—6.

174. Krouse RS, Royal RE, Heywood G, Weintraub BD, White DE, Steinberg SM, Rosenberg SA, Schwartzentruber DJ. Thyroid dysfunction in 281 patients with metastatic melanoma of renal carcinoma treated with interleukin-2 alone. J Immunother 1995;18:272—8.

175. Soni N, Meropol NJ, Porter M, Caligiuri MA. Diabetes mellitus induced by low-dose interleukin-2. Cancer Immunol Immunother 1996;43:59—62.

176. Nakagawa K, Miller FN, Sims DE, Lentsch AB, Miyazaki M, Edwards MJ. Mechanisms of interleukin-2-induced hepatic toxicity. Cancer Res 1996;56:507—10.

177. Asnis LA, Gaspari AA. Cutaneous reactions to recombinant cytokine therapy. J Am Acad Dermatol 1995;33:393—410.

178. Costello R, Blaise D, Jacquemier J, Monges G, Stoppa AM, Viens P, Olive D, Bouabdallah R, Brandely M, Gastaut JA, Maraninchi D. Induction of cutaneous 'graft-versus-host-like' reaction by recombinant IL-2 after autologous bone marrow transplantation. Bone Marrow Transplant 1995;16:199—200.

179. Massumoto C, Benyunes MC, Sale G, Beauchamp M, York A, Thompson JA, Buckner CD, Fefer A. Close simulation of acute graft-versus-host disease by interleukin-2 administered after autologous bone marrow transplantation for hematologic malignancy. Bone Marrow Transplant 1996;17:351—6.

180. Lopez-Jimenez J, Delas-Heras E, Hilara Y, Garcia-Larana J, Perez-Oteyza J, Bellas C, Munoz A, Rocamora A, Nunez M, Odrlozola J. Low-dose interleukin-2 therapy is not associated with cutaneous toxicity after autologous transplantation. Bone Marrow Transplant 1996;18:484—2.

181. Engelhardt M, Rump JA, Hellerich U, Mertelsmann R, Lindemann A. Leukocytoclastic vasculitis and long-term remission in a patient with secondary AML and post-remission treatment with low-dose interleukin-2. Ann Hematol 1995;70:227—30.

182. Esteva-Lorenzo FJ, Janik JE, Fenton RG, Emslie-Smith A, Engel AG, Longo DL. Myositis associated with interleukin-2 therapy in a patient with metastasic renal cell carcinoma. Cancer 1995;76:1219—23.

183. Vadhan-Raj S. PIXY321 (GM-CSF/IL-3 fusion protein): biological and clinical effects of a novel cytokine. Forum Trends Exp Clin Med 1995;5:110—8.

184. Bridges AG, Helm TN, Bergfeld WF, Lawlor KB, Dijkstra J. Interleukin-3-induced urticaria-like eruption. J Am Acad Dermatol 1996;34:1076—8.

185. Scadden DT, Levine JD, Bresnahan J, Gere J, McGrath J, Wang Z, Resta DJ, Young D, Hammer SM. In vivo effects of Interleukin 3 in HIV type 1-infected patients wih cytopenia. AIDS Res Hum Retroviruses 1995;11:731—40.

186. Hurwitz N, Probst A, Zufferey G, Tichelli A, Pless M, Kappos L, Speck B, Gratwohl A. Fatal vascular leak syndrome with extensive hemorrhage, peripheral neuropathy and reactive erythrophagocytosis: an unusual complication of recombinant IL-3 therapy. Leuk Lymphoma 1996;20:337—40.

187. Olencki T, Finke J, Tubbs R, Tuason L, Greene T, McLain D, Swanson SJ, Herzog P, Stanley J, Edinger M, Budd GT, Bukowski RM. Immunomodulatory effects of interleukin-2 and interleukin-4 in patients with malignancy. J Immunother 1996;19:69—80.

188. Vassilopoulou-Sellin R, Thielvodt D, Markowitz AB. Effects of Interleukin-4 administration on endocrine function and lipid profile of patients with malignant diseases. Blood 1996;87:4022—3.

189. Weiss GR, Fehrenkamp SH, Tokaz LK, Sunderland MC. Vitiligo and Graves' disease following treatment of malignant melanoma with recombinant human interleukin 4. Dermatology 1996;192:283—5.

190. Veldhuis GJ, Willemse PHB, Mulder NH, Limburg PC, de Vries EGE. Potential use of recombinant human interleukin-6 in clinical oncology. Leuk Lymphoma 1996;20:373—9.

191. Stouthard JML, Goey H, de Vries EGE, Demulder PH, Groenewegen A, Pronk L, Stoter G, Sauerwein HP, Bakker PJM, Veenhof CHN. Recombinant human interleukin 6 in metastatic cancer: a phase II trial. Br J Cancer 1996;73:789—93.

192. Gordon MS, Nemunaitis J, Hoffman R, Paquette RL, Rosenfeld C, Manfreda S, Isaacs R, Nimer SD. A phase I trial of recombinant human interleukin-6 patients with myelodysplasic syndromes and thrombocytopenia. Blood 1995;85:3066—76.

193. Spath-Schwalbe E, Schrezenmeir H, Bornstein S, Burger K, Porzsolt F, Born J. Endocrine effects of recombinant interleukin 6 in man. Neuroendocrinology 1996;63:237—43.

194. Nieken J, Mulder NH, Buter J, Vellenga E, Limburg PC, Piers DA, deVries EGE. Recombinant human interleukin-6 induces a rapid and reversible anemia in cancer patients. Blood 1995;86:900—5.

195. Huhn RD, Radwanski E, O'Connell SM, Sturgill MG, Clarke L, Cody RP, Affrime MB, Cutler DL. Pharmacokinetics and immunomodulatory properties of intravenously administered recombinant human interleukin-10 in healthy volunteers. Blood 1996;87:699—705.

196. Fuchs AC, Granowitz EV, Shapiro L, Vannier E, Lonnemann G, Angel JB, Kennedy JS, Rabson AR, Radwanski E, Affrime MB, Cutler DL, Grint PC, Dinarello CA. Clinical, hematologic, and immunologic effects of interleukin-10 in humans. J Clin Immunol 1996;16:291—303.

197. Gordon MS, McCaskill-Stevens WJ, Battiato LA, Loewy J, Loesch D, Breeden E, Hoffman R, Beach KJ, Kuca B, Kaye J, Sledge GW. A phase I trial of recombinant human Interleukin-11 (Neumega rhIL-11 growth factor) in women with breast cancer receiving chemotherapy. Blood 1996;9:3615—24.

198. Tepler I, Elias L, Smith JW, Hussein M, Rosen G, Chang AYC, Moore JO, Gordon MS, Kuca B, Beach KJ, Loewy JW, Garnick MB, Kaye JA. A randomized placebo-controlled trial of recombinant human interleukin-11 in cancer patients with severe thrombocytopenia due to chemotherapy. Blood 1996;87:3607—14.

199. Gately MK, Mulqueen MJ. Interleukin-12: potential clinical applications in the treatment and prevention of infectious diseases. Drugs 1996;52 Suppl 2:18—26.

200. Cohen J. IL-12 deaths: explanation and a puzzle. Science 1995;270:908.

201. American Society of Clinical Oncology. Recommendations for the use of hematopoietic colony-stimulating factors: evidence-based, clinical practice guidelines. J Clin Oncol 1994;12:2471—508.

202. Bregni M, Siena S, Di Nicola M, Dodero A, Peccatori F, Ravagnani F, Danesini G, Laffranchi A, Bonadonna G, Gianni AM. Comparative effects of granulocyte-macrophage colony-stimulating factor and granulocyte colony-stimulating factor after high-dose cyclophosphamide cancer therapy. J Clin Oncol 1996;14:628—35.

203. Rosenthal J, Healey T, Ellis R, Gillan E, Cairo MS. A two-year folow-up of neonates with presumed sepsis treated with recombinant human granulocyte colony-stimulating factor during the first week of life. J Pediatr 1996;128:135—7.

204. Kawachi Y, Watanabe A, Uchida T, Yoshizawa K, Kurooka N, Setsu K. Acute arterial thrombosis due to platelet aggregation in a patient receiving granulocyte colony-stimulating factor. Br J Haematol 1996;94:413—6.

205. Kuroiwa M, Okamura T, Kanaji T, Okamura S, Harada M, Niho Y. Effects of granulocyte colony-stimulating factor on the hemostatic system in healthy volunteers. Int J Hematol 1996;63:311—6.

206. Rovelli F, Barni S, Tancini G, Ardizzoia A, Lissoni P. Endocrine effects of granulocyte colony-stimulating factor in cancer patients. Tumori 1995;81:438—9.

207. de Luis DA, Romero E. Reversible thyroid dysfunction with filgastrim. Lancet 1996;348:1595—6.

208. Sandor V, Hassan R, Kohn E. Exacerbation of pseudogout by granulocyte colony-stimulating factor. Ann Intern Med 1996;125:781.

209. deWit R, Verweij J, Bontenbal M, Kruit WHJ, Seynaeve C, Schmitz PIM, Stoter G. Adverse effect on bone marrow protection of prechemotherapy granulocyte colony-stimulating factor support. J Natl Cancer Inst 1996;88:1393—8.

210. Okamoto S, Ishida A, Wakui M, Tanosaki R, Oda A, Ykeda Y. Prolonged thrombocyto-penia after administration of granulocyte colony stimulating factor and leukapheresis in a donor for allogeneic peripheral blood stem cell transplantation. Bone Marrow Transplant 1996;18:482—3.

211. Foster PF, Mital D, Sankary HN, McChesney LP, Marcon J, Koukoulis G, Kociss K, Leurgans S, Whiting JF, Williams JW. The use of granulocyte colony-stimulating factor after liver transplantation. Transplantation 1995;59:1557—63.

212. Hirokawa M, Lee M, Motegi M, Miura AB. Reversible renal impairment during leukocytosis induced by G-CSF in non-Hodgkin's lymphoma. Am J Hematol 1996;51:328—34.

213. Minguez C, Mazuecos A, Ceballos M, Tejuca F, Rivero M. Worsening of renal function in a renal transplant patient treated with granulocyte colony-stimulating factor. Nephrol Dial Transplant 1995;10:2166—7.

214. Narayanan G, Jha R, Shahariah S, Bhoopal R, Jaleel MA. Reversal of leucopenia without precipitating rejection in renal transplant recipients with granulocyte macrophage colongy stimulating factor. J Nephrol 1995;8:276—8.

215. Loraas A, Fossa SD, Franzen S, Saeter G, Rode L. Skin lesions and G-CSF in patients with malignant diseases. Malignancy or cutaneous side-effect? Eur J Cancer 1996;32A:554—5.

216. Glass LL, Fotopoulos T, Messina JL. A generalized cutaneous reaction induced by granulocyte colony-stimulating factor. J Am Acad Dermatol 1996;34:455—9.

217. Garty BZ, Levy I, Nitzan M, Barak Y. Sweet syndrome associated with G-CSF treatment in a child with glycogen storage disease type Ib. Pediatrics 1996;97:401—3.

218. Petit T, Francès C, Marinho E, Herson S, Chosidow O. Lymphoedema-area-restricted Sweet syndrome during G-CSF treatment. Lancet 1996;347:690.

219. Farhey YD, Herman JH. Vasculitis complicating granulocyte colony stimulating factor treatment of leukopenia and infection in Felty's syndrome. J Rheumatol 1995;22:1179—82.

220. McMullin MF, Finch MB. Felty's syndrome treated with rh G-CSF associated with flare of arthritis and skin rash. Clin Rheumatol 1995;14:204—8.

221. Lee PK, Dover JS. Recurrent exacerbation of acne by granulocyte colony-stimulating factor administration. J Am Acad Dermatol 1996;34:855—6.

222. Parkkali T, Volin L, Sirén MK, Ruutu T. Acute iritis induced by granulocyte colony-stimulating factor used for mobilization in a volunteer unrelated peripheral blood progenitor cell donor. Bone Marrow Transplant 1996;17:433—4.

223. Nakashima H, Kawabe K, Ohtsuka T, Hayashida K, Horiuchi T, Nagasawa K, Niho Y. Rheumatoid arthritis exacerbation by G-CSF treatment for bucillamine-induced agranulocytosis. Clin Exp Rheumatol 1995;13:677—8.

224. Martin-Munoz R, Gomez-Bellver M, Na-

varro Pulido AM, Orta Cuevas JC. Probable hypersensitivity reaction to filgrastim. Am J Health-Syst Pharm 1996;53:1607.

225. Laurent D, Schmidberger H, Pradier O, Hess CF. Facial angioedema associated with granulocyte colony-stimulating factor treatment. Onkologie 1996;19:445—6.

226. Harousseau JL, Wu D. The use of GM-CSF and G-CSF in the treatment of acute leukemias. Leuk Lymphoma 1995;18:405—12.

227. Usuki K, Iki S, Endo M, Kitazume K, Ito K, Watanabe M, Urabe A. Granulocyte colony-stimulating factor in acute myeloid leukemia. Stem Cells 1995;13:647—54.

228. Corey SJ, Wollman MR, Deshpande RV. Granulocyte colony-stimulating factor and congenital neutropenia-risk of leukemia? J Pediatr 1996;129:187—8.

229. Hashino S, Imamura M, Tanaka J, Kobayashi S, Musashi M, Kasai M, Asaka M. Transformation of severe aplastic anemia into acute myeloblastic leukemia with monosomy 7. Ann Hematol 1996;72:337—9.

230. Jin JY, Tooze JA, Marsh JCW, Matthey F, Gordon-Smith EC. Myelodysplasia following aplastic anaemia-paroxysmal nocturnal haemoglobinuria syndrome after treatment with immunosuppression and G-CSF: evidence for the emergence of a separate clone. Br J Haematol 1996;94:510—2.

231. Ohsaka A, Sugahara Y, Imai Y, Kikuchi M. Evolution of severe aplastic anemia to myelodysplasia with monosomy 7 following granulocyte colony-stimulating factor, erythropoietin and high-dose methylprednisolone combination therapy. Intern Med 1995;34:892—5.

232. Naparstek E. Granulocyte colony-stimulating factor, congenital neutropenia, and acute myelo6d leukemia. New Eng J Med 1995;333:516—8.

233. Waller CF, Bertz H, Wenger MK, Fetscher S, Hardung M, Engelhardt M, Behringer D, Lange W, Mertelsmann R, Finke J. Mobilization of peripheral blood progenitor cells for allogeneic transplantation: efficacy and toxicity of a high-dose rhG-CSF regimen. Bone Marrow Transplant 1996;18:279—83.

234. Sakamaki S, Matsunaga T, Hirayama Y, Kuga T, Niitsu Y. Haematological study of health volunteers 5 years after G-CSF. Lancet 1995; 346:1432—3.

235. Arici M, Haznedaroglu IC, Erman M, Ozcebe O. Leukoerythroblastosis following the use of G-CSF. Am J Hematol 1996;52:123—4.

236. Petros WP, Rosner GL, Rabinowitz J, Gilbert CL, Coniglio D, Vredenburgh JJ, Ross M, Peters WP. The pharmacologic effects of recombinant, human colony-stimulating factors and their modulation by theophylline. Pharmacotherapy 1996;16:742—8.

237. Astles JR, Petros WP, Peters WP, Sedor FA. Artifactual hypoglycemia associated with hematopoietic cytokines. Arch Pathol Lab Med 1995;119:713—6.

238. Zdanowicz NH, Reynaert CM, Janne PP, Wuulemann PHJ, Chatelain CJ. Mood disorder with manic features in a patient treated with granulocyte-monocyte colony stimulating factor. Psychosomatics 1996;37:305—6.

239. Sarris AH, Majlis A, Dimopoulos MA, Younes A, Swann F, Rodriguez MA, McLaughlin P, Cabanillas F. Rising serum lactate dehydrogenase often caused by granulocyte or granulocyte-macrophage colony stimulating factor and not tumor progression in patients with lymphoma or myeloma. Leuk Lymphoma 1995;17:473—7.

240. Locker GJ, Simonitsch I, Mader RM, Warlamides E, Gnant MFX, Jakesz R, Rainer H, Steger GG. Cutaneous side effects in breast cancer patients treated with cytostatic polychemotherapy and rh GM-CSF: immune phenomena or drug toxicity? Breast Cancer Res Treat 1995;34:231—19.

241. Calderwood S, Doyle JJ, Hitzler JK, Saunders EF, Freedman MH. Administration of recombinant human granulocyte-macrophage colony-stimulating factor after autologous bone marrow transplantation in children with acute myelogenous leukemia: a note of caution. Bone Marrow Transplant 1996;18:87—91.

242. Ganser A, Hoelzer D. Clinical use of hematopoietic growth factors in the myelodysplastic syndromes. Semin Hematol 1996;33:186—95.

243. Yoshida Y, Nakahata T, Shibata A, Takahashi M, Moriyama Y, Kaku K, Masaoka T, Kaneko T, Miwa S. Effects of long-term treatment with recombinant human granulocyte-macrophage colony-stimulating factor in patients with myelodysplastic syndrome. Leuk Lymphoma 1995;18:457—63.

244. Emile JF, Fraitag S, Andry P, Leborgne M, Lellouch-Tubiana A, Brousse N. Expression of GM-CSF receptor by Langerhans' cell histiocytosis cells. Virchows Arch 1995;427:125—9.

245. Weintraub M, Adde MA, Venzon DJ, Shad AT, Horak ID, Neely JE, Seibel NL, Gootenberg J, Arndt C, Nieder ML, Magrath IT. Severe atypical neuropathy associated with administration of hematopoietic colony-stimulating factors and vincristine. J Clin Oncol 1996;14:935—40.

246. Bunn PA, Crowley J, Kelly K, Hazuka MB, Beasley K, Upchurch C, Livingston R. Chemoradiotherapy with or without granulocyte-macrophage colony-stimulating factor in the treatment of limited-stage small-cell lung cancer: a prospective phase III randomized study of the Southwest Oncology Group. J Clin Oncol 1995;13:1632—41.

247. Omura K, Kawamura T, Utsunomiya T, Abe A, Joh K, Sakai O. Development of nephrotic syndrome in a patient with acute myeloblastic leukemia after treatment with macrophage-colony stimulating factor. Am J Kidney Dis 1996; 27:883—7.

248. Wilde MI, Goa KL. Muromonab CD3: a reappraisal of its pharmacology and use as prophylaxis of solid organ transplant rejection. Drugs 1996;51:865—94.

249. Abramowicz D, de Paw L, Le Moine A, Sermon F, Surquin M, Doutrelepont JM, Ickx B,

Depierreux M, Vanherweghem JL, Kinnaert P, Goldman M, Vereerstraeten P. Prevention of OKT3 nephrotoxicity after kidney transplantation. Kidney Int 1996;49 Suppl 53:39—43.

250. Vincenti F, Danovitch GM, Neylan JF, Steiner RW, Everson MP, Gaston RS. Pentoxifylline does not prevent the cytokine-induced first dose reaction following OKT3. A randomized, double-blind placebo-controlled study. Transplantation 1996;61:573—7.

251. Abdallah KA, David-Neto E, Centeno JR, Nahas WC, Arap S. Reversal of the OKT3-related shivering and chest tightness by intravenous meperidine. Transplantation 1996;62:145—6.

252. Jin DC, Kim SY, Lee JM, Koo WS, Choi EJ, Yoon YS, Bang BK. Visual loss complicating OKT3 monoclonal antibody therapy in a renal transplant recipient. Nephrol Dial Transplant 1995;10:2144—6.

253. Embrey RP, Geist LJ. Influenza A pneumonitis following treatment of acute cardiac allograft rejection with murine monoclonal anti-CD3 antibody (OKT3). Chest 1995;108:1456—9.

254. Abramowicz D, Crusiaux A, Niaudet P, Kreis H, Chatenoud L, Goldman M. The IgE humoral response in OKT3-treated patients. Incidence and fine specificity. Transplantation 1996;61:577—81.

255. Bertin D, Haverty T, Sanders M, Daneil D, O'Connor J, Spence S, Starzer-Farrell K, Treichler P, Wu SC. Posttransplant development of lymphoproliferative disorders and other malignancies following orthoclone OKT3 therapy. In: Lieberman R, Mukherjee A, editors. Principles of Drug Development in Transplantation and Autoimmunity 1996;633—41.

256. Stephenson J. Reengineered monoclonal antibodies step up to the plate in cancer studies. J Am Med Assoc 1995;274:1821—2.

257. Gruber R, Holz E, Riethmüller G. Monoclonal antibodies in cancer therapy. Springer Semin Immunopathol 1996;18:243—51.

258. Rankin ECC, Isenberg DA. Monoclonal antibody therapy in rheumatoid arthritis. An update on recent progress. Clin Immunother 1996; 6:143—53.

259. Wang JCY, Beauregard P, Soamboonsrup P, Neame PB. Monoclonal antibodies in the management of acute leukemia. Am J Hematol 1995;50:188—99.

260. Van Gelder T, Zieste R, Mulder AH, Yzermans JNM, Hesse CJ, Vaessen LMB, Weimar W. A double-blind, placebo-controlled study of monoclonal anti-interleukin-2 receptor antibody (BT563) administration to prevent acute rejection after kidney transplantation. Transplantation 1995;60:248—52.

261. Van Gelder T, Balk AHMM, Jonkman FAM, Zieste R, Zondervan P, Hesse CJ, Vaessen LMB, Mochtar B, Weimar W. A randomized trial comparing safety and efficacy of OKT3 and a monoclonal anti-interleukin-2 receptor antibody (BT563) in the prevention of acute rejection after heart transplantation. Transplantation 1996;62: 51—5.

262. Dalesandro MR, Kinney CS, Ghrayeb J. Therapeutic use of a mouse/human chimeric CD4 antibody in rheumatoid arthritis. Methods Companion Methods Enzymol 1995;8:157—65.

263. Moreland LW, Pratt PW, Mayes MD, Postlethwaite A, Weisman MH, Schnitzer T, Lightfoot R, Calabrese L, Zelinger DJ, Woody JN, Koopman WJ. Double-blind, placebo-controlled multicenter trial using chimeric monoclonal anti-CD4 antibody, cM-T412, in rheumatoid arthritis patients receiving concomitant methotrexate. Arthritis Rheum 1995;38:1581—8.

264. Varadi G, Or R, Rund D, Orbach H, Slavin S, Nagler A. Severe migratory polyarthritis following in vivo CAMPATH-1G. Bone Marrow Transplant 1995;16:843—5.

265. Wahrenberger A. Pharmacological immunosuppression: cure or curse? Crit Care Nurs Q 1995;17:27—36.

266. Shoker AS. Immunopharmacologic therapy in renal transplantation. Pharmacotherapy 1996;16:562—75.

267. Morris RE. Mechanisms of action of new immunosuppressive drugs. Kidney Int 1996;49 Suppl 53:26—8.

268. Bouwes Bavinck JN, Hardie DR, Green A, Cutmore S, MacNaught A, O'Sullivan B, Siskind V, Van Der Woude FJ, Hardie IR. The risk of skin cancer in renal transplant recipients in Queensland, Australia. A follow-up study. Transplantation 1996;61:715—21.

269. Mihalov ML, Gattuso P, Abraham K, Holmes EW, Reddy V. Incidence of post-transplant malignancy among 674 solid-organ-transplant recipients at a single center. Clin Transplant 1996;10:248—55.

270. Newell KA, Alonso EM, Whitington PF, Bruce DS, Millis JM, Piper JB, Woodle ES, Kelly SM, Koeppen H, Hart J, Rubin CM, Thistlethwaite JR. Posttransplant lymphoproliferative disease in pediatric liver transplantation: interplay between primary Epstein-Barr virus infection and immunosuppression. Transplantation 1996;62; 370—5.

271. Montagnino G, Lorca E, Tarantino A, Bencini P, Aroldi A, Cesana B, Braga M, Lonati F, Ponticelli C. Cancer incidence in 854 kidney transplant recipients from a single institution: comparison with normal population and with patients under dialytic treatment. Clin Transplant 1996;10:461—9.

272. Sheil AGR. Malignancy in organ transplantation recipients. Transplant Proc 1996;28:1162.

273. Patel R, Snydman DR, Rubin RH, Ho M, Pescovitz M, Martin M, Paya CV. Cytomegalovirus prophylaxis in solid organ transplant recipients. Transplantation 1996;61:1279—89.

274. Singh N, Yu VL. Infections in organ transplant recipients. Curr Opin Infect Dis 1996; 9:223—9.

275. Winston DJ, Emmanouilides C, Busuttil RW. Infections in liver transplant recipients. Clin Infect Dis 1995;21:1077—91.

276. Reis MA, Costa RS, Ferraz AS. Causes of

death in renal transplant recipients: a study of 102 autopsies from 1968 to 1991. J R Soc Med 1995;88:24—7.

277. Bouhnik Y, Lémann M, Mary J-Y, Scemama G, Ta6 R, Matuchansky C, Modigliani R, Rambaud J-C. Long-term follow-up of patients with Crohn's disease treated with azathioprine or 6-mercaptopurine. Lancet 1996;347:215—9.

278. Prujit J, Haanen J, Hollander A, den Ottolandder G. Azathioprine-induced pure red-cell aplasia. Nephrol Dial Transplant 1996;11:1371—3.

279. Kowdley KV, Keeffe EB. Hepatotoxicity of transplant immunosuppressive agents. Gastroenterol Clin N Am 1995;24:991—1001.

280. Pol S, Cavalcanti R, Carnot F, Legendre C, Driss F, Chaix ML, Thervet E, Chkoff N, Brechot C, Berthelot P, Kreis H. Azathioprine hepatitis in kidney transplant recipients. A predisposing role of chronic viral hepatitis. Transplantation 1996;61:1774—6.

281. Kohli HS, Jain D, Sud K, Jha V, Gupta KL, Sakhuja V, Joshi K. Azathioprine-induced hepatic veno-occlusive disease in a renal transplant recipient: histological regression following azathioprine withdrawal. Nephrol Dial Transplant 1996;11:1671—2.

282. Aissaoui M, Mounedji N, Mathelier-Fusade P, Leynadier F. Pancréatite à l'azathioprine: immuno-allergique? Presse Med 1996;25:1650.

283. Tragnone A, Bazzocchi G, Aversa G, Pecorelli MG, Elmi G, Venerato S, Lanfranchi GA. Acute pancreatitis after azathioprine treatment for ulcerative colitis. Ital J Gastroenterol 1996;28:103—4.

284. Kolk A, Horneff G, Wilgenbus KK, Wahn V, Gerharz CD. Acute lethal necrotising pancreatitis in childhood systemic lupus erythematosus. Possible toxicity of immuno-suppressive therapy. Clin Exp Rheumatol 1995;13:399—403.

285. Compton MR, Crosby DL. Rhabdomyolysis associated with azathioprine hypersensitivity syndrome. Arch Dermatol 1996;132:1254—5.

286. Smak Gregoor PJH, Van Saase JLCM, Weimar W, Kramer P. Fever and rigors as sole symptoms of azathioprine hypersensitivity. Neth J Med 1995;47:288—90.

287. Beckett CG, Hill P, Hine KR. Leucocytoclastic vasculitis in a patient with azathioprine hypersensitivity. Postgrad Med J 1996;72:437—8.

288. Blanco R, Martinez-Taboada VM, Gonzalez-Gay MA, Armona J, Fernandez-Sueiro JL, Gonzalez-Vela MC, Rodriguez-Valverde V. Acute febrile toxic reaction in patients with refractory rheumatoid arthritis who are receiving combined therapy with methotrexate and azathioprine. Arthritis Rheum 1996;39:1016—20.

289. Parnham AP, Dittmer I, Mathieson PW, McIver A, Dudley C. Acute allergic reactions associated with azathioprine. Lancet 1996;348:542—3.

290. Kennedy DT, Hayney MS, Lake KD. Azathioprine and allopurinol: the price of an avoidable interaction. Ann Pharmacother 1996;30:951—4.

291. Cummins D, Sekar M, Halil O, Banner N. Myelosuppression associated with azathioprine-allopurinol interaction after heart and lung transplantation. Transplantation 1996;61:1661—2.

292. Van der Pijl JW, Bouwes Bavinck JN, De Fijter JW. Isotretinoin and azathioprin: a synergy that makes hair curl? Lancet 1996;348:622—3.

293. Confavreux C, Saddier P, Grimaud J, Moreau TH, Adeleine P, Aimard G. Risk of cancer from azathioprine therapy in multiple sclerosis: a case-control study. Neurology 1996;46:1607—12.

294. Csuka ME, Hanson GA. Resolution of a soft-tissue sarcoma in a patient with rheumatoid arthritis after discontinuation of azathioprine therapy. Arch Intern Med 1996;156:1573—6.

295. Forbes A, Reading NG. Review article: the risks of malignancy from either immunosuppression or diagnostic radiation in inflammatory bowel disease. Aliment Pharmacol Ther 1995;9:465—70.

296. Gonzalez-Crespo MR, Gomez-Reino JJ, Merino R, Ciruelo E, Gomez-Reino FJ, Muley R, Garcia-Consuegra J, Pinillos V, Rodriguez-Valverde V. Menstrual disorders in girls with systemic lupus erythematous treated with cyclophosphamide. Br J Rheumatol 1995;34:737—41.

297. McDermott EM, Powell RJ. Incidence of ovarian failure in systemic lupus erythematosus after treatment with pulse cyclophosphamide. Ann Rheum Dis 1996;55:224—9.

298. Milford DV, Butler N, Clarke R, Vaid J. Reversible hepatic dysfunction in association with cyclophosphamide therapy. Eur J Pediatr 1995;154:411—2.

299. Assier-Bonnet H, Aractingi S, Cadranel J, Wechsler J, Mayaud C, Saiag P. Stevens-Jonhson syndrome induced by cyclophosphamide: report of two cases. Br J Dermatol 1996;135:864—5.

300. Tumietto F, Raimondi C, Frasca GM, Martello M, DiBiari MA, Costigliola P, Bonomini V, Chiodo F. Disseminated cryptococcosis in a lupus nephritis patient under long-term immunosuppression. Nephrol Dial Transplant 1995;10:896—9.

301. Pryor BD, Bologna SG, Kahl LE. Risk factors for serious infection during treatment with cyclophosphamide and high-dose corticosteroids for systemic lupus erythematosus. Arthritis Rheum 1996;39:1475—82.

302. Talar-Williams C, Hijazi YM, Walther MCM, Linehan WM, Hallahan CW, Lubensky I, Kerr GS, Hoffman GS, Fauci AS, Sneller MC. Cyclophosphamide-induced cystitis and bladder cancer in patients with Wegener granulomatosis. Ann Intern Med 1996;124:477—84.

303. Pasero G, Priolo F, Marubini E, Fantini F, Ferraccioli G, Magaro M, Marcolongo R, Oriente P, Pipitone V, Portioli I, Tirri G, Trotta F, Della Casa Alberighi O. Slow progression of joint damage in early rheumatoid arthritis treated with cyclosporin A. Arthritis Rheum 1996;39:1006—15.

304. Grossman RM, Chevret S, Abirached J, Blanchet F, Dubertret L. Long-term safety of cyclosporine in the treatment of psoriasis. Arch Dermatol 1996;132:623—9.

305. Mrowietz U, Färber L, Henneicke-von Zepelin HH, Bachmann H, Welzel D, Christophers E. Long-term maintenance therapy with cyclosporine and posttreatment survey in severe psoriasis: results of a multicenter study. J Am Acad Dermatol 1995;33:470—5.

306. Kasiske BL, Guijarro C, Massy ZA, Wiederkehr MR, Ma JZ. Cardiovascular disease after renal transplantation. J Am Soc Nephrol 1996;7:158—65.

307. Kronenberg F, Lhotta K, Königsrainer A, König P. Renal artery thromboembolism and immunosuppressive therapy. Nephron 1996;72:101.

308. Hauben M. Cyclosporine neurotoxicity. Pharmacotherapy 1996;16:576—83.

309. Wijdicks EFM, Wiesner RH, Krom RAF. Neurotoxicity in liver transplant recipients with cyclosporine immunosuppression. Neurology 1995;45:1962—4.

310. Aksamit AJ, de Groen PC. Cyclosporine-related leukoencephalopathy and PML in a liver transplant recipient. Transplantation 1995;60:874—90.

311. Rustom R, Moore AP, Bowden AN, Sells RA, Bone JM. Cyclosporin-induced cerebellar syndrome in a pancreatico-renal transplant recipient. Nephrol Dial Transplant 1996;11:1374—5.

312. Nussbaum ES, Maxwell RE, Bitterman PB, Hertz MI, Bula W, Latchaw RE. Cyclosporine A toxicity presenting with acute cerebellar edema and brainstem compression. J Neurosurg 1995;82:1068—70.

313. Edwards LL, Wszolek ZK, Normand MM. Neurophysiologic evaluation of cyclosporine toxicity associated with bone marrow transplantation. Acta Neurol Scand 1995;92:423—9.

314. Memon M, de Magalhaes-Silverman M, Bloom EJ, Lister J, Myers DJ, Pincus SM, Rybka WB, Ball ED. Reversible cyclosporine-induced cortical blindness in allogeneic bone marrow transplant recipients. Bone Marrow Transplant 1995;15:283—6.

315. Esterl RM, Gupta N, Garvin PJ. Permanent blindness after cyclosporin neurotoxicity in a kidney-pancreas transplant recipient. Clin Neuropharmacol 1996;19:259—66.

316. Valldeoriola F, Graus F, Rimola A, Andreu H, Santamaria J, Catafau A, Visa J, Tolosa E, Rodés J. Cyclosporine-associated mutism in liver transplant patients. Neurology 1996;46:252—4.

317. Wasserstein PH, Honig LS. Parkinsonism during cyclosporine treatment. Bone Marrow Transplant 1996;18:649—50.

318. Lorberboym M, Bronster DJ, Lidov M, Pandit N. Reversible cerebral perfusion abnormalities associated with cyclosporine therapy in orthotopic liver transplantation. J Nucl Med 1996;37:467—9.

319. Aakhus S, Dahl K, Wideroe TE. Hyperlipidaemia in renal transplant patients. J Intern Med 1996;239:407—15.

320. Wheeler DC, Morgan R, Thomas DM, Seed M, Rees A, Moore RH. Factors influencing plasma lipid profiles including lipoprotein(a) concentrations in renal transplant recipients. Transplant Int 1996;9:221—6.

321. Arnadottir M, Hultberg B, Vladov V, Nilsson-Ehle P, Thysell H. Hyperhomocysteinemia in cyclosporine-treated renal transplant recipients. Transplantation 1996;61:509—12.

322. Laine J, Holmberg C. Renal and adrenal mechanisms in cyclosporine-induced hyperkalaemia after renal transplantation. Eur J Clin Invest 1995;25:670—6.

323. Morishita E, Nakao S, Asakura H, Jokaji H, Saito M, Uotani C, Kumabashiri I, Yamazaki M, Yoshida T, Takemoto K, Aoshima K, Hashimoto T, Matsuda T. Hypercoagulability and high lipoprotein(a) levels in patients with aplastic anemia receiving cyclosporine. Blood Coagul Fibrinol 1996;7:609—14.

324. Myara A, Cadranel JF, Dorent R, Lunel F, Bouvier E, Gerhardt M, Bernard B, Ghoussoub JJ, Cabrol A, Gandjbakhch I, Opolon P, Trivin F. Cyclosporin A-mediated cholestasis in patients with chronic hepatitis after heart transplantation. Eur J Gastroenterol Hepatol 1996;8:267—71.

325. Actis GC, Debernardi-Venon W, Lagget M, Marzano A, Ottobrelli A, Ponzetto A, Rocca G, Boggio-Bertinet D, Balzola F, Bonino F, Verme G. Hepatotoxicity of intravenous cyclosporin A in patients with acute ulcerative colitis on total parenteral nutrition. Liver 1995;15:320—3.

326. Bennett WM, DeMattos A, Meyer MM, Andoh T, Barry JM. Chronic cyclosporine nephropathy: the Achilles' heel of immunosuppressive therapy. Kidney Int 1996;50:1089—100.

327. Mihatsch MJ, Ryffel B, Gudat F. The differential diagnosis between rejection and cyclosporine toxicity. Kidney Int 1995;48 Suppl 52:63—9.

328. Shihab FS. Cyclosporine nephropathy: pathophysiology and clinical impact. Semin Nephrol 1996;16:536—47.

329. Jacobson SH, Jaremko G, Duraj FF, Wilczek HE. Renal fibrosis in cyclosporin A-treated renal allograft recipients: morphological findings in relation to renal hemodynamics. Transplant Int 1996;9:492—8.

330. Hollander AAMJ, Van Saase JLCM, Koote AMM, Van Dorp WT, Van Bockel J, Van Es LA, van der Woude FJ. Beneficial effects of conversion from cyclosporin to azathioprine after kidney transplantation. Lancet 1995;345:610—4.

331. Rodriguez F, Krayenbühl JC, Harrison WB, Forre O, Dijkmans BAC, Tugwell P, Miescher PA, Mihatsch MJ. Renal biopsy findings and follow-up of renal function in rheumatoid arthritis patients treated with cyclosporin. An update from the International Kidney Biopsy Registry. Arthritis Rheum 1996;39:1491—8.

332. Landewé RBM, Dijkmans BAC, Van der Woude FJ, Breedveld FC, Mihatsch MJ, Bruijn JA. Longterm low dose cyclosporine in patients with rheumatoid arthritis: renal function loss without structural nephropathy. J Rheumatol 1996;23:61—4.

333. Young BA, Marsh CL, Alpers CE, Davis CL. Cyclosporine-associated thrombotic microan-

giopathy/hemolytic uremic syndrome following kidney and kidney-pancreas transplantation. Am J Kidney Dis 1996;28:561—71.

334. Jayamanne DGR, Dayan MR, Porter R. Cyclosporin-induced trichomegaly ofaccessory lashes as a cause of ocular irritation. Nephrol Dialysis Transplant 1996;11:1159—61.

335. El-Shahawy MA, Gadallah MF, Massry SG. Acne: a potential side effect of cyclosporine A therapy. Nephron 1996;72:679—82.

336. Mariani G, Calastrini C, Carinci F, Bergamini L, Calastrini F, Stabellini G. Ultrastructural and histochemical features of the ground substance in cyclosporin A-induced gingival overgrowth. J Periodontol 1996;67:21—7.

337. Thomason JM, Kelly PJ, Seymour RA. The distribution of gingival overgrowth in organ transplant patients. J Clin Periodontol 1996;23:367—71.

338. Nell A, Matejka M, Solar P, Ulm C, S inzinger H. Evidence that cyclosporine inhibits periodontal prostaglandin I2 synthesis. J Period Res 1996;31:131—4.

339. Stevens JM, Hilson AJW, Sweny P. Post-renal transplant distal limb bone pain. An under-recognized complication of transplantation distinct from avascular necrosis of bone? Transplantation 1995;60:305—7.

340. Andant C, Edery J, Fouchard I, Pouchot J, Soulé JC. Syndrome algique poly-articulaire au cours d'un traitement par ciclosporine pour colite aiguë grave. Gastroenterol Clin Biol 1996;20:219—20.

341. Thiébaud D, Krieg MA, Gillard-Berguer D, Jacquet AF, Goy JJ, Burckhardt P. Cyclosporine induced high bone turnover and may contribute to bone loss after heart transplantation. Eur J Clin Invest 1996;26:549—55.

342. Shechter P. Acute tubular necrosis following high-dose cyclosporine A therapy. Eur J Clin Pharmacol 1996;49:521—3,

343. Pesavento TE, Jones PA, Julian BA, Curtis JJ. Amlodipine increases cyclosporine levels in hypertensive renal transplant patients: results of a prospective study. J Am Soc Nephrol 1996;7:831—5.

344. Campana C, Regazzi MB, Buggia I, Molinaro M. Clinically significant drug interactions with cyclosporin. An update. Clin Pharmacokin 1996;30:141—79.

345. Islam SI, Masuda QN, Bolaji OO, Shaheen FM, Sheikh IA. Possible interaction between cyclosporine and glibenclamide in posttransplant diabetic patients. Ther Drug Monit 1996;18:624—6.

346. Helms-Smith KM, Curtis SL, Hatton RC. Apparent interaction between nefazodone and cyclosporine. Ann Intern Med 1996;125:424.

347. Horton RC, Bonser RS. Interaction between cyclosporin and fluoxetine. Br Med J 1995;311:422.

348. Strouse TB, Fairbanks LA, Skotzko CE, Fawzy FI. Fluoxetine and cyclosporine in organ transplantation: failure to detect significant drug interactions or adverse clinical events in depressed organ recipients. Psychosomatics 1996;37:23—30.

349. Gomez E, Sanchez JE, Aguado S, Alvarez Grande J. Interaction between azithromycin and cyclosporin? Nephron 1996;73:724.

350. Boran M, GHnes Z, Doruk E, Gönenç F, Cetin S. Improvement of cyclosporine A associated gingival hyperplasia with azithromycine therapy. Transplant Proc 1996;28:2316.

351. McLellan RA, Drobitch RK, McLellan H, Acott PD, Crocker JFS, Renton KW. Norfloxacin interferes with cyclosporine disposition in pediatric patients undergoing renal transplantation. Clin Pharmacol Ther 1995;58:322—7.

352. Pan SH, Lopez RR, Sher LS, Hoffman AL, Podesta LG, Makowka L, Rosenthal P. Enhanced oral cyclosporine absorption with water-soluble vitamin E early after liver transplantation. Pharmacotherapy 1996;16:59—65.

353. Fernandez-Sola J, Campistol JM, Miro O, Garces N, Soy D, Grau JM. Acute toxic myopathy due to pyrazinamide and cyclosporine therapy. Nephrol Dial Transplant 1996;11:1850—2.

354. Lee HA, Slapak M, Venkat Raman G, Mason JC, Digard N, Wise M. Mizoribine as an alternative to azathioprine in triple therapy immunosuppressant regimens in cadaveric renal transplantation: two successive studies. Transplant Proc 1995;27:1050—1.

355. Fulton B, Markham A. Mycophenolate mofetil: a review of its pharmacodynamic and pharmacokinetic properties and clinical efficacy in renal transplantation. Drugs 1996;51:278—98.

356. Shaw LM, Sollinger HW, Halloran P, Morris RE, Yatscoff RW, Ransom J, Tsina I, Keown P, Holt DW, Lieberman R, Jaklitsch A, Potter J. Mycophenolate mofetil: a report of the consensus panel. Ther Drug Monit 1995;17:690—9.

357. The Three Continental Mycophenolate Mophetil Renal Transplantation Study Group. A blinded, randomized clinical trial of mycophenol ate mophetil for the prevention of acute rejection in cadaveric renal transplantation. Transplantation 1996;61:1029—37.

358. Kenagy DN, Cole BR, Markovitz BP, Graham IL, Lowell JA. One patient's experience with mycophenolic acid. Pediatr Nephrol 1996;10:546—7.

359. Brattström C, Tyden G, Säwe J, Herlenius G, Claesson K, Groth CG. A randomized, double-blind, placebo-controlled study to determine safety, tolerance, and preliminary pharmacokinetics of ascending single doses of orally administered sirolimus (rapamycin) in stable renal transplant recipients. Transplant Proc 1996;28:985—6.

360. Murgia MG, Jordan S, Kahan D. The side effect profile of sirolimus: a phase I study in quiescent cyclosporine-prednisone-treated renal transplant patients. Kidney Int 1996;49:209—16.

361. Jusko WJ, Thomson AW, Fung J, McMaster P, Wong SH, Zylber-Katz E, Christians U, Winkler M, Fitzsimmons WE, Lieberman R, McBride J, Kobayashi M, Warty V, Soldin SJ.

Consensus document: therapeutic monitoring of tacrolimus (FK506). Ther Drug Monit 1995; 17:606—14.

362. Asante-Korang A, Boyle GJ, Webber SA, Miller SA, Fricker FJ. Experience of FK506 immune suppression in pediatric heart transplantation: a study of long-term adverse effects. J Heart Lung Transplant 1996;15:415—22.

363. Pham SM, Kormos RL, Hattler BG, Kawai A, Tsamandas AC, Demetris AJ, Murali S, Fricker FJ, Chang HC, Jain AB, Starzl TE, Hardesty RL, Griffith BP. A prospective trial of tacrolimus (FK 506) in clinical heart transplantation: intermediate-term results. J Thorac Cardiovasc Surg 1996;111:764—72.

364. Hohage H, Brückner D, Arlt M, Buchholz B, Zidek W, Spieker C. Influence of cyclosporine A and FK506 on 24 h blood pressure monitoring in kidney transplant recipients. Clin Nephrol 1996;45:342—4.

365. Baruch Y, Weitzman E, Markiewicz W, Eisenman A, Eid A, Enat R. Anasarca and hypertrophic cardiomyopathy in a liver transplant patient on FK506: relieved after a switch to Neoral. Transplant Proc 1996;28:2250—1.

366. Vincenti F, Laskow DA, Neylan JF, Mendez R, Matas AJ. One-year follow-up of an open-label trial of FK506 for primary kidney transplantation. Transplantation 1996;61:1576—81.

367. Small SL, Fukui MB, Bramblett GT, Eidelman BH. Immunosuppression-induced leukoencephalopathy from tacrolimus (FK506). Ann Neurol 1996;40:575—80.

368. Devine SM, Newman NJ, Siegel JL, Joseph GJ, Geis TC, Schneider JA, Geller RB, Wingard JR. Tacrolimus (FK506)-induced cerebral blindness following bone marrow transplantation. Bone Marrow Transplant 1996;18:569—72.

369. Boeve BF, Kimmel DW, Aronson AE, de Groen PC. Dysarthria and apraxia of speech associated with FK-506 (tacrolimus). Mayo Clin Proc 1996;71:969—72.

370. Furth S, Neu A, Colombani P, Plotnick L, Turner ME, Fivush B. Diabetes as a complication of tacrolimus (FK506) in pediatric renal transplant patients. Pediatr Nephrol 1996;10:64—6.

371. Kanzler S, Lohse AW, Schirmacher P, Otto G, Meyer Zum Büschenfelde KH. Complete reversal of FK506 induced diabetes in a liver transplant recipient by change of immunosuppression to cyclosporin A. Z Gastroenterol 1996;34:128—31.

372. Tanabe K, Koga S, Takahashi K, Sonda K, Tokumoto T, Babazono T, Yagisawa T, Toma H, Kawai T, Fuchinoue S, Teraoka S, Ota K. Diabetes mellitus after renal transplantation under FK 506 (tacrolimus) as primary immunosuppression. Transplant Proc 1996;28:1304—5.

373. Gruessner RWG, Burke GW, Stratta R, Sollinger H, Benedetti E, Marsh C, Stock P, Boudreaux JP, Martin M, Drangstveit MB, Sutherland DER, Gruessner A. A multicenter analysis of the first experience with FK506 for induction and rescue therapy after pancreas transplantation. Transplantation 1996;61:261—73.

374. Gharpure VS, Devine SM, Holland HK, Geller RB, O'Toole K, Wingard JR. Thrombotic thrombocytopenic purpura associated with FK506 following bone marrow transplantation. Bone Marrow Transplant 1995;16:715—6.

375. Mach-Pascual S, Samii K, Beris P. Microangiopathic hemolytic anemia complicating FK506 (tacrolimus) therapy. Am J Hematol 1996; 52:310—2.

376. Suzuki S, Osaka Y, Nakai I, Yasumura T, Omori Y, Yamagata N, Shimazaki C, Oka T. Pure red cell aplasia induced by FK506. Transplantation 1996;61:831—2.

377. Hariharan S, Munda R, Cavallo T, Demmy AM, Schroeder TJ, Alexander JW, First MR. Rescue therapy with tacrolimus after combined kidney/pancreas and isolated pancreas transplantation in patients with severe cyclosporine nephrotoxicity. Transplantation 1996;61:1161—5.

378. Singh N, Gayowski T, Wagener M, Marino IR, Yu VL. Pulmonary infections in liver transplant recipients receiving tacrolimus. Changing pattern of microbial etiologies. Transplantation 1996;61:396—401.

379. Osowski CL, Dix SP, Lin LS, Mullins RE, Geller RB, Wingard JR. Evaluation of the drug interaction between intravenous high-dose fluconazole and cyclosporine or tacrolimus in bone marrow transplant patients. Transplantation 1996;61:1268—72.

380. Moertel CG, Fleming TR, Macdonald JS, Haller DG, Laurie JA, Tangen JM, Ungerleider JS, Emerson WA, Tormey DC, Glick JH, Veeder MH, Mailliard JA. Fluorouracil plus levamisole as effective adjuvant therapy after resection of stage III colon carcinoma: a final report. Ann Intern Med 1995;122:321—6.

381. Moertel CG, Fleming TR, Macdonald JS, Haller DG, Laurie JA, Goodman PJ. Levamisole and fluorouracil for adjuvant therapy of resected colon carcinoma. New Engl J Med 1990;322:352—8.

382. Longrée L, Focani C, Bury J, Beauduin M, Brohee D, Duvivier A, Lecomte M, Markiewicz S, Vindevoghel A, Weerts J. Levamisole adds granulocyte toxicity to 5 FU-based chemotherapies in adjuvant treatment of Dukes-B-C colorectal cancer. A preliminary report. Anticancer Res 1995;15:1561—4.

383. Winquist EW, Lassam NJ. Reversible thrombocytopenia with levamisole. Med Pediatr Oncol 1995;24:262—4.

38

Vitamins

R_x *Safety of antioxidant vitamins*

Since the so-called antioxidant nutrients such as vitamin E, vitamin C and β-carotene are taken by healthy people, it is important that they should be virtually free of toxicity. They are used for disease prevention in dosages that are several-fold higher than the recommended dietary allowances (RDAs), which are based on the amounts necessary to prevent the classic deficiency conditions. The adverse effects of a large range of dosages of vitamin E, vitamin C, and β-carotene have been reviewed (1[R]).

β-Carotene β-Carotene has been characterized by the US Food and Drug Administration as an agent that is 'generally recognised as safe' (GRAS) when used as a coloring compound or a nutritional supplement, on the basis of the Ames test, the mouse hemopoietic micronucleus frequency test, and chronic toxicity studies in rats, rabbits, and dogs. Patients with phototoxicity disorders have been treated with very high dosages of β-carotene without any appreciable adverse effects.

An undesired effect with daily doses of more than about 30 mg for longer than several weeks is a benign yellowing of the skin. Its incidence depends on the dosage and duration of supplementation, and it is reversible. Occasionally mild reversible gastrointestinal distress (gas, bloating) has been reported. Allergic reactions, leukopenia, and retinopathy have been reported anecdotally but not in clinical trials.

Nevertheless the outcome of the Alpha-Tocopherol Beta-Carotene (ATBC) Cancer Prevention Study, conducted in Finland, has raised the question of whether β-carotene supplementation causes an increased incidence of lung cancer (2[C]). In all, 29—133 heavy smokers (20 cigarettes/day for 36 years) aged 50—69 years took α-tocopherol 50 mg/day, or β-caro-

tene 20 mg/day, or both, or placebo. There was a statistically significant 18% increase in the incidence of lung cancer in the men who took β-carotene. This is the only reported finding of this type, and it contrasts with the large amount of epidemiological and other evidence to the contrary. Despite the fact that the study population was somewhat unusual in regard to the heavy tobacco exposure for a long period and that follow-up was relatively short (5—8 years), compared with the many years it takes for carcinogenesis, this finding cannot be ignored, since it is possible that advanced stages of carcinogenesis may be adversely affected by β-carotene.

Ascorbic acid In animal toxicology studies ascorbic acid is extremely well tolerated even in high dosages. In humans, excessive doses are not absorbed by the intestinal tract and can lead to mild diarrhea. The dosage at which this occurs varies from individual to individual.

Reports of the possibility of urinary oxalate stone formation with large dosages of ascorbic acid over prolonged periods lack real clinical concern. Although the urinary excretion of ascorbic acid increases with dose, oxalate excretion does not. Previous reports of high oxalate concentrations in the urine were likely to have been erroneous, because of the conversion of ascorbate to oxalate in alkaline urine samples left standing after collection.

The theoretical concern that increased iron absorption can lead to iron overload states is highly unlikely, since ascorbate intake does not affect iron absorption in healthy, iron replete individuals.

A report of reduced plasma cyanocobalamin concentrations in individuals taking large dosages of ascorbic acid proved to be the result of an analytical error. Further concerns about rebound scurvy after the withdrawal of ascorbic acid were based on uncontrolled studies and have not been confirmed.

Side Effects of Drugs, Annual 20
J.K. Aronson, ed.

β-Tocopherol   *Older reports of animal experiments suggesting that α-tocopherol may have a tumor-promoting effect were most likely incorrect, the activity noted being the result of impurities known to be carcinogenic.*

Interference with coagulation, resulting in a tendency to increased bleeding, has been a concern with high-dosage α-tocopherol. The effects of warfarin can be increased by dosages of α-tocopherol of 100–400 IU/day for some weeks. Reports of the effect of α-tocopherol on blood clotting vary from no effect to significant effects (3[R]). It seems that the greatest effect of α-tocopherol in high dosages occurs in people with pre-existing vitamin K deficiency, such as those taking warfarin. It is therefore recommended that α-tocopherol be avoided in patients with borderline vitamin K deficiency. It is doubtful that vitamin E in dosages up to 800 IU/day, as is usually recommended for prevention of disease, results in any clinically important coagulation abnormalities in subjects with normal coagulation.

In summary, the so-called antioxidant nutrients, α-tocopherol, ascorbic acid, and β-carotene, are well tolerated and virtually free from toxicity, even when used in dosages several-fold higher than the RDA.

VITAMINS OF THE B GROUP

Nicotinic acid (niacin) *(SED-13, 1172; SEDA-17, 439; SEDA-18, 382; SEDA-19, 369)*

The prevalence and nature of adverse effects that occur with the use of ordinary-release and modified-release nicotinic acid have been prospectively investigated (4[C]). Patients were treated for high LDL cholesterol according to the NCEP guidelines. In general, HDL cholesterol concentrations would have to be below 0.78 mmol/l (30 mg/dl) for initiation of nicotinic acid therapy in healthy subjects or below 0.91 mmol/l in patients with coronary artery disease or multiple risk factors for coronary artery disease. In 110 patients who were given 133 separate courses of nicotinic acid over a 5-year period, adverse effects, particularly those severe enough to warrant discontinuation, were monitored.

Only a small percentage of the patients aged 24–48 years had a firm diagnosis of heart disease at the time of the first clinic visit, and most of the patients were classified as being relatively healthy and certainly not severely ill. Patients with hepatic dysfunction, a history of peptic ulcer disease, or diabetes or glucose intolerance (a fasting glucose greater than 6.7 mmol/l (120 mg/dl) were excluded. In all, 63 patients took ordinary-release nicotinic acid and 65 patients modified-release nicotinic acid. Table 1 lists the adverse effects that occurred.

In the 63 patients who took ordinary-release nicotinic acid, 102 occurrences of symptoms were reported. Of those 102 adverse effects, 49 occurred in patients who were forced to stop the drug because of adverse effects. Of the 63 patients who took ordinary-release nicotinic acid 27 (43%) were forced to discontinue the drug because of one or more adverse effects.

In the 65 patients who took modified-release nicotinic acid, there were 80 occurrences of adverse effects, 35 of which were in patients who were forced to stop the drug because of adverse effects.

The average duration of treatment was 24 months. The average length of treatment before adverse effects occurred that were sufficiently severe to warrant stopping treatment was 16.7 months with ordinary-release nicotinic acid and 14.9 months with modified-release nicotinic acid.

The dose-dependency of the incidence of adverse effects was also documented, and the results are listed in Table 2.

The authors concluded that nicotinic acid, in both formulations, causes disturbing adverse effects in over 40% of patients taking the dosages that are generally needed to treat lipid disorders. Such high dosages should be carefully supervised, and physicians who recommend nicotinic acid therapy should give clear instructions on how to take the drug and what possible adverse effects to anticipate. Extended follow-up is important, since adverse effects necessitating withdrawal may not occur until a patient has been taking nicotinic acid for 1 or 2 years.

The feasibility and early toxicity of radiotherapy with carbogen and nicotinamide has been tested in patients with head and neck

Table 1. *Adverse effects in patients taking ordinary- or modified-release nicotinic acid*

Symptoms	Number of reports		Occurrence in patients who discontinued nicotinic acid	
	Ordinary	Modified	Ordinary	Modified
Flushing	18	12	7	5
Abnormal	20	19	11	9
Nausea or vomiting	8	8	6	4
Increased uric acid	15	5	6	1
Headache	2	1	1	1
Rash/welts	7	6	4	4
Ankle swelling	4	0	1	0
Increased serum glucose	11	10	4	2
Fatigue	4	2	2	1
Abdominal pain	10	15	6	7
Itching	2	1	1	0
Dry skin	1	0	0	0
Dysrhythmias	0	1	0	1

Table 2. *Numbers of patients taking ordinary- or modified-release nicotinic acid and the dosages associated with adverse effects*

Dosage (mg/d)	No. of patients treated	No. of patients with adverse effects	No. of patients who discontinued treatment
Ordinary-release			
100—499	3	3	3
500—999	2	1	0
1000	0	0	0
1500	5	3	2
2000	2	2	1
2500	4	4	3
3000	41	30	22
3500	2	2	2
4000	0	0	0
4500	2	2	1
5000	2	1	1
Modified-release			
100—499	1	1	1
500	5	3	2
1000	7	3	2
1500	31	18	14
2000	7	5	5
2500	4	4	3
3000	10	9	6

cancers (5[C]). Nicotinamide was given orally to 42 patients 1.5 h before irradiation. On days when two fractions were given, only one dose of nicotinamide was taken before the first treatment. Initially the daily dose was 6 g. When more pharmacokinetic data became available, this was changed to a weight-adjusted dose of 80 mg/kg, with a maximum of 6 g. The most common adverse effects were nausea and vomiting, reported by 25 (60%) and 15 (36%) of the 42 patients. In 10 patients these adverse effects occurred after the first dose of nicotinamide, and were often unresponsive to antiemetics, including ondanse-tron. Eleven patients discontinued the drug because of severe *nausea* and *vomiting*. In one patient nausea disappeared when the dosage was reduced from 6 to 4 g according to body weight. Apart from this one patient there were no differences in adverse effects between patients taking 6 g and those taking 80 mg/kg. Flushing 0.5—2 h after ingestion was reported by five patients. Signs of *depression* in one patient disappeared within a few days after nicotinamide was discontinued. Two patients complained of nausea and vomiting, and one also had severe diarrhea; nicotinamide (6 and 5.5 g) was discontinued and the patients were admitted to hospital a few days later with dehydration and *renal dysfunction*. The first patient had type 1 diabetes mellitus and hypertension and was taking insulin, lisinopril, bisoprolol, carbasalat calcium, oxazepam, and an antacid. The second was taking metoclopramide, oxazepam, and an antacid; before the start of radiotherapy he received six cycles of cisplatin, 70 mg/m^2/week. Maximum recorded serum creatinine concentrations were 2290 μmol/l in the first patient and 1096 μmol/l in the second. Renal function recovered in both patients with rehydration and bicarbonate administration. In addition both developed *thrombocytopenia* of uncertain origin. The first patient also had moderate transient elevation of *liver enzymes* 2 weeks after discontinuation of nicotinamide; she recovered fully. The second patient had an episode of *ventricular tachycardia*, possibly as a result of electrolyte disturbances.

Special senses In a retrospective survey of 102 patients taking daily doses of nicotinic acid of 3 g or more for hyperlipidemia and 88 control patients who never took nicotinic acid, adverse ocular effects were investigated by means of a questionnaire (6[C]). The frequencies of the adverse effects are summarized in Table 3.

This is the first comprehensive report of ocular adverse effects associated with nicotinic acid, all of which seem to be reversible and dose-related; if the patient wants to continue therapy, it may be feasible to reduce the dosage. Nicotinic acid seems to affect the macula directly; if blurring of vision occurs, *macular edema* should be included in the differential diagnosis and the drug promptly

withdrawn. Aggravation of *sicca symptoms* may be relieved by increasing the frequency of administration of artificial tears. *Periorbital and lid edema or discoloration* also seem to be dose related.

VITAMIN D (CALCIFEROL) AND ANALOGS *(SED-13, 1177; SEDA-17, 440; SEDA-18, 383; SEDA-19, 371)*

Calcitriol (1,25-dihydroxycholecalciferol)

Eleven patients, aged 8—69 years, were hospitalized during a 10-day period after unintentionally using a veterinary vitamin D concentrate (cholecalciferol in peanut oil; 2 million U/g) as a cooking oil. They presented with abdominal cramps, vomiting, and neurological symptoms. They had severe *hypercalcemia*, with mean calcium concentrations of 3.99 mmol/l (7[C]). Although they were treated with a combination of intravenous fluids, diuretics, corticosteroids, and calcitonin, four patients died. In nine patients the serum vitamin D concentrations were determined. Serum concentrations of calcidiol (25-hydroxycholecalciferol) were 847—1652 mmol/l (8—15 times greater than the upper limit of the reference range) and total calcitriol concentrations (mean 106 pmol/l) were increased in only three patients. The percentage of unbound calcitriol (mean 1.02%) was increased in all nine patients in whom it was measured. Unbound calcitriol concentrations (mean 856 fmol/l) were increased in six of the nine patients. Total calcitriol concentrations corre-

Table 3. *The frequencies of ocular effects of nicotinic acid*

	Cases		Controls		
Adverse effects	n	%	n	%	P value
Dry eyes	20	20	6	7	0.011
Blurred vision	26	25	5	6	0.001
Double vision	2	2	0	0	0.500
Discoloration	8	8	3	3	0.227
Swelling	10	10	0	0	0.002
Loss of lashes	2	2	0	0	0.500
Halos	7	7	2	2	0.454
Allergic reactions	3	3	2	2	0.454
Discontinued for ocular reasons	7	7	0	0	0.016
Adverse ocular symptoms	8	8	2	2	0.113
Other adverse effects	63	62	16	16	<0.0001

lated with both concentrations of both calcidiol and unbound calcitriol. Most of the patients had increased concentrations of unbound calcitriol, despite normal or near-normal total calcitriol concentrations. These findings suggest that increased unbound calcitriol concentrations might play a role in the pathogenesis of hypercalcemia in vitamin D toxicity.

There have been increasing numbers of reports of *nephrocalcinosis* diagnosed by renal ultrasound in patients with X-linked hypophosphatemia treated with vitamin D and phosphate (8^C). Since there has been no systematic comparison of treated and untreated patients with X-linked hypophosphatemia with long-term follow-up, 10 adults and four children with no history of medical therapy and 10 adults and eight children who had been treated with phosphate and vitamin D were examined by means of renal ultrasound. None of the untreated patients had nephrocalcinosis; in five treated adults and five treated children the renal ultrasound examination was positive. In three of four treated children, serial renal ultrasounds did not show progression of the nephrocalcinosis. Comparisons of means between treated patients with and without nephrocalcinosis showed statistically significant differences in urine calcium/creatinine and urine phosphorus/creatinine ratios, differences that were not seen between untreated patients and treated patients without nephrocalcinosis. Phosphate dosage, but not vitamin D dosage, was significantly different between the two treated groups (phosphate and vitamin D in patients with nephrocalcinosis 54 and 0.04 mg/kg/day; phosphate and vitamin D in patients with no nephrocalcinosis 29 and 0.02 mg/kg/day). These results point to a convincing role for an association between nephrocalcinosis, as diagnosed by renal ultrasound, and therapy with phosphate and vitamin D.

REFERENCES

1. Gareval HS, Diplock AT. How 'safe' are antioxidant vitamins? Drug Saf 1996;13:8—14.
2. The Alpha-Tocopherol, Beta-Carotene Cancer Prevention Study Group. The effect of vitamin E and β carotene on the incidence of lung cancer and other cancers in male smokers. New Engl J Med 1994;330:1029—35.
3. Kappus H, Diplock AT. Tolerance and safety of vitamin E: a toxicological position report. Free Rad Biol Med 1992;13:55—74.
4. Gibbons LW, Gonzalez V, Gordon N, Grundy S. The prevalence of side effects with regular and sustained-release nicotinic acid. Am J Med 1995;99:378—85.
5. Kaanders JHAM, Pop, LAM, Marre HAM, van der Maazen RWM, van der Kogel AJ, van Daal WAJ. Radiotherapy with carbogen breathing and nicotinamide in head and neck cancer: feasibility and toxicity. Radiother Oncol 1995;37:190—8.
6. Fraunfelder FW, Fraunfelder FT, Ellingworth DR. Adverse ocular effects associated with niacin therapy. Br J Ophthalmol 1995;79:54—6.
7. Pettifor JM, Bikle DD, Cavaleros M, Zachen D, Kamdar MC, Ross FP. Serum concentrations of free 1,25-dihydroxyvitamin D in vitamin D toxicity. Ann Intern Med 1995;122:511—13.
8. Taylor A, Sherman NH, Norman ME. Nephrocalcinosis in X-linked hypophosphatemia: effect of treatment versus disease. Pediatr Nephrol 1995;9:173—5.

39 Corticotrophins and corticosteroids

ACTH *(CORTICOTROPHIN) (SED-13, 1190; SEDA-17, 451; SEDA-18, 386; SEDA-19, 374)*

Infantile spasm is a convulsive disorder almost limited to infants. ACTH is the treatment of choice. The effects of ACTH on brain midline structures have been investigated in seven infants (five boys and two girls, age range 5—10 months) with infantile spasms treated with synthetic ACTH (0.01 mg/kg/day) for 4 weeks (1ᶜ). Changes in midline structures were evaluated by magnetic resonance imaging before and after treatment. The results showed transient brain shrinkage, with volume reductions in the pons, corpus callosum, and cerebellum. These results seem to show that the beneficial effect ACTH in infantile spasms could be due to a direct effect on the brain-stem.

CORTICOSTEROIDS *(SED-13, 1193; SEDA-17, 445; SEDA-18, 386; SEDA-19, 374)*

Cardiovascular Glucocorticoid-induced *hypertension* is defined as a systolic pressure above 160 mmHg and/or a diastolic pressure above 95 mmHg after glucocorticoid administration. To explore the syndrome of glucocorticoid-induced hypertension in the elderly, 35 patients aged over 65 years (12 men, 23 women) who received glucocorticoid therapy have been studied (2ᶜ). Resting blood pressures were under 140/90 mmHg before glucocorticoid therapy, and patients were apparently disease-free, apart from the condition for which the glucocorticoid was prescribed. Glucocorticoid-induced hypertension was seen in 13 patients (37%); all patients with hypertension were taking more than 20 mg/day of prednisolone, and the blood pressure rose rapidly within 1 week of starting treatment. The hypertensive patients did not differ significantly in terms of age, heart rate, blood count, plasma biochemistry, plasma renin activity, plasma aldosterone, routine urinalysis, or urinary electrolytes from patients who did not have hypertension. However, serum total calcium concentrations were significantly lower in the hypertensive patients, both before and after 2 weeks of glucocorticoid therapy. Furthermore, among the hypertensive patients significantly more had a positive family history of essential hypertension. In conclusion, although the detailed mechanisms are as yet uncertain, glucocorticoid-induced hypertension occurs often in elderly patients, and is more common in patients with total serum calcium concentrations below the reference range, and/or in those with a family history of essential hypertension.

Dexamethasone is now often used in the treatment of bronchopulmonary dysplasia. Two premature male babies receiving dexamethasone 0.5 mg/kg/day developed symptomatic reversible steroid-induced *myocardial hypertrophy* with left ventricular outflow tract obstruction, with a mild subaortic gradient, a tachycardia, and an ejection systolic murmur (3ᶜ).

The first neonate began dexamethasone when aged 4 weeks. After 10 days of therapy, echocardiography and Doppler studies showed left ventricular hypertrophy and outflow tract obstruction. Dexamethasone was continued at the full dosage for a further 4 days then withdrawn over 10 days. Two weeks after dexamethasone had been stopped, an echocardiogram showed complete regression of the cardiac changes. Cardiac examination at 4 months of age was normal.

The second neonate received dexamethasone in the same dosage for 6 days from 23 days of age. The drug was then withdrawn over 12 days. A se-

Side Effects of Drugs, Annual 20
J.K. Aronson, ed.

cond course of dexamethasone, in the same dosage as the first course, was started at 47 days of age because of deterioration of bronchopulmonary dysplasia. During withdrawal on this occasion the neonate developed a systolic ejection murmur. An electrocardiogram at 56 days of age showed left ventricular hypertrophy with mild mitral insufficiency. The heart murmur resolved after 30 days and the cardiac changes subsequently returned to normal.

These patients had no known risk factors associated with the development of obstructive hypertrophic cardiomyopathy.

Aortic aneurysms occurred in five women after they had taken corticosteroids for 15–32 years for systemic lupus erythematosus (*n* = 3), Raynaud's phenomenon (one), or rheumatoid arthritis (one). The women, aged 43–75 years, had abdominal aortic aneurysms, and in three a pseudoaneurysm had formed. Marked atherosclerosis was noted at autopsy in two patients who died as a result of ascending aortic dissection with pericardial tamponade and postoperative respiratory failure. The authors suggested that long-term corticosteroid therapy accelerates atherosclerosis and formation of aortic aneurysms, with a high risk of rupture (4[c]).

Respiratory *Voice problems and cough* Local adverse effects are common in asthmatics taking pressurized aerosol, metered-dose, inhaled steroids, as suggested by a survey of the prevalence of throat and voice symptoms in patients with asthma using corticosteroids by metered-dose pressurized aerosol (5[c]). Of 255 consecutive out-patients taking inhaled steroids, 147 (58%) reported dysphonia or throat symptoms, compared with 13% of the 100 controls. Women admitted to symptoms more frequently than men. Throat symptoms were more prevalent in patients using higher doses. Aerosol inhaler-induced cough was reported by 87 patients (34%). Local adverse effects were equally prevalent with beclomethasone dipropionate and budesonide. The use of a large-volume spacing device with either steroid aerosol did not protect against these symptoms.

Nervous system *Epidural lipomatosis* is a rare adverse effect of corticosteroids. A new case has been described in a 42-year-old man who took prednisone (12 mg/day) for more

than a year for rheumatic polyarthritis (6[c]). He was admitted for progressive low back pain radiating into the backs of both thighs. A large amount of fat was surgically removed from the spinal canal.

Psychiatric Glucocorticoids can cause a wide range of psychiatric reactions, including *psychotic symptoms*, *anxiety*, *mania*, and *depression* (SED-13, 1195; SEDA-17, 446; SEDA-18, 387; SEDA-19, 374). New cases of steroid-induced psychosis have recently been published (7[c]). In a recent report (8[c]), a 41-year-old woman treated with long-term high-dosage corticosteroids (prednisone 60 mg/day) for Crohn's disease presented with irritability, racing thoughts, emotional lability, and dysphoria. Her physician decided not to use lithium, in order to avoid gastrointestinal toxicity, and prescribed carbamazepine (800 mg/day), which reversed her symptoms, although she continued to take prednisone. The author explained this by citing the mood-stabilizing properties of carbamazepine.

Endocrine, metabolic *Growth retardation* (SEDA-14, 336; SEDA-15, 420) Poorly controlled severe asthma can lead to growth impairment in childhood. In children with mild asthma, it is less clear whether treatment influences growth or adrenal function. The effect of inhaled beclomethasone dipropionate (400 µg/day for 7 months) on linear growth and adrenal function in 94 children aged 7–9 years has been studied in a randomized, double-blind, placebo-controlled, community-based study (9[c]). Height was measured at least monthly during treatment, and adrenal function was assessed by overnight urinary cortisol at baseline and after 3 and 6 months of treatment. Mean regressed daily growth was significantly reduced during the treatment period in those who took beclomethasone (0.79 vs. 1.14 mm/week). At the end of the 7 months, the beclomethasone-treated children had grown significantly less than the children on placebo (by a mean of 2.66 vs. 3.66 cm). Growth was significantly reduced in both boys and girls. During a washout period of 4 months, there was no significant catch-up growth. Beclomethasone had no effect on overnight urinary cortisol production. Thus, beclomethasone in a dosage taken by many children with mild asthma significantly reduces growth; this effect is unlikely to be mediated via the hypothalamo—pituitary—adrenal axis.

Growth retardation occurred in a 9-year-old boy who had taken an anti-allergic formulation that contained 0.25 mg of betamethasone and 2 mg of *d*-chlorpheniramine maleate per tablet for about 2 years for allergic rhinitis. His growth hormone reserve was slightly reduced (with responses to 3,4-dihydroxyphenylalanine, GH-releasing factor, and insulin of 10.2, 8.1, and 7.6 µg/l respectively); cortisol was undetectable in the serum and urinary excretion of 17-hydroxycorticosteroids was low (0.22—0.31 mg/day). There were no physical or biochemical signs of adrenocortical insufficiency. Catch-up growth occurred when the treatment was withdrawn. This case shows that daily administration of betamethasone 0.25 mg can cause growth retardation and that we should ask about the use of drugs containing corticosteroids in patients who present with short stature (10[c]).

Two children, without a history of diabetes mellitus, were treated with prednisone and died after they developed *hyperosmolar non-ketotic hyperglycemia* (11[c]).

A 12-year-old girl had taken prednisone 30 mg/day for 2 months, tapering to zero over the next 2 months, for systemic lupus erythematosus nephritis, 1 year before presentation. Her condition had relapsed 4 months later and she was treated with prednisone 60—80 mg/day for 2 months followed by 40 mg/day for another 2 months. She noted polyuria and polydipsia 2 weeks before she was hospitalized with seizures, coma, and shock. Her blood pressure was 60/40 mmHg and her pupils were asymmetrical. Her CSF glucose concentration was 24 mmol/l, her serum glucose concentration was 67 mmol/l, and there was glycosuria. She had trace amounts of ketones in her urine, her blood urea nitrogen concentration was 15 mmol/l and her plasma osmolarity was 385 mOsmol/l. She was given intravenous fluids and insulin therapy, but died 17 h after admission.

Eight months before presentation, the second patient, a 14-year-old boy, had taken prednisone 75 mg/day for 4 weeks, tapering gradually to 10 mg every other day, for nephrotic syndrome. Six weeks before he presented with coma, his prednisone dosage had been increased to 60 mg/day, because of proteinuria. The dosage was then increased further to 80 mg/day, and 10 days later he developed frequency and urgency of urination, dysuria, and fever. On admission he was comatose, his blood pressure was undetectable, his blood urea nitrogen concentration was 13 mmol/l, his serum glucose

concentration was over 50 mmol/l, and his plasma osmolarity was 351 mOsmol/l. He was given 300 ml of an isotonic solution but died 2.5 h later. The glucose concentration in a CSF sample taken immediately after death was 40 mmol/l.

A recent case report has confirmed that a single epidural injection of a corticosteroid for lumbar radicular pain may cause *Cushing's syndrome* and *myopathy* (12[c]).

Two to 4 weeks after a 74-year-old woman had been given a epidural low-dose injection of triamcinolone 60 mg, she began to experience progressive proximal muscle weakness, mainly affecting the lower limbs. She had a moon face, a buffalo hump, and truncal obesity, consistent with Cushing's syndrome. She was unable to stand from the sitting position because of muscle weakness. Investigations showed increased excretion of urinary creatinine (124 mg/24 h), and a suppressed serum cortisol concentration (basal concentration 1 µg/100 ml). Her urinary-free cortisol concentration was also reduced (12 µg/24 h). During 16 weeks of follow-up her Cushingoid features resolved partially and her muscle strength returned to normal. Twelve weeks after she had received the epidural triamcinolone, her serum and urinary free cortisol concentrations had normalized.

Another case of iatrogenic Cushing's syndrome occurred in a 28-year-old woman who had taken betamethasone nasal drops (0.1% w/v) for 1 year for allergic rhinitis (13[c]). She presented with weight gain of 11 kg, facial swelling, and livid striae on her thighs and arms. Her 24-h urinary free cortisol was undetectable, as was her baseline 09:00 h plasma cortisol, indicating an exogenous source of corticosteroids as the cause of her Cushing's syndrome. She had used 48 bottles (10 ml of 1 mg/ml solution) of betamethasone over the year. With the use of intranasal drops rather than an aerosol spray, it is possible that significant amounts of the betamethasone were swallowed and absorbed through the gastrointestinal tract.

Severe *vasopressin-resistant polyuria* induced by intravenous administration of a therapeutic dose of dexamethasone has been reported (14[c]).

A 15-year-old girl with a brain tumor was referred for surgery. After induction of anesthesia she received dexamethasone 4 mg intravenously and developed massive polyuria with an hourly diuresis of up to 1250 ml. She did not respond to vasopressin in doses well above those normally used. She did not fulfil any known cause of diabetes insipidus.

Mineral and fluid balance   *Hypocalcemic encephalopathy* occurred in a 35-year-old woman with hypoparathyroidism. She presented with altered sensorium and frequent generalized seizures of short duration 10 h after she had received methylprednisolone 80 mg intramuscularly for an acute exacerbation of rheumatoid arthritis. She was found to have hypoparathyroidism with Albright's osteodystrophy, and it was believed that the administration of methylprednisolone had precipitated severe hypocalcemia which had led to a metabolic encephalopathy (15^c).

Gastrointestinal   *Hypertrophy of the tongue* is a possible adverse effect of inhaled beclomethasone in premature infants, as suggested by the following cases (16^c).

Three infants (one girl and two boys), who had been delivered prematurely at 26—29 weeks of gestation, were given inhaled salbutamol (albuterol) and beclomethasone 50 μg 4—8 times daily for bronchopulmonary dysplasia at the age of 2.5—6 months; all had previously received systemic corticosteroids. Severe hypertrophy of the tongue developed after 1—1.5 months of treatment. The baby girl also had oral candidiasis. Her tongue enlargement caused feeding problems and recurrent apnea. She was changed to systemic corticosteroid therapy and the hypertrophy of her tongue resolved within a month. One of the boys was also changed to systemic corticosteroids. He subsequently died of his pre-existing respiratory complications at the age of 7.5 months. The other boy's dosage of inhaled beclomethasone was gradually tapered over a 2-month period from eight to two inhalations per day. The hypertrophy of his tongue resolved over the next 4 months and his tongue appeared normal when he was seen at 1 year of age.

The author commented that tongue hypertrophy in these infants may have been related to edema of the buccal mucosa and tongue from direct contact with inhaled corticosteroids, infection, glossitis caused by corticosteroid therapy, a direct effect of corticosteroids on the tongue muscle, or excess localized deposition of fat, as is seen in patients given systemic corticosteroids.

Histamine H$_2$ receptor antagonists have been recommended to prevent the gastrointestinal complications of corticosteroids in preterm neonates, even though there is no evidence to support this. Three babies were treated with intravenous cimetidine for the start of dexamethasone therapy for chronic lung disease; they developed gastrointestinal complications (17^c).

Two premature baby boys began a 6-week course of dexamethasone (dosage not stated) on days 9 and 10, along with intravenous cimetidine 10 mg/kg/day. After 3—6 days of treatment, there was abdominal distension and X-rays showed pneumoperitoneum. Dexamethasone was stopped in both cases, but cimetidine was continued. One of the boys had an abdominal drain inserted. He subsequently developed post-hemorrhagic hydrocephalus and his pulmonary disease worsened. He died on day 18. Autopsy showed a jejunal perforation near its junction with the duodenum and there was peritonitis at the site of the perforation. The other boy had a perforation of the bowel and resection and ileostomy were performed. He was extubated at 6 weeks of age and was later discharged. Neither of these neonates had evidence of necrotizing enterocolitis or ischemia. Another baby boy began dexamethasone (dosage not stated) and cimetidine 10 mg/kg/day on day nine. Five days later he developed an acute upper gastrointestinal hemorrhage and 20 ml of blood was aspirated from his stomach. Dexamethasone was stopped, but cimetidine was continued, and he did not experience any further bleeding.

The recommendation that H$_2$ receptor antagonists should be given with steroid therapy may be premature, and requires testing with a randomized controlled trial.

Skin and appendages   In a large case-control study, potential cases of *toxic epidermal necrolysis* and *Stevens-Johnson syndrome* were collected in four European countries (France, Portugal, Italy, and Germany) (18^C). There was a significant relation with corticosteroid use in the preceding week (multivariate analysis relative risk: 4.4, 95% CI 1.9—10), or when prescribed for long-term therapy (crude relative risk for use less than 2 months: 54, 95% CI 23—124). The estimates of excess risks associated with corticoids or sulphonamides (which are well known to cause these syndromes), expressed as the number of cases attributable to the drug per million users in 1 week, were 1.5 and 4.5, respectively. The authors did not have an explanation for this surprising finding, but the association does not appear to be due to underlying diseases for which the drugs were sometimes used or the use of other drugs associated with these syndromes.

Delayed *systemic allergic reactions* to systemic corticosteroids are rare. The literature has been reviewed, with a description of the clinical features and diagnostic procedures in the 24 reported cases (19[R]).

Adverse effects have been reported in two patients who were exposed to corticosteroids by patch-testing.

A 28-year-old woman with a history of intermittent facial reddening was patch-tested with a standard series. She returned 12 days later with localized erythema, papules, and vesiculation at the site of application of tixocortol pivalate 1% (20[c]).

A 16-year-old girl with type II hereditary angio-edema and a history of atopic eczema, was patch-tested for facial dermatitis with the European standard series. Twenty-four hours later she developed angio-edema, with severe swelling of her face. The only positive reaction was to tixocortol pivalate at 2 and 4 days (21[c]).

Allergy is an infrequent adverse reaction to corticosteroids. In some cases the event has not been produced by hypersensitivity but by a non-immune mechanism. Two cases of *pseudo-allergic reactions* have recently been described (22[c]).

One of the patients, a 40-year-old man presented on two occasions with pruritic wheals on his trunk and arms and conjunctival congestion after the administration of single doses of dexamethasone sulphate (2 mg intramuscularly) and paramethasone. The other patient was a 24-year-old woman with a history of water-induced urticaria. She had received an intra-articular injection of paramethasone and mepivacaine and 10 min later presented with coughing, chest pain, wheals, generalized itching, and angio-edema affecting her face, tongue, hands, and feet. Both patients were investigated to determine the possible allergic origin of these reactions. Skin tests (intradermal reaction and prick test) were negative, and IgE—ELISA reactivity to paramethasone was not detected in serum samples. A challenge test was performed with extreme precautions and after obtaining informed consent. The patients received different steroids (prednisone, methylprednisolone, dexamethasone, betamethasone, paramethasone) and excipients contained in the pharmaceutical formulation of paramethasone. The male patient's challenge was only positive to paramethasone, but the female patient responded positively to prednisone, betamethasone, and paramethasone.

The authors considered that these adverse effects had been caused by a pseudo-allergic reaction because of the lack of response to skin tests and ELISA tests.

Special senses With advances in neonatal intensive care, survival of extremely low-birth-weight infants (under 1 kg) has increased significantly over the past decade. Dexamethasone is used increasingly for the prevention and treatment of chronic lung disease in these infants. The impact of dexamethasone therapy on the incidence or severity of *retinopathy of prematurity* remains controversial. A retrospective study of the association between short-term dexamethasone treatment and severe retinopathy of prematurity has been performed in 309 infants of extremely low birth weight from October 1989 to December 1992 (23[c]). In all, 266 infants (86%) survived until hospital discharge; of these, 90 weighed less than 1 kg. Of 90 infants 38 received short-term dexamethasone therapy for chronic lung disease and the other 52 did not. Infants treated with dexamethasone and those not treated with dexamethasone were comparable in birth weight, gestational age, and occurrence of sepsis. Infants treated with dexamethasone required longer periods of mechanical ventilation (44 vs. 26 days), had a longer duration of supplemental oxygen (57 vs. 29 days), had a higher incidence of patent ductus arteriosus (28/38 vs. 18/52), and required surfactant therapy more often for respiratory distress syndrome (17/38 vs. 11/52). Severe retinopathy of prematurity developed in 16 infants (stage III or higher); 12 of these were in the dexamethasone-treated group. Cryotherapy was required in 13 infants, nine from the dexamethasone-treated group. This study has shown an apparent association between the incidence of severe retinopathy of prematurity and dexamethasone therapy. Prospective, randomized, controlled studies are needed to correct for differences in severity of cardiorespiratory disease. Until such studies are available, careful consideration must be given to indications, dosage, time of initiation, and duration of treatment with dexamethasone in infants of extremely low birth weight.

Infectious crystalline keratopathy developed in a 73-year-old woman with non-insulin-dependent diabetes mellitus after the use of topical prednisolone, 1% eye drops, for conjunctival injection over 12 months (24[c]).

Band-shaped keratopathy is caused by the deposition of calcium salts in the basement membrane of the corneal epithelium and superficial stroma. It is typically a chronic process that develops over a period of months and years, and is associated with chronic corneal or intraocular inflammation. Acute-onset calcific band keratopathy has been reported in a woman using topical prednisolone (25[c]).

A 60-year-old woman with severe dry eyes developed a small central calcific band across the left cornea within 72 h of first using topical prednisolone sodium phosphate. The band enlarged progressively to cover the entire cornea over the next 48 h.

Patients with severe keratoconjunctivitis sicca are at definite risk of this complication, and the addition of phosphate-containing eye drops tilted the precariously balanced situation towards precipitation of calcium in the cornea and bandage contact lens. Acetate-containing rather than phosphate-containing steroid eye drops may be a safer alternative in patients with such predisposing factors.

Retinal hemorrhage occurred in four women after they had received epidural methylprednisolone for chronic back and hip pain (26[c]). Three of them experienced visual disturbances immediately after a single epidural injection of methylprednisolone 80 mg.

The first patient, aged 35 years, noticed reduced visual acuity in her left eye associated with scattered paracentral scotomata. The second patient, aged 53 years, reported 'red dots' in the visual field of her left eye, and the third patient, 35 years old, noticed a large 'floater' in her right eye. The fourth woman, aged 81, had reduced visual acuity in both eyes associated with bilateral positive paracentral scotomata immediately after second and third epidural injections of methylprednisolone 80 mg. The hemorrhages resolved in all the patients over several weeks to 3 months. Three of the patients experienced resolution of their visual symptoms over the same period; however, one continued to describe 'blank spots' and the outcome was not stated on the article.

Although there are warnings that corticosteroid tablets and eye drops can cause *cataracts* and *glaucoma*, there is no specific warning that topical steroid ointments may also cause these adverse effects. Long-term topical corticosteroid ointment has now been reported to cause cataracts, glaucoma, and femoral avascular necrosis (27[c]).

A 30-year-old man with discoid eczema on his face, chest, and arm applied topical beclomethasone 0.025% for 4 years on his arms and diflucortolone 0.1% on his face for 1 year, followed by hydrocortisone 2.5% for 3 years. After 5 years he presented with blurred vision. His visual acuities were 6/9 in the right eye and 6/12 in the left. There were cataracts in both eyes and his intraocular pressure was 40 mmHg in both eyes. He was given timolol eye drops, which controlled his intraocular pressure, and he underwent a successful cataract operation on both eyes. Six months later, he presented with a 4-month history of a painful hip. He had steroid-induced femoral avascular necrosis that, at the time of the last assessment, did not require surgery.

The ocular hypertensive response to corticosteroids is well established. However, *increased intraocular pressure* secondary to corticosteroids by nasal spray or inhalation has rarely been reported. Increased ocular hypertension occurred in three patients after treatment with beclomethasone (dosages not stated) by nasal spray and inhalation (28[c]).

A 71-year-old man used a beclomethasone nasal spray for perennial rhinitis. Five months later the intraocular pressure was 37 mmHg in his right eye and 27 mmHg in his left eye. Beclomethasone was stopped and he was treated with timolol and dipivefrine eye drops. After 4 weeks the intraocular pressure was 14 mmHg in his right eye and 16 mm Hg in the left.

A 61-year-old woman used a beclomethasone nasal spray (duration of treatment not stated) for bronchial asthma. The intraocular pressure was 32 mmHg in both eyes. She was treated with dipivefrine eye drops and after 2 weeks the intraocular pressure was 20 mmHg in each eye.

A 60-year-old man had intraocular pressures of 34 mmHg in his right eye and 33 mmHg in his left eye about 3 years after he began using a beclomethasone inhaler for bronchial asthma. The increase in intraocular pressure was corrected with pilocarpine eye drops. He was not able to discontinue beclomethasone owing to his asthma, and so he continued to take pilocarpine to control intraocular pressure.

Patients treated with inhaled and nasal corticosteroids should be under surveillance for intraocular pressure and optic nerve function.

Steroid-induced ocular hypertension is generally attributed to alterations in the trabecular meshwork, reducing aqueous outflow. A patient has been described who had several episodes of steroid-induced ocular hypertension, with unremitting intraocular pressures, above 50 mmHg, despite maximal hypotensive medication. The trabecular meshwork was bypassed with a successful Molteno seton to lower the pressure into the teens. The eye was then challenged with topical steroid on two occasions. The pressure rose, only to fall again with steroid withdrawal. Ocular hypertension was still induced with the application of topical steroid (29[c]).

Injection of slow-release corticosteroids into the posterior space under Tenon's capsule is of value in the treatment of cystoid macular edema secondary to uveitis. Complications of the treatment include cataracts, glaucoma, and blepharoptosis (30[C]) and increased intraocular pressure (31[C]). In a case series, seven patients aged 47—84 years underwent excision of depot triamcinolone in one eye (32[C]). Six of seven eyes required surgical intervention for a medically unresponsive rise in intraocular pressure. Pharmacologically active triamcinolone was identified up to 13 (range 3—13) months after injection. The mean amount in the excised sample was 5.4 (range 2.0—8.8) mg, and the mean percentage of the original sample remaining was 20% (range 4.2—44). Glaucoma was diagnosed a mean of 3 (range 1—6) months after injection. Mean intraocular pressure was 37 mmHg before excision and 16 mmHg after removal. Surgical excision of visible triamcinolone normalized intraocular pressure in six of seven patients without need for glaucoma medication.

Further evidence, from three patients aged 27—53 years, has appeared that systemic corticosteroid treatment may cause severe exacerbation of bullous exudative retinal detachment and lasting visual loss in some patients with idiopathic central serous chorioretinopathy (33[c]). The aims of this report were to emphasize the importance of recognizing the atypical presentation of the condition, to demonstrate that it may include peripheral retinal capillary non-perfusion and retinal neovascularization, and to demonstrate further circumstantial evidence that systemic corticosteroid therapy may have an adverse affect on the severity and course of this

disease. Although the sequence of events in the three subjects of this report has provided circumstantial evidence that corticosteroid treatment had an adverse affect on the course of the pathology, a definite cause and effect relation between corticosteroid use and severity of the disease cannot be established. The treatment of choice in patients with idiopathic central serous chorioretinopathy is laser photocoagulation.

Steroid-induced osteoporosis and osteonecrosis

The use of corticosteroids is associated with reduced bone mineral density, bone loss, osteoporosis, and fractures. These adverse effects have been described during the long-term use of steroids by any route of administration.

Relation to dosage *The effects of long-term inhaled steroids have been evaluated in adults with asthma (26 men and 43 women, 41 of whom were postmenopausal) after treatment with inhaled steroids for 10 (SD 5) years (34[C]). The results showed that the daily dose, but not the duration of use, of inhaled steroids reduced bone density, and that estrogen therapy may offset the bone-depleting effects of corticosteroids in postmenopausal women.*

The possible effects of low-dose glucocorticoids on bone loss are still controversial. In a cohort of elderly Japanese Americans, 1094 women (mean age 64) and 1378 men (mean age 68 years), corticosteroid users (19 women and 21 men) had used glucocorticoids on a regular basis for over 1 month (mean use 2 years, mean dose 5 mg/day of prednisone) (35[C]). The densities of the calcaneus and radius were measured at 1- to 2-year intervals, with an 8-year follow-up. Initial bone density was similar between users of corticosteroids and non-users. Both women and men using corticosteroids had double bone loss rates than controls. The differences persisted after adjustment for confounding variables (age and use of thiazides or estrogens). The authors concluded that low-dosage corticosteroids increase rates of bone loss in both elderly women and men.

A significant reduction of bone mineral den-

sity has been described in 139 patients with rheumatoid arthritis treated with low-dosage corticosteroids (36^C). The patients who took $1-4$ mg/day had the same density as those who were not taking steroids. Patients who took $5-9$ mg/day and those who took more than 10 mg/day had significantly lower bone density (84 and 81% of control values, respectively). Although corticosteroid use seems to be an important factor for low mineral density, sex hormones have also been suggested as an important determinant of bone mineral content.

Mechanisms and risk factors Various mechanisms are involved in the production of steroid-induced osteoporosis (37^R). The major change is a reduction in osteoblast activity that results in a reduced working rate (mean appositional rate), and a reduced active life-span of osteoblasts. The cellular mechanism seems to be related to diminished production of cytokines and other locally acting factors. Increased bone resorption and decreased calcium absorption have also been described.

A sophisticated mathematical model has been used to describe changes in calcium kinetics in patients treated with steroids (38^C). Plasma calcium concentrations were higher than in controls, with a marked reduction in calcium flow into the irreversible stable bone compartment in corticosteroid-treated patients. The authors concluded that prednisone has direct effects on osteoblast function.

The rapid loss of bone mineral after organ and tissue transplant associated with immunosuppressive therapy is widely recognised. Losses of 7 and 9% at 6 and 12 months have been reported in the lumbar spine. The long-term effects of immunosuppressive therapy on bone density has been determined in 25 cardiac transplant patients (39^C). As expected, there was rapid bone loss in the spine during the first year, but this was not maintained during the second and third years of transplant, despite continuing maintenance immunosuppression with prednisolone. Only four patients, all of whom were hypogonadal, continued to lose bone. It seems that if therapy to reduce the rapid loss is begun soon after transplantation, prolonged treatment may not be necessary.

Bone mineral density and sex hormone status have been studied in 99 men with rheu-matoid arthritis and 68 age-matched controls (40^C). There were significant reductions in lumbar and femoral density, and salivary testosterone, androstenedione, and dehydroepiandrosterone in rheumatoid patients. Salivary testosterone correlated with femoral density. By multiple regression analysis, weight, serum testosterone concentrations, and cumulative dose of corticosteroid were significant predictors of lumbar bone density. Weight, age, androstenedione concentrations, and cumulative dose of corticosteroids were significant predictors of femoral bone density.

Patients with inflammatory bowel disease have reduced bone mineral content and density that can result in osteoporosis. The prevalence and risk factors for low bone mineral density have been assessed in 152 patients with inflammatory bowel disease in comparison with 73 healthy controls (41^C). Corticosteroid use was a clear risk factor, especially in those whose lifetime corticosteroid dose was over 10 g. The patients who had never taken oral steroids did not have reduced bone mineral density.

The frequency of musculoskeletal damage, including avascular necrosis of bone, osteoporosis, and fractures, has been determined in a cohort of 407 patients with systemic lupus erythematosus (42^C). Prednisolone in dosages over 20 mg/day increased the risk of avascular necrosis (odds ratio 2.3; 95% CI $1.16-4.57$); other predictors were the presence of vasculitis and Raynaud's phenomenon. Higher dosages of prednisone acted as a predictor for the appearance of osteoporosis. Predictors of fracture were age, prednisone (both cumulative and highest dose), avascular necrosis, postmenopausal status, and prior identification of osteopenia.

In a cross-sectional study, bone mineral densities at the ultradistal and midshaft radius, hip, and lumbar spine of 1677 community controls (aged $56-91$ years) were compared with those of 34 users of inhaled and 44 users of oral corticosteroids (43^C). Women who used oral corticosteroids had significantly lower bone density in midshaft radius, hip and spine than never-users. Women who used inhaled steroids had bone densities at ultradistal radius and spine that were intermediate between those of oral corticosteroid users and those of *never-users. Bone mineral density did not vary significantly in male corticosteroid users.*

Complications   *The most severe complication of osteoporosis is the appearance of fractures. Some studies have investigated the relation between the use of corticosteroids and the risks of hip and vertebral fractures in rheumatoid arthritis. A population-based case−control comparison has been carried out in 300 consecutive patients with hip fracture aged 50 years and over and 600 age- and sex-matched controls (44[C]). The results showed that the risk of hip fracture was increased in patients with rheumatoid arthritis (OR 2.1, 95% CI 1.0−4.7). The use of corticosteroids increased the risk in patients who did not have rheumatoid arthritis (OR 2.8, CI 95% 1.2−6.5), and in those who did (OR 2.9, 95% CI 0.6−15).*

Patients with rheumatoid arthritis either currently using (n = 52) or not using (n = 55) corticosteroids have been evaluated by X-radiology of the thoracic and lumbar vertebral spine and clinical symptoms related to fractures (45[C]). Seven of the patients taking corticosteroids had vertebral fractures versus one in the control group. There was no correlation between deformity scores and the cumulative dose of prednisone.

The prevalence of vertebral fractures has been determined in 76 postmenopausal women (aged 59−79 years) with steroid-treated rheumatoid arthritis, and 347 age-matched women (46[C]). Patients were assessed using spinal radiography and lumbar spine bone mineral density measurements. Vertebral fracture was more common in the women with rheumatoid arthritis (OR 6.2, 95% CI 3.2−12.3); the bone density measure was a bad predictor of vertebral fractures.

Management   *The management of corticosteroid-induced osteoporosis has recently been reviewed by the UK Consensus Group Meeting on Osteoporosis (37[R]).*

The efficacy of different drugs in the treatment or prophylaxis of steroid-induced osteoporosis has been assessed in some recent studies. Cyclical etidronate (400 mg/day for 2 weeks every 3 months) plus ergocalciferol (0.5 mg/week) has been given to 15 postmenopausal women (mean age 63 years) starting corticosteroid therapy (prednisone 5−20 mg/day)

(47[C]). A control group of 11 postmenopausal women (mean age 60 years) with corticosteroid-induced osteoporosis were treated with calcium supplements only (1 g/day). Lumbar spine and femoral neck bone mineral densities were measured at baseline and at 12 and 24 months of glucocorticoid therapy. During the first year, the cyclical regimen significantly increased lumbar and femoral neck bone density compared with placebo (7 and 2.5%, respectively for spine and femur). After the second year of cyclical therapy, femoral neck bone density continued to increase while lumbar spine density remained stable.

Fluoride is a potent stimulator of trabecular bone formation. Sodium monofluorophosphate has been given to 48 patients with osteoporosis due to corticosteroids (more than 10 mg of prednisone equivalents/day) (48[C]). Patients were randomly allocated to 1 g of calcium carbonate (control) or 200 mg of sodium monofluorophosphate plus 1 g of calcium carbonate for 18 months. At the end of the study lumbar spine bone density had increased by 7.8% in the fluoride group vs. 3.3% in the controls. There were no changes in femoral neck density.

Growth hormone is a potent anabolic agent that stimulates protein synthesis, cell growth, and osteoblast activity. Recombinant human growth hormone has been used in patients taking long-term corticosteroid treatment with suppressed endogenous growth hormone responses to GH-releasing hormone (49[C]). A single daily dose of 0.1 IU/kg of human growth hormone was given subcutaneously to nine non-obese patients (seven women and two men, mean age 61 years, mean dosage of prednisone 7.8 mg/day). There was a significant increase in nitrogen balance, osteocalcin, carboxy-terminal propeptide of type I procollagen, and carboxy-terminal telopeptide of type I collagen. Growth hormone also lowered total high-density lipoprotein, and low-density lipoprotein cholesterol. These preliminary data suggest that growth hormone could ameliorate some adverse effects induced by long-term glucocorticoids.

Infections and infestations   There is a well-known association between systemic corticosteroid use and an increased risk of infections, including those produced by rare pathogens. A case of acute disseminated *Aspergillus fumigatus* sepsis has been described in a 39-year-old woman treated with corticosteroids for systemic lupus erythematosus (50[c]).

Severe varicella has been described in an immunocompetent 5-year-old girl treated with inhaled beclomethasone dipropionate for asthma (51[c]). She required hospitalization and intravenous acyclovir. Although there are few descriptions of chickenpox in patients treated with aerosolized corticosteroids, the author recommended that when possible aerosolized corticosteroids should be discontinued in asthmatic patients after exposure to chickenpox.

It has been suggested that *Varicella zoster* immunoglobulin should be given to patients in contact with chicken-pox if they have taken steroids in dosages over 0.5 mg/kg/day during the preceding 3 months, in the context of near-fatal chickenpox in a child receiving prednisolone (52[cr]) (see also SEDA-19, 378).

There is some concern about the use of corticosteroids as adjunctive therapy for patients with AIDS who develop *Pneumocystis carinii* pneumonia. The immunosuppressant properties of steroids have been reported to enhance the risk of tuberculosis and other AIDS-related diseases (e.g. Kaposi's sarcoma or cytomegalovirus infection). In a retrospective study, corticosteroid use during *Pneumocystis carinii* pneumonia (mean total dose methylprednisolone 420 mg, mean treatment duration 12 days) did not enhance the risk of development or relapse of tuberculosis or other AIDS-related diseases (53[c]). The study included 129 patients (72 who took steroids and 57 who did not) who were followed up at 6, 12, 18, and 24 months of steroid therapy. The rates of infections were similar in both groups, and the cumulative rate of developing tuberculosis at 2 years was 12—13%.

A case of *Pneumocystis carinii* pneumonia has been described in a 3.5-year-old asthmatic boy treated with inhaled triamcinolone (54[c]). He had a 1-week history of intermittent wheezing and dyspnea, and was admitted to the intensive care unit for respiratory failure. Bronchoscopic lavage fluid was positive for *Pneumocystis carinii*. Immune studies showed immunocompetence. This seems to have been the first description of *Pneumocystis carinii*

pneumonia in an immunocompetent patient treated with inhaled corticosteroids.

Reactivation of *tuberculous peritonitis* after corticosteroid therapy has been reported in a 41-year-old woman who was given methylprednisolone 32 mg/day for 4 weeks for acute alcoholic hepatitis, and 3 months later developed peritonitis (55[c]).

Symptoms of *bronchial asthma* worsened in four patients after treatment with parenteral corticosteroids, due to superinfection with the nematode *Strongyloides stercoralis* (56[c]). The patients suffered a new attack or exacerbation of asthma that appeared to be precipitated by systemic corticosteroids. Paradoxical worsening of asthma after corticosteroid treatment was the major pulmonary manifestation of *Strongyloides* superinfection. The subjects had eosinophilia, high IgE concentrations, and *Strongyloides* in the stools. When the infection was diagnosed, the symptoms of asthma improved when corticosteroids (oral or parenteral) were withheld or the dosages reduced. After treatment with thiabendazole, an inappropriate response to corticosteroids during subsequent episodes of asthma was no longer observed.

Miscellaneous Significant differences in the pharmacokinetics of methylprednisolone have been described in black and white renal transplant patients (57[C]). The authors selected nine patients of each race, with similar demographic and pathological characteristics, who received the same daily dose of methylprednisolone (11 mg/day). Black patients had a slower clearance rate and a lower apparent volume of distribution. Blacks had higher cortisol concentrations throughout the day, with higher nadir concentrations. Most of the patients had moon face (nine black, eight white). While five of the black patients had steroid-associated diabetes, no white patients did. Further studies are needed to define the differences between the races.

Use in pregnancy Corticosteroids have been recommended in pregnancy to prevent respiratory distress syndrome in the neonate. A meta-analysis of 15 trials, involving 1780 patients treated with corticosteroids and 1780 controls, has demonstrated a lower risk of contracting the syndrome, and a substantial reduction in neonatal mortality (OR 0.60, 95% CI 0.48—0.76), without a higher risk of infection in the mother or maternal pulmonary edema (58[R]).

Preterm labor   The effects of corticosteroids on uterine activity and preterm labor in high-order multiple gestations have been retrospectively reviewed (59[C]). In 15 women with triplet or quadruplet pregnancies, 17/57 courses of betamethasone were associated with episodes of significant *contractions* requiring tocolytic intervention; 11 of these episodes were associated with cervical change and four resulted in premature delivery. The authors did not recommend the use of corticosteroids if patients have more than 3.5 contractions per hour.

SPECIAL FORMS OF ADMINISTRATION
(SED-13, 1204; SEDA-17, 449; SEDA-18, 391; SEDA-19, 379)

Epidural corticosteroids

Epidural steroids are often used in the treatment of low back pain, but their effects can be seen in the endocrine system. A recent case report (12[c]) has been discussed above in the section on endocrine effects.

The occurrence of *facial flushing* after intra-articular steroid administration for the management of capsulitis of the shoulder and after cervical epidural steroid injection has been reported. However, facial flushing and erythema after lumbar epidural steroid administration have not previously been reported. Of 1399 epidural steroid injections for patients with chronic radicular pain, 1021 were performed at the lumbar level and the remaining 378 were cervical epidural injections; there was facial flushing and/or generalized erythema in 12 patients, aged 24—86 years, after the epidural administration of triamcinolone diacetate 80 or 120 mg (60[C]). The mean time to onset of reaction was 27 h after injection. The reactions were typically described as a 'sunburn' or generalized redness. Once a reaction had occurred, an average of 72 h was required for complete resolution.

REFERENCES

1. Konishi Y, Hayakawa K, Kuriyama M, Saito M, Fujiii Y, Sudo M. Effects of ACTH on brain midline structures in infants with infantile spasms. Pediatr Neurol 1995;13:134—6.
2. Sato A, Funder JW, Okubo M, Kubota E, Saruta T. Glucocorticoid-induced hypertension in the elderly. Relation to serum calcium and family history of essential hypertension. Am J Hypertens 1995;8:823—8.
3. Haney I, Lachance C, van Doesburg NH, Fouron JC. Reversible steroid-induced hypertrophic cardiomyopathy with left ventricular outflow tract obstruction in two newborns. Am J Perinatol 1995;12:271—4.
4. Sato O, Takagi A, Miyata T, Takayama Y. Aortic aneurysms in patients with autoimmune disorders treated with corticosteroids. Eur J Vasc Endovasc Surg 1995;10:366—9.
5. Williamson IJ, Matusiewicz SP, Brown PH, Greening AP, Crompton GK. Frequency of voice problems and cough in patients using pressurized aerosol inhaled steroid preparations. Eur Respir J 1995;8:590—2.
6. Zentner J, Buchbender K, Vahlensieck M. Spinal epidural lipomatosis as a complication of prolonged corticosteroid therapy. J Neurosurg Sci 1995;39:81—5.

7. Silva RG, Tolstunov L. Steroid-induced psychosis: report of case. J Oral Maxillofac Surg 1995;53:183—6.
8. Lynn DJ. Lithium in steroid-induced depression. Br J Psychiatry 1995;166:264.
9. Doull IJ, Freezer NJ, Holgate ST. Growth of prepubertal children with mild asthma treated with inhaled beclomethasone dipropionate. Am J Respir Crit Care Med 1995;151:1715—9.
10. Nishikawa M, Hikosaka M, Yonemoto T, Gondou A, Tabata S, Ogawa Y, Kanasaki M, Miyake Y, Shimizu H, Shouzu A, Inada M. A case of iatrogenic growth retardation induced by a corticosteroid-containing anti-allergic drug. Horm Metab Res 1995;27:376—8.
11. Yang JY, Cui XL, He XJ. Non-ketotic hyperosmolar coma complicating steroid treatment in childhood nephrosis. Pediatr Nephrol 1995;9:621—2.
12. Boonen S, van Distel G, Westhovens R, Dequeker J. Steroid myopathy induced by epidural triamcinolone injection. Br J Rheumatol 1995;34:385—6.
13. Nutting CM, Page SR. Iatrogenic Cushing's syndrome due to nasal betamethasone: a problem not to be sniffed at! Postgrad Med J 1995;71:231—2.

14. Toftegaard M, Knudsen F. Massive vasopressin-resistant polyuria induced by dexamethasone. Intensive Care Med 1995;21:238—40.

15. Handa R, Wali JP, Singh RI, Aggarwal P. Corticosteroids precipitating hypocalcemic encephalopathy in hypoparathyroidism. Ann Emerg Med 1995;26:241—2.

16. Linder N, Kuint J, German B, Lubin D, Loewenthal R. Hypertrophy of the tongue associated with inhaled corticosteroid therapy in premature infants. J Pediatr 1995;127:651—3.

17. McDonnell M, Evans N. Upper and lower gastrointestinal complications with dexamethasone despite H_2 antagonists. J Paediatr Child Health 1995;31:152—4.

18. Roujeau JC, Kelly JP, Naldi L, Rzany B, Stern RS, Anderson T, Auquier A, Bastuji-Garin S, Correia O, Locati F, Mockenhaupt M, Paoletti C, Shapiro S, Shear N, SchHpf E, Kaufman DW. Medication use and risk of Stevens-Johnson syndrome or toxic epidermal necrolysis. New Engl J Med 1995;333:1600—7.

19. Withmore SE. Delayed systemic allergic reactions to corticosteroids. Contact Dermatitis 1995;32:193—8.

20. Goldsmith PC, White IR, Rycroft RJG, Mc Fadden JP. Probable active sensitization to tixocortol pivalate. Contact Dermatitis 1995;33:429.

21. Parry EJ, Lever RS. An unusual complication of patch testing. Contact Dermatitis 1995;32:179.

22. Valdivieso R, Subiza J, Subiza JL, Narganes MJ, Cabrera M. Pseudo-allergic reactions to corticosteroids: diagnosis and alternatives. J Invest Allergol Clin Immunol 1995;5:171—4.

23. Ramanathan R, Siassi B, de Lemos RA. Severe retinopathy of prematurity in extremely low birth weight infants after short-term dexamethasone therapy. J Perinatol 1995;15:178—82.

24. Apel A, Campbell I, Rootman DS. Infectious crystalline keratopathy following trabeculectomy and low-dose topical steroids. Cornea 1995;14:321—3.

25. Rao GP, O'Brien C, Hicky-Dwyer M, Patterson A. Rapid onset bilateral calcific band keratopathy associated with phosphate-containing steroid eye drops. Eur J Implant Refractive Surg 1995;7:251—2.

26. Kushner FH, Olson JC. Retinal hemorrhage as a consequence of epidural steroid injection. Arch Ophthalmol 1995;113:309—13.

27. McLean CJ, Lobo RFJ, Brazier DJ. Cataracts, glaucoma, and femoral avascular necrosis caused by topical corticosteroid ointment. Lancet 1995;345:330.

28. Opatowsky I, Feldman RM, Gross R, Feldman ST. Intraocular pressure elevation associated with inhalation and nasal corticosteroids. Ophthalmology 1995;102:177—9.

29. Muecke J, Brian G. Steroid-induced ocular hypertension in the presence of a functioning Molteno seton. Aust NZ J Ophthalmol 1995;23:67—8.

30. Yoshikawa K, Kotake S, Ichiishi A, Sasamoto Y, Kosaka S, Matsuda H. Posterior sub-Tenon injections of repository corticosteroids in uveitis patients with cystoid macular edema. Jpn J Ophthalmol 1995;39:71—6.

31. Helm CJ, Holland GN. The effects of posterior subtenon injection of triamcinolone acetonide in patients with intermediate uveitis. Am J Ophthalmol 1995;120:55—64.

32. Kalina PH, Erie JC, Rosenbaum L. Biochemical quantification of triamcinolone in subconjunctival depots. Arch Ophthalmol 1995;113:867—9.

33. Gass JD, Little H. Bilateral bullous exudative retinal detachment complicating idiopathic central serous chorioretinopathy during systemic corticosteroid therapy. Ophthalmology 1995;102:737—47.

34. Toogod JH, Baskerville JC, Markov AE, Hodsman AB, Fraher LJ, Jennings B, Haddad RG, Drost D. Bone mineral density and the risk of fracture in patients receiving long-term inhaled steroid therapy for asthma. J Allergy Clin Immunol 1995;96:157—66.

35. Saito JK, Davis JW, Wasnich RD, Ross PD. Users of low-dose glucocorticoids have increased bone loss rates: a longitudinal study. Calcif Tissue Int 1995;57:115—9.

36. Buckley LM, Leib ES, Cartularo KS, Vacek PM, Cooper SM. Effects of low dose corticosteroids on the bone mineral density of patients with rheumatoid arthritis. J Rheumatol 1995;22:1055—9.

37. Eastel R, on behalf of a UK Consensus Group Meeting on Osteoporosis. Management of corticosteroid-induced osteoporosis. J Intern Med 1995;237:419—47.

38. Goans RE, Weiss GH, Abrams SA, Perez MD, Yergey AL. Calcium tracer kinetics show decreased irreversible flow to bone in glucocorticoid treated patients. Calcif Tissue Int 1995;56:533—5.

39. Henderson NK, Sambrook PN, Kelly PJ, MacDonald P, Kcogh AM, Spratt P, Eisman JA. Bone mineral loss and recovery after cardiac transplantation. Lancet 1995;346:905.

40. Mateo L, Nolla JM, Bonnin MR, Navarro MA, Roig-Escofet D. Sex hormone status and bone mineral density in men with rheumatoid arthritis. J Rheumatol 1995;22:1455—60.

41. Silvennoinen JA, Karttunen TJ, Niemel SE, Manelius JJ, Lehtola JK. A controlled study of bone mineral density in patients with inflammatory bowel disease. Gut 1995;37:71—6.

42. Petri M. Musculoskeletal complications of systemic lupus erythematosus in the Hopkins lupus cohort: an update. Arthritis Care Res 1995;8:137—45.

43. Marystone JF, Barrett-Connor EL, Morton DJ. Inhaled and oral corticosteroids: their effects on bone mineral density in older adults. Am J Public Health 1995;85:1693—5.

44. Cooper C, Coupland C, Mitchell M. Rheuma-

toid arthritis, corticosteroid therapy and hip fracture. Ann Rheum Dis 1995;54:49—52.

45. Lems WF, Zahangier ZN, Jacobs JWG, Bulsma JWJ. Vertebral fractures in patients with rheumatoid arthritis treated with corticosteroids. Clin Exp Rheumatol 1995;13:293—7.

46. Peel NFA, Moore DJ, Barrington NA, Bax DE, Eastell R. Risk of vertebral fracture and relationship to bone mineral density in steroid treated rheumatoid arthritis. Ann Rheum Dis 1995;54:801—6.

47. Diamond T, McGuigan L, Bargallo S, Bryant C. Cyclical etidronate plus ergocalciferol prevents glucocorticoid-induced bone loss in postmenopausal women. Am J Med 1995;98:459—63.

48. Rizzoli R, Chevaley T, Slosman DO, Bonjour JP. Sodium monofluorophosphate increases vertebral bone mineral density in patients with corticosteroid-induced osteoporosis. Osteoporosis Int 1995;5:39—45.

49. Giustina A, Bussi AR, Jacobello C, Weherenberg WB. Effects of recombinant human growth hormone (GH) on bone and intermediary metabolism in patients receiving chronic glucocorticoid treatment with suppressed endogenous GH response to GH-releasing hormone. J Clin Endocrinol Metab 1995;80:122—9.

50. Nenoff P, Horn LC, Mierzwa M, Leonhart R, Weidenbach H, Lehman I, Haustein UF. Peracute disseminated fatal *Aspergillus fumigatus* sepsis as a complication of corticoid-treated systemic lupus erythematosus. Mycoses 1995;38:467—71.

51. Choong K, Zwaigenhaum L, Onyett H. Severe varicella after low dose inhaled corticosteroids. Pediatr Infect Dis J 1995;14:809—11.

52. Burnett I. Severe chickenpox during treatment with corticosteroids. Immunoglobulin should be given if steroid dosage was > or =0.5 mg/kg/day in preceding three months. Br Med J 1995;310:327 (erratum 534).

53. Martos A, Podzamczer D, Mart7nez-Lacasa J, Rufi G, Santin M, Gudiol F. Steroids do not enhance the risk of developing tuberculosis or other AIDS-related diseases in HIV-infected patients treated for *Pneumocystis carinii* pneumonia. AIDS 1995;9:1037—41.

54. Lilibeth MT, Chin TW, Nussbaum E. *Pneumocystis carinii* pneumonia associated with inhaled corticosteroids in an immunocompetent child with asthma. J Pediatr 1995;127:1000—2.

55. Korula J. Tuberculous peritonitis complicating corticosteroid therapy for acute alcoholic hepatitis. Dig Dis Sci 1995;40:2119—20.

56. Sen P, Gil C, Estrellas B, Middleton JR. Corticosteroid-induced asthma: a manifestation of limited hyperinfection syndrome due to *Strongyloides stercoralis*. Southern Med J 1995;88:923—7.

57. Tornatore KM, Biocevich DM, Reed K, Tousley K, Peter-Singh J, Venuto RC. Methylprednisolone pharmacokinetics, cortisol response, and adverse effects in blacks, and white renal transplant recipients. Transplantation 1995;59:729—36.

58. Crowley PA. Antenatal corticosteroid therapy: a meta-analysis of the randomized trials, 1972 to 1994. Am J Obstet Gynecol 1995;173:322—35.

59. Elliott JP, Radin TG. The effect of corticosteroid administration on uterine activity and preterm labour in high-order multiple gestations. Obstet Gynecol 1995;85:250—4.

60. DeSio JM, Kahn CH, Warfield CA. Facial flushing and/or generalized erythema after epidural steroid injection. Anesth Analg 1995;80:617—9.

A. Buitenhuis and C.J. van Boxtel

40 Sex hormones and related compounds, including hormonal contraceptives

ESTROGENS AND PROGESTOGENS

Estrogens *(SED-13, 1255; SEDA-17, 462; SEDA-18, 394; SEDA-19, 386)*

Endocrine, metabolic *Cholestatic jaundice* has been reported with oral estrogens and is probably related to an effect on the permeability of the canalicular membrane (1[cr]). The first case of cholestatic jaundice induced by a subcutaneous estrogen implant in the absence of any other cause of liver disease has been reported (1[cr]). At presentation the implant was removed and found to have spontaneously fragmented. After removal the patient's symptoms resolved. The authors' explanation was that fragmentation of the implant led to the release of excessive amounts of estradiol.

Hormone replacement therapy (HRT)

On the ground of the balance of benefits and risks of estrogen HRT the American College of Physicians has recommended that all postmenopausal women be considered for treatment and that the decision to treat or not to treat should be made on individual grounds (2[R]).

Cardiovascular Estrogen replacement in HRT reduces cardiovascular risk by about 50% in postmenopausal women (2[R]), (3[C]). The greatest improvement in total mortality occurs in women with significant coronary stenosis, in women whose serum cholesterol concentrations are over 6 mmol/l (235 mg/dl),

and in non-smokers. In women with severe coronary stenoses the 10-year survival was 97% in users and 60% in non-users, a statistically significant difference (2[R]). The most important predictor of occlusion was total plasma cholesterol; there was a significant benefit from HRT in non-smoking women with lower cholesterol concentrations. In women smokers whose cholesterol concentrations were less than 6 mmol/l (235 mg/dl) there was no significant benefit.

In a group of 2268 women undergoing coronary arteriography, 446 had no detectable coronary artery disease, and differences in 5- and 10-year survival between estrogen users and non-users were not statistically significant (2[R]). In 644 women with mild-to-moderate disease 10-year survival was 96% in the users and 85% in the non-users, a statistically significant difference. It is not yet known how the cardiovascular benefit of estrogen HRT is affected by the addition of a progestogen in women with a uterus.

No more than 30—50% of the cardioprotective effect of estrogen HRT can be explained by improvements in serum lipids, i.e. increased concentrations of HDL cholesterol and triglycerides and reduced concentrations of LDL and total cholesterol. Unopposed estrogen is the optimal regimen for increasing HDL cholesterol (3[C]). It is very likely that vasodilatation also plays a significant role in the cardioprotective effect of estrogen HRT. This vasodilatation is mediated by the endothelial production of prostaglandin I_2. Other plausible mechanisms are effects on coagulation factors and endothelial function. For women with a uterus most of the favorable effects of estrogen can be preserved by adding micronized progesterone (3[C]).

Nervous system   In 54 women estrogen therapy was associated with better performance on a variety of intellectual tests (4[C]). Estrogen may therefore protect against postmenopausal intellectual decline. Exogenous estrogen is also involved not only in the control of reproductive behavior but also in problem solving, cognitive function, and mood. This holds not only for exogenous estrogens but also for variations in estrogen across the natural menstrual cycle. The effects of exogenous estrogens on mood last for only a short time after the start of therapy (4[C]).

Musculoskeletal   Estrogen-related bone loss, resulting in *osteoporosis*, occurs especially during the first 5 years after the menopause (5[R]). However, bone mineral content is maintained when women take estrogen HRT. If there are no contraindications (thromboembolic disease, thrombophlebitis, estrogen-dependent tumors, pregnancy, and abnormal genital bleeding without a diagnosis), estrogen HRT should be given as soon after the menopause as possible. The earlier a women begins taking estrogen the less bone mass she is likely to lose. If she has an intact uterus a progestogen should also be prescribed.

How long estrogen HRT should be continued for is a question of debate and depends on the indication.

- For relief of vasomotor symptoms therapy may be as short as 6—12 months and may be gradually tapered off to prevent recurrence of symptoms (5[R]).
- For prevention of osteoporosis some experts have recommended life-long use of estrogen; when women taking estrogen plus progestogen are switched to placebo bone mineral content is reduced (5[R]).
- For cardiovascular benefits women may require lifelong ERT (5[R]).

Women smokers may have increased activity of the hepatic estrogen-metabolizing enzymes. These women are at an increased risk of an early menopause and may not benefit as much from the effects of estrogen HRT as non-smokers (5[R]). In addition to smoking, other exogenous risk factors for osteoporosis are: excessive alcohol use, a low level of weight-bearing exercise, excessive caffeine ingestion, and a low calcium intake.

The effect of combined therapy with estrogen and etidronate on bone mineral density in the hip and vertebrae has been studied in a 4-year, prospective, randomized study in 58 early postmenopausal patients randomly allocated to four treatment groups (6[C]). All received 1.0 g/day of elemental calcium, and in addition group 1 received percutaneous estrogen and oral micronized progesterone (HRT), group 2 intermittent cyclical etidronate (ICE), group 3 HRT and ICE, and group 4 calcium alone. In patients treated with HRT and calcium there was a positive effect on hip and vertebral bone. Patients treated with ICE and calcium had a similar effect in vertebral bone but only a small increase in bone mineral density, in the hip. In addition mineralization defects were observed in the bones of patients treated with etidronate. These defects could not be prevented with the addition of 1.0 g/day of elemental calcium (the manufacturer's currently recommended regimen). This means that bone strength at the femoral neck may be compromised in postmenopausal women treated with long-term etidronate. The effect of combined treatment (group 3) was additive in increasing bone mineral density over 4 years in vertebral bone (11%) and in the hip (7%). Treatment with HRT and calcium had a significantly smaller effect compared with combined therapy. Adverse effects were minor and partly due to the calcium rather than the HRT.

The increase in bone mass has been studied in 32 postmenopausal woman over 60 years of age with low mineral bone density after 1 year of percutaneous estradiol implants (75 mg). In addition, 14 women with an intact uterus were given cyclical dydrogesterone 10 mg for the first 12 days of each calendar month in order to prevent endometrial hyperplasia (7[C]). The median increase in mineral bone density was 13% in the lumbar spine and 5% in the total hip. The increase in vertebral bone density was greatest in women with low initial bone density and in those with highest treatment estradiol concentrations. The increase in bone mass was dose dependent. Adverse effects were the return of the monthly withdrawal bleed, increased urinary frequency and incontinence, weight gain, and transient mastalgia.

Other hormonal replacement therapy (HRT)

An alternative method of HRT has been described, using the three natural types of sex steroids synthesized by the ovary: androgens, progestogens, and estrogens (8^R). Androgens maintain muscle mass and strength, bone density, skin and libido. Sex steroids should be given in doses that achieve premenopausal concentrations of the deficient hormones. Natural estradiol and progesterone and micronized testosterone with or without dehydroepiandrosterone, an androgen precursor hormone secreted by the adrenals, are preferred because of potential disadvantages of the synthetic derivatives.

Combined estrogen–progestogen replacement therapy

Progestogens alone help to prevent osteoporosis. Adding a progestogen to adequate dosages of estrogen promotes new bone formation, restores bone that has been lost, reduces the risk of carcinoma of the breast, and (in the long term) does not reduce HDL cholesterol (9^R).

The most important adverse effect of the progestogen component is withdrawal bleeding (97% of patients up to age 60). The estrogen component can cause premenstrual syndrome-like symptoms, bloating, edema, breast tenderness, and a feeling of abdominal pressure (9^R). These symptoms are caused by estrogen-related fluid retention and can be at least 50% relieved by a mild diuretic, given for 7–10 days before the menses or during the last days of added progestogen.

Cardiovascular Six patients with intracranial venous thrombosis related to oral contraceptives have been described (10^{cr}). One had been given an estrogen-containing formulation (Metrulen-M) for menopausal symptoms. A further case of *thrombosis of the straight sinus* has been reported in a patient taking HRT (Estraderm TTS 100) (10^{cr}). There was no family history of clotting disorders. There were no other risk factors for sinus thrombosis, such as head injury, infection, dehydration, diabetes, or congenital heart disease. The authors suggested that dural sinus throm-

bosis is a rare but dangerous complication of HRT. The patient was discharged completely well after 14 days and was advised not to restart HRT.

Bleeding in patients with the diffuse form of antral vascular ectasia can be treated with an estrogen/progestogen combination (11^c). This therapy is recommended before considering endoscopic thermoablation or surgical antrectomy. Patients (women or men) can for example be treated with ethinylestradiol 0.05 mg plus norethindrone acetate 1 mg/day. The only adverse effect is mild *gynecomastia*, which can be controlled with danazol. This therapy does not eradicate the vascular malformations, but only stops the bleeding, as has been shown in a controlled clinical trial of 10 patients bleeding from angiodysplasias in the upper and lower gastrointestinal tract; discontinuation of the hormone therapy resulted in recurrence of the bleeding (11^c).

Transdermal estrogen therapy

Transdermal estrogen therapy is at least as effective in relieving climacteric symptoms as oral estrogen (12^C)r. The efficacy and tolerability of Menorest 50 and Estraderm TTS 50 have been compared in a randomized, multicenter, parallel-group study of 205 patients (12^C)r. The two treatments were therapeutically equivalent, and there were no statistically significant differences between the two formulations as assessed by either investigator or patient. Most of the adverse effects were mild to moderate. Five patients in the Menorest group and five in the reservoir transdermal patch group experienced severe adverse events. In the Menorest group the adverse events were *skin reactions at the site of application, depression, migraine, nausea, vomiting, edema*, and *sleep disorders*, and in the transdermal patch group bone pain, *allergic reactions, weakness, back pain, arthralgia*, and *reactions at the site of application*. No adverse events were life-threatening or required hospitalization. Menorest has better local tolerability, due in part to the absence of alcohol as a solvent in the adhesive matrix system.

Nervous system During the menopause many women become depressed and irritable, and transdermal estradiol has a mood-lifting effect (13[CR]). However, data supporting the assumption that estrogen deprivation is the root cause of this depression are equivocal. The antidepressant and vigilance-promoting properties of transdermal estrogen have been studied in post-menopausal depression in a 3-month, double-blind, placebo-controlled study in 69 women (13[CR]). In the placebo group estradiol and follicle-stimulating hormone (FSH) remained unchanged. In the group treated with Estraderm TTS (ETTS, 50 g twice weekly) estradiol rose and FSH fell significantly. There was no inter-group difference in the Hamilton Depression Rating scale. EEG mapping showed significant inter-drug differences in brain function, suggesting improved vigilance from estrogen, previously referred to as 'mental tonic' or 'mood lifting' effect. Additional evidence for this is that ovariectomized women who take estrogen have better short-term memory than those who take placebo and that improved vigilance is correlated with better memory. The authors found a significant correlation between estradiol concentrations and vigilance: the lower the estradiol concentrations, the lower the α activity, the higher the β activity, and the higher the centroid of the α and of the total power spectrum. In the treatment group 82% of the 27 patients had no adverse effects. Adverse effects in the others were *petechiae, reactions at the site of application, redness, itchiness*, and *allergy*.

Estradiol can be used in combination with other psychotherapeutic drugs for the medical management of physically aggressive patients with dementia. The frequency of aggressive behavior, agitation, hallucinations, and suspiciousness in five men with dementia fell during treatment with transdermal estradiol from almost daily to one episode per week (14[c]). They were able to discontinue or reduce other medications being used to control their behavior, medications that have more serious adverse effects than transdermal estradiol (for example, parkinsonism, tardive dyskinesia, and postural hypotension).

Progestogens *(SED-13; 1262; SEDA-17, 466)*

In a multicenter, prospective, double-blind, randomized, parallel-group study undertaken by 45 general practitioners to compare progesterone pessaries with placebo in the relief of symptoms of premenstrual syndrome, spontaneous reports of adverse events were recorded (15[C]). In all, 281 patients were screened for premenstrual syndrome; of these, 141 patients were randomized to treatment or placebo groups. The response to progesterone was significantly greater than to placebo during each cycle. Patients taking active therapy reported more frequent *irregularity of menstruation, vaginal pruritus*, and *headache*.

Medroxyprogesterone acetate *(SED-13, 1263)*

The use of depot medroxyprogesterone has been studied in the management of benign prostatic hyperplasia in 80 patients in a double-blind, placebo-controlled study (16[C]). The patients were randomized to placebo or medroxyprogesterone 150 mg as a single intramuscular injection. After 3 months the following changes were seen with medroxyprogesterone:

- serum testosterone reached castration concentrations within 3 days but did not change in the placebo group;
- prostatic volume was reduced by 25% (3% with placebo);
- maximum urinary flow rates increased by 3.7 ml/s (from 9.5 to 13.2) compared with placebo (9.4—9.5);
- total urinary symptom scores fell by 4.9 points compared with a non-significant fall with placebo.

Medroxyprogesterone improved the quality of life, since it did not produce hot flushes. Important adverse effects, which occurred more often than with placebo, were *impotence, reduced libido*, and *a reduced volume of ejaculate*.

Oral contraceptives *(SED-13, 1211; SEDA-17, 459; SEDA-19, 381)*

Cardiovascular The risks of cardiovascular illness in otherwise healthy women exposed to one of three oral contraceptives containing less than 35 µg of estrogen plus levonorgestrel, desogestrel, or gestodene have been compared (17[C]). There were 15 cases of *unexpected cardiovascular death* among 303 470 women. The estimated incidence rates were

4.3 per 100 000 women-years at risk for users of combined oral contraceptives containing levonorgestrel, 1.5 per 100 000 for desogestrel users, and 4.8 per 100 000 for gestodene users. The relative risk estimates compared with levonorgestrel were 0.4 (95% CI 0.1—2.1) and 1.4 (0.5—4.5) for desogestrel and gestodene, respectively.

In the same study (17[C]) there were 80 cases of *non-fatal venous thromboembolism* among 238 130 women. The estimated incidence rates per 100 000 women-years were 16.1 for levonorgestrel, 29.3 for desogestrel, and 28.1 for gestodene. The adjusted relative risk estimates from the cohort analysis compared with levonorgestrel were 1.9 (1.1—3.2) and 1.8 (1.0—3.2) for desogestrel and gestodene, respectively. The excess risk for non-fatal venous thromboembolism associated with the new generation of combined oral contraceptives containing low-dose estrogen and the progestogens desogestrel and gestodene compared with levonorgestrel is estimated to be 16 per 100 000 woman-years.

Neurological The effects of Microgynon and Diane-35, two sub-50-µg ovulation inhibitors, on voice function in women have been studied in 91 patients over a period of 1 year (18[C]). Adverse effects on the voice were not demonstrated. Women taking Diane-35 had less intracycle bleeding and amenorrhea. Acne was more favorably affected by Diane-35 (which contains cyproterone acetate), perhaps partly due to its pronounced anti-androgenic effect. Blood pressure remained unchanged during the study.

Endocrine, metabolic The effect of a combination of ethinylestradiol plus drospirenone (a progestogen with natriuretic properties) on body weight, blood pressure, the renin—aldosterone system, atrial natriuretic factor, plasma lipids, and glucose tolerance have been investigated (19[C]) in four groups of 20 women aged 18—34 years who each took for 6 months: (A) 30 µg ethinylestradiol plus 3 mg drospirenone; (B) 20 µg ethinylestradiol plus 3 mg drospirenone; (C) 15 µg ethinylestradiol plus 3 mg drospirenone; (D) 30 µg ethinylestradiol plus 150 mg levonorgestrel (Microgynon).

Mean body weight fell by 0.8—1.7 kg in groups A, B, and C and rose by 0.7 kg in group D. Systolic and diastolic blood pressures fell by 1—4 mmHg in groups A, B, and C and increased by 1—2 mmHg in group D. Plasma renin activity and plasma aldosterone rose significantly in the drospirenone groups, presumably due to sodium loss. In these groups HDL cholesterol rose, in contrast to group D. LDL cholesterol fell slightly, whereas triglyceride concentrations rose more in the drospirenone groups than in group D. The most frequently reported adverse effects were headache and breast tenderness, more in group D than in the drospirenone groups.

In the comparison of Microgynon and Diane cited above (18[C]) *weight gain* occurred more often in the women who took Diane-35.

Gastrointestinal Reversible *ischemic colitis* has been described in 17 young women, with evidence for an association with oral contraceptives (20[C]). Ischemic colitis occurs uncommonly in younger people. The authors described 18 young adults (mean age 29, range 17—39 years) with spontaneous ischemic colitis, 17 of whom were women. The median duration of illness was 2.1 days (range 1—4 days). All recovered with supportive care. Ten women (59%) were using low-dose estrogenic oral contraceptive agents, compared with the 1988 US average of 18.5% oral contraceptive users among women aged 15—44 years. The odds ratio showed a greater than six-fold relative risk for the occurrence of ischemic colitis among oral contraceptive users. Among the 18 young patients with reversible, left-sided, segmental ischemic colitis, sites of involvement included the distal transverse colon ($n = 3$), left colonic flexure ($n = 3$), descending colon ($n = 5$), and sigmoid colon ($n = 7$).

Second-generation effects *Use in pregnancy* Oral contraceptives are taken inadvertently by 2—5% of women in early pregnancy (21[R]). Fear of adverse fetal effects secondary to sex hormone exposure leads many women to consider terminating otherwise wanted pregnancies. A meta-analysis has been performed to determine if exposure during the first trimester of pregnancy to sex hormones in general, and to oral contraceptives in particular, is associated with an increased risk of external genital malformations in the fetus. Seven cohort studies and seven case-control studies, involving 65 567 women, met the criteria for meta-analysis. The overall summary odds ratio was 1.09 (95% CI 0.90—1.32); subanalysis of oral contraceptive exposure identified an odds ratio of 0.98 (95% CI 0.24—3.94). The authors concluded that there was no association between first trimester exposure to sex hormones generally (or to oral contraceptives specifically) and external genital malformations. Thus, women exposed to sex hormones after conception may be assured that there is no increased risk of fetal sexual malformation. This study was limited to the first trimester, because the sexual differentiation of internal genital ducts and external genitalia along either male or female lines is complete by 12—14 weeks gestation.

ANDROGENIC AND ANABOLIC STEROIDS AND RELATED COMPOUNDS (SED-13, 1265)

The effects of testosterone enanthate or placebo on regional fat distribution and health risk factors have been compared in 30 obese middle-aged men undergoing weight loss by dietary means (22[C]). An oral anabolic steroid (oxandrolone) reduced subcutaneous abdominal fat more than testosterone or weight loss alone. Both steroid treatments were well tolerated, with minimal adverse effects, for example *increased energy*, *reduced appetite*, *irritability*, *gastrointestinal adverse effects*, and *sleeplessness*.

Cyproterone acetate-containing formulations (SED-13, 1267)

The beneficial and adverse effects of long-term treatment with cyproterone acetate have been described (23[C]). The degree of androgenization was assessed in 143 of 188 women treated since 1968. The results were good to very good in 75% of patients with hirsutism and in more than 90% of patients with acne. Adverse events were recorded in 23% of cases. Most were mild and transient and required withdrawal in only 9% of patients. The adverse effects were: *weakness*, *depression*,

irritability headache (6%); *increased body weight* (5%); *mastodynia, galactorrhea* (4%); *amenorrhea, breakthrough bleeding* (4%); *nausea and other gastrointestinal complaints* (1%); *reduced libido* (1%); *chloasma* (1%); *thrombophlebitis* (one case); *hypertension* (one case).

Danazol (SED-13, 1267; SEDA-18, 399)

The current management of endometriosis has been reviewed (24[R]). Danazol, which is used in this disease, inhibits the secretion of follicle-stimulating hormone (FSH) and luteinizing hormone (LH). These effects reduce the secretion of estrogen and progesterone from the ovary and thereby remove hormonal support of endometriotic implants. Adverse effects occur in up to 80% of patients, and include *weight gain, fluid retention, acne, reduced breast size, atrophic vaginitis, hot flushes, muscle cramps*, and *emotional lability*.

The effect of danazol-induced chronic hyperglucagonemia on glucose tolerance and turnover has been studied in six patients before and after treatment with danazol for immune thrombocytopenia (25[c]). Plasma glucagon concentrations rose significantly from 88 pg/ml before to 683 pg/ml after therapy. Glucose concentrations during an oral glucose tolerance test were not significantly different before and after therapy. Glucose-stimulated insulin secretion at 60 and 120 min and the area under the curve for insulin during the oral glucose tolerance test were significantly increased after danazol compared with pre-treatment values. The authors concluded that chronic glucagon excess leads to a *reduction in peripheral and hepatic insulin action*, accompanied by an *increase in insulin secretion*. Attention was subsequently drawn to the fact that danazol often causes liver damage in patients with idiopathic thrombocytopenic purpura that fails to respond to glucocorticoids and splenectomy (26[C])r. The frequency of liver damage in patients with endometriosis is markedly lower (15%) than in patients with idiopathic thrombocytopenic purpura (85%). These findings suggest that glucocorticoids increase the incidence of liver disease due to danazol.

Insulin-like growth factor-I

Long-term growth hormone treatment of healthy elderly men with low concentrations of insulin-like growth factor-I (IGF-I) is associated with a high incidence of adverse effects: of 62 patients, *carpal tunnel syndrome* occurred in 10, *gynecomastia* in four, and *hyperglycemia* in three (27[R]). The authors suggested that adverse effects might be minimized by carefully monitoring the dose of growth hormone and adjusting it to produce optimum IGF-I concentrations. Long-term growth hormone treatment of healthy elderly women is also accompanied by frequent adverse effects: *arthralgia, joint swelling, carpal tunnel swelling* and *fluid retention*. IGF-I has acute insulin-like effects and long-term anabolic effects on lean body tissues. Its adverse effects are mild and give no reason for interrupting therapy. Prominent adverse effects were *hypoglycemia* in four of six patients, *parotid tenderness* in two of six, and *headache* in 10 of 13 patients.

Testosterone supplementation in older men with low-normal testosterone concentrations can produce apparent benefits, for example an increase in lean body mass by 3%, an increase in urinary creatinine excretion of 12%, increased libido, and an enhanced sense of well-being. Adverse effects of testosterone supplementation are *rising concentrations of prostate specific antigen*, suggesting prostate stimulation and the appearance of prostate carcinoma, *worsening of the symptoms of obstructive uropathy*, and *an increased number of strokes and transient ischemic attacks*. Patients should be screened to rule out prostate cancer before treatment and carefully followed to detect signs of prostate complications and an abnormally high hematocrit during treatment.

ANTIANDROGENS *(SED-13, 1267)*

Antiandrogens are used in the treatment of hyperandrogenic conditions in women, for example polycystic ovary syndrome, idiopathic hirsutism, acne, seborrhea, and hair loss. In men they are used in the treatment of prostatic cancer. Antiandrogens may cause significant adverse effects because of interactions with androgen receptors, but also with receptors for progesterone, glucocorticoids, and mineralocorticoids, and because of their various enzyme activities (28[R]).

Endocrine, metabolic   Androgens may explain the higher prevalence of *atherosclerosis* in men than in women. Hyperandrogenemia in women is associated with an increase in LDL cholesterol, due to increased hepatic lipase activity, which enhances the catabolism of VLDL cholesterol by the liver. Androgens may also cause increased degradation and reduced serum concentrations of HDL cholesterol, resulting in an unfavorable LDL/HDL ratio.

Finasteride *(SEDA-18, 321)*

The effects of finasteride and placebo on quality of life have been evaluated for 12 months in a diverse population of 2342 men with benign prostatic hyperplasia (29[C]). Symptom scores fell significantly at month three in those taking finasteride and continued to improve throughout the study. The incidence of drug-related *sexual adverse experiences* was significantly higher in the finasteride group, but led to withdrawal in only 1.5% of patients.

The effects of finasteride for 9 months on hirsutism and serum concentrations of basal gonadotropin, androgens, estrogen, and sex hormone-binding globulin have been in studied 18 women with idiopathic hirsutism (30[C]). Nine hirsute patients took oral finasteride 7.5 mg/day, the other nine placebo. Hirsutism and the laboratory measurements were evaluated in all patients before and every 3 months during treatment. Hirsutism improved significantly with finasteride after 6 and 9 months; there were no significant effects with placebo. Adverse effects were *headache* and *modest depression* during the first month. Libido did not change. Hirsute patients treated with finasteride had a marked fall in dihydrotestosterone from the third month and a significant increase in serum testosterone concentrations from the sixth month of treatment.

Sexual function   The commonest adverse effect of finasteride is *erectile impotence* (5% of patients) (31[R]). A few men complain of *decreased ejaculatory volume*. It seems wise to avoid the use in men who actively want to father a child.

Interference with diagnostic routines Finasteride causes a 45% *fall in prostate-specific antigen concentrations* (31[R]).

Flutamide *(SED 13, 1269)*

Flutamide is the only antiandrogen that specifically blocks the androgen receptor. In a comparison of the safety and efficacy of oral flutamide (125 mg bd) alone and in combination with a triphasic oral contraceptive in 33 women with idiopathic hirsutism, there was a statistically significant reduction in hirsutism after 3 months with flutamide alone or flutamide with an oral contraceptive (32[C]). Flutamide alone did not change the serum lipoprotein concentrations, but in combination with a triphasic formulation it significantly increased HDL cholesterol. The major adverse effects were *skin dryness* (54%) and *increased appetite* (22%) without associated weight gain.

The effectiveness of the antiandrogen flutamide has also been studied for a period of 24 months in 25 patients with polycystic ovary syndrome and severe hirsutism (33[C]). There was marked reduction of hirsutism. No important hormonal changes or adverse effects were observed.

Liver In a 12-month study in 18 women with hirsutism, flutamide was well tolerated, except by one woman, who had an *increase in serum aspartate aminotransferase and alanine aminotransferase* to three times the upper limits of the reference ranges in the absence of other plausible causes of liver damage (34[C]). These alterations reversed completely within 3 months of withdrawal.

Hematological A patient with flutamide-induced *methemoglobinemia* has been described (35[c]).

Spironolactone *(SED-13, 575; SEDA-19, 162, 218, 219, 326)*

Besides being an aldosterone antagonist, spironolactone is also a potent antiandrogen and has a direct inhibitory effect on 5α-reductase. Initially it may cause *polyuria, polydipsia, weakness*, and *fatigue*, but its diuretic ef-

fects are usually limited to the first few days of treatment. Its long-term adverse effects are usually minor but may occur often (91% of patients) and include *menstrual disturbances* (22%), *breast enlargement and tenderness* (26%), and *dizziness* (26%).

GONADOTROPHINS AND OVULATION-INDUCING DRUGS *(SED-13, 1259)*

The development and uses of antagonists of luteinizing hormone-releasing hormone (LHRH) in the treatment of infertility have been reviewed (36[R]). LHRH binds to specific transmembrane receptors in gonadotrophic cells, causing a micro-aggregation of these receptors and complex formation. This complex formation is crucial for the action of LHRH. LHRH is liberated in a pulsatile manner at intervals of 70—90 min, and circulating LHRH has a half-life of 2—5 min. Because of this short half-life, hypothalamic pulses of LHRH are recognized as single events by the pituitary receptors. This mechanism is important in the maintenance of normal ovarian function. LHRH agonists have a 100—200 times higher binding affinity for LHRH receptors. These agonists initially liberate large amounts of FSH and LH (the undesirable flare-up effect) and up-regulate LHRH receptors. If they are used continuously they cause down-regulation of LHRH receptors as a result of degradation of the agonist/receptor complex by lysosomal enzymes. The pituitary becomes refractory to LHRH, resulting in reduced concentrations of LH and FSH and arrest of follicular development. The fall in LH and FSH is followed by a fall of sex steroid concentrations to the castrate range. This pituitary blockade reverses after withdrawal. A normal menstrual cycle is re-established after about 6 weeks.

LHRH antagonists produce an immediate effect by competitive blockade of LHRH receptors, resulting in a fall in LH and FSH. Withdrawal causes a surge of LH, followed by a postovulatory rise in progesterone in all women. The LH surges can be blocked by injecting LHRH antagonists during the periovulatory period. This suggests that endogenous LHRH is required for the estradiol-induced surge of LH.

Endocrine, metabolic In contrast to LHRH agonists, LHRH antagonists do not cause exhaustion of the pituitary, resulting in an almost immediate response to an adequate stimulus, for example in patients pretreated with the LHRH antagonist cetrorelix in an IVF program (36[R]). Cetrorelix has a half-life of 30 h after a single dose and about 80 h after multiple injections. Subcutaneous injection of 3 mg of cetrorelix in female volunteers resulted in spotting in three subjects but no systemic adverse effects. The injection of other antagonists occasionally gave considerable *local inflammation, subcutaneous induration* for up to 3 weeks, and *local erythema* lasting for up to 2 days (36[R]). Cetrorelix is not teratogenic.

Recombinant and urinary follicle-stimulating hormone have been compared in an in vitro fertilization program in a randomized, assessor-blind, multicenter study (37[C]). The subjects received recombinant FSH ($n = 585$) or urinary FSH ($n = 396$). Significantly more oocytes were retrieved after recombinant FSH treatment (10.8 vs. 9.0). With respect to safety there were no clinically relevant differences between recombinant and urinary FSH and no cases of ovarian hyperstimulation syndrome.

Ovarian stimulation has been studied in women undergoing in vitro fertilization and embryo transfer using recombinant human follicle-stimulating hormone (GONAL-F) in non-down-regulated cycles in 71 patients (38[C]). There was a pregnancy rate of 24% per transfer. The dominant adverse effect was mild *pain at the site of injection* in under 20% of patients. There were two cases of *ovarian hyperstimulation syndrome*. In under 10% of patients *redness, swelling, or bruising* were reported. One patient developed *headache*. In conclusion, recombinant FSH is very attractive to patients in non-down-regulated cycles, because it does not come from a human source and it can be self-administered subcutaneously.

'Prolonged coasting', a method for preventing ovarian hyperstimulation syndrome, has been studied in 51 women who were inadvertently severely overstimulated with menotrophins, with peak plasma estradiol concentrations of over 6000 pg/ml (39[C]). Prolonged coasting involved withholding the menotrophins and human chorionic gonadotrophin and continuing a gonadotrophin-releasing hormone agonist until the plasma estradiol concentration fell to below 3000 pg/ml. The reported adverse effects were two spontaneous abortions and four multiple gestations. None of the women developed severe ovarian hyperstimulation syndrome. There were 21 pregnancies resulting in 19 births.

Immunological and hypersensitivity reactions
Some adverse effects of the LHRH antagonists are due to the existence of LHRH receptors on mast cells, which degranulate after binding of basic antagonists, producing *general edema, induration, local erythema,* and *anaphylactoid reactions*. These allergic effects and the hydrophobicity of some antagonists, which results in gel formation after the injection, have hampered the development of antagonists. Some of the LHRH antagonists (for example, Nal-Glu) combine continuous suppression of LH with delay in ovulation, without a significant effect on FSH. This might be advantageous in the treatment of polycystic ovarian disease, which is often associated with an unfavorable LH/FSH ratio (36[R]).

Cabergoline *(SED-13, 360; SEDA-17, 169)*

Cabergoline has a high affinity for dopamine D_2 receptors and is a very long-acting inhibitor of prolactin secretion (40[R]). It can be used for treating hyperprolactinemic amenorrhea (in which it restores ovulatory cycles in 72% of women) and for the prevention or suppression of puerperal lactation. It appears to be better tolerated than bromocriptine in both patients with hyperprolactinemia and post-partum women.

Adverse events have been reported in up to 68% of patients with hyperprolactinemia and in 16% of puerperal women.

Nervous system: *nausea/vomiting* (35%), *headache/migraine* (30%), *dizziness/vertigo* (25%), *drowsiness, somnolence, paresthesia*.

Hematological: *hemoglobin concentrations fell slightly* during cabergoline therapy in a significant proportion of 162 patients (41[C]). This adverse effect is almost certainly related to restoration of the menses.

Miscellaneous: *diarrhea, dyspnea, a sensation of suffocation, epistaxis, pleuropulmonary disease* (three cases).

The severity of adverse events was

generally mild to moderate, but 14% were classified as severe. Because of adverse events 3% of patients stopped cabergoline therapy.

Second-generation effects A total of 82 cabergoline-associated pregnancies have been reported in published literature and a further 140 in unpublished studies. The outcome of 199 evaluable pregnancies was as follows: normal births, 68%; elective abortion, 14%; spontaneous abortion, 12%; abnormalities at birth, 3.5%; therapeutic abortions, 2.0%; fetal death in utero, 0.5%.

In addition there have been three cases of *major congenital malformations* and one *tubal pregnancy*.

These figures are consistent with the incidence of malformations observed in the general population and in bromocriptine-associated pregnancies.

Clomiphene *(SED-13, 1260; SEDA-17, 466)*

The possible teratogenic effects of periconceptional use of clomiphene citrate has been reviewed in a pooled analysis of controlled epidemiological studies (42[R]). The estimated summary prevalence ratio was 1.08 (95% CI 0.76 and 1.51). The authors concluded that their analysis suggested that an increase in the risk of *neural tube defects* due to clomiphene citrate cannot be ruled out, but that any such increase seems likely to be less than two-fold and there may be no increase at all.

Clomiphene citrate increases endogenous production of testosterone in men, an effect that has been empirically used in the treatment of infertility. The development of *non-bacterial pyospermia* has been studied in 42 non-pyospermic men with low serum testosterone concentrations treated with clomiphene citrate 25 mg/day (43[C]). The men were retrospectively compared with 27 untreated non-pyospermic men referred for evaluation of infertility. Spontaneous non-bacterial pyospermia developed more often in the treated men (14 vs. 7%). Serum testosterone increased in all the treated men. Only the treated, non-pyospermic men had improvement in sperm characteristics. The results suggested that clomiphene citrate-associated pyospermia has a negative effect on male fertility. This adverse effect occurs more often in men aged over 35 years and may be due to an adverse effect of leukocytes on sperm motility and function.

REFERENCES

1. Bowling TE, Al-Adnani M, Silk DBA. Cholestatic jaundice induced by spontaneous disruption of an oestrogen implant. Eur J Gastroenterol Hepatol 1995;7:85—6.

2. Sullivan JM. Coronary arteriography in estrogen treated postmenopausal women. Progr Cardiovasc Dis 1995;38:211—22.

3. The writing group for the postmenopausal estrogen/progestin interventions (PEPI) trial. Effects of estrogen or estrogen/progestin regimens on heart disease risk factors in post-menopausal women. J Am Med Assoc 1995;273:199—208.

4. Kimura D. Estrogen replacement therapy may protect against intellectual decline in postmenopausal women. Horm Behav 1995;29:312—21.

5. Sograves R. Estrogen therapy for postmenopausal symptoms and prevention of osteoporosis. J Clin Pharmacol 1995;35:2S—10S.

6. Wimalawansa SJ. Combined therapy with estrogen and etidronate has an additive effect on bone mineral density in the hip and vertebrae: four-year randomized study. Am J Med 1995; 99:36—42.

7. Holland EFN, Leather AT, Studd JWW. Increase in bone mass of older postmenopausal women with low mineral bone density after one year of percutaneous oestradiol implants. Br J Obstet Gynaecol 1995;102:238—42.

8. Hargrove JT, Osteen KG. An alternative method of hormone replacement therapy using the natural sex steroids. Infert Reprod Med Clin North Am 1995;6:653—674.

9. Gambrell RD. Progestogens in estrogen-replacement therapy. Clin Obstet Gynecol 1995; 38:890—901.

10. Strachan R, Hughes D, Cowie R. Thrombosis of the straight sinus complicating hormone replacement therapy. Br J Neurosurg 1995;9:805—8.

11. Manning RJ. Estrogen/progesterone treatment of diffuse antral vascular ectasia. Am J Gastroenterol 1995;90:154—6.

12. Pornel B, Genazzani AR, Costes D, Dain MP, Lelann L, Van de Pol C. Efficacy and tolerability of Menorest® 50 compared with Estraderm® TTS 50 in the treatment of postmenopausal symptoms. A randomized, multicenter, parallel group study. Maturitas 1995;22:207—18.

13. Saletu B, Brandstätter N, Metka M, Stamenkovic M, Anderer P, Semlitsch HV, Heytmanek

G, Huber J, Grunberger J, Linzmayer L, Kurz CH, Decker K, Binder G, Knogler W, Koll B. Double-blind, placebo-controlled, hormonal, syndromal and EEG mapping studies with transdermal oestradiol therapy in menopausal depression. Psychopharmacol Berlin 1995;122:321—9.

14. Kay PAJ, Yurkow J, Forman LJ, Chopra A, Cavalieri T. Transdermal estradiol in the management of aggressive behaviors in male patients with dementia. Clin Gerontol 1995;15:54—8.

15. Magill PJ. Investigation of the efficacy of progesterone pessaries in the relief of symptoms of premenstrual syndrome. Br J Gen Pract 1995; 45:589—93.

16. Onu PE. Depot medroxyprogesterone in the management of benign prostatic hyperplasia. Eur Urol 1995;28:229—35.

17. Jick H, Jick SS, Gurewich V, Wald Mijers M, Vasilakis C. Risk of idiopathic cardiovascular death and non fatal venous thromboembolism in women using oral contraceptives with differing progestogen components. Lancet 1995;346: 1589—93.

18. Wendler J, Sieger TC, Schelhorn P, Klinger G, Gurr S, Kaufmann J, Aydinlik S, Braunschweig T. The influence of Microgynon and Diane-35, two sub-fifty ovulation inhibitors, on voice function in women. Contraception 1995;52:343—8.

19. Oelkers W, Foidart JM, Dombrovicz N, Welter A, Heithecker R. Effects of a new oral contraceptive containing an antimineralocorticoid progestogen, drospirenone on the renin-aldosterone system, body weight, blood pressure, glucose tolerance and lipid metabolism. J Clin Endocrinol Metab 1995;80:1816—21.

20. Deana DG, Dean PJ. Reversibel ischemic colitis in young women. Association with oral contraceptive use. Am J Surg Pathol 1995;19:454—62.

21. Raman-Wilms L, Tseng AL, Wighardt S, Einarson TR, Koren G. Fetal genital effects of first-trimester sex hormone exposure: a meta-analysis. Obstet Gynecol 1995;85:141—9.

22. Lovejoy JC, Bray GA, Greeson CS, Klemperer M, Morris J, Partington C, Tulley R. Oral anabolic steroid treatment, but not parenteral androgen treatment, decreases abdominal fat in obese older man. Int J Obesity 1995;19:614—24.

23. van Wayjen RGA, van den Ende A. Experience in the long-term treatment of patients with hirsutism and/or acne with cyproterone acetate containing preparations: efficacy, metabolic and endocrine effects. Exp Clin Endocrinol 1995; 103:241—51.

24. Lu PY, Ory SJ. Endometriosis: current management. Mayo Clin Proc 1995;70:453—63.

25. Kotzmann H, Linkesch M, Ludvik B, Clodi M, Luger A, Schernthaner G, Prager R, Klauser R. Effect of danazol-induced chronic hyperglucagonaemia on glucose tolerance and turnover. Eur J Clin Invest 1995;25:942—7.

26. Sakuma A, Tsuboi I, Morimoto K, Sawadu U, Horie T. Liver damage after danazol and glucocorticoids for chronic idiopathic thrombocytopenic purpura (ITP). Int Med 1995;34:69.

27. Carter WJ. Effect of anabolic hormones and insulin-like growth factor-I on muscle mass and strength in elderly persons. Clin Geriatr Med 1995;11:735—48.

28. Diamanti-Kandarakis E, Tolis G, Duleba AJ. Androgens and therapeutic aspects of antiandrogens in women. J Soc Gynecol Invest 1995; 2:577—92.

29. Byrnes CA, Morton AS, Liss CL, Lippert MC, Gillenwater JY. Efficacy, tolerability, and effect on health-related quality of life of finasteride versus placebo in men with symptomatic benign prostatic hyperplasia: a community based study. CUSP Investigators. Community based study of Proscar. Clin Ther 1995;17:956—69.

30. Ciotta L, Cianci A, Calogero AE, Palumbo MA, Marletta E, Sciuto A, Palumbo G. Clinical and endocrine effects of finasteride, a 5α-reductase inhibitor in women with idiopathic hirsutism. Fertil Steril 1995;64:299—306.

31. Neal DE. Drugs in focus: finasteride. Presc J 1995;35:89—95.

32. Dodin S, Faure N, Cedrin I, Mechain C, Turcot-Lemay L, Guy J, Lemay A. Clinical efficacy and safety of low-dose flutamide alone and combined with an oral contraceptive for the treatment of idiopathic hirsutism. Clin Endocrinol 1995; 43:575—82.

33. Pucci E, Genazzani AD, Monzani F, Lippi F, Angelini F, Gargani M, Barletta D, Luisi M, Genazzani AR. Prolonged treatment of hirsutism with flutamide alone in patients affected by polycystic ovary syndrome. Gynecol Endocrinol 1995;9:221—8.

34. Moghetti P, Castello R, Negri C, Tosi F, Magnani CM, Fontanaro SAMC, Armanini D, Muggeo M. Flutamide in the treatment of hirsutism: long-term clinical effects, endocrine changes and androgen receptor behavior. Fertil Steril 1995; 64:511—17.

35. Jackson SH, Barker SJ. Methemoglobinemia in a patient receiving flutamide. Anesthesiology 1995;28:1065—7.

36. Reissmann TH, Felberbaum R, Diedrich K, Engel J, Comaru-Schally AM, Schally AV. Development and applications of luteinizing hormone-releasing hormone antagonists in the treatment of infertility: an overview. Hum Reprod 1995: 10:1974—81.

37. Out HJ, Mannaerts BMJL, Driessen SGAJ, Coeling H, Bennink HJT. A prospective, randomized, assessor-blind, multicentre study comparing recombinant and urinary follicle stimulating hormone (Puregon versus Metrodin) in invitro fertilization. Hum Reprod 1995;10:2534—40.

38. Strowitzki T, Kentenich H, Kiesel L, Neulen J, Bilger W. Ovarian stimulation in women undergoing in vitro-fertilization and embryo transfer using recombinant human follicle stimulating hormone (Gonal-F) in non-down-regulated cycles. Hum Reprod 1995;10:3097—101.

39. Sher G, Zouves C, Feinman M, Maassarani G. Prolonged coasting: an effective method for preventing severe ovarian hyperstimulation syndrome in patients undergoing in-vitro fertilization. Hum Reprod 1995;10:3107—9.

40. Rains CP, Bryson HM, Fitton A. Cabergoline. A review of its pharmacological properties and therapeutic potential in the treatment of hyperprolactinaemia and inhibition of lactation. Drugs 1995;49:255—79.

41. Webster J, Piscitelli G, Polli A, D'Alberton A, Falsetti L, Ferrari C, Fioretti P, Giordano G, L'Hermite M, Ciccarelli E et al. The efficacy and tolerability of long-term cabergoline therapy in hyperprolactinaemic disorders: an open, uncontrolled, multicentre study. European Multicentre Cabergoline Study Group. Clin Endocrinol 1993;39:323—9.

42. Greenland S, Ackerman DL. Clomiphene citrate and neural tube defects: a pooled analysis of controlled epidemiologic studies and recommendations for future studies. Fertil Steril 1995; 64:936—41.

43. Matthews GJ, Goldstein M, Henry JM, Schlegel PN. Non bacterial pyospermia: a consequence of clomiphene citrate therapy. Int J Fertil 1995;40:187—91.

J.A. Franklyn

41   Thyroid hormones and antithyroid drugs

THYROID HORMONES *(SED-13, 1275; SEDA-17, 473; SEDA-18, 406; SEDA-19, 391)*

Problems of dosage The literature continues to focus on the question of whether therapy with thyroxine (one of the most commonly prescribed drugs in the West), especially in dosages that suppress serum concentrations of thyrotrophin (TSH) to below normal, are associated with adverse effects, particularly on the heart and bone.

Cardiovascular There is increasing evidence of an adverse effect of thyroxine on the heart, especially in dosages that suppress serum TSH to below normal. The effects of TSH-suppressive therapy for 3—9 years in 25 patients have been compared with findings in 20 controls (1[C]). The thyroxine-treated patients had an *increase in left ventricular mass*, together with *prolongation of the isovolumic relaxation time* and a *reduction in diastolic filling*. These findings are in accord with those of our own studies (2[C]), which showed a marked increase in left ventricular size in patients taking long-term thyroxine. More recently, the same group (3[C]) has reported the use of radionuclide angiography to assess left ventricular function at rest and during exercise in subjects taking thyroxine. Ventricular diastolic filling, although not left ventricular systolic function, was impaired at rest. During exercise, left ventricular systolic function fell in the thyroxine-treated patients, mainly because of increased end-systolic left ventricular volume. Exercise capacity was also markedly reduced. In the light of evidence that left ventricular hypertrophy is an independent risk factor for cardiovascular morbidity, these data highlight

the need for large prospective studies of the frequency of cardiac events, including mortality, in patients taking long-term thyroxine.

Musculoskeletal A recent study in 50 women treated with thyroxine in TSH-suppressive dosages for a mean of 11 years showed no significant difference from controls in *bone mineral density* and no significant changes in bone mass 1.5 years later (4[C]).

While this report has supported previous failures to show an adverse effect of thyroxine on bone mineral density, a recent meta-analysis of 41 studies (involving 1250 patients) of the effect of thyroxine on bone mass has served to highlight the conflicting results in the literature (5[CR]). Sources of heterogeneity between studies were identified, including replacement or suppressive thyroxine therapy, menopausal status, site of bone mineral density measurement (for example, the femur or lumbar spine), and a history of hyperthyroidism (which has itself been found to be an independent risk factor for fracture of the femur in a large epidemiological study (6[C])). It was also noted that controls had often not been matched with cases for many factors that affect bone mineral density, such as body weight, ages of menarche and menopause, dietary calcium, smoking habits, alcohol consumption, and exercise. Taking these problems into account, the authors concluded that there was evidence of an adverse effect of thyroxine treatment in TSH-suppressive dosages on bone mineral density in postmenopausal women alone, whereas, surprisingly, non-suppressive dosages were associated with reductions in bone mineral density in the spine and hip in premenopausal women alone. It is clear that a large prospective study of bone mineral density at several sites and of the rates of fracture at these sites is required to settle the issue of whether thyroxine therapy causes significant morbidity via an effect upon bone metabolism.

ANTITHYROID DRUGS *(SED-13, 1279; SEDA-17, 474; SEDA-18, 406; SEDA-19, 391)*

Propylthiouracil

There have been several small series of published cases of *vasculitis* associated with propylthiouracil therapy (SEDA-17, 474). Three subjects with Graves' hyperthyroidism treated with propylthiouracil had a flu-like illness and several weeks later developed proteinuria, hematuria, and a modest degree of renal failure due to crescentic glomerulonephritis associated with antineutrophil cytoplasmic antibodies (ANCA) (7[C]). Renal failure was rapidly corrected by withdrawal of propylthiouracil and immunosuppressive therapy. While the development of ANCA-associated renal problems may be a manifestation of an underlying autoimmune disorder and Graves' disease, these case reports are similar to cases of ANCA-associated vasculitis that have previously been described (8[C]), and lend support to the view that propylthiouracil may be a factor in the development of vasculitis in a small number of patients.

IODINE AND THE IODIDES *(SED-13, 1281; SEDA-17, 475; SEDA-18, 407; SEDA-19, 392)*

Radioactive iodine (radioiodine; 131I)

Radioiodine is increasingly recommended as first-line therapy for patients with thyrotoxicosis, regardless of age and sex. Despite evidence in support of the efficacy and safety of radioiodine, doubts persist regarding the long-term risks of carcinogenesis and teratogenesis. The *fertility* of 627 women of child-bearing age who had received radioiodine for differ-

entiated thyroid cancer (in a higher dose than that used for hyperthyroidism) has been compared with the fertility of 187 women with the same diagnosis who did not receive radioiodine (9[CR]). There were no significant differences in fertility rate, birth weight, or prematurity. There was only one case of a ventricular septal defect in a child born to a mother treated with radioiodine. Furthermore, the incidence of second tumors was not higher in those who had received radioiodine therapy. While the length of follow up in this study was relatively short (only 50% of cases were more than 3 years from treatment), these data are reassuring in the context of the treatment of hyperthyroidism with radioiodine in women of child-bearing age.

The use of radioiodine has also been advocated in children with hyperthyroidism, in whom management is often difficult because of problems with drug compliance, relapse or failure to control hyperthyroidism, and adverse drug effects (10[CR]). A report of the use of radioiodine in 35 cases of childhood hyperthyroidism, which had not been cured by antithyroid drug therapy, has confirmed its efficacy, in accord with the results of previous studies (summarized in the paper). Mild radiation-induced *thyroiditis* occurred in only one case and *benign thyroid nodules* in two; 86% of the patients required only one treatment dose to control hyperthyroidism, although *hypothyroidism* ensued in nearly all by 300 days after treatment.

Iodine excess in neonates from the use of iodine-containing antiseptics is a well-known cause of transient hypothyroidism, especially in iodine-deficient areas. The use of povidone iodine to disinfect maternal skin during labor and vaginal lacerations after delivery has now been reported to cause an increase in breast-milk iodine concentrations, and in turn an increase in serum TSH concentrations in the neonates (11[C]). Alternatives to povidone iodine should therefore be sought in both the delivery room and the neonatal ward.

REFERENCES

1. Fazio S, Biondi B, Carella C, Sabatini D, Cittadini A, Panza N, Lombardi G, Sacca L. Diastolic dysfunction in patients in thyroid-stimulating hormone suppressive therapy with levothyroxine: beneficial effect of β-blockade. J Clin Endocrinol Metab 1995;80:2222—6.

2. Ching GW, Franklyn JA, Stallard TJ, Daykin J, Sheppard MC, Gammage MD. Cardiac hypertrophy as a result of long-term thyroxine therapy and thyrotoxicosis. Heart 1996;75:363—8.

3. Biondi B, Fazio S, Cuocolo A, Sabatini D, Nicolai E, Lombardi G, Salvatore M, Sacca L. Impaired cardiac reserve and exercise capacity in patients receiving long-term thyrotropin suppressive therapy with levothyroxine. J Clin Endocrinol Metab 1996;81:4224—8.

4. Muller C, Bayley A, Harrison JE, Tsang R. Possible limited bone loss with suppressive thyroxine therapy is unlikely to have clinical relevance. Thyroid 1995;5:81—7

5. Uzzan B, Campos J, Cucherat M, Nony P, Boissel JP, Perret GY. Effects on bone mass of long term treatment with thyroid hormones: a meta-analysis. J Clin Endocrinol Metab 1996; 81:4278—89.

6. Cummings SR, Nevitt MC, Browner WS. Risk factors for hip fracture in white women. New Engl J Med 1995;332:767—73.

7. Tanemoto M, Miyakawa H, Hanai J, Yago M, Kitaoka M, Uchida S. Myeloperoxidase-antineutrophil cytoplasmic antibody-positive crescentic glomerulonephritis complicating the course of Graves' disease: report of three adult cases. Am J Kidney Dis 1995;26:774—80

8. Dolman KM, Gans ROB, Vervaat TJ, Zevenbergen G, Maingay D, Nikkels RE, Donker AJM, von dem Borne AEGK, Goldschmeding R. Vasculitis and antineutrophil cytoplasmic antibodies associated with propylthiouracil therapy. Lancet 1993;342:651—2.

9. Dottorini ME, Lomuscio G, Mazzucchelli L, Vignati A, Colombo L. Assessment of female fertility and carcinogenesis after iodine-131 therapy for differentiated thyroid carcinoma. J Nucl Med 1994;36:21—7

10. Clark JD, Gelfand MJ, Elgazzar AH. Iodine-131 therapy of hyperthyroidism in pediatric patients. J Nucl Med 1995;36:442—5.

11. Koga Y, Sano H, Kikukawa Y, Ishigouoka T, Kawamura M. Affect on neonatal thyroid function of povidone-iodine used on mothers during neonatal period. J Obstet Gynaecol 1995; 21:581—5.

H.M.J. Krans

42 Insulin, glucagon, and hypoglycemic drugs

INSULIN *(SED-13, 1290; SEDA-17, 477; SEDA-18, 409; SEDA-19, 393)*

Endocrine, metabolic *Severe hypoglycemia* Severe hypoglycemia (blood glucose concentration below 1 mmol/l) with bilateral cortical blindness and cerebral infarction [1] has been reported in a 22-year-old woman, in whom blood glucose control had never been tight. Apneic periods necessitated mechanical ventilation. After 2 months she could walk with help. A CT scan after 4 months showed gross global cerebral atrophy and she remained disabled owing to the neurological defects.

Bilateral cortical blindness has also been reported in a 22-year-old woman with severe hypoglycemia [2]. It improved slightly after 2 weeks but normal vision was restored only after 5 months. Temporary blindness after hypoglycemia has been reported before in children [3], [4].

Awareness of hypoglycemia The relation between frequent attacks of hypoglycemia and unawareness of hypoglycemia is still being intensively debated. Hyperinsulinemic hypoglycemic clamps with blood glucose concentrations of 2.2—4.7 mmol/l in healthy people have shown that neuroendocrine responses and symptoms of hypoglycemia, but not cognitive dysfunction, are shifted to lower plasma glucose concentrations after recent antecedent hypoglycemia [5]. There were no differences in autonomic neuropathy or catecholamine response on tilting after hypoglycemia had been instituted gradually in insulin-using patients with and without awareness [6]. The warning symptoms occurred at lower blood glucose concentrations (1.74 vs

2.54 mmol/l), and the reaction of hormones under the control of the hypothalamus was delayed in the unaware group, suggesting less well functioning hypothalamic glucoreceptors. Currently available methods for measuring neuropsychological functions are not sufficiently precise and are partly responsible for variable and contradictory results on the effect of hypoglycemia in impairing brain function [7].

When intensive injection therapy was changed to continuous subcutaneous insulin infusion the frequency of serious hypoglycemia fell from 138 events to 22 events per 100 patient years [8]. In a 1-year crossover study the numbers of instances of mild or severe hypoglycemia did not significantly increase after transfer from conventional to intensive multiple injection therapy or continuous subcutaneous infusion therapy [9], although HbA_{1c} concentrations were significantly lower during continuous subcutaneous infusion therapy. During intensive therapy, attacks of hypoglycemia (blood glucose below 3.0 mmol/l) often occur in the early or late night and rarely around 03:00 h, the time when patients on intensive treatment are asked to check their nightly blood glucose [10].

A recent 3-month, double-blind, crossover study with human and porcine insulins showed no differences in awareness of hypoglycemia [11], as has been reported before (SEDA-17, 479; SEDA-18, 411).

Immunological and hypersensitivity reactions *Immediate local reactions* and general *urticaria* developed gradually in a 20-year-old man after the institution of human regular (i.e. soluble) insulin and human NPH insulin [12]. Three weeks after desensitization urticaria reappeared after insulin had been injected into the abdominal wall. This cleared

Side Effects of Drugs, Annual 20
J.K. Aronson, ed.

after a few hours. He was able to use insulin by avoiding the abdominal wall, although he continued to have local reactions of less than 10 mm.

Specific IgE antibodies against insulin were found in a 63-year-old man who had never been in contact with insulin (13[C]). He developed *erythema* and a *wheal* (larger than 10 mm) within 15 min after injection of various types of insulin without further late reactions. Insulin components or other substances in the injection fluid did not produce the reaction. Desensitization was not very effective, but combined with oral antihistamines the situation improved.

A description of latex allergy in a 13-year-old boy (14[C]) has prompted a plea that latex-free materials (vial tops, syringes) should be available for diabetics.

Insulin-induced *lipoatrophy* has been reported in a patient who had never used insulins other than human insulin (15[c]). It improved when human insulin therapy was continued. Successful treatment of lipoatrophy with a jet-injection device has been reported (16[C]).

Continuous insulin delivery The incidence and determinants of insulin underdelivery in intraperitoneal infusion of insulin with implanted pumps (Minimed 2001) (17[r]) have been studied over a period of 3 years in 47 patients, a total of 103 patient years. When delivery was reduced to less than 15% the following actions were taken:

- rinsing of the catheters with 0.01 mol/l NaOH;
- surgical examination and eventual replacement of blocked catheters;
- finally rinsing the pump with 0.01 mol/l NaOH.

Various batches of Hoechst 21 pH-neutral semisynthetic insulin 400 U/ml were used. The number of obstructions increased during the study. This appeared not to be related to the duration of pump implantation, but the insulin was formulated with regard to new regulations of the *European Pharmacopoeia*, intended to improve insulin stability and to reduce the presence of undesirable insulin derivatives (to below 2%). However, this resulted in more frequent clogging and aggregation in the pumps, although investigation of the catheter never showed massive aggregates. It may be that aggregated insulin from the chamber induces adverse reactions in the peritoneum, including fibrin formation and encapsulation.

Pump pocket complications (SEDA-18, 412; SEDA-19, 395) have again been described, at a rate of 24 per 100 patient years (18[r]). The results were subsequently compared with the results with 117 pumps in 137 patients in 16 centers (435 patient years) (19[r]). The authors of this report warned against vigorous exercise when a pump has just been implanted.

Novel routes of administration Nasal insulin (SEDA-18, 413) had a low systemic availability and a high rate of failure in 31 patients with type I diabetes mellitus (20[C])r. However, the number of instances of *hypoglycemia* was comparable to subcutaneous insulin. There was transient *nasal irritation* in 16 patients, but there were no changes in mucociliary function or acoustic rhinometry.

Structural changes in the insulin molecule Lispro insulin, an analog in which the 28th and 29th amino acid of the B chain are interchanged, does not differ in antigenicity compared with recombinant human insulin (21[r]).

An insulin analog, in which proline on the B28 site was substituted with arginine, was faster absorbed and gave less hyperinsulinemia than regular short-acting insulin, as has previously been reported for other analogues. It did not clearly reduce hypoglycemic events (22[r]).

Insulin-like growth factor I (IGF-I)

Recently the use of insulin-like growth factor I (IGF-I) in type I and type II diabetics with extreme insulin resistance has been reviewed (23[R]). Recombinant IGF-I is now available. The structures of IGF-I and its receptor are comparable to those of insulin and the insulin receptor, although the affinity of binding of IGF-I to the insulin receptor is only 1—5% of that of insulin. The adverse effects that were reported included *hypoglycemia, parotid gland tenderness, increased heart rate, fluid retention and facial edema, arthralgias, myalgias, flushing, dyspnea,* and *burning at the site of injection.*

COMBINATIONS OF INSULIN AND ORAL DRUGS

The American Diabetic Association has recently published a consensus statement on the pharmacological treatment of hyperglycemia in type II diabetes (24[R]), including the question of when to start combined therapy.

The interactions of hypoglycemic drugs with other drugs including that of insulin and oral hypoglycemic drugs of other classes has been reviewed (25[R]).

There has been a progress report of the first 6 years of the UK Prospective Diabetes Study (26[r]), the object of which is to determine whether improved blood glucose control can prevent or delay the development of the secondary complications of type II diabetes. Five types of treatment are being studied: intensive sulfonylurea therapy, intensive insulin therapy, conventional therapy, metformin, and diet alone. Major hypoglycemic episodes occurred in 3.3, 11.2, 0.15, 0.3, and 0.1% and any hypoglycemic episodes in 45, 76, 3, 5, and 1%, respectively. There were mean increases in body weight of 6 and 4 kg in patients treated with intensive sulfonylurea or insulin therapy, and only 2 kg in the group using conventional therapy. In two groups of obese patients treated with metformin or diet alone body weight increased by 1 kg.

ORAL HYPOGLYCEMIC DRUGS

SULFONYLUREAS *(SED-13, 1297; SEDA-17, 484; SEDA-18, 413; SEDA-19, 395)*

The role of sulfonylureas in cardiovascular problems in type II diabetes has recently been reviewed (27[R]). New findings on the role of sulfonylurea derivatives on ATP-sensitive potassium (K_{ATP}) channels during ischemic periods may shed new light on the finding of increased numbers of cardiovascular deaths during tolbutamide in the UGDP study (SEDA-4, 301-3).

Glibenclamide

A new case of fatal *intrahepatic cholestasis with hepatorenal syndrome* due to glibenclamide has been reported.

A 69-year-old woman had taken glibenclamide 10 mg/day for 7 years, but an increase in dosage to 15 mg/day resulted in fever and jaundice (28[c]). There was no history of alcoholism or evidence of hepatitis or other virus infections. A liver biopsy 7 days after withdrawal of glibenclamide showed intrahepatic cholestasis; there was no evidence of alcoholism, no duct defects were demonstrable on ultrasonography, and all viral serology was negative. She died after 43 days, and a post-mortem examination was refused.

Glimepiride   A new sulfonylurea, glimepiride, with a different binding site on the K_{ATP} channel to the conventional sulfonylureas, should act more rapidly and have a more sustained effect. It has been called a third-generation sulfonylurea. Dosages of 1, 4, and 8 mg/day for 14 weeks have been compared in 231 patients (29[C]). The hypoglycemic effects of 4 and 8 mg were almost identical. Symptomatic hypoglycemia occurred in 12—23% of the patients (5.4% in the placebo group); there were no fasting plasma glucose concentrations below 3.3 mmol/l. Other adverse effects were: *dizziness, nausea, abdominal pain, tremor, abnormal vision, anorexia, aphasia, dry mouth, headache, pruritus, rash,* and *vasodilatation*; the following occurred only in the placebo group: insomnia, blurred vision, and anxiety; weakness occurred in both groups. In another study 4 mg bd, 8 mg od, 8 mg bd, 16 mg od, and placebo were compared in 417 patients after a 3-week placebo wash-out period (30[r]). There was no laboratory-documented hypoglycemia. Four patients withdrew because of subjective hypoglycemic symptoms. In the 16 mg group one patient withdrew because of *abnormal liver function tests* and one because of *anorexia*.

BIGUANIDES *(SED-13, 1301; SEDA-17, 488; SEDA-18, 415; SEDA-19, 396)*

Metformin, which was registered in the US in 1995, has been reviewed, and the problem of *lactic acidosis* discussed (31[R]). Exclusion criteria are: increased plasma creatinine concentrations (over 130 µmol/l), liver disease, alcohol abuse, a history of lactic acidosis, severe infections, or respiratory or circulatory insufficiency leading to central hypoxia or reduced peripheral perfusion. Whether metformin can be given to older patients has been discussed (32[r]). The authors thought that it could, provided that renal function is regularly assessed and that metformin is withdrawn or not given when renal function is abnormal.

Gastrointestinal The incidence of gastrointestinal symptoms has been studied in 324 middle-aged non-diabetics who took metformin 850 mg/day or a matched placebo for 1 year. *Diarrhea*, and to a much lesser extent *nausea and vomiting*, were more often reported in those who had a waist-to-hip ratio of ≥ 0.95 (in men) or ≥ 0.80 (in women) and were free from cardiovascular complaints (33[r]). Adverse effects caused 11 patients in the treated group and five in the placebo group to withdraw.

Metabolic Although phenformin has been withdrawn in many countries, it is still available in some. A non-lethal case of *lactic acidotic coma* (34[R]) has been reported in the US in a 67-year-old man who had been given phenformin 25 mg tds and glibenclamide 5 mg tds in China. With increasing travel, adverse effects of drugs that are no longer registered in a country may still be seen when the drug is prescribed elsewhere.

Interactions *Acarbose* reduces the systemic availability of metformin (25[P]).

Iodinated contrast agents can impair renal function, and in nine or 10 cases lactic acidosis has been reported in patients who were also taking metformin (35[r]). The authors recommended that metformin be withheld 48 h before an iodinated contrast agent is used and that renal function should be checked after such an investigation.

α-GLUCOSIDASE INHIBITORS *(SED-13, 1302; SEDA-17, 489; SEDA-18, 416; SEDA-19, 397)*

A 39-year-old Japanese woman (36[c]) developed *ileus* when taking acarbose 100 mg tds. It subsided spontaneously after 2 days of treatment with intravenous fluids and the withdrawal of all food and drugs. No previous or subsequent gastrointestinal symptoms were reported. The authors drew attention to a Japanese report of six patients over 60 years of age or with preceding abdominal surgery who developed ileus (with one death) when given acarbose or voglibose, a different glucose oxidase inhibitor (37[c]).

THIAZOLIDINEDIONES *(SED-13, 1302; SEDA-19, 398)*

This new group of insulin sensitizers has been recently reviewed (38[R]). They reduce insulin resistance, an important factor in type II diabetes, but their mechanism of action is not clear. Reports of better availability of Glut 4 (39[r]) have not been confirmed. The thiazolidinediones may interact with a family of nuclear receptors known as peroxisome proliferator-activated receptors. They reduce lipid availability (40[r]), and englitazone prevents the glucose transport defect without changes in glucose transporter content (41[r]).

Troglitazone (42[r]) reduces fasting blood glucose and HbA_{1c}. In a multicenter study of 145 patients treated with troglitazone 200 mg bd there was subjective *hypoglycemia* in 10 cases, twice as many as in 139 patients treated with placebo. There were four cases of *dizziness* in the treated group and one in the placebo group, and *edema* occurred three times on the treated group. Troglitazone improved glucose tolerance and insulin resistance in non-diabetic obese patients (43[r]) and increased insulin responsiveness in Werner's syndrome (44[r]). In patients judged stable but unsatisfactorily treated with a sulfonylurea, either troglitazone ($n = 145$) or placebo ($n = 146$) was added for 12 weeks (45[r]). There were no serious adverse events. Subjective hypoglycemia occurred only with troglitazone (3.6%). Other treatment-related adverse effects occurred equally in the placebo and the troglitazone group. In a multicenter study 330 patients, previously treated with diet or oral hypoglycemic drugs, were treated for 12 weeks with troglitazone (200, 400, 600, or 800 mg/day or 200 or 400 mg bd) after a run-in period of 2 weeks (46[r]). One patient had a bout of dizziness that might have been due to hypoglycemia, but was not supported by blood glucose measurements, and 9—20% of the patients taking troglitazone had a fall in neutrophil count to below 0.9% of the lower limit of normal, with the highest incidence in the highest dosage group. The same occurred in 9% of the patients taking placebo. Other adverse effects were not more common in the treated groups.

ALDOSE REDUCTASE INHIBITORS

(SED-13, 1302; SEDA-17, 489; SEDA-18, 417; SEDA-19, 398)

A meta-analysis of three randomized clinical trials of tolrestat (738 patients) has shown that the only more frequently observed adverse effect compared with placebo was *increased alanine aminotransferase (AlT) and aspartate aminotransferase (AsT) activity*, to greater than three times the upper limit of normal, in about 9% of over 3700 patients (47[r]).

In a multicenter study of epalrestat 120 patients received 50 mg tds of epalrestat for 12 weeks. One patient got *blisters* in the skin of the extremities, in one *AlT activity rose* from 17 to 40 units, and in one *serum creatinine rose* to 1300 μmol/l (48[r]).

REFERENCES

1. Gold AE, Marshall SM. Cortical blindness and cerebral infarction associated with severe hypoglycemia. Diabetes Care 1996;19:1001—3.
2. Odeh M, Oliven A. Hypoglycemia and bilateral cortical blindness. Diabetes Care 1996; 19:272—3.
3. Mukamel M, Weitz R, Nissenkorn I, Yassur I, Varsano I. Acute cortical blindness associated with hypoglycemia. J Pediatr 1981;98:583—4.
4. Garty BZ, Dinari G, Nitzan M. Transient acute cortical blindness associated with hypoglycemia. Pediatr Neurol 1987;3:169—70.
5. Hvidberg A, Fanelli CG, Hershey T, Terkamp C, Craft S, Cryer PE. Impact of recent hypoglycemia on hypoglycemic cognitive dysfunction in nondiabetic humans. Diabetes 1996;46:1030—6.
6. Bacatselos SO, Karamitsos DT, Kourtoglou GI, Zambulis CX, Yovos JG, Vytzantiadis AT. Hypoglycaemia unawareness in Type I diabetic patients under conventional insulin treatment. Diabetes Nutr Metab 1995;8:267—75.
7. Heller SR, MacDonald IA. The measurement of cognitive function during acute hypoglycaemia: experimental limitations and their effect on the studies of hypoglycaemia unawareness. Diabetic Med 1996;13:607—15.
8. Bode BW, Steed RD, Davidson PC. Reduction in severe hypoglycemia with long-term continuous subcutaneous insulin infusion in type I diabetes. Diabetes Care 1996;19:324—27.
9. Kerum G, Bozikov V, Metelko Z. Frequency of hypoglycemic episodes during intensive therapy with human insulin. Diabetes Care 1996;19:181—2.
10. Vervoort G, Goldschmidt HMG, van Doorn LG. Nocturnal blood glucose profiles with type 1 diabetes mellitus on multiple (−4) daily injection regimens. Diabetic Med 1996;13:794—9.
11. MacLeod K, Gold AE, Frier BM. A comparative study of responses of acute hypoglycemia induced by human and porcine insulins in patients with type I diabetes. Diabetic Med 1996;13:346—57.

12. Chng HH, Leong KP, Loh KC. Primary systemic allergy to human insulin: recurrence of generalized urticaria after successful desensitization. Allergy 1995;50:984—7.
13. Takuma H, Kawagishi T, Kyogoku I, Okuno Y, Nishizawa Y, Morii H. A case of primary and generalized allergy to human insulin with no history of any prior insulin exposure. Diabetes Res Clin Pract 1995;30:69—73.
14. MacCracken J, Stenger P, Jackson T. Latex allergy in diabetic patients. Diabetes Care 1996; 19:184.
15. Jaap AJ, Horn HM, Tidman MJ, Walker JD. Lipoatrophy with human insulin. Diabetes Care 1996;19:1289—90.
16. Logwin S, Conget I, Jansa M, Vidal M, Nicolau C, Gomis R. Human insulin-induced lipoatrophy; succesful treatment using a jet-injection device. Diabetes Care 1996;19:255—6.
17. Renard E, Boutelau S, Jacques-Apostol J, Lauton D, Gibert-Boulet F, Costalat G, Bringer J, Jaffiol J. Insulin undelivery from implanted pumps using peritoneal route; determinant role of insulin pump compability. Diabetes Care 1996; 19:812—7.
18. Renard E, Bringer J, Jacques-Apostol J, Lauton D, Mestre C, Costalat G, Jaffiol J. Complications of the pump pocket may represent a significant cause of incidents with implanted system for insulin delivery. Diabetes Care 1994;17:1064—6.
19. Scavini M, Christallo M, Sarmiento M, Dunn FL. Pump-pocket complications during long-term insulin delivery using an implanted programmable pump. Diabetes Care 1996;19:384—5.
20. Hilsted J, Madsbad S, Hvidberg A, Rasmusen MH, Krarup T, Ipsen H, Hansen B, Pedersen M, Djurup R, Oxenboll B. Intranasal insulin therapy: the clinical realities. Diabetologia 1995;38:680—4.
21. Fineberg NS, Fineberg SE, Anderson JH, Birkett MA, Gibson RG, Hufferd S. Imunologic effects of insulin lispro [Lys (B28), Pro (B29) human insulin] in IDDM and NIDDM patients

previously treated with insulin. Diabetes 1996;
45:1750—4.

22. Wiefels K, Hübinger A, Dannehl K, Gries
FA. Insulin kinetic and -dynamic in diabetic patients under insulin pump therapy after injections
of human insulin or the insulin analogue
(B28Asp). Horm Metab Res 1995;27:421—4.

23. Cusi K, DeFronzo RA. Treatment of
NIDDM, IDDM, and other insulin- resistant
states with IGF-I. Diabetes Rev 1995;3:206—36.

24. Consensus statement. The pharmacological
treatment of hyperglycemia in NIDDM. Diabetes
Care 1995;18:1510—8.

25. Scheen AJ, Lefèbvre PJ. Antihyperglycaemic
agents; drug interactions and clinical importance.
Drug Saf 1995;12:32—45.

26. UK Prospective Diabetes Study Group. Overview of 6 years' therapy of type II diabetes: a
progressive disease. Diabetes 1995;44:1249—58
(correction in Diabetes 1996;45:1655).

27. Leibowitz G, Cerasi E. Sulphonylurea treatment of NIDDM patients with vascular disease: a
mixed blessing? Diabetologia 1996;39:503—14.

28. Krivoy N, Zaher A, Yaacov B, Alroy G. Fatal
toxic intrahepatic cholestasis secondary to glibenclamide. Diabetes Care 1996;19:385—6.

29. Goldberg RB, Sherman MH, Schneider J. A
dose response study of glimepiride in patients with
NIDDM who have previously received sulfonylurea agents. Diabetes Care 1996;19:849—56.

30. Rosenstock J, Samols E, Muchmore DB,
Schneider J, the Glimepiride Study Group. Gli-
mepiride, a new once-daily sulfonylurea. Diabetes
Care 1996;19:1194—9.

31. Bailey CJ, Turner RC. Metformin. New Engl
J Med 1996;334:574—9.

32. Gregorio F, Ambrosi F, Filipponi P, Manfrini
S, Testa I. Is metformin safe enough for ageing
type 2 diabetic patients? Diabetes Metab
1996;22:43—50.

33. Fontbonne A, Charles MA, Juhan-Vague I,
Bard J-M, André P Isnard F, Cohen J-M, Grand-
mottet P, Safar ME, Eschwège E, the BIGPRO
Study Group. The effect of metformin on the
metabolic abnormalities associated with up-
perbody fat distribution. Diabetes Care 1996;
19:920—6.

34. Lu HC, Parikh PP, Lorber DL. Phenformin-
associated lactic acidosis due to imported phenformin. Diabetes Care 1996;19:1449—50.

35. Dachman H. New contraindication to intravascular iodinated contrast material. Radiology
1995;197:545.

36. Nishii Y, Aizawa T, Hashizume K. Ileus: a
rare side effect of acarbose. Diabetes Care
1996;19:1033.

37. Ohno T. Gastrointestinal side effects of alpha-

glucosidase inhibitors with special reference to
ileus. Shinyaku to Rinsho 1995;44:144—6.

38. Saltiel AR, Olefsky JM. Thiazolidinediones in
the treatment of insulin resistance and type II
diabetes. Diabetes 1996, 45:1661—9.

39. Young PW, Cawthorne MA, Coyle PJ,
Holder JC, Holman GD, Kozka IJ, Kirkham DM,
Lister CA, Smith SA. Repeat treatment of obese
mice with BRL 49653, a potent insulin sensitizer,
enhances insulin action in white adipocytes. Diabetes 1995;44:1087—92.

40. Oakes ND, Kennedy CJ, Jenkins AB, Laybutt
DS, Chisholm DJ, Kraegen EW. A new antidia-
betic agent, BRL 49653, reduces lipid availability
and improves insulin action and glucoregulation
in the rat. Diabetes 1994;43:1203—10.

41. Stevenson RW, McPherson RK, Persson LM,
Genereux PE, Swick AG, Spitzer J, Herbst JJ,
Andrews KM, Kreutter DK, Gibbs EM. The anti-
hyperglycemic agent englitazone prevents the de-
fect in glucose transport in rats fed a high-fat diet.
Diabetes 1996;45:60—6.

42. Iwamoto T, Kosako K, Kuzuya T, Akanuma
Y, Shigeta Y, Kaneko T. Effects of troglitazone.
Diabetes Care 1996;19:151—6.

43. Nolan JJ, Ludvik B, Beerdsen P, Joyce M,
Olefsky J. Improvement in glucose tolerance and
insulin resistance in obese subjects treated with
troglitazone. New Engl J Med 1996;331:1188—93.

44. Takino J, Okuno S, Uotani S, Yano M, Matsumoto K, Kawasaki E, Takao Y, Yamasaki H,
Yamaguchi Y, Akazawa S, Nagataki S. Increased
insulin responsiveness after CS-045 treatment associated with Werner's syndrome. Diabetes Res
Clin Pract 1994;24:167—72.

45. Iwamoto Y, Kosaka K, Kuzuya T, Akanuma
Y, Shigeta Y, Kaneko T. Effect of combination
therapy of troglitazone and sulphonylureas in patients with type 2 diabetes who were poorly controlled by sulphonylurea therapy alone. Diabetic
Med 1996;13:365—70.

46. Kumar S, Boulton AJM, Beck-Nielsen H,
Berthezene, Muggeo M, Persson B, Spinas GA,
Donoghue S, Lettis S, Stewart-Long P, for Trogli-
tazone Study Group. Troglitazone, an insulin ac-
tion enhancer, improves metabolic control in
NIDDM patients. Diabetologia 1996;39:701—9.

47. Nicolucci A, Carinci F, Graepel JG, Hohman
TC, Ferris F, Lachin JM. The efficacy of tolrestat
in the treatment of diabetic peripheral neuropathy. Diabetes Care 1996;19:1091—6.

48. Goto Y, Hotta N, Shigeta Y, Sakamoto N,
Kikkawa R. Effect of an aldose reductase inhibitor, epalrestat, on diabetic neuropathy. Clinical
benefit and indication for the drug assessed from
the results of a placebo-controlled double-blind
study. Biomed Pharmacother 1995;49:269—77.

43 Miscellaneous hormones and prostaglandins

Calcitonin and analogues *(SED-13, 1307; SEDA-17, 494; SEDA-19, 402)*

Recent large studies have confirmed that both intranasal salmon calcitonin (1[C]) and intramuscular eel calcitonin (2[C]) reverse bone loss in established osteoporosis. However, the use of a similar dosage (200 i.u./day) of intranasal salmon calcitonin in an add-back regimen (3[C]) was insufficient to prevent bone loss during gonadotrophin-releasing hormone (GnRH) agonist treatment. Adverse effects were as previously documented (SEDA-17, 494; (4[R])). In 150 women who took part in a trial of salmon calcitonin given by rectal suppository there was a 40% withdrawal rate because of local intolerance in both placebo and treatment groups (5[C]).

Parathyroid hormone *(SED-13, 1307; SEDA-17, 494; SEDA-19, 402)*

Parathyroid hormone is one of several agents currently being promoted to prevent the osteoporosis associated with gonadotrophin-releasing hormone (GnRH) analog treatment in women. PTH(1–34) administered subcutaneously in a dose of 40 µg/day completely inhibited the 3% fall in lumbar bone density seen during 6 months of treatment with nafarelin (200 µg bd intranasally) (6[C]). There were no significant adverse effects, in keeping with previous experience of acute administration (7[C]).

Human growth hormone (hGH, somatotrophin) *(SED-13, 1307; SEDA-17, 494; SEDA-18, 421; SEDA-19, 402)*

As experience with long-term hGH treatment or replacement increases, the pattern of adverse effects is becoming clearer. In children the overall frequency of events per patient-year of treatment was 2.3% (210 events in 151 of 2922 subjects) (8[R]). Problems associated with fluid retention were less common than in adults, but musculoskeletal problems (slipped epiphyses, kyphoscoliosis) were more common. There was a higher frequency of adverse effects in children who had been previously treated for leukemia and craniopharyngioma and lower rates in those treated for idiopathic short stature. Benign intracranial hypertension (pseudotumor cerebri), associated with papilledema, remains the most significant subacute onset effect (9[C]).

The recurrence of malignancy in children subsequently treated with hGH remains unsubstantiated (8[R]), (10[C]). A possible reason for the apparent association between leukemia and hGH treatment (11[C]) may be undiagnosed Fanconi's anemia in children with short stature (12[C]). The incidence of type I diabetes in a large cohort of children treated with growth hormone is no greater than expected by chance (13[CR]). A report suggesting an association between poor outcome in children receiving hGH after kidney transplantation is of low scientific value (14[c]).

In adults with hypopituitarism, hGH was associated with an 18% incidence of adverse effects related to fluid retention during the first 2 months of treatment (15[C]). However, this large study suggested a progressive fall in the incidence and prevalence of such effects over the 1-year treatment period. A higher incidence of adverse effects may be predicted (16[C]) by age, greater body mass index, better pre-treatment GH reserve (as measured on provocative testing), and a supraphysiological response of insulin-like growth factor I to initial treatment. Caution is recommended in elderly patients (17[C]). Longer-term studies of hGH replacement have shown no adverse effects on cardiovascular structure or function (18[C]). Greater susceptibility to osteoarthrosis remains a theoretical risk with time (19[R]), (20[C]).

Insulin-like growth factor I (hIGF-I)
(SEDA-19, 402)

Recombinant human IGF-I, although currently unlicensed, has been used in a variety of clinical settings (21[R]). It is the peptide through which GH exerts most of its growth-promoting effects, and it causes reduced endogenous secretion of GH and insulin, with increased insulin sensitivity (22[C]). In healthy individuals and in type II diabetes it improves glucose tolerance, increases lipid oxidation, and reduces LDL cholesterol and VLDL triglycerides (23[C]), (24[C]). In combination with hGH its anabolic effects are synergistic (25[C]).

Possible clinical uses of IGF-I have been described in diabetes, to overcome insulin resistance (26[C]), in AIDS-associated cachexia (27[C]), in growth hormone insensitivity (28[C]), and in elderly people (29[R]).

Acute adverse effects include hypoglycemia, which is dose related, and fluid retention at days 3—4 (30[R]). Pseudotumor cerebri has been reported, as with hGH (31[C]). Bilateral parotid pain on eating (25[C]) occurs frequently, as do hypoglycemia (28[C]) and tachycardia and flushing (26[C]). Although the frequency of adverse effects compelled the last authors to suspend their study before completing their 8-week trial of subcutaneous treatment, others have suggested that the adverse effects are less limiting (29[R]), (32[CR]).

Growth hormone release-inhibiting hormone (somatostatin) and analogues *(SED-13, 1309; SEDA-17, 496; SEDA-18, 42; SEDA-19, 403)*

The early indications for and the use of somatostatin and its analogs have been summarized elsewhere (SEDA-17, 496; (33[R]), (34[R])). Experience is increasing, with larger numbers of acromegalic patients treated (35[C]). Lack of effect in AIDS-related diarrhea has been reported (36[C]). There is a suggestion of benefit in low grade non-Hodgkin's lymphoma (37[C]) and, in combination with tamoxifen, improved outcome has been reported in adenocarcinoma of the pancreas (38[C]). The adverse effects are those previously described, primarily local gastrointestinal symptoms and cholelithiasis. The incidence of gallstones increases to almost 60% in patients with resistant acromegaly treated with dosages up to 1.5 mg/day (39[C]). The debate continues about the magnitude of effect on glucose tolerance and lipid metabolism in treated acromegaly (40[C]), (41[C]).

The requirement for multiple daily subcutaneous doses of octreotide appears to have been overcome by the development of the longer-acting octapeptide lanreotide (42[R]), with an injection frequency of 1—2 weeks. Studies of the use of lanreotide in acromegaly (43[C]) and the carcinoid syndrome (44[C]) have shown that its efficacy and adverse effect profile are comparable with those of octreotide. A modified-release microencapsulated formulation of Sandostatin may be equally effective, with even longer dosage intervals possible (45[C]), (46[C]).

Vasopressin and analogs *(SED-13, 1310; SEDA-17, 497; SEDA-18, 42; SEDA-19, 403)*

The difficulties of administering vasopressin, and its potential for adverse effects related to hypertension and vasoconstriction, have favored its replacement by DDAVP (1-D-amino-8-D-arginine vasopressin, or desmopressin). This is a synthetic analog with a prolonged duration of action and antidiuretic properties but little vasoconstrictor effect (47[R]). Hyponatremia and convulsions are increasingly reported, both with standard doses of DDAVP (48[C]), (49[C]), and in its combined use with imipramine for nocturnal enuresis (50[C]). The introduction of an oral formulation of desmopressin has coincided with renewed interest in its use for nocturnal enuresis. In two studies in a total of 60 children and adolescents treated for 6—12 weeks two-thirds of individuals responded positively. There were no instances of water intoxication (51^C), (52^C) and other adverse effects are rare.

Desmospressin also has hemostatic properties because it increases plasma concentrations of von Willebrand factor antigen 2- to 4-fold. It can therefore replace cryoprecipitate in some patients with factor IX deficiency (53^C). However not all patients respond equally well (54^C), and tachyphylaxis (55^C) or thrombocytopenia (56^C) may develop.

A retrospective study has suggested that DDAVP is not teratogenic (57^C).

Gonadotrophin-releasing hormone (gonadorelin, GnRH) and analogs *(SED-13, 1311; SEDA-17, 498; SEDA-18, 422; SEDA-19, 403)*

The hypothalamic releasing factor for both luteinizing hormone and follicle-stimulating hormone is a decapeptide, widely used in testing hypothalamic–pituitary–gonadal function. Several superagonist analogs with or without prolonged durations of action have been synthesized (58^R), (59^R). The therapeutic indications for use of these agents have been summarized elsewhere (SEDA-17, 498).

Cumulative experience in large numbers of patients (60^R) has suggested that in the treatment of benign gynecological conditions, apart from the incidence of predictable hypoestrogenic effects, gonadorelin agonists are associated with few acute adverse effects.

Endocrine, metabolic The most frequent adverse effects are symptoms of hypo-estrogenism (hot flushes in almost all patients) and less often vaginal dryness, reduced libido and breast discomfort, initial headache, and bleeding. Severe flushing, which is not uncommon, can be treated with either clonidine (61^C) or the dopamine receptor antagonist veralipride (62^C). Ovarian hyperstimulation is less frequent than with gonadotrophin treatment in amenorrheic woman (63^C), (64^R), and there appear to be no differences in the effects of different analogs in inducing follicle cyst formation (65^C).

Two cases of pituitary apoplexy precipitated by GnRH agonist analogs have been reported in patients with undiagnosed nonfunctioning pituitary adenomas (66^c), (67^c).

Hematological There has been a report of thrombocytopenia in a patient with systemic lupus erythematosus (68^c).

Urinary system There has been a report of obstructive renal failure due to ureteric fibrosis in a woman treated for endometriosis (69^c).

Musculoskeletal Osteoporosis, in the form of reduction of trabecular bone density, has been regularly observed with chronic GnRH agonist treatment, but was initially reported to be reversible within 6 months of withdrawal, and was not considered a contraindication (70^C). Later reports, however, have suggested a more rapid onset during treatment and less complete reversal of bone loss after withdrawal of GnRH (71^C), (72^C). The prospect of routine 'add-back' concurrent treatment to prevent osteoporotic bone loss in this setting is increasing (73^{CR}), (74^R). Estrogens alone are not effective (75^C). Other more promising candidates include combinations of etidronate and norethindrone (76^C), parathyroid hormone (6^C), tibolone (77^C), and the non-hormone agent ipriflavone (78^C).

Thyrotrophin-releasing hormone (protirelin, TRH) *(SED-13, 1311; SEDA-17, 498)*

Early studies suggesting that TRH had a synergistic effect with corticosteroids to increase fetal lung maturation led to its increased use in obstetrics (79^R), (80^C). However, its clinical efficacy has not been confirmed in recent trials (81^C). Adverse effects include facial flushing, increased urinary frequency, vaginal sensations, nausea, chest pain, and altered taste sensation (82^C). Transient hypertension may be of more significance in pre-eclampsia (83^C), (84^C).

REFERENCES

1. Overgaard K, Hansen MA, Jensen SB, Christiansen C. Effect of salcatonin given intranasally on bone mass and fracture rates in established osteoporosis: a dose-response study. Br Med J 1992;305:556−61.

2. Jimenez FE, Albizuri JMA, Alier JMA, Soto JJM, Canales AG. Effectiveness and safety of medium- and long-term elcatonin use in the prevention and treatment of bone mass loss. Curr Ther Res 1995;56:385−99.

3. Roux C, Pelissier C, Listrat V, Kolta S, Simonetta C, Guignard M, Dougados M, Amor B. Bone loss during gonadotropin releasing hormone agonist treatment and use of nasal calcitonin. Osteoporosis 1995;5:185−90.

4. Avioli LV. Calcitonin therapy in osteoporotic syndromes. Rheum Dis Clin North Am 1994; 20:777−85.

5. Reginster JY, Jupsin I, Deroisy R, Biquet I, Franchimont N, Franchimont P Prevention of postmenopausal bone loss by rectal calcitonin. Calcif Tissue Int 1995;56:539−42.

6. Finkelstein JS, Klibanski A, Schaefer EH, Hornstein MS, Schiff I, Neer RM. Parathyroid hormone for the prevention of bone loss induced by estrogen deficiency. New Engl J Med 1994; 331:1618−23.

7. Mallette LE. Synthetic human parathyroid hormone 1−34 fragment for diagnostic testing. Ann Intern Med 1988;109:800−4.

8. Cowell CT, Dietsch S. Adverse events during growth hormone therapy. J Pediatr Endocrinol Metab 1995;8:243−52.

9. Malozowksi S, Tanner LA, Wysowski D, Fleming GA. Growth hormone insulin-like factor I and benign intracranial hypertension. New Engl J Med 1993;329:665−6.

10. Ogilvy Stuart AL, Ryder WD, Gattamaneni HR, Clayton PE, Shalet SM. Growth hormone and tumour recurrence. Br Med J 1992; 304:1601−5.

11. Fisher DA, Job JC, Preece M, Underwood LE. Leukaemia in patients treated with growth hormone. Lancet 1988;1:1159−60.

12. Butturini A, Bernasconi S, Izzi G, Gertner JM, Gale RP. Short stature, Fanconi's anaemia, and risk of leukaemia after growth hormone therapy. Lancet 1994;343:1576.

13. Czernichow P, Albertsson-Wikland K, Tuvemo T, Gunnarsson R. Growth hormone treatment and diabetes: survey of the Kabi Pharmacia International Growth Study. Acta Paediatr Scand 1991;379 Suppl: 104−7.

14. Chavers BM, Doherty L, Nevins TE, Cook M, Sane K. Effects of growth hormone on kidney function in pediatric transplant recipients. Pediatr Nephrol 1995;9:176−81.

15. Mardh G, Lindeberg A. Growth hormone replacement therapy in adult hypopituitary patients with growth hormone deficiency: combined clinical safety data from clinical trials in 665 patients. Endocrinol Metab 1995;2 Suppl B:11−16.

16. Holmes SJ, Shalet SM. Which adults develop side effects of growth hormone replacement? Clin Endocrinol 1995;43:143−9.

17. Powrie J, Weissberger A, Skonsen P. Growth hormone replacement therapy for growth hormone-deficient adults. Drugs 1995;49:656−63.

18. Beshyah SA, Shahi M, Foale R, Johnston DG. Cardiovascular effects of prolonged growth hormone replacement in adults. J Intern Med 1995;237:35−42.

19. Lamberts SWJ, Valk NK, Binnerts A. The use of growth hormone in adults: a changing scene. Clin Endocrinol 1992;37:111−15.

20. Bagge E, Eden S, Rosen T, Bengtsson BA. The prevalence of radiographic osteoarthritis is low in elderly patients with growth hormone deficiency. Acta Endocrinol 1993;129:296−300.

21. Froesch ER, Zenobi PD, Hussain M. Metabolic and therapeutic effects of insulin-like growth factor I. Horm Res 1994;42:66−71.

22. Guler HP, Schmid C, Zapf J, Froesch ER. Effects of recombinant insulin-like growth factor I on insulin secretion and renal function in normal human subjects. Proc Natl Acad Sci USA 1989; 86:2868−72.

23. Zenobi PD, Jaeggi-Groisman SE, Riesen W, Roder M, Froesch ER. Insulin-like growth factor I improves glucose and lipid metabolism in type 2 diabetes mellitus. J Clin Invest 1992;90:2234−41.

24. Zenobi PD, Graf S, Ursprung H, Froesch ER. Effects of insulin-like growth factor I on glucose tolerance, insulin levels, and insulin secretion. J Clin Invest 1992;89:1908−13.

25. Kupfer SR, Underwood LE, Baxter RC, Clemmons DR. Enhancement of the anabolic effects of growth hormone and insulin-like growth factor I by use of both agents simultaneously. J Clin Invest 1993;91:391−6.

26. Jabri N, Schalch DS, Schwartz SL, Fischer JS, Kipnes MS, Radnik BJ, Turman NJ, Marcsisin VS, Guler HP. Adverse effects of recombinant human insulin-like growth factor I in obese insulin-resistant type II diabetic patients. Diabetes 1994;43:369−74.

27. Lieberman SA, Butterfield GE, Harrison D, Hoffman AR. Anabolic effects of recombinant insulin-like growth factor-I in cachectic patients with the acquired immunodeficiency syndrome. J Clin Endocrinol Metab 1994;78:404−10.

28. Ranke MB, Savage MO, Chatelain PG, Preece MA, Rosenfeld RG, Blum WF, Wilton P. Insulin-like growth factor I improves height in growth hormone insensitivity: two years' results. Horm Res 1995;44:253−64.

29. Carter WJ. Effect of anabolic hormones and insulin-like growth factor-I on muscle mass and strength in elderly persons. Clin Geriatr Med 1995;11:735−48.

30. Froesch ER, Hussain M. Metabolic effects of insulin-like growth factor-I with special reference

to diabetes. Acta Paediatr 1994;399 Suppl:165—70.

31. Lordereau-Richard I, Roger M, Chaussain JL. Transient bilateral papilloedema in a 10 year old boy treated with recombinant insulin-like growth factor I for growth hormone receptor deficiency. Acta Paediatr 1994;399 Suppl:152.

32. Ranke MB, Wilton P. Adverse events during treatment with recombinant insulin-like growth factor I in patients with growth hormone insensitivity. Acta Paediatr 1994;399 Suppl:143—5.

33. Tauber MT, Harris AG, Rochiccioli P. Clinical use of the long acting somatostatin analogue octreotide in pediatrics. Eur J Pediatr 1994; 153:304—10.

34. Oberg K. Treatment of neuroendocrine tumors. Cancer Treat Rev 1994;20:331—55.

35. Arosio M, Macchelli S, Rossi CM, Casati G, Biella O, Faglia G and Italian Multicenter Octreotide Study Group. Effects of treatment with octreotide in acromegalic patients—a multicenter Italian study. Eur J Endocrinol 1995;133:430—9.

36. Simon DM, Cello JP, Valenzuela J, Levy R, Dickerson G, Goodgame R, Brown M, Lyche K, Fessel WJ, Grendell J et al. Multicenter trial of octreotide in patients with refractory acquired immunodeficiency syndrome-associated diarrhea. Gastroenterology 1995;108:1753—60 (erratum in 1995;109:1024).

37. Witzig TE, Letendre L, Gertsner, J, Schroeder G, Mailliard JA, Colon-Otero G, Marschke RF, Windschitl HE. Evaluation of a somatostatin analog in the treatment of lymphoproliferative disorders: results of a phase II North Central Cancer Treatment Group Trial. J Clin Oncol 1995;13:2012—15.

38. Rosenberg L, Barkun AN, Denis MH, Pollak M. Low dose octreotide and tamoxifen in the treatment of adenocarcinoma of the pancreas. Cancer 1995;75:23—8.

39. McKnight JA, McCance DR, Sheridan B, Atkinson AB. Four years' treatment of resistant acromegaly with octreotide. Eur J Endocrinol 1995;132:429—32.

40. Koop BL, Harris AG, Ezzat S. Effect of octreotide on glucose tolerance in acromegaly. Eur J Endocrinol 1994;130:581—6.

41. Benito P, Calanas A, Galvez MA, Corpas MS. Effect of octreotide on plasma lipid metabolism on acromegaly. Ann Pharmacother 1994;28:1198.

42. Robinson C, Castaner J. Lanreotide acetate. Drugs Future 1994;19:992—9.

43. Marek J, Hana V, Krsek M, Justova V, Catus F, Thomas F. Long term treatment of acromegaly with the slow-release somatostatin analogue lanreotide. Eur J Endocrinol 1994;131:20—6.

44. Scherubl H, Widenmann B, Riecken EO, Thomas F, Bohme E, Rath U. Treatment of carcinoid syndrome with a depot formulation of the somatostatin analogue lanreotide. Eur J Cancer 1994;30A:1591—2.

45. Flogstad AV, Halse J, Haldorsen T, Lancranjan I, Marbach P, Bruns C, Jervell J. Sandostatin LAR in acromegalic patients: a dose-range study. J Clin Endocrinol Metab 1995;80:3601—7.

46. Stewart PM, Kane KF, Stewart SE, Lancranjan I, Sheppard MC. Depot long-acting somatostatin analog (Sandostatin-LAR) is an effective treatment for acromegaly. J Clin Endocrinol Metab 1995;80:3267—72.

47. Richardson DW, Robinson AG. Desmopressin. Ann Intern Med 1985;103:228—39.

48. Humphries JE, Siragy H. Significant hyponatremia following DDAVP administration in a healthy adult. Am J Hematol 1993;44:12—15.

49. Suchowersky O, Furtado S, Rohs G. Beneficial effect of intranasal desmopressin for nocturnal polyuria in Parkinson's disease. Mov Disord 1995;10:337—40.

50. Hamed M, Mitchell H, Clow DJ. Hyponatraemic convulsion associated with desmopressin and imipramine treatment. Br Med J 1993;306:1169.

51. Stenberg A, Lackgren G. Desmopressin tablets in the treatment of severe nocturnal enuresis in adolescents. Pediatrics 1994;94:841—6.

52. Matthiesen TB, Rittig S, Djurhuus JC, Norgaard JP. A dose titration, and an open 6-week efficacy and safety study of desmopressin tablets in the management of nocturnal enuresis. J Urol 1994;151:460—3.

53. Nieuwenhuis HK, Sixma JJ. 1-Desamino-8-D-arginine vasopressin (desmopressin) shortens the bleeding time in storage pool deficiency. Ann Intern Med 1988;108:65—7.

54. Casonato A, Pontara E, Dannhaeuser D, Bertomoro A, Sartori MT, Zerbinati P, Girolami A. Re-evaluation of the therapeutic efficacy of DDAVP in type IIB von Willebrand's disease. Blood Coagul Fibrinolysis 1994;5:959—64.

55. Mannucci PM, Bettega D, Cattaneo M. Patterns of development of tachyphylaxis in patients with haemophilia and von Willebrand disease after repeated doses of desmopressin (DDAVP). Br J Haematol 1992;82:87—93.

56. Castaman G, Rodeghiero F, Lattuada A, Mannucci PM. Desmopressin-induced thrombocytopenia in type 1 platelet discordant von Willebrand disease. Am J Hematol 1993;43:5—9.

57. Kallen AJB, Carlsson SS, Bengtsson KAB. Diabetes insipidus and use of desmopressin (Minirin) during pregnancy. Eur J Endocrinol 1995; 132:144—6.

58. Barbieri RL. Clinical applications of GnRH and its analogues. Trends Endocrinol Metab 1992;3:30—4.

59. Friedman AJ The biochemistry, physiology, and pharmacology of gonadotropin releasing hormone (GnRH) and GnRh analogs. In: Barbieri RL, Friedman AJ, editors. Gonadotropin Releasing Hormone Analogs: Applications in Gynecology. New York: Chapman-Hall, 1991.

60. Miller RM, Frank RA. Zoladex (goserelin) in the treatment of benign gynaecological disorders: an overview of safety and efficacy. Br J Obstet Gynaecol 1992;99 Suppl 7:37—41.

61. Bressler LR, Murphy CM, Shevrin DH, Warren RF. Use of clonidine to treat hot flushes secondary to leuprolide or goserelin. Ann Pharmacother 1993;27:182—5.

62. Vercellini P, Sacerdote P, Trespidi L, Manfredi B, Panerai AE, Crosignani PG. Veralipride for hot flushes induced by a gonadotropin-releasing hormone agonist: a controlled study. Fertil Steril 1994;62:938—42.

63. Shalev E, Geslevich Y, Matilsky M, Ben-Ami M. Induction of pre-ovulatory gonadotrophin surge with gonadotrophin-releasing hormone agonist compared to pre-ovulatory injection of human chorionic gonadotrophins for ovulation induction in intrauterine insemination treatment cycles. Hum Reprod 1995;10:2244—7.

64. Rizk B, Smitz J. Ovarian hyperstimulation syndrome after superovulation using GnRH agonists for IVF and related procedures. Hum Reprod 1992;7:320—7.

65. Tarlatzis BC, Bili H, Bontis J, Lagos S, Vatev I, Mantalenakis S. Follicle cyst formation after administration of different gonadotrophin releasing hormone analogues for assisted reproduction. Hum Reprod 1994;9:1983—6.

66. Ando S, Hoshino T, Mihara S. Pituitary apoplexy after goserelin. Lancet 1995;345:458.

67. Chanson P, Schaison G. Pituitary apoplexy caused by GnRH agonist treatment revealing gonadotroph adenoma. J Endocrinol Metab 1995; 80:2267—68.

68. Miyagawa S, Shirai T, Shimamoto I, Ichijo M, Ueki H. Worsening of systemic lupus erythematous associated thrombocytopenia after administration of gonadotropin-releasing hormone analog. Arthritis Rheum 1994;37:1708—9.

69. Barrington JW, Roberts A. Acute renal failure precipitated by lutenizing hormone releasing hormone analogue for the treatment of endometriosis. Br J Urol 1994;74:672.

70. Matta WH, Shaw RH, Hesp R, Evans R. Reversible trabecular bone density loss following induced hypo-oestrogenism with the GnRH analogue buserelin in premenopausal women. Clin Endocrinol 1988;29:45—51.

71. Orwoll ES, Yuzpe AA, Burry KA, Heinrichs L, Buttram VC Jr, Hornstein MD. Nafarelin therapy in endometriosis: long-term effects on bone mineral density. Am J Obstet Gynecol 1994; 71:1221—5.

72. Maillefert JF, Sibilia, J, Kuntz JL, Tavernier C. Gonadotrophin-releasing hormone agonists induce osteoporosis. Br J Rheumatol 1994;33:12.

73. Adashi EY. Long term gonadotrophin releasing hormone agonist therapy: the evolving issue of steroidal 'add back' paradigms. Hum Reprod 1994;9:1380—97.

74. Lemay A, Surrey ES, Friedman AJ. Extending the use of gonadotrophin-releasing hormone agonists: the emerging role of steroidal and non steroidal agents. Fertil Steril 1994;61:21—34.

75. Leather AT, Studd JWW, Watson NR, Holland EFN. The prevention of bone loss in young women treated with GnRH analogues with 'add-back' estrogen therapy. Obstet Gynecol 1993; 81:104—7.

76. Surrey ES, Fournet N, Voigt B, Judd HL. Effects of sodium etidronate in combination with low-dose norethindrone in patients administered a long-acting GnRH agonist: a preliminary report. Obstet Gynecol 1993;81:581—6.

77. Compston JE, Yamaguchi K, Croucher PI, Garrahan NJ, Lindsay PC, Shaw RW. The effects of gonadotrophin releasing hormone agonists on iliac crest cancellous bone structure in women with endometriosis. Bone 1995;16:261—7.

78. Gambacciani M, Spinetti A, Piaggesi L, Cappagli B, Taponeco F, Manetti P, Weiss C, Teti GC, La Commare P, Facchini V. Ipriflavone prevents the bone mass reduction in premenopausal women treated with gonadotropin hormone releasing hormone agonists. Bone Miner 1994; 26:19—26.

79. Shennan A, Peek MJ. The use of thyrotophin releasing hormone to enhance fetal lung maturity. Contemp Rev Obstet Gynaecol 1995;7:77—82.

80. Knight DB, Liggins GC, Wealthall SR. A randomised, controlled trial of antepartum thyrotropin-releasing hormone and betamethasone in the prevention of respiratory disease in preterm infants. Am J Obstet Gynecol 1994;171:11—16.

81. Actobat Study Group. Australian collaborative trial of antenatal thyrotopin-releasing hormone (ACTOBAT) for prevention of neonatal respiratory disease. Lancet 1995;345:877—82.

82. Dolva LO, Riddervold F, Thorsen RK. Side effects of thyrotropin releasing hormone Br Med J 1993;287:532.

83. Crowther C, Haslam R, Hiller J, McGee T, Ryall R, Robinson J. Thyrotropin-releasing hormone: does two hundred micrograms provide effective stimulation to the preterm fetal pituitary gland compared with four hundred micrograms? Am J Obstet Gynecol 1995:173:719—23.

84. Peek MJ, Bajoria R, Shennan AH, Dalzell F, de Swiet M, Fisk NM. Hypertensive effect of antenatal thyrotropin releasing hormone in preeclampsia. Lancet 1995;345:793.

44   Drugs affecting lipid metabolism

GENERAL *(SED-13, 1324; SEDA-17, 510; SEDA-18, 426; SEDA-19, 407)*

The beneficial effects of cholesterol-lowering drugs have been demonstrated both with quantitative angiography of coronary vessels and clinically in terms of reduced morbidity and mortality (SEDA-19, 407). These drugs have generally good safety and tolerability. Concern has been raised, however, about their potential for *carcinogenicity*. All members of the two most popular classes of lipid-lowering drugs (the fibrates and the statins) cause cancer in rodents (1). Notably, in the CARE study, breast cancer occurred in one of the 2078 patients in the control group and 12 of the 2081 patients in the pravastatin group (2[C]). Otherwise the frequencies of cancers in clinical studies and up to 9 years after have been reassuring (3[R]).

Rhabdomyolysis is a problem with several of the lipid-lowering drugs, and the co-administration of various hypolipidemic drugs and of hypolipidemic drugs with other drugs (for example, lovastatin with gemfibrozil, bezafibrate with furosemide) increases the risk (SED-13, 1325; SEDA-8, 426).

ION-EXCHANGE RESINS *(SED-13, 1326; SEDA-17, 510; SEDA-18, 427)*

As ion-exchange resins do not cause systemic adverse effects, all of their untoward effects are related to effects on the gastrointestinal tract or to the binding of other substances in the gastrointestinal tract.

Interactions There was increased elimination of *meloxicam*, a non-steroidal anti-inflammatory drug, after intravenous injection in patients taking oral cholestyramine. This effect was assumed to have been due to the binding of meloxicam during enterohepatic or enteroenteric circulation (4[C]).

HMG COENZYME-A REDUCTASE INHIBITORS *(SED-13, 1327; SEDA-17, 511; SEDA-18, 427; SEDA-19, 408)*

It is the general impression that the four currently available statins (fluvastatin, lovastatin, pravastatin, and simvastatin) have similar safety and tolerability, as has recently been reviewed (5[R]). However, there may be some differences (e.g. see 'Interactions' below).

Psychiatric In a study of 17 244 individuals *depression* occurred in 289; the prevalence ratio for absence from work as a result was 1.83 (95% CI 1.30—2.58) for those who took an antihyperlipidemic diet and 2.18 (95% CI 1.18—4.03) for the 376 individuals taking simvastatin (6[C]).

A comparison of lovastatin and pravastatin has previously shown that neither affected nocturnal sleep, although lovastatin affected daytime performance (SEDA-18, 427). It has been argued that although lovastatin, as opposed to the more water-soluble pravastatin, has access to the cerebrospinal fluid, its concentrations there are extremely low and that its central adverse effects may not be as common as might be expected (7[R]).

Musculoskeletal system Musculoskeletal symptoms develop in about 0.5% of individuals within a month of starting therapy with a statin, and most cases develop within 3 months. Most patients recover after withdrawal. The predominant symptoms are *stiffness and tenderness of proximal limb muscles* and *difficulty* *in rising from a low chair* (8[C]). In a series of 15 patients, of whom 12 were women over the age of 60 years, there were no major increases in serum creatine kinase activity, all values being less than twice the upper limit of the reference range (8[C]).

There were *increases in serum myoglobin concentration and creatine kinase activity* shortly after a standardized ergometer muscle provocation test in patients with heterozygous familial hypercholesterolemia compared with healthy subjects, regardless of whether the patients were taking simvastatin or no drugs (9[C]). The authors concluded that some of the markers of muscle damage observed in cohorts taking lipid-lowering drugs are due to the underlying disease and not to the treatment.

A detailed comparison of exercise-induced muscle pathology in 24 patients taking simvastatin and pravastatin did not show any changes after 18 weeks and no differences between the two drugs (10[C]).

Interactions   Interactions with inhibitors of HMG coenzyme-A reductase have recently been reviewed (11[R]). The various inhibitors have different potentials for drug interactions, probably because of their different pharmacokinetic characteristics. It has been claimed that the combination of pravastatin with gemfibrozil carries a lower risk of myopathy than the combination of lovastatin with gemfibrozil. However, this conclusion has been criticized as being based on historical controls, and it has been pointed out that all package inserts for statins contain warnings against concomitant use with fibrates (7[R]). However, when fluvastatin was compared with gemfibrozil for evidence of muscle damage, there was no difference, and in patients who took both drugs there was a statistically significant *reduction* in creatine kinase activity compared with each of the drugs alone (12[C]).

The metabolic clearance of simvastatin was reduced in a small series of heart transplant patients taking *cyclosporin*; as a result plasma concentrations of the β-hydroxy acid metabolite of simvastatin were higher (12.1 vs. 6.8 ng/ml) than in a non-transplant control group (13[C]).

Atorvastatin

Although there is as yet little experience with this drug, it appears to have a promisingly low risk of adverse effects. Among 78 patients in a 6-week double-blind study, there were dose-related *increases in liver enzymes* (AsT and AlT) in 15 patients (up to twice the upper limit of the reference range), comparable to findings with other statins. There were adverse effects in 30 patients, compared with 34 among the 81 patients who took placebo. In one patient taking atorvastatin liver enzymes increased to 3—4 times the upper limit of the reference range, and one had an *increase in serum creatine kinase* (14[C]).

Fluvastatin

Like pravastatin, fluvastatin does not cross the blood—brain barrier, but this has not been shown to have clinical significance as regards the occurrence of adverse effects. It has also been suggested that the pharmacokinetics of fluvastatin, including extensive biliary excretion and no circulating active metabolites, might be advantageous. However, long-term experience with this drug is limited.

Gastrointestinal   As with other statins, there is a tendency towards increased reporting of gastrointestinal adverse effects compared with placebo (SEDA-19, 408). This effect increases when fluvastatin is combined with cholestyramine, but it has been pointed out that patients treated with cholestyramine alone suffer to a greater extent from gastrointestinal symptoms (15[C]).

Liver   The effects of fluvastatin on liver enzymes are similar to those of other statins. The proportion of patients who had *increases in serum transaminase activities* leading to discontinuation of therapy in controlled trials was 0.5% with fluvastatin compared with 0.3% with placebo (15[C]).

Musculoskeletal system   There have been no reports of myopathy with fluvastatin in any studies. Some cases of *myalgia* have been reported, mainly after exercise, but the increases in creatine kinase activity were less than 3 times the upper limit of the reference range, rather than the 10-fold increase that is used to define myopathy. However, in one patient the creatine kinase activity was transiently more than 10 times increased after exercise (15^C).

NICOTINIC ACID DERIVATIVES
(SED-13, 1329; SEDA-17, 512; SEDA-18, 428; SEDA-19, 409)

Many patients discontinue niacin because of adverse drug reactions or abnormal laboratory results, but fewer of those who take modified-release compared with immediate-release formulations (SEDA-19, 409). The high withdrawal rate has been confirmed in a study of 110 patients, but the difference between modified-release and regular formulations is perhaps over-rated (16^C). Moreover, adverse effects can occur after therapy for 1 or 2 years.

Special senses Niacin has previously been suspected of causing ocular changes, and this has been confirmed in a retrospective study (17^C) Altogether 7% of those taking niacin discontinued treatment because of ocular adverse effects. From spontaneous reporting systems, niacin in high dosages has been associated with *decreased vision*, *cystoid macular edema*, *sicca-like syndromes*, *discoloration of the eyelids*, and *superficial punctuate keratitis*, all these effects being dose-dependent and reversible on discontinuation (17^C).

REFERENCES

1. Newman TB, Hulley SB. Carcinogenicity of lipid-lowering drugs. J Am Med Assoc 1996;275:55—60.
2. Sacks FM, Pfeffer MA, Moye LA, Rouleau JL, Rutherford JD, Cole TG, Brown L, Warnica JW, Arnold JM, Wun CC, Davis BR, Braunwald E. The effect of pravastatin on coronary events after myocardial infarction in patients with average cholesterol levels. New Engl J Med 1996;335:1001—9.
3. Dalen JE, Dalton WS. Does lowering cholesterol cause cancer? J Am Med Assoc 1996;275:67—9.
4. Busch U, Heinzel G, Narjes H. The effect of cholestyramine on the pharmacokinetics of meloxicam, a new non-steroidal anti-inflammatory drug (NSAID), in man. Eur J Clin Pharmacol 1995;48:269—72.
5. Hsu I, Spinler SA, Johnson NE. Comparative evaluation of the safety and efficacy of HMG-CoA reductase inhibitor monotherapy in the treatment of primary hypercholesterolemia. Ann Pharmacother 1995;29:743—59.
6. Boumendil E, Tubert-Bitter P. Depression-induced absenteeism in relation to antihyperlipidemic treatment: A study using GAZEL cohort data. Epidemiology 1995;6:322—5.
7. Tobert JA. Lovastatin-associated sleep and mood disturbances. Am J Med 1995;99:108—9.
8. England JDF, Walsh JC, Stewart P, Boyd I, Rohan A, Halmagyi GM. Mitochondrial myopathy developing on treatment with the HMG CoA reductase inhibitors-simvastatin and pravastatin. Aust NZ J Med 1995;25:374—5.
9. Smit JWA, Bär PR, Geerdink RA, Erkelens DW. Heterozygous familial hypercholesterolaemia is associated with pathological exercise-induced leakage of muscle proteins, which is not aggravated by simvastatin therapy. Eur J Clin Invest 1995;25:79—84.
10. Contermans J, Smit JWA, Bär PR, Erkelens DW. A comparison of the effects of simvastatin and pravastatin monotherapy on muscle histology and permeability in hypercholesterolaemic patients. Br J Clin Pharmacol 1995;39:135—41.
11. Garnett WR. Interactions with hydroxymethylglutaryl-coenzyme A reductase inhibitors. Am J Health-Syst Pharm 1995;52:1639—45.
12. Smit JWA, Jansen GH, de Bruin TWA, Erkelens DW. Treatment of combined hyperlipidemia with fluvastatin and gemfibrozil, alone or in combination, does not induce muscle damage. Am J Cardiol 1995;76:126A—128A.
13. Campana C, Iacona I, Regazzi MB, Gavazzi A, Perani G, Raddato V, Montemartini C, Vigano M. Efficacy and pharmacokinetics of simvastatin in heart transplant recipients. Ann Pharmacother 1995;29:235—9.
14. Nawrocki JW, Weiss SR, Davidson MH, Sprecher DL, Schwartz SL, Lupien PJ, Jones PH, Haber HE, Black DM. Reduction of LDL cholesterol by 25% to 60% in patients with primary hypercholesterolemia by atorvastatin, a new HMG-CoA reductase inhibitor. Arterioscleros Thromb Vasc Biol 1995;15:678—82.
15. Deslypere JP. The role of HMG-CoA reductase inhibitors in the treatment of hyperlipidemia: a review of fluvastatin. Curr Ther Res 1995;56:111—28.
16. Gibbons LW, Gonzalez V, Gordon N, Grundy S. The prevalence of side effects with regular and sustained-release nicotinic acid. Am J Med 1995;99:378—85.
17. Fraunfelder FW, Fraunfelder FT, Illingworth DR. Adverse ocular effects associated with niacin therapy. Br J Ophthalmol 1995;79:54—6.

Andrew Stanley

45 Cytostatic drugs

Author's note: *The wide range of cytostatic drugs, the multitude of their toxic effects, and the fact that they are generally used in combinations of several agents all make it impossible to provide as detailed an overview of adverse reactions in this field as the annual gives in others. For this reason, in this chapter I present only salient points that appear to provide entirely new data, or increase the understanding of known but uncommon adverse effects. I have paid particular attention to incidents in which it seems possible to attribute particular effects to individual agents. In Table 1 are listed some review articles (either of individual cytostatic drugs or of specific toxicity across the whole range) that contribute to our overall understanding of cytostatic drug toxicity and its occurrence, significance, and management $(1^R)-(7^R)$, $(8^C)-(13^C)$.*

Because of the methods used to identify toxic effects for inclusion, far fewer potential sources of information have been reviewed; thus, the information in this year's chapter may not be as comprehensive as before.

Finally, I should like to thank those clinicians and researchers who have sent me copies of their original research papers.

DOSING VARIABLES AND PATIENT CHARACTERISTICS

While cancer is not being cured with existing cytostatic drugs (and in certain cases just about all possible active combinations have been tested), some authors are examining the effects of different doses or dosage schedules on both response and toxicity. Consequently, there are several recent papers that help to develop our understanding of the mechanism, nature, or course of a particular toxic effect, by examining the effects that different doses or dosage schedules have on the efficacy or toxicity of treatment, even though they have not reported new toxic effects or quantified or characterized known toxic effects. All of these papers allow us to see how such factors affect or leave unaltered the adverse effects profiles of the established antineoplastic drugs (see Table 2).

A final group of papers should also be mentioned here, for while they have not directly described toxic effects of the cytostatic drugs, they have discussed the use of drugs allied to oncology. These, because they are associated with particular adverse effects, often give good qualitative and quantitative descriptions of a specific adverse effect or range of effects. Two such papers cover the antioxidant and chemopreventive properties of N-acetylcysteine and glutathione with special reference to lung cancer (14^R) and inhibitors of hemopoiesis and their potential clinical relevance (15^R).

CARDIOVASCULAR

A case of *atrial fibrillation* has been attributed to ifosfamide after a dose of only 1800 mg/m^2, with mesna, in a regimen for metastatic breast cancer (16^c).

Pain along the vein occurred in five of 43 patients receiving vinorelbine 30 mg/m^2/week; none of these patients developed extravasation, but their symptoms were very similar (17^C). A similar rate of toxicity, 4.5%, has been reported in a review of the use of vinorelbine in 321 patients with breast cancer (18^R).

Orthostatic hypotension has been reported in 'several' of 126 patients given cisplatin 50 mg/m^2 on days 1, 8, 29, and 36 as part of treatment for lung cancer in combination with etoposide and chest radiotherapy (19^C).

RESPIRATORY

A fatal case of mitomycin C-induced *pneumonitis* has been reported in a radiotherapy/chemotherapy trial in 43 patients (20^C). The dose was 8 mg/m^2 on days 1 and 29, radiother-

Table 1. *Articles on adverse effects of cytostatic drugs*

Review articles for individual drugs
The prevention of cisplatin-associated neurotoxicity ([1R])
Comparative toxicity and mutagenic effects of platinum anticancer drugs ([2R])
A phase II study of flurouracil and its modulation in advanced colorectal cancer ([3R])
The use of tamoxifen for breast cancer ([4R])

Review articles for specific diseases
Present and future prospects in the treatment of metastatic breast cancer ([5R])
A topical perspective on hormone therapy for prostate cancer ([6R])
Single-agent and combination chemotherapy for advanced soft tissue sarcomas ([7R])

Drug resistance
The expression and prognostic significance of P-glycoprotein in adult solid tumors ([8R])

Table 2. *Articles on the effects of different doses and dosage regimens*

Dose range
An extension of the continual reassessment method, using a preliminary up-and-down design in a dose-
  finding study in cancer patients, in order to investigate a greater range of doses ([9R])

Total dose
Optimal number of chemotherapy courses in advanced non-seminomatous testicular carcinomas ([10R])

Dosage schedule
Elimination of dose-limiting toxic effects of cisplatin, 5-fluorouracil, and leucovorin using a weekly 24-
  hour infusion schedule in patients with nasophayngeal carcinoma ([11R])
Infusion chemotherapy in patients with refractory or relapsed lymphoma ([12R])
Schedule dependency of 21-day oral versus 3-day intravenous etoposide in combination with intravenous
  cisplatin in extensive stage small cell lung cancer ([13R])

apy and vindesine being given on the intervening days.

Severe morbidity has been reported after the use of bleomycin-containing therapies: 10% of patients developed *adult respiratory distress syndrome* and a further 9% needed prolonged ventilation ([21C]). The authors thought that these rates were higher than expected and attributed this to a combination of the toxic effects of bleomycin on the lung and a large retroperitoneal and/or pulmonary tumor burden.

NERVOUS SYSTEM

The vinca alkaloids have long been associated with both *peripheral and autonomic neuropathy*. However, the incidence of these complications with the newest member of the group, vinorelbine, has not yet been established. Incidence rates of 1.3% for peripheral neuropathy (mainly loss of deep tendon reflexes) and 4.1% for autonomic neuropathies

(manifested by constipation) have been reported from a European overview of 321 patients ([18R]).

In another study, in which vincristine 0.625 mg/m^2/week was given to 264 patients for a maximum of 10 weeks, the incidence of grade III/IV neuropathy rate was 7%, suggesting that dose intensity rather than total dose may be important for determining the severity of this toxic effect; the rate of grade I—IV neuropathy was 56% ([22C]).

LIVER

Hepatotoxicity, either *hyperbilirubinemia* or *increased alkaline phosphatase activity*, occurred in 36% of 14 patients in a trial of cytarabine 200 mg/m^2/day for 9 days by continuous infusion and daunorubicin 70 mg/m^2/day for 3 days ([23C]).

URINARY SYSTEM

A lot has been written about the effects of cisplatin on the kidneys. However, in 39 patients given low-dose continuous 5-fluorouracil and cisplatin 20 mg/m^2/week for 8 weeks there was a very low incidence of renal toxicity, although the incidence of electrolyte abnormalities, particularly hyponatremia and hypomagnesemia, was as expected (24[C]).

A patient with no other risk factors developed irreversible nephrotoxicity after four cycles of carboplatin 300 mg/m^2 and methotrexate 50 mg/m^2 (25[c]). This appears to have been an additive effect of drugs that are not individually nephrotoxic until much higher doses.

The risk factors associated with chronic ifosfamide nephrotoxicity up to 28 months after treatment have been studied in 23 children. The authors concluded that cumulative doses of 100 g/m^2 or higher should be avoided in children with cancer (26[C]).

The incidence of *cystitis* and/or *dysuria* was only 8% in 531 women with breast cancer who were given oral cyclophosphamide 60 mg/m^2/day for 1 year; the majority of cases were only grade I (22[C]).

SKIN AND APPENDAGES

Maculopapular eruptions and *desquamation* of hands and/or feet occurred in 35% of patients with non-small cell lung cancers given docetaxel (27[C]).

IMMUNOLOGICAL AND HYPERSENSITIVITY REACTIONS

A case of life-threatening allergy to cisplatin has been reported after 16 doses of cisplatin 20 mg/m^2/week (24[c]).

A 25% incidence of grade 2 or more severe immunological reactions to docetaxel has been reported after the use of oral prednisone (100 mg orally before treatment and 50 mg once on the morning of treatment and the following 2 days) in 20 patients with non-small-cell lung cancers (27[C]). No other premedications were given routinely. If infusion-related symptoms occurred, the infusion was interrupted and diphenhydramine was given. On subsequent cycles those patients then were routinely premedicated with diphenhydramine 25 or 50 mg intravenously and cimetidine 300 mg intravenously.

TUMOR-INDUCING EFFECTS

The National Wilms' Tumor Study Group has reported the incidence of second malignant neoplasms in 5278 patients treated over 22 years (28[C]). There were 43 second malignant neoplasms, whereas only five were expected. Fifteen years after the diagnosis of Wilms' tumor, the cumulative incidence of a second malignant neoplasm was 1.6% and was increasing steadily. Abdominal irradiation, given as part of the initial therapy, increased the risk and doxorubicin potentiated the radiation effect. Among 234 patients who received doxorubicin and over 35 Gy of abdominal radiation, eight second malignant neoplasms were observed, whereas only 0.22 were expected. Treatment for relapse further increased the risk by a factor of 4—5.

REFERENCES

1. Alberts DS, Noel JK. Cisplatin-associated neurotoxicity: can it be prevented? Anticancer Drugs 1995;6:369—83.

2. Yarema KJ. Comparative toxicities and mutagenics of platinum anticancer drugs. Drug Inf J 1995;29:1633s—1644s.

3. Leichman CG, Fleming TR, Muggia FM, Tangen CM, Ardalan B, Doroshow JH, Meyers FJ, Holcombe RF, Weiss GR, Mangalik A et al. Phase II study of fluorouracil and its modulation in advanced colorectal cancer: a Southwest Oncology Group study. J Clin Oncol 1995;13:1303—11.

4. Jaiyesimi IA, Buzdar AU, Decker DA, Hortobagyi GN. Use of tamoxifen for breast cancer: twenty-eight years later. J Clin Oncol 1995;13:513—29.

5. Hayes DF, Henderson IC, Shapiro CL. Treatment of metastatic breast cancer: present and future prospects. Semin Oncol 1995;22 Suppl 5:5—21.

6.   Klein EA. Hormone therapy for prostate cancer: a topical perspective. Urology 1996;47 Suppl 1A:3—12.

7.   Demetri GD, Elias AD. Results of single-agent and combination chemotherapy for advanced soft tissue sarcomas. Implications for decision making in the clinic. Hematol Oncol Clin North Am 1995;9:765—85.

8.   Leighton JC Jr, Goldstein LJ. P-glycoprotein in adult solid tumours. Expression and prognostic significance. Hematol Oncol Clin North Am 1995;9:251—73.

9.   Moller S. An extension of the continual reassessment method using a preliminary up-and-down design in a dose finding study in cancer patients, in order to investigate a greater range of doses. Stat Med 1995;14:911—22.

10.   Kennedy BJ, Torkelson J, Fraley EE. Optimal number of chemotherapy courses in advanced nonseminomatous testicular carcinomas. Am J Clin Oncol 1995;18:463—8.

11.   Chi KH, Chan WK, Shu CH, Law CK, Chen SY, Yen SH, Chen KY. Elimination of dose limiting toxicities of cisplatin, 5-fluorouracil, and leucovorin using a weekly 24-hour infusion schedule for the treatment of patients with nasopharyngeal carcinoma. Cancer 1995;76:2186—92.

12.   Carrion JR, Garcia-Arroyo FR, Salinas P. Infusional chemotherapy (EPOCH) in patients with refractory or relapsed lymphoma. Am J Clin Oncol 1995;18:44—6.

13.   Miller AA, Herndon JE 2nd, Hollis DR, Ellerton J, Langleben A, Richards F 2nd, Green MR. Schedule dependency of 21-day oral versus 3-day intravenous etoposide in combination with intravenous cisplatin in extensive-stage small-cell lung cancer: a randomised phase III study of the Cancer and Leukaemia Group B. Br J Clin Oncol 1995;13:1871—9.

14.   van Zandwijk N. *N*-Acetylcysteine (NAC) and glutathione (GSH): antioxidant and chemopreventive properties, with special reference to lung cancer. J Cell Biochem Suppl 1995;22:24—32.

15.   Parker AN, Pragnell IB. Inhibitors of haemopoiesis and their potential clinical relevance. Blood Rev 1995;9:226—33.

16.   Ingle JN, Krook JE, Mailliard JA, Hartmann LC, Wieand HS. Evaluation of ifosfamide plus mesna as first-line chemotherapy in women with metastatic breast cancer. Am J Clin Oncol 1995; 18:498—501.

17.   Frasci G, Comella G, Comella P, Salzano F, Cremone L, Della-Volpe N, Imbriani A, Persico G. Mitoxantrone plus vinorelbine with granulocyte-colony stimulating factor (G-CSF) support in advanced breast cancer patients. A dose and schedule finding study. Breast Cancer Res Treat 1995;35:147—56.

18.   Fumoleau P, Delozier T, Extra JM, Canobbio L, Delgado FM, Hurteloup P. Vinorelbine (Navelbine) in the treatment of breast cancer: the European experience. Semin Oncol 1995;22 Suppl 5:22—8.

19.   Albain KS, Rusch VW, Crowley JJ, Rice TW, Turrisi AT 3rd, Weick JK, Lonchyna VA, Presant CA, McKenna RJ, Gandara DR et al. Concurrent cisplatin/etoposide plus chest radiotherapy followed by surgery for stage IIIaA (N2) and IIIB non-small-cell lung cancer: mature results of Southwest Oncology Group Phase II Study 8805. J Clin Oncol 1995;13:1880—92.

20.   Furuse K, Kubota K, Kawahara M, Kodama N, Ogawara M, Akira M, Nakajima S, Takada M, Kusunoki Y, Negoro S et al. Phase II study of concurrent radiotherapy and chemotherapy for unresectable stage III non-small-cell lung cancer. Southern Osaka Lung Cancer Study Group. J Clin Oncol 1995;13:869—75.

21.   Baniel J, Foster RS, Rowland RG, Bihrle R, Donohue JP. Complications of post chemotherapy retroperitoneal lymph node dissection. J Urol 1995;153:976—80.

22.   Budd GT, Green S, O'Bryan RM, Martino S, Abeloff MD, Rinehart JJ, Hahn R, Harris J, Tormey D, O'Sullivan J et al. Short-course FAC-M versus 1 year of CMFVP in node-positive, hormone receptor-negative breast cancer: an intergroup study. J Clin Oncol 1995;13:831—9.

23.   Kouides PA, Rowe JM. A dose intensive regimen of cytosine arabinoside and daunorubicin for chronic myelogenous leukemia in blast crisis. Leuk Res 1995;19:763—70.

24.   Williamson SK, Tangen CM, Maddox AM, Spiridonidis CH, Macdonald JS. Phase II evaluation of low-dose continuous 5-fluorouracil and weekly cisplatin in advanced adenocarcinoma of the stomach. A Southwest Oncology Group study. Am J Clin Oncol 1995;18:484—7.

25.   Dogliotti L, Bertetto O, Berruti A, Clerico M, Fanchini L, Sicora W, Faggiuolo R. Combination chemotherapy with carboplatin and methotrexate in the treatment of advanced urothelial carcinoma. A phase II study. Am J Clin Oncol 1995; 18:78—82

26.   Skinner R, Pearson AD, English MW, Price L, Wyllie R, Coulthard MG, Craft AW. Risk factors for ifosfamide nephrotoxicity in children. Lancet 1996;348:578—80.

27.   Miller VA, Rigas JR, Francis PA, Grant SC, Pisters KM, Venkatraman ES, Woolley K, Heelan RT, Kris MG. Phase II trial of 75-mg/m^2 dose of docetaxel with prednisone premedication for patients with advanced non-small cell lung cancer. Cancer 1995;75:968—72.

28.   Breslow NE, Takashima JR, Whitton JA, Moksness J, D'Angio GJ, Green DM. Second malignant neoplasms following treatment for Wilms' tumor: a report from the National Wilms' Tumor Study Group. J Clin Oncol 1995;13:1851—9.

Peter Dawson

46 Radiological contrast agents

Contrast enhancing agents for use with X-rays, magnetic resonance imaging (MRI), and (more recently) ultrasound imaging, are among the most frequently used pharmaceuticals. While they are associated with a very low incidence of significant adverse effects, they are used on such a large scale that problems are not uncommon.

The spectrum of adverse events with the iodinated X-ray contrast agents, from mild to life-threatening, has been extremely well documented and in recent years the greater safety of the newer non-ionic contrast agents has been established. One area of increased interest recently is that of delayed reactions to contrast agents, discussed below. There has been little if any progress in understanding the mechanisms of adverse reactions to such contrast agents, though some new ideas on mediators and markers of allergic reactions are being explored.

The most widely used by far of the limited number of MRI contrast enhancing agents, the gadolinium chelates, are associated with significant adverse effects and major reactions only rarely, but documentation of their clinical use continues.

Various types of ultrasound echo-enhancing agents are being explored and developed, but their use has so far been limited. An update on this is provided.

DELAYED REACTIONS

There have recently been several anecdotal reports of delayed reactions of various kinds (usually defined as reactions that occur more than 24 h after exposure) in patients who have undergone radiological examinations with X-ray contrast agents. It must be said that many of the symptoms described are vague, such as *flu-like illness*, *malaise*, *aches and pains*, *headache*, and various *skin reactions*, some of which are among the mostly commonly encountered in general practice. Furthermore, in some studies there has been an element of asking patients leading questions. However, there is still a persisting impression that there may be a real effect here, and more objective phenomena, such as salivary gland swelling, have occasionally been reported.

A case of '*iodide mumps*' after a CT examination enhanced with a non-ionic contrast agent has been reported from Japan (1[c]).

A 70-year-old woman with a history of a right nephrectomy for renal carcinoma underwent CT examination to explore local recurrence and abdominal metastasis. Three hours after the examination she complained of nausea, vomiting, facial flushing, bilateral jaw pain, and fever. The laboratory findings 12 h after CT examination showed increased white blood cell count and serum amylase. Amylase fractionation showed that 86% originated from the salivary glands and she was admitted to hospital. The symptoms continued for 4 days with decreasing severity. Unspecified anti-inflammatory therapy was given and she was discharged well 6 days after the event.

The authors noted that swelling of the salivary glands after contrast injection is a rare but well established adverse reaction. The patient in this case had impaired renal function, which may be relevant, since higher plasma and tissue concentrations will have been achieved for a longer time than usual.

Acute anaphylactoid reactions after the injection of a non-ionic contrast agent, iohexol, for urography or CT have been studied in 321 Finnish children (2[c]). Follow-up was only for up to 24 h, but late reactions were recorded in about 6% of the patients. The late reactions included urticaria, facial edema, congested nose and sneezing, swelling of the eyelids, and redness of the eyes. The authors suggested that the short follow-up period was adequate because of the rapid excretion of iohexol. However, this is not a valid suggestion, in view of the observations of others that such reactions may occur over a period of a few days.

A case of *delayed hypersensitivity reaction* after contrast injection for an intravenous urogram has been reported (3[cr]).

A 67-year-old man was developed mild urticaria of the trunk and extremities 12 h after administration of the non-ionic contrast agent iohexol. This rapidly settled spontaneously, but 5 days later the patient presented to the emergency room with a diffuse, erythematous, severely pruritic, maculopapular rash on the arms, legs, trunk, and face. He was treated with antihistamines and settled over the next 3—5 days.

The authors wrote that the true incidence of immune-mediated delayed adverse reactions to intravenous contrast material is difficult to define, because of the usual lack of follow up; literature reports suggest something between 5 and 8%. Many reactions are vague, and include headache, fatigue, flu-like illness, which are unlikely to have any kind of allergic basis. The reported incidence of urticaria as a delayed adverse response was difficult to ascertain from the literature, but it has certainly been described in a number of series. The literature suggests no difference between ionic and non-ionic contrast agents in this respect.

An important point to note is that the latest type of iodinated X-ray contrast agent to be developed, the non-ionic dimer, has been anecdotally noted to be associated with an unusually high incidence of delayed, usually urticarial, skin reactions. More data are currently being collected on this issue.

INTRAVENOUS CHOLANGIOGRAPHY
(SED-13, 1391)

The use of intravenous cholangiography has fallen dramatically in Europe and the US in recent years, largely because of the advent of new and safer techniques for imaging the biliary tree, including high-quality ultrasound. Conversion to these new techniques has certainly been given extra impetus by the relatively poor tolerance and relatively high risk associated with the use of agents for intravenous cholangiography compared with general angiographic agents. However, the introduction of laparoscopic cholecystectomy has led

surgeons to demand that radiologists restore the technique, largely in order to explore preoperatively the presence of any anatomical anomalies that might lead to surgical problems.

The most modern of the agents for intravenous cholangiography is meglumine iotroxate (Biliscopin, Schering AG Berlin). An Australian group (4[c]) has reported on 405 intravenous cholangiographic examinations of their own, and 611 performed in private hospitals, giving a total of 1061. Patients with asthma, hay fever, or atopy were always given an antihistamine before the examination. Seven of their own 405 patients and four of the 611 others, making a total of 11 out of 1061 patients, had any kind of reaction, and only one developed mild bronchospasm. The authors concluded that intravenous cholangiography, at least with this modern agent, was acceptably safe. They also cited a comparison of this with two other agents for intravenous cholangiography (5[c]). Reactions with all agents were trivial, but occurred least often with Biliscopin. They also cited a large study by Nilsson (6[c]), in which the three agents were studied in 2492 patients. Adverse events were minor. The authors argued that, contrary to popular opinion, reactions are apparently no more frequent with agents for intravenous cholangiography than with angiographic agents, and that their use for the performance of intravenous cholangiography before laparoscopic cholecystectomy is acceptably safe.

ENDOSCOPIC RETROGRADE CHOLANGIOPANCREATOGRAPHY (ERCP) *(SED-13, 1392; SEDA-17, 535)*

Pancreatitis (SEDA-19, 425) is a not uncommon complication of ERCP, and the contrast agent itself is held to be a significant factor, among others, implicated in this serious complication (7[c]). One strategy for minimizing the risk of pancreatitis has been to use non-ionic/low osmolality contrast agents. Another recommendation has been not to use too high an injection pressure, thereby reducing risk of extraductile extravasation. A multicenter study in the US has recently been undertaken to evaluate the role that contrast material plays in the development of pancreatitis after ERCP (7[C]). It involved nearly 2000 patients, 1659 of whom had pancreatic duct injections and were divided into subgroups according to the complexity of the ERCP. Throughout the study, patients were randomized to receive injections of either a non-ionic/low osmolality agent or an ionic/high osmolality agent. The findings were surprising, in that the incidence of pancreatitis depended far more on the complexity of the procedure than on anything else. Simple diagnostic ERCP had the lowest incidence (5.6%) and therapeutic procedures in general a higher incidence (12%). Sphincter of Oddi manometry had an even higher rate (15%). There was no statistically significant difference between ionic agents (10%) and non-ionic agents (10%). This finding has cost implications and also supports the impression obtained from other areas of medical imaging that, while contrast agents may certainly be associated with a number of problems, the nature of the study, the technique used, and the condition of the patient are sometimes insufficiently taken into account in discussing complications.

INTRAVENOUS UROGRAPHY *(SED-13, 1393; SEDA-17, 535)*

The use of intravenous urography has been in decline in the West for some years, principally following the advent of high-quality real-time ultrasound techniques, but it is still used on a significant scale. Anxieties about adverse reactions to contrast agents in urography are therefore still widespread. Undoubtedly the non-ionic contrast agents have rendered urography better tolerated and safer, and yet more new agents of this design continue to appear. Two such are iomeprol and iobitridol. Studies of the incidence of problems with iomeprol (8[C]) and iobitridol (9[C]) have been published, but in quite small numbers of patients. In both cases there has been a low incidence of reactions, with no serious reactions at all. Studies of this kind in small numbers of patients serve only to establish routine tolerance, rather than the incidence of the rarer more severe reactions. It seems likely that newer and very similar non-ionic contrast agents will, in terms of safety, turn

out to be similar to the established non-ionic agents.

A multicenter study has been performed in Norway, Belgium, France, and the UK of intravenous urography with the same non-ionic contrast agent (iohexol), but supplied in polypropylene containers as opposed to the more routinely used glass vials, emphasizing the incidence of allergic adverse events (10[C]). The authors have argued that polypropylene is a pure plastic material with practically no additives and should therefore be as acceptable as glass, but with greater convenience. Indeed, they found no difference in the incidence of allergic reactions between the two groups (some 740 patients in each).

By way of background, it may be noted in this context that some have argued that at least a proportion of adverse reactions to contrast agents, in both intravascular and intrathecal procedures, may be due not to the agents themselves but to impurities in the solutions. One hypothesis that has gained some currency is that contamination from plastic and/or rubber in syringes or bottles may play a role. Little serious research has been done in this potentially important field.

MYELOGRAPHY *(SED-13, 1400; SEDA-17, 538; SEDA-18, 445; SEDA-19, 430)*

Myelography is performed less often now than in the past, because of the availability of CT scanning and MRI technology, but in some parts of the world large numbers of procedures continue to be carried out. Contrast agent nephrotoxicity in this context remains an important issue.

Nervous system   The complications of myelography have recently been reported from the UK, including a case of *sixth nerve palsy* after myelography, the disability lasting for several months (11[c]).

A 47-year-old woman underwent myelography for the investigation of low back pain. She had reduced sensation at L5 and S1. Myelography (radiculography) was performed using 10 ml of iopamidol (a non-ionic contrast agent) into the L3/4 intervertebral space. This showed amputation of the right nerve root sheath at L5/S1, due to bilateral disc prolapse. She complained of headache after the procedure and also had nausea, vomiting, and dizziness, which improved over the next few days. However, on the sixth day after the procedure she developed diplopia. Two days later she had an epidural injection of bupivacaine and depomedrone between L4 and L5 to relieve her continuing back ache. Four days later the diplopia was still present and examination showed a right lateral rectus palsy. A CT scan of the brain was normal. The diplopia resolved 4 months after the procedure and a detailed examination at 8 months showed no abnormality.

Headache, *nausea*, and *vomiting* are common complications reported with myelography with any contrast agents. *Sixth nerve palsy* and severe *meningeal irritation* have been reported in myelography and radiculography, and although they can occur with lumbar puncture alone they are more frequent when a contrast agent is injected. The authors cited a previous report of two cases of sixth nerve palsy out of 1138 myelograms with iopamidol. The mechanism is not known. Adhesive arachnoiditis, which has been reported after myelography with water-soluble contrast agents, may be implicated, but is very rare. A direct neurotoxic effect on the nucleus of the nerve is possible, but in this case it would have been anticipated to be bilateral. Leakage of CSF through the lumbar puncture site could have caused a caudal brain shift and hence traction on the sixth cranial nerve. Bearing this possibility in mind, the point made in the report on pancreatitis and ERCP is worth repeating, namely that problems apparently associated with a contrast agent may not necessarily be due to the contrast agent.

That contrast agents, particularly the ionic ones, have neurotoxic potential has been illustrated by a report of *focal seizures* in an 11-year-old girl after intraoperative visualization of a cervical syringoperitoneal shunt with diatrizoate meglumine (an ionic contrast agent of high osmolality) (12[c]). Feingold, commenting on the case (13[c]), recorded that he had published a similar report of a near catastrophe as long ago as 1970, and thought it remarkable that such an avoidable complication might still occur. He called for clear protocols to be established so that mistakes of this kind in the choice of contrast agent should not be made in simple ignorance.

COMPUTED TOMOGRAPHY (CT)

Contrast-enhanced CT is the radiological examination second only to angiography in its use of large volumes of contrast agents in many patients. Anaphylactoid reactions and various aspects of dose-related systemic and organ-specific toxic effects may occur

Both immediate and delayed adverse effects have been sought in a study of two different iodine concentrations (240 and 320 mg/ml) of the same non-ionic contrast agent in enhanced dynamic CT (14[c]). While there was greater opacification with the higher concentration, there was no difference in the diagnostic yield. Fewer patients were affected by immediate minor complications with the lower concentration. The number of patients affected by delayed adverse effects (see above) was similar in the two groups. The authors argued that, in the interest of greater patient tolerance with no loss of diagnostic power, lower concentrations than those typically used should be considered in CT.

Since the number of patients in this study was small, since there were no serious adverse effects, and since such dose-dependent adverse effects of contrast agents as nephrotoxicity were not studied, this report is of limited value. However, it has raised the general issue of whether in many procedures greater concentrations and/or greater total doses of contrast agents than necessary are being used.

ULTRASOUND CONTRAST AGENTS

A considerable amount of work has been done by several pharmaceutical companies and in clinical trials, leading to the commercial availability of at least two products in various parts of the world for the enhancement of ultrasound images and Doppler studies. One of these products, Levovist (Schering AG, Berlin), is a galactose-based material consisting of microbubbles less than 8 μm in size. After injection it crosses the lung and enters the systemic circulation. Its efficacy and adverse effects have been studied in 27 patients in Japan (15[c]) and 30 patients in California (16[c]). Given the anxieties about the injection of any kind of particulate or 'bubble' agent into the circulation, the lack of any adverse effects in either study is reassuring and in line with results from earlier studies and clinical trials.

℞ Contrast agents used in magnetic resonance imaging

In the last decade or so intravenous contrast agents for use in magnetic resonance imaging (MRI), first of the central nervous system and later of other organs, have become widely available (SED-13, 1407; SEDA-17, 538; SEDA-18, 446). A considerable research investment has been made by the pharmaceutical industry, and there is promise of a great variety of agents, some targeted at specific applications.

Gadolinium chelates

The most extensively used agents in MRI are gadolinium chelates, which are available from at least four manufacturers in various countries.

The strong impression gained anecdotally and from wide-scale formal and informal monitoring of their use is that the gadolinium chelates ('Magnevist', gadolinium-DTPA, Schering AG, Berlin, and 'Omniscan', Nycomed AS, Oslo) are significantly safer in every respect than even the non-ionic X-ray agents. A US study in some 15 000 patients has provided further confirmation of this view (17[C]). The rate of adverse reactions was only 2.4% overall, and the symptoms abated spontaneously within 24 h in 95% of cases. There were only two serious adverse reactions and those were attributed to the underlying disease: one patient with metastatic brain lesions died of tentorial herniation of the brain during the 24-h follow-up period and the other required hospitalization for severe vertigo after the procedure. The rate of adverse reactions in patients with a history of asthma or allergy was marginally higher, at 3.7%. Patients with a history of a previous reaction to an MRI or iodinated X-ray contrast agent had adverse reaction rates of 21 and 6%, respectively. There was a marginal difference between slow and fast administration reaction rates.

Two gadolinium chelates, 'Magnevist' and 'Omniscan', have been compared in 60 Swe-dish patients (18[C]). There were only three adverse events attributable to the contrast agent (5%) and all were mild.

The safety and tolerance of another chelate (gadolinium-DOTA, 'Dotarem') has been compared with the longest established agent (gadolinium-DTPA) in 1038 patients (19[C]). Non-serious adverse reactions occurred in only 0.97 and 0.77%, respectively.

Super-paramagnetic iron oxide (SPIO) contrast agents

Super-paramagnetic iron oxide (SPIO) contrast agents are used intravenously to enhance liver imaging. Their efficacy and safety have been studied in the context of patients with cirrhotic livers (20[C]). Low back pain was observed in two patients during the infusion, but was transient, lasting only some 5 min and requiring no treatment. There were no other adverse effects. The efficacy and safety of an experimental SPIO agent have been examined in a US multicenter study of 208 patients with known or suspected focal hepatic lesions (21[C]). All had extensive clinical and laboratory assessments before and after the contrast-enhanced MRI study. There were no serious adverse reactions. The reported adverse events were mild to moderate in all cases, except for severe back pain in two and severe flushing in one. All symptoms resolved without sequelae; 15% had a total of 47 adverse reactions, including vomiting and diarrhea (three), back pain (nine), urticaria (two), flushing (five), dizziness (two), and muscle spasm (two).

Clearly the incidence of adverse effects is significantly higher with these particulate iron oxide agents than it is with the very well-tolerated gadolinium chelates, but that is not a great cause for concern. Few of the reactions are severe and all are self-limiting. Nevertheless, as the authors concluded, longer term assessment of their use in clinical practice is necessary.

We shall undoubtedly see contrast agents being used more extensively in MRI and a number of variants of existing agents and some entirely new agents will emerge. Even given an assumption of a low incidence of adverse events with all these materials, their use on a wide scale will, as with the X-ray contrast agents, lead to a significant number of problems.

ORGAN-SPECIFIC EFFECTS

Cardiovascular *(SED-13, 1384; SEDA-17, 536; SEDA-18, 443)* Many factors have been identified in the adverse effects of contrast agents on cardiac pump function and electrophysiology. These include osmolality, chemotoxicity, and additives such as a number of varieties of EDTA (22[R]). Calcium is essential for normal cardiac physiology and some salts of EDTA can bind calcium. It has been long established that this was a significant factor in the toxic effects of some early ionic contrast agents, including transient impairment of pump function, bradycardia, and prolongation of the PR interval.

Two formulations of the same contrast agent (Hypaque 76, a conventional high-osmolality ionic agent), one with and one without a calcium-binding additive, have been studied in 223 consecutive patients, who were randomly given one or the other (23[C]). Electrocardiographic and hemodynamic changes related to coronary angiography and left ventriculography were measured, and any complications that required intervention were recorded. There were more complications in the patients who received the contrast agent with the calcium-binding additive: arterial pressures fell more, the QT interval increased more, and the heart rate fell more.

It should be noted that financial considerations underpinned the perceived need for this study. The non-ionic contrast agents do not routinely contain a calcium-binding additive and do not themselves significantly bind calcium. It is only if the cheaper conventional ionic agents, which do bind calcium, are considered for cardiac angiography that these considerations of the impact of different calcium-binding associated with different agents needs to be considered.

Endocrine, metabolic (SED-13, 1385; SEDA-18, 443) During an iodine balance study of 24-h intake and urinary excretion of iodine in 107 premature infants at different postnatal ages, 13 excreted far more iodine than was available through food, whereas most of the others excreted less iodine in urine than daily intake (24[C]). This was unexpected, as iodinated disinfectants were not used and infants undergoing radiological examinations had been excluded. It was then discovered that parenteral feeding via a percutaneous non-radio-opaque silastic catheter of 0.6 mm diameter had involved the injection of a small amount of an iodinated X-ray contrast agent (Hexabrix) to assist with positioning. The authors therefore undertook a careful study of iodine balance in these children and in 24 age-matched premature control infants who received formula milk. No infant in either group was identified as having congenital hypothyroidism and there was no difference between the groups in either the frequency of neonatal complications generally or measures of age of gestation at birth. The infants were studied during the first week of life and every 15 days up to 4 months (group 1) or 2 months (group 2). Serum tri-iodothyronine and thyroxine were lower and serum TSH higher in group 1 than in group 2.

It is well known that an iodine load can alter thyroid function and cause *hypothyroidism*. Contrast agents contain very large amounts of iodine, though it is in a bound form. The dose delivered to a neonate at the time of injection may be as high as 1.8—12.5 g. There is little absorption of iodine from the normal gut, but the authors noted that even topical disinfectants that contain iodine in concentrations below 10 mg/ml as a single application to the skin of neonates may result in the excretion of as much as 30 mg/l of iodine in the urine on the first day after use. The minimum amount of iodine that may impair thyroid function in premature babies and neonates has never been clearly defined, as it obviously depends on several factors, but the data support the view that thyroid complications should be suspected in any premature infant with a urinary iodine concentration greater than 200 μg/l. These results emphasize that great caution should be undertaken during radiological examinations in infants.

Urinary system *(SED-13, 1385; SEDA-17, 537; SEDA-18, 444; SEDA-19, 427)* Intravascular X-ray contrast agents have long been believed to be nephrotoxic. The effect is deemed to be more likely, and more severe, if the patient has pre-existing renal failure, if the dose is large, if the patient is diabetic, and (most important of all) if there is dehydration. Although generally accepted, it should be said that the evidence for all this is not overwhelming, largely because of a lack of controls in most of the studies and because of the anecdotal nature of some of the evidence. The problem is made more difficult by the lack of a convincing hypothesis for the underlying mechanisms and of an animal model for experimental study.

Supposed nephrotoxic events associated with both ionic and non-ionic contrast agents have been investigated in a randomized multi-center US study in 1196 patients (25[C]). If we take it as an established fact that contrast agents are nephrotoxic, one can ask whether non-ionic contrast agents, which are less toxic and better tolerated in every other respect, might be better tolerated by the kidneys. It is this question that the authors set out to examine, by carefully monitoring several measures of renal physiology before, during, and after contrast examinations in this very carefully designed study. They noted that no difference has emerged in several previous studies, but that those all involved small numbers of subjects, usually with pre-existing renal insufficiency, alone or combined with diabetes, thereby limiting confidence in their conclusions

The study showed that the non-ionic contrast agent iohexol was associated with significantly less nephrotoxicity than the ionic agent diatrizoate in high-risk uremic patients undergoing elective cardiac angiography. In addition, there was no evidence of reduced nephrotoxicity in non-uraemic patients, regardless of the presence or absence of diabetes mellitus, by the non-ionic agent. The authors' overall conclusion was that iohexol offers advantages in uraemic patients but not otherwise. Interestingly, 15 patients developed acute nephrotoxicity of more marked severity, with oliguria requiring acute dialysis, or an increase in the serum creatinine of sufficient magnitude for dialysis to be considered. Nine of the patients received the ionic agent and six the non-ionic agent. Whether fewer patients will be tipped into severe renal

failure by non-ionic contrast agents than by ionic agents remains unclear.

The effects of ionic and non-ionic contrast agents on renal function have been studied in 38 children (26[C]). The context was intravenous urography and the patients were divided into three groups according to their pre-study glomerular filtration rate. Urine specific gravity, protein/creatinine ratios, and serum sodium and creatinine concentrations were monitored. Only the specific gravity of the urine changed outside normal limits and there was no significant difference in any of the effects of the ionic and non-ionic agents. The value of this study was severely limited because of the few patients studied.

As mentioned above, there is no single convincing hypothesis that explains the nephrotoxic effect of contrast agents. However, investigators continue to measure what they can, such as urinary tubular enzyme excretion, to monitor the effects of different contrast agents. Thus, plasma creatinine concentration, creatinine clearance, plasma and urine osmolality, fractional sodium excretion, and urinary ratios of AST:creatinine, AlT:creatinine, and LDH:creatinine have been measured in children undergoing cardiac angiography with the non-ionic contrast agent iopromide (27[C]). There were no significant changes.

A possible role of endothelin in nephrotoxic events associated with contrast agents has been studied in 77 children who underwent cardiac angiography for the investigation of congenital cardiac disease (28[C]). There was increased endothelin excretion and significant increases in markers of tubular toxicity. The changes in endothelin excretion were correlated with changes in the tubular enzymes α_1-microglobulin and N-acetyl-β-D-glucosaminidase (NAG) in all children, but particularly in those aged under 1 year. Tubular damage was not correlated with the dosage of contrast agent and contrast agents of high and low osmolarity did not differ.

Endothelin is a very potent vasoconstricting hormone. It reduces transepithelial transport in the distal tubular cells of the kidney and is particularly hazardous in pre-injured cells. A strategy of inhibiting the nephrotoxic effects of contrast agent by interfering with intrarenal endothelin production seems a promising strategy. Preliminary studies with an oral endothelin receptor antagonist have showed promising results (29[C]).

R̥ *Anaphylactoid and allergic reactions to contrast agents*

Anaphylactoid and allergic reactions to contrast agents (SEDA-17, 536; SEDA-18, 441), although reduced several-fold in incidence with the modern non-ionic contrast agents, cause the greatest anxiety during X-ray procedures. The conventional ionic agents were associated with an incidence variously reported as 1:5000 to 1:130 000 administrations.

Incidence   Recently, 30 cases of fatal drug-induced anaphylactic shock, identified between 1968 and 1990, have been notified to the Danish Committee on Adverse Drug Reactions and the Central Death Register (30[C]). The most frequent causes were contrast agents, antibiotics, and extracts of allergens. Contrast agents accounted for eight of the 30 deaths. The authors concluded that fatal drug-induced anaphylactic and anaphylactoid reactions are rare (0.3 cases per million inhabitants per year in the Danish experience), but that X-ray contrast agents make a significant contribution.

The rates of various causes of anaphylactic and anaphylactoid reactions in a voluntary hospital emergency room in the US have been reported (31[C]). Of 326 cases analysed, 72 (22%) were drug-related; most (32%) were due to antibiotics and only four were due to X-ray contrast agents. This is slightly more reassuring, in that only 1.2% of major anaphylactoid and anaphylactic events were related to contrast agents. However, it should be noted that this was in an emergency room—most patients who have anaphylactoid reactions to contrast agents naturally present in the X-ray department, and so these figures may be falsely low.

The incidence of allergic adverse events among 142 atopic and asthmatic patients undergoing cardiac angiography in Detroit has been reported in a study of a non-ionic agent, iopamidol, versus the sole low-osmolality ionic agent, ioxaglate (32[C]). The expectation that the incidence of 'allergic' reactions (such as urti-caria, bronchospasm, conjunctival and periorbital edema, and angio-edema) should be lower in patients receiving the non-ionic agent was confirmed, a finding that is in line with the results of other studies and with anecdotal observations.

Risk of repeated exposure   If a patient has a history of a prior idiosyncratic reactions to ionic contrast agents, what is the risk of a further reaction on repeated exposure and what premedication should be used? These questions have been tackled by Dyer and Cohan (33[r]), who have argued that one of the clear indications for the use of a non-ionic contrast agent is a previous idiosyncratic reaction and that the use of such an agent should reduce the overall incidence significantly, although major reactions, and some fatalities, continue to be reported. He has correctly stated that most radiologists would use some form of premedication, such as corticosteroids and occasionally antihistamines, but that the foundation for this practice is based on shifting sands. I have elsewhere reviewed the evidence for the use of corticosteroid prophylaxis in such patients and found it wanting (34[R]). This subject remains a surprisingly contentious one. Evidence for the effectiveness of any of the regimens that are frequently used is lacking, but the widespread belief that they may be of some efficacy perhaps frames the medicolegal context in which radiologists have to work.

Markers of allergic reactions to contrast agents   Two groups (35[C]) and (36[C]) have reported on the use of serum concentration measurements of tryptase and eosinophil cationic protein in patients who have allergic reactions. In a group of 20 subjects tryptase and histamine were increased, although not in all cases for both markers, but there was no clear association with eosinophil cationic protein either at 2 or 24 h after the allergic episode (35[C]). The results suggested that mast cells participate in adverse reactions, but the role of eosinophils could not be established. These markers were also studied in 13 subjects who had immediate allergic reactions to a variety of drugs, and the results also suggested that tryptase was involved and that eosinophil cationic protein was not (36[C]). Only one patient in one of the studies had a reaction to a contrast agent.

Clearly this is a promising field of investigation, for both the understanding and the monitoring of major allergic drug reactions, and work is needed specifically in the field of contrast agent reactions.

ALTERNATIVES TO IODINATED CONTRAST AGENTS

Iodinated X-ray contrast agents of the safer non-ionic type are expensive, and alternatives have been sought. One investigated and used in a number of centers around the world is carbon dioxide, a highly soluble gas, which is therefore relatively safe to inject into the circulation. It displaces blood and reduces X-ray absorption, acting as a negative contrast agent. Two groups from Korea (37[C]) and the UK (38[C]) have assessed the use of carbon dioxide as a contrast medium in arteriography, the former in image-guided placement of peripherally inserted central venous catheters and the latter in aortography and peripheral arteriography; there were 30 patients in the UK study and 41 in the Korean study. No complication of any kind was observed. It may at first sight seem surprising that this natural and apparently safe contrast agent should not have been more widely adopted by radiologists. The explanation probably lies in deep-seated anxieties about injecting gas into the circulation, which are uninfluenced by any logical discussion about the important distinction between, say, air and carbon dioxide.

RADIOACTIVE SUBSTANCES OF HISTORICAL INTEREST *(SED-13, 1409; SEDA-18, 446; SEDA-19, 431)*

Thorium dioxide (Thorotrast)

The long redundant contrast agent Thorotrast is a 20% colloidal solution of thorium dioxide, an α emitter that is not excreted from the body but is taken up and stored in the reticuloendothelial system. It was used in the 1930s and 1940s in Europe, North America, and Japan for a variety of intra-arterial and intrathecal investigations. The induction of *malignancy* is the hallmark of thorium dioxide and, though its use is historical, its legacy is still with us. The Danish Thorotrast Study now has a collection of 1003 patients who were exposed to Thorotrast (39[C]). The following leukemias and related hematological disorders occurred (numbers in parentheses): acute myeloblastic leukemia (16), chronic myelocytic leukemia (three), acute lymphoblastic leukemia (one), chronic lymphocytic leukemia (two), myelodysplastic syndrome (eight), myelofibrosis (two), multiple myeloma (two), non-Hodgkin's lymphoma (four). The expected number of leukemias was under 2.5 and, except for the cases of chronic lymphocytic leukemia, it was thought that all were probably secondary to Thorotrast. The authors reported that the findings in German, Japanese, Portuguese, and Danish studies are all very similar.

Similarly, 99 Japanese cases of angiosarcoma in a variety of body sites have ben reviewed (40[C]). In five (29%) of 17 patients with hepatic angiosarcoma Thorotrast had been used.

The incidence of malignant mesothelioma and lung carcinoma has been studied in Danish patients exposed to Thorotrast (41[C]). In a previous registry-based survey of 999 patients given Thorotrast the authors had identified increased risks of lung carcinoma and malignant mesothelioma. This was presumably because injected Thorotrast, retained life-long in the liver, spleen, and lymph nodes, irradiates the mesothelial surfaces of these organs continuously. Patients given Thorotrast also exhale radon, a thorium daughter product, and may thereby provide data on the carcinogenicity of radon, a current public health concern, as well as on the pathogenesis of malignant mesothelioma. The cumulative risk for lung cancer was 11%, based on 20 confirmed cases. The risk for malignant mesothelioma was 2.5% based on seven cases. The actuarial risk of malignant mesothelioma for patients given more than 20 ml of Thorotrast was 7.8% compared with 1.4% for patients given smaller amounts.

REFERENCES

1. Kuwatsuru R, Katayama H, Minowa O, Tsukada K. Iodide mumps after contrast enhanced CT with iopamidol: a case report. Radiat Med 1995;13:147—8.

2. Mikkonen R, Kontkanen T, Kivisaari L. Late and acute adverse reactions to iohexol in a pediatric population. Pediatr Radiol 1995;25:350—2.

3. Stovsky MD, Seftel AD, Resnick MI. Delayed hypersensitivity reaction after infusion of nonionic intravenous contrast material for an excretory urogram: a case report and review of the literature. J Urol 1995;153:1641—3.

4. Sacharias N. Safety of biliscopin. Australas Radiol 1995;39:101.

5. Taenzer V, Volkhardt V. Double blind comparison of meglumine iotroxate (Biliscopin), meglumine iodoxamate (Endobil), and meglumine ioglycamate (Biligram). Am J Roentgenol 1979; 132:55—8.

6. Nilsson U. Adverse reactions to iotroxate at intravenous cholangiography. A prospective clinical investigation and review of the literature. Acta Radiol 1987;28:571—5.

7. Johnson GK, Geenen JE, Bedford RA, Johanson J, Cass O, Sherman S, Hogan WJ, Ryan M, Silverman W, Edmundowicz S et al. Midwest Pancreaticobiliary Study Group. A comparison of nonionic versus ionic contrast media: results of prospective, multicentre study. Gastrointest Endosc 1995;42:312—16.

8. Harding JR, Bertazzoli M, Spinazzi A. A randomized, double-blind, parallel group trial of iomeprol, iohexol and iopamidol in intravenous urography. Br J Radiol 1995;68:712—15.

9. Taylor W, Moseley I. Assessment of the safety and efficacy of iobitridol, an iodinated contrast medium (30% iodine), in cranial CT. Eur J Radiol 1995;20:57—60.

10. Tveit K, Dardenne AN, Svihus R, Fairhurst J, Jenssen G, Lemaitre L, Grellet J, Brekke O, Skinningsrud K. Iohexol in patients undergoing urography: a comparison of polypropylene containers (Unique Soft Pack) and glass vials. Clin Radiol 1995;50:44—8.

11. Dinakaran S, Desai SP, Corney CE. Case report: sixth nerve palsy following radiculography. Br J Radiol 1995;68:424.

12. Karl HW, Talbott GA, Roberts TS. Intraoperative administration of radiologic contrast agents: potential neurotoxicity. Anesthesiology 1994;81:1068—71.

13. Feingold A. Neurotoxicity of contrast agents. Anesthesiology 1995;82:1302—3.

14. Wang R, Birchall IW, Hanson J. Reducing the concentration of contrast medium in dynamic computed tomography of the neck: consequences for image quality, side effects and cost. Can Assoc Radiol J 1995;46:27—31.

15. Tanaka S, Kitamra T, Yoshioka F, Kitamura S, Yamamoto K, Ooura Y, Imaoka T. Effectiveness of galactose-based intravenous contrast medium on color Doppler sonography of deeply located hepatocellular carcinoma. Ultrasound Med Biol 1995;21:157—60.

16. Otis S, Rush M, Boyajian R. Contrast-enhanced transcranial imaging. Results of an American phase-two study. Stroke 1995;26:203—9.

17. Nelson KL, Gifford LM, Lauber-Huber C, Gross CA, Lasser TA. Clinical safety of gadopentetate dimeglumine. Radiology 1995;196:439—43.

18. Akeson P, Jonsson E, Haugen I, Holtas S. Contrast-enhanced MRI of the central nervous system: comparison between gadodiamide injection and gadolinium-DTPA. Neuroradiology 1995;37:229—33.

19. Oudkerk M, Sijens PE, Van Beek EJR, Kuijpers TJA. Safety and efficacy of Dotarem (Gd-DOTA) versus Magnevist (Gd-DTPA) in magnetic resonance imaging of the central nervous system. Invest Radiol 1995;30:75—8.

20. Yamamoto H, Yamashita Y, Yoshimatsu S, Baba Y, Hatanaka YO, Murakami R, Nishiharu T, Takahashi M, Higashida Y, Moribe N. Hepatocellular carcinoma in cirrhotic livers: detection with unenhanced and iron oxide-enhanced MR imaging. Radiology 1995;195:106—12.

21. Ros PR, Freeny PC, Harms SE, Seltzer SE, Davis PL, Chan TW, Stillman AE, Muroff LR, Runge VM, Nissenbaum MA, Jacobs PM. Hepatic MR imaging with ferumoxides: a multicenter clincal trial of the safety and efficacy in the detection of focal hepatic lesions. Radiology 1995; 196:481—8.

22. Dawson P. Cardiovascular effects of contrast agents. Am J Cardiol 1989;64:2E-9E.

23. Matthai WH Jr, Groh WC, Waxman HL, Kurnik PB. Adverse effects of calcium binding contrast agents in diagnostic cardiac angiography. A comparison between formulations with and without calcium binding additives. Invest Radiol 1995;30:663—8.

24. Ares S, Pastor I, Quero J, Morreale de Escobar G. Thyroid complications, including overt hypothyroidism, related to the use of non-radiopaque silastic catheters for parenteral feeding in prematures requiring injection of small amounts of an iodinated contrast medium. Acta Paediatr 1995;84:579—81.

25. Rudnick MR, Goldfarb S, Wexler L, Ludbrook PA, Murphy MJ, Halpern EF, Hill JA, Winniford M, Cohen MB, VanFossen DB. Nephrotoxicity of ionic and nonionic contrast media in 1196 patients: a randomized trial. The Iohexol Cooperative Study. Kidney Int 1995;47:254—61.

26. Buyan N, Arab M, Hasanoglu E, Gokcora N, Ercan S. The effects of contrast media on renal function in children: comparison of ionic and nonionic agents. Turk J Pediatr 1995;37:305—13.

27. Kavukcu S, Tavli V, Fadiloglu M, Akhunlar H, Oran B, Akcoral A. Urinary enzyme changes in children undergoing cineangiographic evalu-

ation using iopromid. Int Urol Nephrol 1995;
27:131—5.

28. Hentschel M, Gildein P, Brandis M, Zimmer-
hackl LB. Endothelin (ET-1) is involved in the
contrast media induced nephrotoxicity in children
with congenital heart disease. Clin Nephrol
1995;43 Suppl 1:S12—15.

29. Clozel M, Breu V, Burri K, Cassal J-M,
Fischli W, Gray GA, Hirth G, Loffler BM, Muller
M, Neidhart W, et-al. Pathophysiological role of
endothelin revealed by first orally active endothelin receptor antagonist. Nature 1993;365:759—
61.

30. Lenler-Petersen P, Hansen D, Andersen M,
Sorensen HT, Bille H. Drug-related fatal anaphylactic shock in Denmark 1968—1990. A study
based on notifications to the Committee on Adverse Drug Reactions. J Clin Epidemiol 1995;
48:1185—8.

31. Schwartz HJ. Acute allergic disease in a hospital emergency room: a retrospective evaluation of
one year's experience. Allergy Proc 1995;16:
247—50.

32. Simon MR. Allergic-type adverse reactions to
low osmolality contrast media in patients with a
history of allergy or asthma. Invest Radiol
1995;30:285—90.

33. Dyer R, Cohan RH. What is the risk of reaction on repeat exposure to contrast material, and
how should the patients be premedicated? Am J
Roentgenol 1995;165:1543.

34. Dawson P, Sidhu PS. Is there a role of corticosteroid prophylaxis in patients at increased risk of

adverse reactions to intravascular contrast agents?
Clin Radiol 1993;48:225—6.

35. Moreno F, Blanca M, Fernandez J, Ferrer A,
Mayorga C, del Cano A, Aguilar F, Juarez C,
Garcia J. Determination of inflammatory markers
in allergic reactions to drugs. Allergy Proc
1995;16:119—22.

36. Fernandez J, Blanca M, Moreno F, Garcia
J, Segurado E, del Cano A, Aguilar F. Role of
tryptase, eosinophil cationic protein and histamine in immediate allergic reactions to drugs. Int
Arch Allergy Immunol 1995;107:160—2.

37. Hahn ST, Pfammatter T, Cho KJ. Carbon
dioxide gas as a venous contrast agent to guide
upper-arm insertion of central venous catheters.
Cardiovasc Intervent Radiol 1995;18;146—9.

38. Yusuf SW, Whitaker SC, Hinwood D, Henderson MJ, Gregson RHS, Wenham PW, Hop-
kinson BR, Makin GS. Carbon dioxide: an alternative to iodinated contrast media. Eur J Vasc
Endovasc Surg 1995;10:156—61,

39. Visfeldt J, Andersson M. Pathoanatomical aspects of malignant haematological disorders
among Danish patients exposed to thorium dioxide. APMIS 1995;103:29—36.

40. Naka N, Ohsawa M, Tomita Y, Kanno H,
Uchida A, Aozasa K. Angiosarcoma in Japan. A
review of 99 cases. Cancer 1995;75:989—96.

41. Andersson M, Wallin H, Jonsson M, Nielsen
LL, Visfeldt J, Vyberg M, Bennett WP, De Benedetti VMG, Travis LB, Storm HH. Lung carcinoma and malignant mesothelioma in patients exposed to Thorotrast: incidence, histology and p53
status. Int J Cancer 1995;63:330—6.

B.C.P. Polak

47 Drugs used in ocular treatment

ANTIGLAUCOMATOUS DRUGS *(SED-13, 1418, 1421—4; SEDA-19, 433)*

Primary open angle-glaucoma is commonly treated with long-term hypotensive drugs. When this approach becomes inadequate, surgery is used. Short- and long-term topical medical therapy of primary open-angle glaucoma may give rise to morphological changes in the conjunctival and subconjunctival tissues. For this reason surgery should be considered as an alternative to long-term medical therapy as first choice in the treatment of primary open-angle glaucoma.

Biopsy specimens from glaucomatous patients treated with timolol and pilocarpine eye-drops for various periods of time and control patients without conjunctival pathology or topical treatment have been compared (1[C]). Morphometric analysis of histological sections and immunohistochemistry (anti-fibronectin antibody) in patients using medium- and long-term therapy showed significant increases in the thickness and number of epithelial cell layers, significant increases in the fibroblast density in both subepithelial and deep connective tissue, and a more compact connective tissue with some inflammatory elements. These findings were confirmed by ultrastructural analysis. In the same patients the other immunohistochemical parameters investigated (anti HLA-DR, anti-CD1a, anti-6D4, anti-CD8, and anti-IL2, and anti-C3b antibodies) showed a tendency to chronic inflammation. After specific surgery this tendency manifested itself in a diffuse immune response, especially in patients who had taken medium- and long-term drug therapy.

β-Adrenoceptor antagonists *(SED-13, 1418)*

Alopecia and nail pigmentary changes have been reported after ocular timolol. Recently three cases have suggested that periocular cutaneous changes may be secondary to local instillation of betaxolol (Betoptic) (2[c]).

A 47-year-old black man with primary open-angle glaucoma started to use betaxolol 0.5% in both eyes. Bilateral hypopigmentation of the eyelids was first documented nearly 7 years later. Betaxolol was discontinued, and 3 years later the pigmentation had returned to normal.
A 4-month-old white boy with unilateral primary infantile glaucoma started to use betaxolol 0.25% in the left eye and developed left lower eyelid hypopigmentation 7 months later. Betaxolol was discontinued and the pigmentation returned to normal.
A 75-year-old black man with primary open-angle glaucoma started to use betaxolol 0.5% in both eyes. In the following year hyperpigmentation of the eyelids was seen bilaterally. Betaxolol was discontinued and 2 years later the pigmentation had returned to normal.

Carbonic anhydrase inhibitors *(SED-13, 1423; SEDA-19, 433)*

Carbonic anhydrase inhibitors cause a reduction in aqueous formation. They should be used with caution in the long-term control of glaucoma because of their serious systemic adverse effects (see also Chapter 21).

The safety profile and efficacy of 2% dorzolamide hydrochloride eye-drops (3[r]), administered three times daily for up to 1 year, have been compared with 0.5% timolol maleate and 0.5% betaxolol hydrochloride, each administered twice daily. In addition, the effects of adding dorzolamide to timolol or betaxolol in patients with inadequate ocular hypotensive efficacy and the effects of adding timolol in patients using dorzolamide have been evaluated in a double-masked, randomized, parallel comparison in 523 patients with open-angle glaucoma or ocular hypertension in a multicenter trial in 34 international sites for up to 1 year (4[C]). The ocular hypotensive efficacy of 2% dorzolamide tds was comparable with that of 0.5% betaxolol bd. Long-term use of dorzolamide was not associated with important electrolyte disturbances or the systemic adverse effects commonly observed with oral carbonic anhydrase inhibitors, but there is as yet no information on its effects on plasma potassium during the first few weeks of treatment.

Dorzolamide 2% bd has been compared with pilocarpine 2% qds in a 4-week, randomized, crossover study, in which quality of life and preference were studied in 92 patients concurrently using 0.5% timolol bd (5[c]). The patients reported less interference with quality of life with dorzolamide than pilocarpine, particularly in regard to limitations in their ability to drive, read, and perform moderate activities. In addition, they reported missing fewer doses of medication when using dorzolamide. There was no difference in bitter/unusual taste between the treatment groups, despite a higher frequency reported by patients using dorzolamide. Dorzolamide and pilocarpine were equally effective in lowering intraocular pressure. The patients preferred dorzolamide to pilocarpine in a ratio of over 7:1.

Apraclonidine hydrochloride *(SEDA-19, 433)*

Apraclonidine, an oral antihypertensive agent, appears to be safe and efficacious when used topically in the eye to lower intraocular pressure. The most common ocular complications are conjunctival hyperemia, itching, foreign body sensation, and lacrimation. The most frequent non-ocular adverse events related to apraclonidine are dry mouth and unusual taste perception (6[c]), (7[c]), (8[R]).

ANTI-INFLAMMATORY DRUGS

Corticosteroids *(SED-13, 1419; SEDA-18, 450)*

Locally or systemically administered corticosteroids may cause cataract, glaucoma, papilledema, pseudotumor cerebri, activation of corneal infections, superficial keratitis, ptosis, pupillary dilatation, conjunctival palpebral petechiae, uveitis, and scleromalacia.

Phosphate-containing steroid eye-drops may cause calcific band keratopathy and the use of acetate- rather than phosphate-containing steroid eye-drops is suggested in patients with factors, e.g. dry eyes, that predispose to band keratopathy.

A patient with severely dry eyes developed calcific band keratopathy on two different occasions within 72 h after starting phosphate-containing steroid eye-drops (9[c]).

REFERENCES

1. Nuzzi R, Vercelli A, Finazzo C, Cracco C. Conjunctival and subconjunctival tissue in primary open-angle glaucoma after long-term topical treatment: an immunohistochemical and ultrastructural study. Graefe Arch Clin Exp Ophthalmol 1995;233:154—62.
2. Arnoult L, Bowman ZL, Kimbrough RL, Stewart RH. Periocular changes associated with topical betaxolol. J Glaucoma 1995;4:263—7.
3. Palmberg P. A topical carbonic anhydrase inhibitor finally arrives. Arch Ophthalmol 1995; 113:985—6.
4. Strahlman E, Tipping R, Vogel R. A double-masked, randomized 1-year study comparing dorzolamide (Trusopt), timolol and betaxolol. Arch Ophthalmol 1995;113:1009—16.
5. Laibovitz R, Strahlman ER, Barber BL, Strohmaier KM. Comparison of quality of life and patient preference of dorzolamide and pilocarpine as adjunctive therapy to timolol in the treatment of glaucoma. J Glaucoma 1995;4:306—13.
6. Aroujo SV, Bond JB, Wilson RP, Moster MR, Schmidt Jr CM, Spaeth GL. Long term effect of apraclonidine. Br J Ophthalmol 1995; 79:1098—101.
7. Robin AL, Ritch R, Shin D, Smythe B, Mundorf T, Lehmann RP, Spaeth GL. Topical apraclonidine hydrochloride in eyes with poorly controlled glaucoma. Trans Am Ophthalmol Soc 1995;93:421—41.
8. Robin AL, Ritch R, Shin DH, Smythe B, Mundorf T, Lehmann RP, The Apraclonidine Maximum-Tolerated Medical Therapy Study Group. Short-term efficacy of apraclonidine hydrochloride added to maximum-tolerated medical therapy for glaucoma. Am J Ophthalmol 1995; 120:423—32.
9. Prasad-Rao G, O'Brien C, Hicky-Dwyer M, Patterson A. Rapid onset bilateral calcific band keratopathy associated with phosphate-containing steroid eye drops. Eur J Implant Refractive Surg 1995;7:251—2.

E. Ernst

48 Treatments used in complementary medicine

Complementary medicine is a booming business. In the US, for instance, sales of herbal remedies have grown from practically zero 20 years ago to a $1.5 billion industry today. The expected annual growth is currently about 15%. If this sounds impressive, one should consider that the US sales amount to merely one-third of the European market (1[R]).

Complementary medicine is not totally safe. Most remedies are associated with direct hazards (2. In addition there are the risks of exploitation, particularly of desperate patients (3[r]) and the potential for medical incompetence in inadequately trained practitioners (4).

However, adverse reactions to complementary treatments are under-investigated. The common notion that such therapies are inherently safe is a prime motivator for patients to try them, yet it is also dangerously wrong. There are few safeguards: herbal remedies can be marketed as food supplements, thus escaping licensing. Consequently, data on efficacy, safety, and quality are not required. This is unsatisfactory to many, and a special licensing procedure with minimal requirements, for example product quality, has been suggested as one way forward (5).

ACUPUNCTURE *(SED-13, 1447; SEDA-18, 456; SEDA-19, 438)*

The potential complications of acupuncture have recently been reviewed by two independent groups (6[R]), (7[R]). The most frequent adverse reactions are listed in Table 1. In a survey of 1135 Norwegian doctors and 197 acupuncturists, a total of 403 adverse effects were reported. Some of these were serious (Table 1) (8[C]).

Cardiovascular Another case of *cardiac tamponade* occurred when an acupuncturist accidentally pushed a needle through a foramen in the sternum; the patient was dead on arrival at the hospital (9[c]). Furthermore, needles that have been left subcutaneously in situ can migrate to the peritoneal cavity, stomach, liver, colon, or urinary bladder (10[c]).

Nervous system Paraspinal acupuncture has led to a *transverse myelopathy* in a 43-year-old man treated for low back pain (11[c]).

Skin and appendages The stimulation of acupuncture points by heat is known as moxibustion. This may cause *burns*, and at least five such cases have been reported (8[c]), (12[c]). One was a patient with painful diabetic neuropathy who sought help from an acupuncturist; moxibustion resulted in a badly healing wound on the endangered leg (12[c]).

Musculoskeletal In a 29-year-old man acupuncture was followed by *increased bone metabolism* in those regions of the skull in which needles had been inserted (13[c]).

HERBAL TREATMENTS (PHYTOTHERAPY) *(SED-13, 1428; SEDA-17, 546; SEDA-18, 453; SEDA-19, 436)*

Nervous system A 28-year-old woman complained of severe headache, nausea, and vomiting after ingesting a bowl of ginseng extract made from about 60 slices of ginseng root (14[c]). A cerebral angiogram showed *arteritis* in the anterior and posterior cerebral arteries and the cerebellar artery. No other

Side Effects of Drugs, Annual 20
J.K. Aronson, ed.

Table 1. *Frequent, serious adverse reactions to acupuncture*

Nature of event	Number of cases documented
Drowsiness/syncope/fainting	274
Hepatitis	127
Other infections (endocarditis, osteomyelitis, septicemia, perichondritis, skin infection etc.)	100
Pneumothorax	65
Increased pain	70
Cardiac trauma	7

Combined data from (27[C]) and (29[C]).

plausible cause was found and the authors felt that a causal relation was 'most likely'.

Liver   The potential of medicinal plants to cause liver damage has recently been reviewed (15[R]). Amongst others, the following popular remedies have been implicated: germander, mistletoe, senna, skullcap, valerian.

Two reports of *fulminant liver failure* have been associated with Chinese herbal preparations taken as a tea (16[c]), (17[c]). In both cases, the product was called 'eternal life'. Enquiries about the composition of this product led to the information that it does not always contain the same herbs, but that each prescription is tailor-made to suit the patient's needs.

Another traditional Chinese herbal remedy, Syo-saiko-to, has apparently been used in China for thousands of years to treat the common cold. More recently, it has been used in Japan to treat chronic liver disease. Japanese authors have described four patients in whom it caused *acute liver injury* and *chole stasis* (18[cr]). They also mentioned that they had seen 40 similar cases.

A further 11 cases of liver damage have been described after the ingestion of Chinese herbal remedies (19[c]). In two cases there was compelling evidence for a causal link, based on withdrawal/rechallenge. In two other cases a causal relation was thought likely. Several Chinese herbs were implicated. The effects seem to be idiosyncratic and not dose-related.

Chaparral is being promoted as a free-radical scavenger. A 60-year-old woman who had taken chaparral for 10 months was brought to hospital with severe *hepatitis* (20[cr]). Chaparral appeared to be the only possible cause. Her condition deteriorated and she required liver transplantation, after which she recovered. Similar cases implicating chaparral as the cause of severe liver damage have been reported previously.

Kombucha 'mushroom' has been used medicinally for thousands of years. Today it is marketed as a 'fountain of youth' and a virtual panacea. It is in fact not a mushroom but a symbiotic yeast/bacteria aggregate surrounded by a permeable membrane. A 53-year-old college professor has been reported to have developed liver damage after ingesting Kombucha tea (21[c]). No other cause of the liver problem could be found. The patient recovered after withdrawal.

Gastrointestinal   A 37-year-old Saudi Arabian man was admitted to hospital with *vomiting, colicky pain*, and *bloody diarrhea* after self-medication with *Citrullus colocynthis* (bitter apple) (22[c]). The remedy is popular in Arab and African countries as a treatment for constipation. It can cause severe intestinal damage, presenting as acute colitis indistinguishable from infectious colitis.

Urinary system   There has been a follow-up of the series of people in Belgium who developed *nephropathy* after taking a Chinese herbal mixture prescribed by a slimming clinic (23[C])r. The Chinese remedy was supposed to contain *Stephania terandra* and *Magnolia officinalis*. However, subsequent analysis showed that it contained *Aristolochia fangchi*, which suggests that aristolochic acid was the cause of the disaster. More than 80 women have been affected in Belgium alone. About half of them later required renal replacement therapy. Even more worrying is the discovery of extensive cellular atypias in some of the patients; one patient was diagnosed as suffering from a *urothelial carcinoma*.

Hypersensitivity and immunological reactions   Allergic reactions are possible with virtually any herbal product. They can vary from a mild skin rash to anaphylactic shock.

Balsam of Peru is derived from *Myroxolon balsamum* and has been used in medicinal and cosmetic ointments for centuries. It can cause allergic reactions, and some 500 articles have been published on the matter. Balsam of Peru contains about 25 different substances. Experiments on guinea-pigs have shown that they have a weak sensitization capacity; several new sensitizing constituents have been found by various analytical techniques (24.

Sunscreens are often associated with strong allergenic properties. A 15-year-old boy experienced *photo-distributed skin eruptions* after applying a sunscreen containing camphor. Camphor allergy was subsequently confirmed by patch test (25^c).

In the UK and elsewhere, aromatherapy is gaining in popularity. One case of allergic airborne *contact dermatitis* has been observed. A 53-year-old man had relapsing itching eczema on uncovered areas of the skin, resistant to routine treatment (26^c). Patch testing showed allergies to the essential oils of lavender, jasmin, and rosewood. The patient had previously used these oils for aromatherapy. Owing to the persistence of these volatile oils in the patient's home, complete renewal of the interior of the patient's flat was needed for complete recovery.

In the course of a 10-week trial of psyllium for hypercholesterolemia in 49 patients, one *anaphylactic reaction* occurred (27^c). The authors were confident that the reaction was caused by psyllium.

A traditional Japanese Kampo medicine containing the climbing stems of *Sinomenium acutum Rehder et Wilson* is used for its alleged analgesic and anti-inflammatory properties. A 41-year-old woman was admitted to hospital with a severe *edematous erythema* that turned out to be caused by this medicine, which she had taken as a decoction for about 3 weeks (28^c). She was completely cured in about 2 weeks after withdrawal. The authors provided a list of 29 similar published cases related to Kampo medicines.

Interactions   A patient taking *warfarin* presented with an abnormally long bleeding time and melena (29^c). On the recommendation of a Chinese herbalist he had taken a decoction of *Salvia miltiorrhiza Bge*. This reduced the elimination of warfarin.

In a cross-over study in healthy volunteers, Chinese herbs containing glycyrrhizin (Shosaiko-Tok, Sai-boku-To, and Sairei-To) affected *prednisolone* pharmacokinetics, albeit in a non-uniform fashion (30^C). The authors suggested that glycyrrhizin, which is a major constituent of liquorice, acts on unknown enzyme modifiers as inhibitors or promoters of metabolism.

Adulteration   The absence of quality control for many herbal remedies opens the door to adulteration with organic or non-organic compounds. The adulteration of a Chinese herbal preparation with mefenamic acid resulted in acute renal failure in a 51-year-old woman (31^c). She required hemodialysis and subsequently improved. Another eight patients presented with various symptoms after taking Chinese herbal drugs; subsequent analysis of the remedies showed that all the pills analysed contained *mefenamic acid* and *diazepam* (32^c).

Some herbal remedies are adulterated with *heavy metals*. Ayurvedic (traditional Indian) herbal drugs have repeatedly been shown to contain undeclared toxic compounds. A British poisons information center identified five such cases during 7 years. The preparations concerned contained lead (up to 60% by weight) zinc, mercury, arsenic, aluminium, or tin. In the individuals who had ingested these contaminated herbals, blood concentrations of these heavy metals were 2—10-times higher than the upper limit of normal physiological values (33^c). One Chinese remedy contained toxic amounts of arsenic and mercury (34.

In Oman and the United Arab Emirates bint al dhahab ('daughter of gold') is used medicinally in neonates and small children for stomach ailments. It has been shown to consist mainly of lead oxide, and cases of lead encephalitis are on record. The Omani Government has banned its import. A bulk analysis has shown that 100 g of bint al dhahab contains 91 g of lead monoxide, 600 mg of antimony oxide, and 50 mg of cadmium (35).

Relative safety   Unquestionably, herbal remedies can be safer than their synthetic competitors. Recently, two examples of this have been published. St John's wort (*Hypericum perforatum*) may be as effective as standard antidepressants for mild to moderate depression, but it is associated with significantly fewer adverse effects (36[R]). Similarly, a herbal expectorant mixture was associated with adverse effects in 0.8% of treated cases, whereas ambroxol and acetylcysteine were associated with adverse effects in 1.0 and 4.3% of patients, respectively (37[R]).

HOMEOPATHY *(SED-13, 1443; SEDA-19, 438)*

Homeopathic remedies are predominantly highly dilute preparations of the original material (the 'mother tincture') and are therefore generally considered to be inherently safe. However, there is concern over the fact that homeopaths may advise against immunization. A survey of all registered homeopaths in the Exeter area has shown that most of the medically trained homeopaths advised in favor of immunization while the lay homeopaths invariably did not (38). On a large scale, this advice would not only endanger the patients it is given to, but it could also jeopardize herd immunity in the entire population.

SPINAL MANIPULATION *(SED-13, 1448; SEDA-19, 438)*

Spinal manipulation therapy, i.e. chiropractic and osteopathy, is a therapeutic technique predominantly (but by no means exclusively) used for back problems. Its risks have been reviewed in a book for the general reader (39[R]).

A survey of 177 members of the American Academy of Neurology aimed to find out how many adverse events related to chiropractic had been noted by these doctors within a 2-year period. Chiropractic interventions were associated with 55 *strokes*, 16 *myelopathies*, and 30 *radiculopathies* (40[C]).

In contrast to these worrying findings, a review of the literature has provided reassurance of the relative safety of spinal manipulation (41[R]). When serious adverse effects of non-steroidal anti-inflammatory drugs were compared with those of spinal manipulation, both used for neck pain, manipulation emerged as being safer by more than two orders of magnitude.

The frequency with which chiropractors use X-rays of the spine might be cause for concern. Among Dutch chiropractors, 40% have been reported to use X-rays 'often or always' (42). In the US, 96.3% of chiropractors use X-rays routinely on all new patients, and 80% use them on follow-ups (43[R]).

REFERENCES

1. Marwick C. Growing use of medicinal botanicals forces assessment by drug regulators. J Am Med Assoc 1995;273:607—9.
2. Ernst E. Bitter pills of nature: safety issues in complementary medicine. Pain 1995;60:237—8.
3. Ernst E. Complementary cancer treatments: Hope or hazard? Clin Oncol 1995;7:259—63.
4. Ernst E. Competence in complementary medicine. Comp Ther Med 1995;3:6—8.
5. De Smet PAGM. Should herbal medicine-like products be licensed as medicines? Br Med J 1995;310:1023.
6. Rampes H, James R. Complications of acupuncture. Acupunct Med 1995;13:26—33.
7. Ernst E. The risks of acupuncture. Int J Risk Saf Med 1995;6:179—86.
8. Norheim AJ, Fønnebø V. Adverse effects of acupuncture. Lancet 1995;345:1576.
9. Halvorsen TB, Anda SS, Naess AB, Levang OW. Fatal cardiac tamponade after acupuncture through congenital sternal foramen. Lancet 1995;345:1175.
10. Gerard PS, Wilck E, Schiano T. Images in clinical medicine: acupuncture-needle fragments. New Engl J Med 1995;332:1792—3.
11. Ilhan A, Adanir M. Transverse myelopathy after acupuncture therapy: a case report. Acupunct Electro-Ther Res 1995;20:191—4.
12. Clark MH, Jowett NI. Diabetic peripheral neuropathy, acupuncture and moxibustion. Pract Diabetes Int 1995;12:139—40.
13. Kuno RC, Cerqueira MD. Enhanced bone metabolism induced by acupuncture. J Nucl Med 1995;36:2246—7.
14. Ryu S-J, Chien Y-Y. Ginseng-associated cerebral arteritis. Neurology 1995;45:829—30.
15. Larrey D, Pageaux GP. Hepatotoxicity of herbal remedies and mushrooms. Semin Liver Dis 1995;15:183—8.
16. Vautier G, Spiller RC. Safety of complemen-

tary medicines should be monitored. Br Med J 1995;311:633.

17. Sanders D, Kennedy N, McKendrick MW. Monitoring the safety of herbal remedies: herbal remedies have a heterogeneous nature. Br Med J 1995;311:1569.

18. Itoh S, Marutani K, Nishijima T, Matsuo S, Itabashi M. Liver injuries induced by herbal medicine, Syo-saiko-to (xiao-chai-hu-tang). Dig Dis Sci 1995;40:1845—8.

19. Perharic L, Shaw D, Leon C, De Smet PAGM, Murray VSG. Possible association of liver damage with the use of Chinese herbal medicine for skin disease. Vet Hum Toxicol 1995; 37:562—6.

20. Gordon DW, Rosenthal G, Hart J, Sirota R, Baker AL. Chaparral ingestion: the broadening spectrum of liver injury caused by herbal medications. J Am Med Assoc 1995;273:489—90.

21. Perron AD, Patterson JA, Yanofsky NN. Kombucha 'mushroom' hepatotoxicity. Ann Emerg Med 1995;26:660—1.

22. Al Faraj S. Haemorrhagic colitis induced by *Citrullus colocynthis*. Ann Trop Med Parasitol 1995;89:695—6.

23. van Ypersele de Strihou C, Vanherweghem JL. The tragic paradigm of Chinese herbs nephropathy. Nephrol Dial Transplant 1995;10:157—9.

24. Hausen BM, Simatupang T, Bruhn G, Evers P, Koenig WA. Identification of new allergenic constituents and proof of evidence for coniferyl benzoate in balsam of Peru. Am J Contact Dermatitis 1995;6:199—208.

25. Marguery MC, Rakotondrazafy J, El Sayed F, Bayle-Lebey P, Journe F, Bazex J. Contact allergy to 3-(4'-methylbenzylidene) camphor and contact and photocontact allergy to 4-isopropyl dibenzoylmethane. Photodermatol Photoimmunol Photomed 1995;11:209—12.

26. Schaller M, Korting HC. Allergic airborne contact dermatitis from essential oils used in aromatherapy. Clin Exp Dermatol 1995;20:143—5.

27. Spence JD, Huff MW, Heidenheim P, Viswanatha A, Munoz C, Lindsay R, Wolfe B, Mills D. Combination therapy with colestipol and psyllium mucilloid in patients with hyperlipidemia. Ann Intern Med 1995;123:493—9.

28. Okuda T, Umezawa Y, Ichikawa M, Hirata M, Oh-i T, Koga M. A case of drug eruption caused by the crude drug Boi® (Sinomenium Stem/Sinomeni Caulis et Rhizoma). J Dermatol 1995;22:795—800.

29. Tam LS, Chan TYK, Leung WK, Critchley JAJH. Warfarin interactions with Chinese traditional medicines: danshen and methyl salicylate medicated oil. Aust NZ J Med 1995;25:258.

30. Homma M, Oka K, Ikeshima K, Takahashi N, Niitsuma T, Fukuda T, Itoh H. Different effects of traditional Chinese medicines containing similar herbal constituents on prednisolone pharmacokinetics. J Pharm Pharmacol 1995;47:687—92.

31. Abt AB, Oh JY, Huntington RA, Burkhart KK. Chinese herbal medicine induced acute renal failure. Arch Intern Med 1995;155:211—12.

32. Gertner E, Marshall PS, Filandrinos D, Potek AS, Smith TM. Complications resulting from the use of Chinese herbal medications containing undeclared prescription drugs. Arthritis Rheum 1995;38:614—7.

33. Bayly GR, Braithwaite RA, Sheehan TMT, Dyer NH, Grimley C, Ferner RE. Lead poisoning from Asian traditional remedies in the West Midlands—report of a series of five cases. Hum Exp Toxicol 1995;14:24—8.

34. Espinoza EO, Mann M-J, Bleasdell B. Arsenic and mercury in traditional Chinese herbal balls. New Engl J Med 1995;333:803—4.

35. Worthing MA, Sutherland HH, Al-Riyami K. New information on the composition of bint al dhahab, a mixed lead monoxide used as a traditional medicine in Oman and the United Arab Emirates. J Trop Pediatr 1995;41:246—7.

36. Ernst E. St John's wort, an anti-depressant? Phytomedicine 1995;2:67—71.

37. Ernst E, Siedler Ch, März R. Adverse drug reactions to herbal and synthetic expectorants. Int J Risk Saf Med 1995;7:219—25.

38. Ernst E, White AR. Homoeopathy and immunization. Br J Gen Pract 1995;45:629—30.

39. Magner G, Barrett S, editors. Chiropractic: the victim's perspective. Amherst NY: Prometheus Books, 1995.

40. Lee KP, Carlini WG, McCormick GF, Albers GW. Neurologic complications following chiropractic manipulation: a survey of Californian neurologists. Neurology 1995;45:1213—5.

41. Dabbs V, Lauretti WJ. A risk assessment of cervical manipulation vs NSAIDs for the treatment of neck pain. J Manip Physiol Ther 1995; 18:530—6.

42. Assendelft WJJ, Pfeifle CE, Bouter LM. Chiropractic in the Netherlands: a survey of Dutch chiropractors. J Manip Physiol Ther 1995;18:129—34.

43. Plamondon RL. Summary of 1994 ACA Annual Statistical Study. J Am Chiropract Assoc 1995;32:57—63.

49 Miscellaneous drugs, materials, and medical devices

CATHETERS *(SED-13, 1002; SEDA-19, 447)*

Central venous catheters

Infections In a prospective study of infection associated with central venous catheters in a general hospital in Australia, systemic catheter-related infection and local infection at the catheter exit site were studied in relation to 479 central venous catheters in 311 patients (68[C]). Local infection developed in association with 54 catheters (11%) and systemic infection with 32 (6.7%). Local infection was predictive of systemic infection, but its absence did not exclude systemic infection. Local complications included entry-site abscesses, local cellulitis, and septic thrombophlebitis. Hemodialysis catheters were responsible for a higher systemic infection rate than other catheter types. The most common organism responsible was methicillin-resistant *Staphylococcus aureus*. Of all bacteremias (33/160) detected in the hospital, 20% occurred in patients with a central venous catheter and 24 of these (73%) were definitely or probably due to the catheter. Staphylococci were the predominant isolates, and 40% of the methicillin-resistant *S. aureus* bacteremias were due to catheter-related infection. Infection complications were few: three patients developed local abscesses, one developed endocarditis, and two died. Infective endocarditis has complicated 20% of systemic catheter-related infections in other surveys, but it occurred only once in this study. It is possible that the short duration of this study (5 months) resulted in an underestimation of the real incidence of late complications of catheter-related infections. The authors concluded that empirical antibiotic treatment should include at least antistaphylococcal cover, as staphylococci were the predominant isolates; infection with Gram-negative bacteria was uncommon. It is clear from this study that apparently innocuous in situ catheters can be responsible for systemic infection.

There is some disagreement as to whether infectious complications differ with use of different types of chronic central venous access devices in cancer patients. One group (69[C]) has concluded that there was no significant difference in the risk of infection between subcutaneous ports and external catheters, but this has been disputed by Hidalgo (70[r]), who has pointed out that in children with cancer a lower infection rate is observed using subcutaneous ports compared with external catheters. According to Hidalgo, the advantage of a subcutaneous port in adult patients is unclear, but that may be explained by the small size of the studies on which the conclusions are based. The differences between the studies and the conclusions reached may be the result of their size and design, rather than real differences.

Catheter-related bacteremia due to *Pseudomonas paucimobilis* has been reported in two patients with cancer-associated neutropenia (71[C]). This organism has rarely been implicated in community-acquired and nosocomial infections. Both of the patients had been undergoing intensive chemotherapy, and both required removal of the catheter to eradicate the infection. Adequate antibiotic treatment may not eradicate the infection in cases of severe prolonged neutropenia, and the catheter is likely to have to be removed if bacteremia due to *P. paucimobilis* persists or recurs despite 48 h of appropriate therapy.

Non-infectious complications A 53-year-old woman developed a serious air embolism from the central venous catheter tract, after lung transplantation, at the time of removal of the catheter (72^c). Lung transplant patients appear to be at increased risk of this complication, perhaps because of the considerable negative intrathoracic pressure that may develop when the diseased lung is replaced with a normal lung. Also, lung transplant patients are often emaciated and have little subcutaneous tissue, allowing for a short tract from the central venous line insertion site to the opening of the central vein. The authors referred in their report to four other cases of air embolism in lung transplant patients.

There has been a report of fracture of a central venous catheter due to compression between the clavicle and the adjacent first rib (73^c). A 'pinched-off sign' on X-ray indicates the need to remove the catheter, because of a significant risk of subsequent fracture of the catheter, which has an incidence of 0.9%. Catheters lying anterior to the subclavian vein between the clavicle and the first rib are liable to be compressed and subsequently to fracture. This is a potentially life-threatening complication that can be averted by correct placing of the central venous catheter and by immediate chest radiography to search for any evidence of catheter kinking or compression, the latter of which should prompt its immediate removal. Catheters that are oval in cross-section are more likely to adapt to a confined space.

Intrathecal catheters (7)—(9)

Complications have been described after the insertion of 157 intrathecal catheters in 142 patients (10^R). In most cases problems were related to the placement procedure, with subsequent neurological complications. Clinically unsuspected *degeneration of the posterior columns*, perhaps related to intraspinal infusion of morphine or to a paraneoplastic effect, has been observed post mortem in two patients with implanted pumps (11^c).

Paraplegia has also been reported (12^c).

A 42-year-old woman had a history of previous lumbosacral spinal operations. Spinal cord stimulation had been attempted twice, at midthoracic and upper thoracic levels, without lasting benefit. A programmable infusion pump (SynchroMed, Medtronic) and an intrathecal catheter were implanted at T11 to infuse morphine, because of persistent low back and lower limb pain. Two months later she developed progressive paraparesis, culminating in paraplegia and incontinence 1 month later. There was no sensation to pinprick below T11 on the left side and T10 on the right and the legs were flaccid and areflexic with bilateral extensor plantar responses. A myelogram showed a nearly complete block of flow at T10—11, and a CT scan showed extensive arachnoid fibrosis without evidence of extradural compression. At laminectomy a darkly pigmented partly liquefied mass measuring 6 × 8 × 40 mm was identified; it communicated with an intramedullary cavity containing a creamy fluid.

Another case of paraplegia has been reported in a 73-year-old man with an intrathecal catheter and a spinal cord stimulator (13^c).

The Landmark company has received reports of adverse events either during or within 30 min of placement of the Landmark midline catheter (14^r). These events ranged from minor signs and symptoms to occasional life-threatening incidents. The most frequently reported were: *facial flushing*, which may progress to the neck and torso; *pain*, including chest pain or tightness, abdominal pain, and back pain; *breathing difficulties*, including shortness of breath, respiratory distress, and throat tightness; *sweating*; *urticaria* or other types of rash; *cyanosis*; *alterations in vision*. The company has emphasized that slower insertion with constant flushing during the time when the catheter is being advanced may minimize the risk of adverse events, whose cause is not currently known.

SURGICAL AND DENTAL MATERIALS AND DEVICES

Acrylate glue embolization *(SED-13, 1455)*

Embolization of brain vascular malformations with the cyanoacrylate glues isobutyl-2-cyanoacrylate (IBCA) and *n*-butyl-2-cyanoacrylate (NBCA) has been performed for two decades (1^R), (2^R). Various complications resulting from this type of therapy have been described, usually affecting the nervous system (3^c). An infrequently documented complication involves *embolization* of cyanoacrylate to the lung. Asymptomatic embolization of IBCA to the lungs has been described (4[c]) and there has been a report of a death from respiratory failure caused by pulmonary emboli after IBCA embolization of a nasopharyngeal arteriovenous malformation (5[r]).

Systemic pulmonary complications have been sought in the clinical records of 182 patients embolized with acrylate glue since 1978 for the treatment of brain arteriovenous malformations (6[C]). Three patients had pulmonary symptoms within 48 h of injection. One patient with a left frontal cerebral arteriovenous malformation had embolization with a mixture of IBCA, pantopaque, and acetic acid and developed severe *pleuritic pain* 2 days later. One patient with a left temporal and one with a left cerebellar arteriovenous malformation had embolization with a mixture of NBCA and lipiodol, and developed *cough*, *pleuritic pain*, and *hemoptysis* within 24 h. Two patients had a significant drop in P_aO_2. No flow-arrest techniques were used for any of the injections in these patients. All had significant changes on chest X-ray and CT scans of the chest. All were treated conservatively and recovered spontaneously.

Cementless hip arthroplasty

Patients with avascular necrosis of the femoral head have a higher rate of failure of total hip prostheses (15[R]). Because osteonecrosis most commonly occurs in the third to fifth decades of life, a functional and durable hip operation is required. In younger patients, the incidence of failure of cemented hip prostheses is reported to be even higher (16[r]), (17[r]).

Cementless porous-coated prostheses may cause more problems than cemented total hip arthroplasty using contemporary techniques, judging from a study of 61 patients (78 hips) who were followed for an average of 7.2 (range 6—9) years after they had primary cementless porous-coated total hip arthroplasty and who had avascular necrosis of the femoral head (18[C]). The average age of the patients at the time of surgery was 48 (range 20—73) years. The average preoperative hip score was 46 (range 28—75) points, which improved to 90 (range 34—100) points at the 7.2-year follow-up examination. Sixteen of 78 arthroplasties failed during the period of follow-up,

with an overall failure rate of 21%. Of the failed hips, 11 had femoral component loosening, four had femoral and acetabular component loosening, and one had excessive wear in the polyethylene liner. Four femoral components and five acetabular components were revised. Twenty-one of the 78 hips (27%) had an average of 5.6 (range 3—9) mm of wear in the polyethylene liner. Sixteen (21%) of the 78 hips had acetabular and femoral periprosthetic osteolysis, and 22 (28%) hips had femoral periprosthetic osteolysis only.

Electric heating pads

The FDA and the Consumer Product Safety Commission (CPSC) have received many reports of injuries and deaths from *burns*, *electric shocks*, and *fires* associated with the use of electric heating pads (19[r]). These incidents have occurred in nursing homes, hospitals, and at home. Those at particular risk are infants, as well as people who may be unable to feel pain because of advanced age, diabetes, spinal cord injury, or medications. Prolonged use on one area of the body can cause a severe burn, even when the pad is set at a low temperature. In most cases, these incidents could have been avoided by careful inspection and proper use of the heating pads.

Hair implants

Artificial hair implantation, to remedy baldness, involves implanting colored plastic or resin fibers into the scalp. This process has been reported to cause serious complications. There have been varying degrees of *foreign body reaction* and the fibers may act as a conduit for bacteria. *Infections*, sometimes severe, will eventually occur in most people who have undergone this procedure. Systemic spread of the infection may result in distant sepsis, such as endocarditis and brain abscess. Infection with Gram-negative organisms, including *Pseudomonas aeruginosa*, has been reported. This procedure has been prohibited in the US since 1983, but it is still performed in other countries, including the UK and Australia.

The New Zealand Ministry of Health has received reports about the potential health risks to recipients of artificial hair implants

(20[r]). Implant recipients are instructed to seek medical advice and it is recommended that recipients be regularly monitored by their doctor for signs of sepsis. Recipients of artificial hair implants require counselling on the health risks. However, they may be resistant to treatment and not act objectively; care when counselling is recommended to ensure that appropriate action is taken, as patients may prefer not to deal with the issues. Based on the advice of a doctor who has been treating these patients, the Ministry has recommended that if there is evidence of sepsis swabs should be taken for culture, antibiotic treatment should be given as required, and the patient should be referred to a dermatologist or plastic surgeon. The extent of tissue damage can be assessed by biopsy. The artificial fibers should be removed and surgery may be required to repair the scalp.

Latex *(SED-13, 1463)*

Regulatory changes have been proposed in Australia for the labelling and safety requirements of latex-containing devices that directly or indirectly come into contact with body tissues, after an increasing number of reports of *allergic reactions* (21[c]). The majority of latex-containing devices are in this category, and include tubes, catheters, empty containers, syringes, medical gloves, and devices such as condoms and diaphragms. Pending the adoption of the new regulations, the Therapeutic Goods Administration has indicated that all users of latex-containing devices must be made aware of the current situation, must be familiar with methods for avoiding the problems, and must be able to deal effectively with them when they occur.

Health care workers have become aware of a marked worldwide increase in reactions to latex during the past decade. These reactions have been shown to be due to either or both:

- The formulation chemicals (vulcanizers, stabilizers, preservatives). These cause mainly local delayed hypersensitivity reactions. However, some of these chemicals are also carcinogenic, and may therefore have more serious and not immediately apparent consequences.
- Proteins in the latex. These can cause generalized systemic allergic reactions,

including anaphylactic shock, which can be very severe and life-threatening. The two major contributing factors to anaphylactic shock appear to be a hereditary disposition and occupational exposure. The latter has increased rapidly owing to progress in medical technology, the associated increase in the use of medical devices, and increased awareness among health-care professionals of the need to wear protective gloves during health-care procedures. This increased exposure has meant that a growing number of people have become sensitized to latex proteins. Particularly high-risk circumstances appear to be direct contact of a latex device or air-borne particles from a latex device (e.g. corn starch carrying latex proteins) with mucous membranes, or with tissues exposed as a result of surgical procedures. It has recently been estimated that about 1% of the general population, up to 17% of hospital staff, and up to 40% of people with chronic mucous membrane exposure to latex devices (e.g. spina bifida sufferers) are now sensitive to latex.

Severe anaphylactic reactions have been reported in response to dental work (latex dental dams), barium enemas (latex enema devices), and numerous surgical procedures involving mainly latex gloves and catheters.

Silicone gel breast implants *(SED-13, 1458; SEDA-16, 555; SEDA-17, 555; SEDA-18, 462)*

One of the frequent uses of silicone is in breast cosmetic and reconstructive surgery. Since the early 1980s there have been case reports and, more recently, series of small numbers of patients, detailing the possible association of silicone breast implants and underlying connective tissue diseases (22[c]) — (24[c]). In an evaluation of the frequency and clinical characteristics of the underlying connective tissue disorders that occur in association with silicone breast implants, 300 consecutive women with silicone breast implants, referred to an arthritis clinic have been studied (25[C]). A complete history was taken and a physical examination was performed, as well as laboratory testing for C reactive protein, rheumatoid factor, and autoantibody determination by indirect immunofluorescence and immunodiffusion. Criteria for fibromyalgia and/or chronic fatigue syndrome were met by 54%, connective tissue diseases were detected in 11% and undifferentiated connective tissue disease or human adjuvant disease in 10.6%, and a variety of disorders, such as angioedema, frozen shoulder, and a multiple sclerosis-like syndrome, were also found. Several other miscellaneous conditions, including recurrent and unexplained low-grade fever, hair loss, skin rash, symptoms of the sicca syndrome, Raynaud's phenomenon, carpal tunnel syndrome, memory loss, headaches, chest pain, and shortness of breath were also seen accompanying specific and non-specific conditions. Of 93 patients who underwent explantation, 70% reported improvement in their systemic symptoms.

DIETARY INGREDIENTS AND SWEETENERS

Monosodium glutamate

Monosodium glutamate is used as a flavor enhancer in a variety of foods. Its use has become controversial in the past 30 years because of reports of adverse reactions in people who have eaten foods that contain it. Research on the role in the nervous system of the glutamate-a group of chemicals (which includes monosodium glutamate) has also raised questions about its safety (26[r]).

Glutamate is an amino acid neurotransmitter in the brain, and there are glutamate-responsive tissues in other parts of the body as well. Abnormal function of glutamate receptors has been linked with certain neurological diseases, such as Alzheimer's disease and Huntington's chorea. Injections of glutamate in laboratory animals have resulted in damage to nerve cells in the brain, but consuming glutamate in food does not have this effect. Although people normally consume dietary glutamate in large amounts, and the body can make and metabolize glutamate efficiently, the results of animal studies conducted in the 1980s raised a significant question: can monosodium glutamate and possibly some other glutamates harm the nervous system?

A 1995 report from the Federation of American Societies for Experimental Biology (FASEB), an independent body of scientists, has helped to put these safety concerns into perspective and has reaffirmed the FDA's belief that monosodium glutamate and related substances are safe food ingredients for most people when eaten in usual amounts.

MISCELLANEOUS ORGANIC COMPOUNDS

Alcohol *(SEDA-18, 459; SEDA-19, 441)*

The subarachnoid administration of alcohol for neurolysis is a valuable means of providing relief for intractable malignant pain (27[r]). Pain impulses enter the spinal cord via the posterior roots, and these roots can be blocked by injection of an alcohol solution percutaneously.

The effect of alcohol on nerve tissue has been examined in animal models and in postmortem specimens from patients who received neurolytic blocks (28[c]), (29[c]). In general, alcohol causes destruction of nerve fibers, with subsequent Wallerian degeneration. The basal lamina around the Schwann cell usually remains intact. This leaves a tract available for axon regeneration without the formation of a neuroma. If the cell bodies are completely destroyed, regeneration will not occur.

Contact of alcohol with unintended nerve roots underlies many of the more serious complications. Involvement of anterior rootlets sufficient to interrupt motor nerve function will result in *muscle weakness or paralysis*. Interruption of parasympathetic fibers in the anterior roots of the three middle sacral segments may result in *bowel and bladder dysfunction* and can cause urinary retention and anal sphincter paralysis.

Finally, it has been concluded that alcohol causes less serious complications, such as *vomiting*, *headache*, and *paresthesia*, which are relatively common but fortunately of limited duration, while *loss of proprioception* and profound *numbness* are disconcerting but almost always preferable to the pain that the alcohol injection has relieved (30[R]).

Diethylene glycol

Diethylene glycol is a highly toxic organic solvent that causes acute renal failure and death when ingested (31[r]), (32[r]). It is still occasionally found in medical formulations or foods, although rarely in lethal concentrations (33[r]), (34[r])

A large, initially unexplained epidemic of *acute renal failure* that was due to diethylene glycol poisoning has been investigated (35[R]). From January 1990 to December 1992, 429 children with acute renal failure were admitted to a renal unit. The cause of the renal failure was identified in 90 cases (21%): 40 (44%) had the hemolytic—uremic syndrome, 49 (55%) had acute tubular necrosis following severe dehydration or shock, and one had poststreptococcal glomerulonephritis. The cause of renal failure in the remaining 339 (79%) patients could not be identified initially. The affected patients were older and better nourished and more often had hepatomegaly, generalised edema, and hypertension. They also had higher mean serum creatinine and hemoglobin concentrations on admission, but a lower serum bicarbonate concentration and white cell count. When compared with the 90 patients with an identified cause of renal failure, a significantly higher proportion of the 339 patients with no identified cause had been given a medicine for fever or an elixir known to contain paracetamol. Of these, 67 (20%) had taken a brand of elixir subsequently found to contain diethylene glycol; none of the 90 patients with an identified cause for their renal failure had done so. The clinical features of 272 patients with unexplained renal failure in whom ingestion of one of these brands could not be documented were similar to the features in these 67 patients.

Ethanolamine

Recently, tissue adhesive material has been used to improve the initial control of bleeding from huge esophagogastric varices and to prevent them from rebleeding. The value of the combination of the tissue adhesive substance *N*-butyl-2-cyanoacrylate with ethanolamine oleate 5% in the management of bleeding esophagogastric varices has recently been assessed in 114 patients with documented active variceal bleeding at the time of endoscopy (36[C]). The patients were randomized into two groups, 58 patients who underwent combined injection with cyanoacrylate for large esophageal and gastric varices and a sclerosant, ethanolamine oleate, for the remaining varices, and 56 patients who underwent injection with ethanolamine oleate only.

Most of the patients experienced tolerable *chest pain* and *dysphagia* after sclerotherapy, but severe chest pain developed in 17 (29%) and 38 patients (68%) in the combined therapy group and the ethanolamine group, respectively. Permanent troublesome dysphagia requiring re-endoscopy occurred in five patients in the combined therapy group and six in the ethanolamine group. In two patients in the combined group, the esophagus was completely obstructed by the Histoacryl material, which was easily removed at endoscopy. The other three patients had esophageal strictures and experienced permanent relief of dysphagia following the passage of an endoscope.

In the ethanolamine group, tight *esophageal strictures* requiring repeated endoscopic dilatation were reported in three of six cases; one patient had an esophageal stricture and two had marked mucosal inflammation and sloughing, with complete obstruction of the esophageal lumen, secondary to injection therapy. These last two patients were treated conservatively and by insertion of a Ryle's tube for feeding for 48 h; thereafter the dysphagia gradually regressed. Prolonged high *fever* (above 38°C and lasting for more than 24 h) developed in 17 (29%) and 30 cases (54%) in the combined therapy group and the ethanolamine group, respectively. One patient developed prolonged fever unresponsive to treatment. He was diagnosed as having portal bacteremia following extension of the injected Histoacryl from the site of injection into the portal vein; he died of hepatic failure. During the period of follow-up, four patients (7%) died in the combined group compared with 10 patients (18%) in the ethanolamine group.

Glycine *(SEDA-18, 460)*

Systemic absorption of the fluid used for bladder irrigation during transurethral resection of the prostate may cause a variety of disturbances of the circulatory and nervous systems, which are often referred to as the *transurethral resection syndrome*. A number of such cases probably occur in most hospitals, but they tend to be ascribed to advanced age, medications, and excessive blood loss. The lack of a consistent definition and varying degrees of awareness of mild forms of this complication probably explain the different figures given for the incidence of the syndrome in prospective studies, varying from 2 to 10% of all transurethral resections performed. Many urologists claim they have not encountered the transurethral resection syndrome for many years (38[r]),(39[c]), (40[c]).

However, the incidence and severity of symptoms of the transurethral resection syndrome on absorption of increasing volumes of glycine solution have now been described (37[r]). The signs and symptoms of the transurethral resection syndrome were evaluated and recorded during and after 273 transurethral prostatic resections performed at two hospitals between 1984 and 1993. Glycine solution was used as the irrigant and ethanol served as a tracer for fluid absorption. The incidence and severity of symptoms that could possibly be related to the syndrome increased progressively as more glycine solution was absorbed. Patients who absorbed up to 300 ml of glycine solution had an average of 1.3 such symptoms. This number increased to 2.3 when 1000—2000 ml were absorbed, 3.1 when 2000—3000 ml were absorbed, and 5.8 for volumes greater than 3000 ml. Nausea and vomiting occurred significantly more often when 1000—2000 ml were absorbed compared with no absorption. Confusion and arterial hypotension were other prominent signs of fluid absorption, whereas hypertension was not. The severity of symptoms was markedly aggravated when more than 3000 ml were absorbed. Extravasation resulted in higher risks of bradycardia, hypotension, and failed spontaneous diuresis postoperatively than absorption by the intravascular route.

Nicotine *(SED-13, 1468; SEDA-17, 554; SEDA-18, 461; SEDA-19, 443)*

The introduction of nicotine transdermal systems is a significant advance in the treatment of nicotine addiction. This therapy reduces the severity of nicotine withdrawal symptoms during smoking abstinence and improves smoking cessation rates. However, there are adverse reactions. In a recent study of the pharmacokinetics of nicotine transdermal systems it was found that although the adverse effects were not serious, a number of users experienced *headache* and transient *itching* at the site of application (41[r]). In another study of 37 subjects three reported itching and headache, while one who was allergic to the patch was advised to change the site of application and successfully continued to wear it (42[c]).

While there is a reasonable body of evidence regarding the efficacy of nicotine patches in outpatients, there have hitherto been no data on the use of transdermal nicotine in hospitalized patients. Now the safety, tolerability, and efficacy of transdermal nicotine in highly addicted, hospitalized patients with significant medical problems, and its effect on concomitant medications has been reported in an open noncomparative study of 80 smokers (42 men and 38 women) who used 24-h nicotine patches and received simple support for 12 weeks and were followed for up to 26 weeks (43[R]). Smoking was assessed by interview, carbon monoxide in the expired air, and blood cotinine concentration. The adverse effects observed included *itch* and local *erythema, insomnia*, and *abnormal taste sensation*. Two subjects withdrew because of adverse effects. At 12 weeks, 17 were non-smokers. At 26 weeks, 19 were non-smokers and a further 14 had reduced their use of cigarettes significantly.

Transdermal nicotine has also been used as maintenance therapy for ulcerative colitis (44[r]). *Nausea, light-headedness*, and *itching* were reported.

Finally, there has been a report of a woman who developed *hallucinations*, and *cerebral arterial narrowing* following the use of nicotine patches (45[c]). In another case delusions and hallucinations occurred when a woman who had been using nicotine to try to stop smoking took a cigarette (46[c]).

Nicotine has also been administered in a nasal spray. In a study of 255 patients, 128 of whom were randomly assigned to nicotine nasal spray and 127 to placebo, there were nine cases of *sinusitis* (five nicotine and four placebo) and two of *nose bleeding* and occasional spots of blood from the nostrils (one in each group) (47[r]), while in another study of 15 healthy smokers, aged 20—40 years, *sneezing, irritation in the throat,* and *headache* were reported (48[r]). Vapor inhalers have also been used for the relief of tobacco withdrawal symptoms in 15 subjects (49[C]). The most frequently reported adverse effects were *irritated throat* (four events), *hiccups, heartburn, bad taste sensation, dry mouth,* and *dizziness.*

Polidocanol

Polidocanol was developed in the early 1950s as a local anesthetic, and the active substance is the topical anesthetic hydroxypolyethoxydodecane. In more recent years, polidocanol has been introduced as a sclerosant (50[r]), (51[r]) in concentrations of less than 1% for the treatment of spider nevi, while concentrations of 1—3% have been used to treat varicose veins.

More recently (52[R]) a study of the safety, possible complications, and effectiveness of polidocanol has been performed in Australia, in which 16 804 limbs were injected over a 2-year period. There were no deaths or anaphylactic reactions. There were 34 reported complications that although not necessarily due to the polidocanol itself, could possibly be construed as indicative of *allergic reactions,* a frequency of 0.20%. These complications included *urticaria* that was more marked than is normally seen with sclerotherapy (12 patients; 0.07%). Four patients (0.02%) fainted on injection (*vasovagal reaction*).

There were three cases of *deep vein thrombosis* (0.02%). One was a major thrombosis that occurred in a 55-year-old woman who was taking hormone replacement therapy. She had two injections in the affected leg 5 weeks apart. On the second occasion she had a total injection of 4 ml of 0.5% polidocanol, was given support hose to wear, and was fully mobile. She complained of severe pain and swelling of the leg a week after the second injection and a deep vein thrombosis was diagnosed. The second patient had a minor thrombosis in the soleal sinus, diagnosed by venography 3 days after a second injection of 4 ml of 0.5% polidocanol. The third patient had a peroneal vein clot on duplex scan 2 days after an injection of 0.5 ml of 1% of polidocanol; it had disappeared on rescanning 1 week later.

A total of 43 *ulcers* were reported at injection sites in 32 legs (0.2%). Various concentrations of polidocanol were used, including 0.5% in four legs and 1% in 10 legs. *Thrombophlebitis* that was more severe than would normally be expected was reported in 14 legs (0.08%). Residual marked *discoloration of the skin* was reported in 30 legs that had hyperpigmentation (0.2) and in seven legs that had telangiectatic matting (0.06%).

Polyethylene glycol

For the past decade peroral orthograde polyethylene glycol—electrolyte lavage solutions, such as Colyte® and GoLYTELY® (Braintree Laboratories Inc, Braintree, MA,

Table 1. *Miscellaneous reports*

Drug/Material	Adverse effect(s)	Reference
Bisphosphonate	Ototoxicity	58[c]
Cobalt chloride	Contact allergies	59[r]
Dental amalgam fillings	Allergies	60[c]
Electrode lead wires	Hazardous electrical connections	61[r]
Fumaric acid (alkyl ester)	Leukopenia, eosinophilia	62[r]
Gelatin-containing injectables	Anaphylactoid reactions	63[r]
Glycerol	Vomiting	64[c]
Nickel sulfate	Contact allergies	59[r]
Pamidronate	Asymptomatic hypocalcemia	65[c]
Potassium dichromate	Contact allergies	59[r]
Para-phenylenediamine	Contact allergies	59[r]
Statin/fibrate combination	Myositis	67[r]
Thiuram mix	Contact allergies	59[r]

USA), have been the preferred bowel-cleansing agents before diagnostic and therapeutic procedures on the colon and rectum. Numerous studies have shown that these agents are safe and effective, and when compared with traditional 2-day mechanical cleansing regimens consisting of dietary restriction, laxatives, and enemas, offer enhanced patient compliance and cost-effectiveness (53ʳ)—(55ʳ). Despite these advantages, problems still remain with discomfort, inconvenience, and patient compliance. The large volume and unpalatability of these solutions lead many patients to experience troubling adverse effects, such as *nausea, vomiting, bloating, abdominal cramps*, and *loss of sleep*. In consequence, many patients are unable to complete a course of treatment, which can result in a poorly prepared colon and an inadequate procedure.

In a recent study, 329 patients undergoing elective ambulatory colonoscopy were prospectively randomized to one of three bowel preparation regimens (56ᶜ). Groups 1 and 2 received 4 l of polyethylene glycol—electrolyte lavage solution ($n = 124$) and group 2 also received oral metoclopramide ($n = 99$).

Group 3 received oral sodium phosphate ($n = 106$). All the groups were matched for age and sex. A complete course was taken by 91% of the patients. There were no differences among the three groups in the incidence of nausea, vomiting, abdominal cramps, anal irritation, or quality of bowel preparation. Oral sodium phosphate was better tolerated than the other regimens: more patients completed the course, fewer complained of abdominal fullness, and more were willing to repeat the treatment.

In another study (57ᶜ) polyethylene glycol-L-asparaginase was used as single-agent induction therapy for a 35-day investigational window in 21 patients under the age of 21 years. Mild reactions were observed after the first, second, or third dose of polyethylene glycol-L-asparaginase in five of the 21 patients and consisted of *local discomfort* at the site of injection, *rash*, and *urticaria*.

MISCELLANEOUS

Other reports on some adverse effects of a variety of miscellaneous drugs and materials are given in Table 1.

REFERENCES

1.   Zanetti P, Sherman F. Experimental evaluation of a tissue adhesive as an agent for the treatment of aneurysms and arteriovenous anomalies. J Neurosurg 1972;36:72—9.
2.   Berenstein AB, Krall R, Choi IS. Embolization with *n*-butyl cyanoacrylate in management of CNS lesions (a). Am J Neuroradiol 1989; 10:883—9.
3.   Lownie SP. Clinical and technical complications of endovascular therapy in the central nervous system. Semin Intervent Radiol 1993; 10:243—53.
4.   Takasugi JE, Shaw C. Inadvertent bucrylate pulmonary embolization: a case report. J Thorac Imaging 1989;4:71—3.
5.   Goldman ML, Philip PK, Sarrafizadeh MS, Marar HG, Singh N. Transcatheter embolization with bucrylate (in 100 patients). Radiographics 1982;2:340—75.
6.   Pelz DM, Lownie SP, Fox AJ, Hutton LC. Symptomatic pulmonary complications from liquid acrylate embolization of brain arteriovenous malformations. Am J Neuroradiol 1995; 16:19—26.

7.   Wang JK, Naus LA, Thomas JE. Pain relief by intrathecally applied morphine in man. Anesthesiology 1979;50:149—51.
8.   Brezenor GA: Long term intrathecal administration of morphine: a comparison of bolus injection via reservoir with continuous infusion by implanted pump. Neurology 1987;21:484—91.
9.   Arner S, Rawal N, Gustafsson LL. Clinical experience of long-term treatment with epidural and intrathecal opioids. A nationwide survey. Acta Anaesthesiol Scand 1988;32:253—9.
10.   Nitescu P, Appelgren L, Hultman E, Linder LE, Sjoberg M, Curelaru I. Long-term, open catheterization of the spinal subarachnoid space for continuous infusion of narcotic and bupivacaine in patients with 'refractory' cancer pain: a technique of catheterization and its problems and complications. Clin J Pain 1984;7:143—61.
11.   Coombs DW, Fratkin JD, Meier FA, Nierenberg DW, Saunders RL. Neuropathologic lesions and CSF morphine concentrations during chronic continuous intraspinal morphine infusion: a clinical and post-mortem study. Pain 1985;22:337—51.
12.   North RB, Cutchis PN, Epstein JA, Long

DM. Spinal cord compression complicating subarachnoid infusion of morphine: case report and laboratory experience. Neurosurgery 1991; 29:778—84.

13. Aldrete JA, Vascello LA, Ghaly R, Tomlin D. Paraplegia in a patient with an intrathecal catheter and a spinal cord stimulator. Anesthesiology 1994;81:1542—5.

14. Anonymous. Onset of adverse patient responses during the placement of LANDMARK Midline Catheters. FDA Med Bull 1966;26:5.

15. Chandler HP, Reineck FT, Wixson RL, McCarthy JC. Total hip replacement in patients younger than thirty years old. A five-year follow-up study. J Bone Joint Surg 1981;63A:1426—34.

16. Charnley J, Cupic F. The nine and ten year results of the low friction arthroplasty of the hip. Clin Orthop 1973;95:9—25.

17. Bisla RS, Inglis AE, Ranawat CS. Joint replacement surgery in patients under thirty. J Bone Joint Surg 1976;58A:1098—104.

18. Kim YH, Oh JH, Oh SH. Cementless total hip arthroplasty in patients with osteonecrosis of the femoral head. Clin Orthop 1995;320:73—84.

19. Anonymous. Hazards associated with the use of electric heating pads. FDA Med Bull 1996; 26/2:5.

20. Anonymous. Artificial hair implants-potential risks. WHO Pharm Newslett 1995;5/6:18.

21. Anonymous. Latex in devices-regulations concerning health and safety. WHO Pharm Newslett 1995;5/6:19.

22. Spiera H, Kerr LD. Scleroderma following silicone implantation: a cumulative experience of 11 cases. J Rheumatol 1993;20:958—61.

23. Gutierrez FJ, Espinoza LR. Progressive systemic sclerosis complicated by severe hypertension. Reversal after silicone implant removal. Am J Med 1990;89:390—2.

24. Endo LP, Lawrence EN, Longley S, Corman LC, Panush RS. Silicone and rheumatic diseases. Semin Arthritis Rheum 1987;17:112—18.

25. Cuellar ML, Gluck O, Molina JF, Gutierrez S, Garcia C, Espinoza R. Silicone breast implant-associated musculoskeletal manifestations. Clin Rheumatol 1995;14:667—72.

26. Anonymous. Monosodium glutamate. FDA Med Bull 1966;26/1:3.

27. Swerdlow M. Complications of neurolytic neural blockade. In: Cousins MJ, Bridenbaugh PO, editors. Neural Blockade in Clinical Anesthesia and Management of Pain, 2nd Edn. Philadelphia: Lippincott, 1988;719—33.

28. Merrick RL. Degeneration and recovery of autonomic neurons following alcoholic block. Ann Surg 1941;113:298—305.

29. Woolsey RM, Taylor JJ, Nagel JH. Acute effects of topical ethylalcohol on the sciatic nerve of the mouse. Arch Phys Med Rehab 1972; 53:410—14.

30. Kemp JR, Kilbride MJ, Winnie AP. Intrathecal alcohol neurolysis for the treatment of injectable pain. Pain Digest 1995;5:186—91.

31. Windholz M, Budavari S, Blumetti RF, Otterbein ES, editors. The Merck Index, 10th Edn. Rahway, NJ: Merck, 1983;453.

32. Andrews LS, Snyder R. Toxic effects of solvents and vapors. In: Amdur MO, Doull J, Klassen CD, editors. Casarett and Doull's Toxicology, 4th Edn. New York: Pergamon, 1991: 704—5.

33. Van Leusen R, Uges DRA. A patient with acute necrosis of the renal tubules due to consumption of wine containing diethylene glycol. Ned Tijdschr Geneeskd 1987;131:768—71.

34. Cantarell MC, Fort J, Camps J, Sans M, Piera I. Acute intoxication due to topical application of diethylene glycol. Ann Intern Med 1987; 106:478—9.

35. Hanif M, Mobarak RM, Ronan A, Rahman D, Donovan J. Fatal renal failure caused by diethylene glycol in paracetamol elixir: the Bangladesh epidemic. Br Med J 1995;311:88—91.

36. Thakeb F, Salama H, Raouf TA, Kader SA, Hamid HA. The value of combined use of N-butyl-2-cyanoacrylate and ethanolamine oleate in the management of bleeding esophagogastric varices. Endoscopy 1995;27:358—64.

37. Olsson J, Nilsson A, Hahn RG. Symptoms of the transurethral resection syndrome using glycine as the irrigant. J Urol 1995;154:123—8.

38. Mebust WK, Holtgrewe HL, Cockett ATK, Peters PC, and Writing Committee. Transurethral prostatectomy: immediate and postoperative complications. A cooperative study of 13 participating institutions evaluating 3,885 patients. J Urol 1989;141:243—7.

39. Olsson J, Rentzhog L, Hjertberg H, Hahn RG. Reliability of clinical assessment of fluid absorption in transurethral prostatic resection. Eur Urol 1993;24:262—6.

40. Hahn RG, Stalberg HP, Gustafsson SA. Intravenous infusion of irrigating fluids containing glycine or mannitol with and without ethanol. J Urol 1989;142:1102—5.

41. Gupta SK, Okerhalm RA, Eller M, Wei G, Rolf CN, Gorslione J. Comparison of the pharmacokinetics of two nicotine transdermal systems: Nicoderm and Habitol. J Clin Pharmacol 1995; 35:493—8.

42. Saenghirunvattana S. Trial of transdermal nicotine patch in smoking cessation. J Med Assoc Thailand 1995;78:466—8.

43. Martin PD, Robinson GM. The safety, tolerability and efficacy of transdermal nicotine (Nicotinell TTS) in initially hospitalised patients. New Zealand Med J 1995;108:6—8.

44. Thomas GAO, Rhodes J, Mani V, Williams GT, Newcombe RG, Russell MAH, Feyerabend C. Transdermal nicotine as maintenance therapy for ulcerative colitis New Engl J Med 1995; 332:988—92.

45. Jackson M. Cerebral arterial narrowing with nicotine patch. Lancet 1993;342:236—7.

46. Foulds J, Toone B. A case of nicotine psychosis? Addiction 1995;90:435—7.

47. Schneider NG, Olmstead R, Mody FV, Doan K, Franzon M, Jarvik ME, Steinberg C. Efficacy

of a nicotine nasal spray in smoking cessation: a placebo-controlled, double-blind trial. Addiction 1995;90:1671—82.

48.   Lunell E, Molander L, Anderson M. Relative bioavailability of nicotine from a nasal spray in infectious rhinitis and after use of a topical decongestant. Eur J Clin Pharmacol 1995;48:71—5.

49.   Lunell E, Molander L, Leischow SJ, Fagerstrom KO. Effect of nicotine vapour inhalation on the relief of tobacco withdrawal symptoms. Eur J Clin Pharmacol 1995;48:235—40.

50.   Eichenberger H. Resultäte der Varizenverodung mit Hydroxypolyäthoxy-Dodecan. Zentralbl Phlebol 1969;8:181—3.

51.   Ouvry P, Chaudet A, Guillerot E. L'Aetoxisclerol: premières impressions. Phlébologie 1978; 31:75—7.

52.   Conrad P, Malouf GM, Stacey MC. The Australian polidocanol (aethoxysklerol) study. Results at 2 years. Dermatol Surg 1995;21:334—6.

53.   DiPalma JA, Brady CE. Colon cleansing for diagnostic and surgical procedures: polyethylene glycol-electrolyte lavage solution. Am J Gastroenterol 1989;84:1008—16.

54.   Wolf BG, Beart RW, Dozois RR. A new bowel preparation for elective colon and rectal surgery: a prospective, randomized clinical trial. Arch Surg 1988;123:895—900.

55.   Burke DA, Manning AP, Murphy L, Axon AT. Oral bowel lavage preparation for colonoscopy. Postgrad Med J 1988;64:772—4.

56.   Golub RW, Kerner BA, Wise WE Jr, Meesig DM, Hartmann RF, Khanduja KS, Aguilar PS. Colonoscopic bowel preparations. Which one? A blinded, prospective, randomized trial. Dis Colon Rectum 1995;38:594—9.

57.   Ettinger LJ, Kurtzberg J, Voute PA, Jurgens H, Halpern SL. An open-label, multicenter study of polyethylene glycol L asparaginase for the treatment of acute lymphoblastic leukemia. Cancer 1995;75:1176—81.

58.   Reid IR, Mills DAJ, Wattie DJ. Ototoxicity associated with intravenous bisphosphonate administration. Calcif Tissue Int 1995;56:584—5.

59.   Geier J, Schnuch A. A comparison of contact allergies among construction and non-construction workers in Germany. Am J Contact Dermatitis 1995;6:86—94.

60.   Anonymous. Dental analgam fillings-review of safety. WHO Pharm Newslett 1966;1:9.

61.   Anonymous. Electrode lead wires-proposed performance standard. WHO Pharm Newslett 1995;10:6.

62.   Anonymous. Fumaric acid (alkyl esters): blood dyscrasias. WHO Pharm Newslett 1996;2:1.

63.   Anonymous. Gelatin-containing injectable preparations. WHO Pharm Newslett 1966;3:4.

64.   Kilpi T, Peltola H, Jauhiainen T, Kallio MJT. Oral glycerol and intravenous dexamethasone in preventing neurologic and acidiologic sequelae of childhood bacterial meningitis. Pediatr Infect Dis J 1995;14:270—8.

65.   Liote F, Boral-Boizard B, Fritz P, Kuntz D. Lymphocyte subsets in pamidronate-induced lymphopenia. Br J Rheumatol 1995;34:991—5.

67.   Feher MD, Foxton J, Banks D, Lant AF, Wray R. Long-term safety of statin-fibrate combination treatment in the management of hypercholesterolaemia in patients with coronary artery disease. Br Heart J 1995;14:14—17.

68.   Gosbell IB, Duggan D, Breust M, Mulholland K, Gottlieb T, Bradbury R. Infection associated with central venous catheters: a prospective study. Med J Aust 1995;162:210—13.

69.   Keung YK, Watkins K, Chen SC, Groshen S, Silberman H, Dovar D. Comparative study of infectious complications of different types of chronic central venous access devices. Cancer 1994;73:2832—7.

70.   Hidalgo M. Comparative study of infectious complications of different types of chronic central venous access devices. Cancer 1995;75:132.

71.   Salazar R, Martino R, Sureda A, Brunet S, Subira M, Domingo-Albos A. Catheter-related bacteremia due to *Pseudomonas paucimobilis* in neutropenic cancer patients: report of two cases. Clin Infect Dis 1995;20:1573—4.

72.   McCarthy PM, Wang N, Birchfield F, Mehta AC. Air embolism in single-lung transplant patients after central venous catheter removal. Chest 1995;107:1178—9.

73.   Ramsden WH, Cohen AT, Blanshard KS. Case report: central venous catheter fracture due to compression between the clavicle and first rib. Clin Radiol 1995;50:59—60.

International drug monitoring*

For nearly 30 years an international collaboration in monitoring adverse drug reactions, under the auspices of the World Health Organization, has been in operation. The program started in 1968 as a pilot project with the participation of 10 countries. The intent was to develop international collaboration to make it easier to detect adverse drug reactions, not revealed during clinical trials. Some years later, the Swedish government assumed operational and financial responsibility for technical aspects of the program and a WHO Collaborating Centre for International Drug Monitoring was created in Uppsala (the Uppsala Monitoring Centre (UMC)).

Now the system is based on interchange of adverse reactions information between national drug monitoring centres in 47 countries (listed on pp. 472–477). Collectively these centres annually provide 150 000–200 000 individual reports of reactions suspected of being drug-induced. The cumulative database that has been constructed from these reports now comprises over 1.7 million records (Fig. 1). In addition to the full members of the Program, there are contacts with drug safety professionals in other countries who are active in developing drug monitoring facilities. About 10 of these collaborators are close to being recognised as 'national centres' by their own governments, and consequently by WHO when a formal application has been made and they can comply with the basic technical requirements.

In each country it is the national centre which processes and evaluates adverse reaction reports, sent to them either directly from health professionals and/or, in some countries, from pharmaceutical manufacturers. Information obtained from these reports is passed back to the medical profession on a national basis, but also contributes to drug experience at the international level.

The summarized case material is collected in the WHO database, which is updated in a weekly routine. It is screened using agreed output routines 4 times a year for new and serious reactions, as well as the reporting frequencies of associations of particular interest chosen by national centres or by Uppsala Monitoring Centre Staff. In addition, the national centres receive an annual reference document containing summary data on all suspected reactions reported to the WHO program.

The main aim of the international program, i.e. the early identification of new adverse reactions, has been re-emphasized during the last few years. At the start of the program it was hoped that by applying carefully designed statistical analysis to the large amount of data available, it would be possible to identify new, unexpected reactions of medical significance. In spite of a good deal of effort, with the state of knowledge at that time, it was impossible to realise the goal of automated signal generation. It was thought that the heterogeneous nature of the data collected, and the frequency of missing data would not allow such an approach. Recently, a pilot study, in collaboration with a research unit at Stockholm's Royal Institute of Technology, has shown that the use of a Bayesian neural network may be successful in automated support for signal generation. In principle, the neural network can generate a priori probabilities and correlations for the relationships between any data elements (or combinations thereof) in the total data base reports or selected parts of the data base. It is possible to compare any selected data against such backgrounds. For example, the probabilities

*Contributed by Prof. I.R. Edwards, Director, on behalf of the WHO Collaborating Centre for International Drug Monitoring, Uppsala, Sweden (Uppsala Monitoring Centre).

444

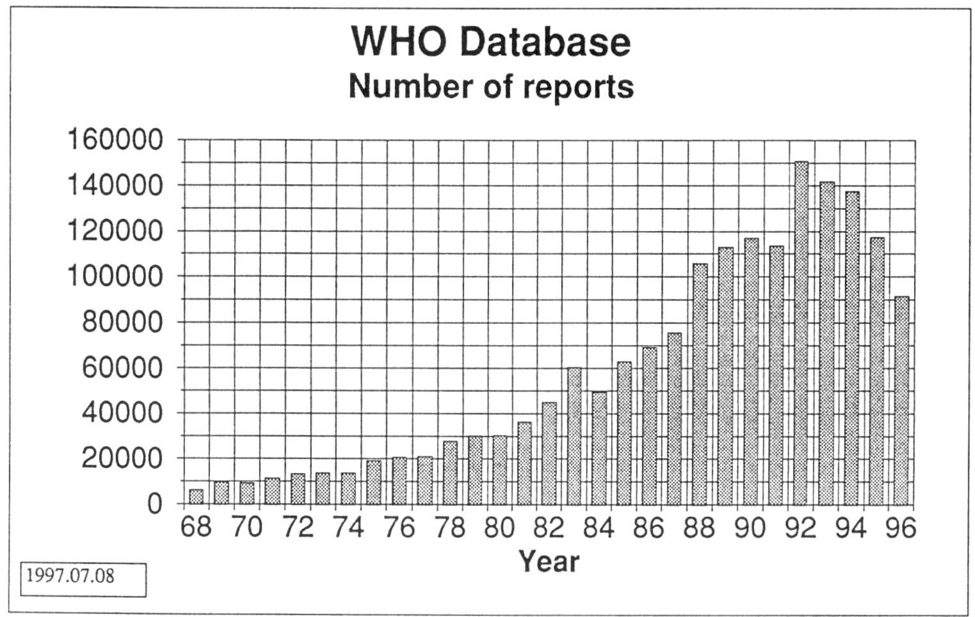

Fig. 1. *Number of individual case reports submitted regularly from national drug monitoring centres to the WHO Collaborating Centre located in Uppsala Sweden 1.7 million (June 1997) are stored in the database INTDIS (International Drug Information System).*

and strengths of correlation for new drugs, their reported doses, the type of ADR and patient characteristics and concomitant medication can be compared with all drugs in the data base or drugs in the same therapeutic or other class. Apart from using state-of-the-art technology, the routine comparison of different aspects of reported drug risk with the background of reports is a novel approach, essentially answering the question 'Are the ADRs reported with the selected drug (or patient group etc.) significantly different from our background reporting experience?' The neural network approach is robust from the point of view of incomplete and heterogeneous data. Work is proceeding to automate the process for routine use.

The review of adverse reaction signals has been intensified during the last 10 years by the appointment of reviewers in national centres to analyze reactions pertaining to particular body systems. Short summaries of their findings are circulated to participating national centres in a memorandum called 'Signal'. In order not to miss important signals, reports of adverse drug reaction associations that are new adverse reactions are reviewed by Centre staff every 3 months for critical adverse reaction terms. Any signal based on 3 or more good quality reports that are not already in the readily available international literature are also reported to participating centres in 'Signal'. This provides a back-up for the reviews performed by national centres' experts. The success of the signalling function is also dependent on a speedy input of reports from national centres to the UMC. One of the main objectives at the moment is to reduce delay in this input as much as possible. Whilst few centres take advantage of the facility at the moment it is possible for any national centre to use file transfer of cases via computer networks to the WHO data base.

Apart from rapidity of transfer, capture of more information is possible using automated systems. The UMC has a working data model, based on the CIOMS 1a report (obtainable from the Council for International Organisations of Medical Sciences, WHO, Geneva), which allows for much more data to be stored at the same time being compatible with the current WHO data-base and that being proposed by ICH (see below). The UMC will encourage industry to use this facility, parallel to, and not in place of, the national centres' data bases. This will ensure that all spontaneous reports are in the international arena, though users will need to be aware that duplications will occur between the two sets of data.

Increased communication between national centres during the past few years has resulted in a number of publications in medical journals. The focal point of the analyses behind many of these publications is the WHO database. There are always opportunities to intensify research activities on the basis of the WHO register. There are opportunities for researchers to stay at the UMC for short periods to study specific drug related problems, though funding issues need to be discussed with each situation.

There is a general need to quantify adverse drug reactions information. Under-reporting of adverse drug reactions in routine monitoring is the norm. There is, however, a considerable difference in the degree from time-to-time, place-to-place and between drugs. Publicity and the novelty of the drug or reaction are but two of the reasons for changes in reporting rate. The UMC is working jointly with IMS International, who have a variety of drug use data from most of the countries that are also in the WHO Program. This allows national differences in reporting rates to be further analyzed for reasons that may be due to differences in indications for use, medical practice and demographics, amongst many others. The EU's BIOMED Program is funding a research project in this area, and already the data have been useful in dealing with a drug safety signal, as well as raising a new issue for consideration. This project was called the ADR Signals Analysis Project (ASAP). It is now clear that it bridges the gap between having raw numbers of spontaneous reports, as the earliest signal of a problem with a drug, and the expensive and time consuming efforts that are entailed by observational and, certainly, interventional studies.

The aim was to provide more definition to an ADR signal as quickly as possible (thus the acronym ASAP—as soon as possible). Speed is important, since, if a signal is of a serious nature, an early decision must be made on whether a formal study is needed and what features in its design are necessary to give the best result. It is also necessary to provide as much information as quickly as possible to all the players in the drug safety field.

Two questions which the ASAP may be able to answer for any given signal are:
is there an urgent public health concern or not? e.g. is the reporting rate high or low? is there a consistent international picture? are there obvious confounding variables which provide alternative explanations for the signal other than the drug in question?

if there could be a problem what type of further investigation is needed? e.g. does the reporting rate and type of reaction suggest a problem that can be studied by a case control or cohort method or other? What kind of investigation should be done of an at risk group? is a mechanistic study indicated?

In short the objective of ASAP is to focus the gaze of pharmacovigilance on the more important issues for follow up.

An important part of the Centre's activities is also to act in other ways as a communication centre – a clearing house for information on drug safety at the service of drug regulatory agencies. In view of the current trends in pharmacoepidemiology, the Centre is also trying to increase its collaboration with groups involved with databases which may be useful in pharmacovigilance. The EU has supported an important initiative in the creation of a European Pharmacovigilance Working Group. This has allowed regulators and drug safety specialists from a variety of European countries to come together to plan co-ordinated drug safety exercises. This approach may pave the way for a much more logical development and investigation of drug safety signals world wide.

Requests for special database searches and investigations are also accepted by the Centre from participating national centres. Through searches in the WHO register, direct communication can be established between centres with a similar drug problem. The fastest way for a national centre to gain access to international experience is through an on-line connection to the WHO Centre computer.

There is also a continuous flow of external enquiries from parties outside the Collaborative Program concerning the pooled international data, and flexible search programs are available to allow for the most complex of these enquiries. Online access, within confidentiality limits agreed by the Program members, also allows a range of do-it-yourself searches. Some countries maintain the right to refuse release of their own information if they so wish. Use of the information released is subject to a caveat document as to its proper use. At present 150–160 queries from parties outside the programme are processed annually. In addition about 15 external users subscribe to on-line access to information from the approximately 30 countries that agree to general release of data without prior consultation.

Since 1982, the UMC has been distributing an *Adverse Reactions Newsletter* to participating centres, with reviews of national adverse reaction bulletins and news of drug problems being investigated in the various countries, supplemented with figures from the WHO register.

The WHO program has assumed responsibility for developing a standardized adverse reaction terminology (WHO-ART) and a comprehensive index of reported drugs (WHO-DD), both of which have a utility beyond their importance to the monitoring system. These tools are used in the pre-marketing safety area, as well as for post-marketing studies, by many pharmaceutical companies. WHO-ART has also been adopted by the International Program on Chemical Safety as the medical terminology used to describe poisoning incidents. The WHO-ART has been continuously developed over the almost 30 years of the Program and is in need of some renovation. Discussions are being undertaken with the International Committee on Harmonisation (ICH), comprising regulators and industry representatives from Japan, the EU and the USA on the development of a new terminology. This will be a difficult task, raising as it does, complicated problems of definition and hierarchical relationships that must be acceptable to Program member states with differing kinds of medical practice and language. Throughout the world, there has been concern over the introduction of a new medical terminology. The UMC is committed to maintain the WHO-ART for as long as it is required and to try to work with the managers of the new terminology to ensure as much compatibility as possible. Now, there is an arrangement whereby updates of terms in the two terminologies are exchanged. The WHO-DD is unique in its coverage of drugs marketed throughout the world, but the Centre is trying to develop it further with the co-operation of industry users. There is now a working data model of a new Drug Dictionary which will allow the entry of many more details about drugs e.g. dosage forms, strengths and licence holders.

The Collaborating Centre is developing new tools for drug safety use on a continuous basis. New logic systems are under preparation for the examination of the database for new types of signal, and new output documents will enhance the ability of experts to evaluate the data.

There are new challenges in the drug safety arena. One is the increasing use of herbal preparations in western countries. In other countries the dangers of the use of the wrong or badly prepared herbs are better known; in western countries, 'herbal' or 'natural' remedies are synonymous with safety. The Collaborating Centre has over 5000 adverse reaction reports involving herbals, but the vast majority are impossible to interpret because of uncertainty over the contents of what are frequently multiple-ingredient, unregistered products. The Centre is discussing, with a variety of authorities throughout the world, better ways of collecting and classifying information. It is clear that international co-operation is vital, since these drugs are marketed with little control throughout the world. Much work has been done to improve the recording of herbal products in the data-base consistently. A new joint project is proposed with the Royal Botanical Gardens, Kew, London, and the Department of Complementary Health Studies, University of Exeter, England and Dr. Peter de Smet in The Netherlands. This will also link with known projects in S. Africa, Kenya and Zimbabwe. Other countries are actively being contacted and the project is also linked with the International Programme on Chemical Safety project on poisonous plants.

Poisoning from drugs (and other chemicals) has not fallen within the scope of 'adverse drug reactions'. Indeed, the widely used WHO definition of an ADR specifically excludes doses outside the normal therapeutic range: 'A response to a drug which is noxious and unintended, and which occurs at doses normally used in man for the prophylaxis, diagnosis, or therapy of disease, or for the modification of physiological function' (WHO Technical Report No. 498 (1972). This definition has always begged the question of what is 'normal', particularly for a new drug, but it has also meant that useful information on drug safety from overdose situations may not have been collected. Many overdose patients are treated by poison control centres, or, with their advice, by general physicians and intensive care experts. Their records are not usually sent to national ADR centres. The Collaborating Centre has been involved in a pilot exercise with several poison control centres throughout the world to capture information on poisoned patients. This has been a successful study and has included much physiological data from the most severely affected patients, which will improve the understanding of dose-related ADRs and aid in the treatment of overdose patients.

The UMC is particularly conscious of the need to consider the benefit to risk balance in relationship to drug safety. This requires, amongst other things, the ability to balance the risk of the disease being treated together with the likely benefit of the drug against the risks of the drug, using similar measures. The merits of the use of a particular drug (or other therapy) are context dependant. Different indications for use, individuals with varieties of concurrent diseases are just two examples of such different contexts. Some overall public health view of a drug's merits seems desirable and this is another very different situation. Some of these issues have been aired in a joint publication and are the subject of new work with CIOMS.

Both this activity, and others that have broader implications in the general area of pharmacovigilance, are being pursued in collaboration with other interested parties. It is likely that co-operation with groups interested in developing early signals of significance will broaden within the scope of this important WHO program. Development of pharmacoepidemiology is one area where this can occur, and also in the area of risk-benefit assessment. The role of CIOMS (Council for International Organizations of Medical Sciences) is pivotal in bringing interested parties together to mount various collaborative projects, as also has ISPE (International Society for Pharmacoepidemiology). These organizations are specifically interested in the science of pharmacovigilance, whereas many others, such as HAI (Health Action International), INRUD (International Network for the Rational Use of Drugs), the IFPMA (International Federation of Pharmaceutical Manufacturers Associations), and the DIA (Drug Information Association), have a broader interest in the area of drug use.

These possibilities for co-operation are exciting since they have in prospect a more rational, cost-effective, and safe drug therapy, but the negative potential for duplication of both effort and dialog must be avoided, since patient safety is at stake.

In order to foster education and communication in pharmacovigilance in general, the Centre now offers an annual course, which is increasingly popular. The course is in 3 consecutive modules. The first offers some insight into the clinical aspects and diagnosis of adverse drug reactions; the second is about the Collaborating Program and also gives 'hands on' experience in using the Collaborating Centre's database; and the final module is an introduction to wider issues in pharmacoepidemiology.

There has also been an increasing trend towards both local and regional meetings in pharmacovigilance. Attendance by Centre staff at such meetings is increasingly requested, but it is to those meetings in developing countries that the Centre gives its priority. Regional meetings have been particularly useful in showing the links between pharmacovigilance, toxicovigilance, drug information, and drug regulation. In many countries developing these kind of activities, it has been possible to suggest considerable savings using shared staff and resources.

Finally, the needs of the general public must not be forgotten. It is clear from some publications, and many discussions with consumer groups, that issues of drug safety and risk and benefit in clinical care are not well understood. This is not surprising, since they are complex and often not considered by an individual until illness supervenes and they change from person to patient. The threat of illness must make it difficult to objectively contemplate different therapeutic management proposals, even if they are offered to the patient by the physician. Thus, the empowerment of patients to be involved in decisions that affect their lives seems to be a nearly impossible task, given the variety of intelligence, knowledge, and attitudes displayed by patients. One effort that has met with success, if sales are anything to judge by, is the provision of a 'Patient Pharmacopoeia'. This is the most widely selling publication in Sweden. A meeting in Verona, Italy, was recently organised by the UMC, the Department of Clinical Pharmacology, University of Verona and Equus Training, Marketing and Business Services (UK). Both the World Health Organisation (Division of Drug Management and Policy) and the Council for International Organisations of Medical Sciences (CIOMS) were sponsors.

The meeting was of professionals reflecting the major groups of players concerned with drug safety issues: consumers, health professionals, the pharmaceutical industry, drug regulators, health professional teachers, clinical pharmacology researchers, the professional media, the legal profession as well as the organisations mentioned above. It was thought essential to involve all the players in a dialogue in order to achieve greater maturity and effectiveness through greater understanding of themselves and others. A general communications model was proposed for examination which should be used to test communications traffic between the players.

The focus of communication in drug safety should be towards the empowerment of consumers and patients to make realistic decisions on their therapy.

Further meetings are being planned, under the CIOMS umbrella, to discuss several issues in more detail. A larger, more global meeting is proposed, under the WHO umbrella, to ensure that pharmacovigilance communications principles and practices can be developed which will benefit all cultures and countries.

Address list of national centres participating in the WHO drug monitoring programme

Argentina
Dr. Mabel Teresa Foppiano
Tel. +54-1-340 0866
Fax +54-1-40 0866

Administración Nacional de Medicamentos,
  Alimentos y Tecnologia Medica (ANMAT)
Departamento de Farmacovigilancia
Avenida de Mayo 869, piso 11o
(1084) BUENOS AIRES
Argentina

Australia
Dr. Ian Boyd
Tel. +61-6-89 8671
Fax +61-6-32 8392
E-mail: ian.boyd@health.gov.au

Therapeutic Goods Administration
Department of Community Services and Health
P.O. Box 100
WODEN, A.C.T. 2606
Australia

Austria
Ms. Eva Hofbauer
Tel. +43-1-711 72, ext. 4641
Fax +43-1-12 0823
E-mail: eva.hofbauer@bmgsk.ada.at

Federal Ministry of Health and Consumer Protection
Pharmacovigilance Department II/A/3
Radetzkystraße 2
A-1030 VIENNA
Austria

Belgium
Mr. Thierry Roisin
Tel. +32-2-210 4909
Fax +32-2-210 4909

Ministry of Health
Pharmacy General Inspectorate
Centre National de Pharmacovigilance
Vesale Building, 20 rue Montague de l'Oratoire
B-1010 BRUSSELS
Belgium

Bulgaria
Dr. Jasmina Mircheva
Director
Tel. +359-2-446 566, 434 71
Fax +359-2-442 697
E-mail: ndi@bulmail.sprint.com

National Drug Institute
Committee on Adverse Drug Reactions
26, Yanko Sakazov Boulevard
BC-1504 SOFIA
Bulgaria

Canada
Dr. Philippe Duclos
Tel. +1-613-957 0325
Fax +1-613-998 6413
E-mail: pduclos@hpb.hwc.ca

Health Canada
Division of Immunization
Laboratory Centre for Disease Control (LCDC)
OTTAWA, Ontario K1A 0L2
Canada

Dr. L. Bruce Rowsell
Director
Tel. +1-613-957 0337, 954 6522
Fax +1-613-957 0335, 952 7738

Health Canada
Bureau of Drug Surveillance
ADR Monitoring Division
OTTAWA, Ontario K1A 1B9
Canada

Chile
Dr. Q.F. Cecilia Morgado-Cadiz
Tel. +56-2-239 8769, 1105
Fax +56-2-239 8760, 6960
E-mail: cmorgado@ispch.cl

Instituto de Salud Publica de Chile
Centro Nacional de Información de Medicamentos y
  Farmacovigilancia CENIMEF
Avenida Marathon 1000
Ñuñoa-Casilla 48
SANTIAGO
Chile

Costa Rica
Dr. Albin Chaves Matamoros
Coordinador
Tel. +506-222 1878
Fax +506-257 7004

Caja Costarricense de Seguro Social
Centro Nacional de Farmacovigilancia
Apartado 10-105
SAN JODE 1000
Costa Rica

Croatia
Prof. Bozidar Vrhovac
Tel. +385-1-213 861
Fax +385-1-213 861
E-mail: vrhovac@rebro.met.hr

National ADR Monitoring Centre
Section of Clinical Pharmacology
Department of Medicine
University Hospital Centre
12 Kispaticeva
41000 ZAGREB
Croatia

Cuba
Dr. Carlos Dotres Martinez
Fax +53-7-333 299

Ministerio de Salud Publica
Calle 23 esq. N. Vedado
C.P. 10 400
CIUDAD DE LA HABANA
Cuba

Czech Republic
MUDr. Dana Stolbova
Tel. +42-2-670 828 17
Fax +42-2-744 944
E-mail: sukl@sukl.anet.cz

State Institute for Drug Control
Státni ústav pro Kontrolu Léciv
Committee on Adverse Drug Reactions
Srobárova 48, post. prihr. 87
100 41 PRAHA 10
Czech Republic

Denmark
Mrs. Kirsten G. Astrup   Lægemiddelstyrelsen
Head   378, Frederikssundsvej
Tel. +45-4-488 9111   DK-2700 BRØNSHØJ
Fax +45-4-284 7077   Denmark
E-mail: lma@sumlma.dk

Finland
Dr. Erkki Palva   National Agency for Medicines (NAM)
Research Director   Lääkelaitos
Tel. +358-9-396 725 18   Drug Information Centre
Fax +358-9-396 725 11   P.O. Box 278
E-mail: erkki.palva@ll.nam.fi   Siltasaarenkatu 18 A
                                               SF-00531 HELSINKI
                                               Finland

France
Dr. Anne Castot   Agence du Médicament
Tel. +33-1-481 322 85   Unité de Pharmacovigilance
Fax +33-1-481 322 83   143–145, boulevard Anatole France
                                               F-93285 SAINT-DENIS, Cedex
                                               France

Dr. Claude Larousse   CHR Institut de Biologie
Tel. +33-240-084 096   Centre Regional Pharmacovigilance
Fax +33-240-084 097   BP 1005
                                               F-44035 NANTES, Cedex
                                               France

Germany
Dr. Jürgen Beckmann   Federal Institute for Drugs and Medical Devices
Tel +49-30-454 830 00   Bundesinstitut für Arzneimittel und Medizinprodukte
Fax +49-30-454 832 07   Seestraße 10
                                               D-13353 BERLIN
                                               Germany

Dr. Karl-Heinz Munter   Drug Commission of the German Medical Profession
Secretary-General   P.O. Box 41 01 25, Aachener Straße 233–237
Tel. +49-221-400 4525   D-50931 KÖLN
Fax +49-221-400 4510, 400 4539   Germany

Greece
Ms. Antonia Pandouvaki   National Drug Organization (EOF)
Tel. +30-1-654 9585   Adverse Drug Reactions Section
Fax +30-1-654 5535   284 Messogion Av.
                                               GR-155 62 HOLARGOS
                                               Greece

Hungary
Dr. János Borvendég
Tel. +36-1-215 8977
Fax +36-1-215 8977

National Institute of Pharmacy
Adverse Drug Reactions Monitoring Centre
Zrínyi u. 3, Box 450
H-1372 BUDAPEST
Hungary

Iceland
Dr. Olafur Olafsson
Director
Tel. +354-5-627 555
Fax +354-5-623 716

Director General of Public Health
Landlæknir
Laugavegi 116
IS-150 REYKJAVIK
Iceland

Indonesia
Dra Andajaningsih
Chairman
Tel. +62-21-424 5459
Fax +62-21-424 3605

Ministry of Health
Directorate General of Drug and Food Control
National Centre for Monitoring of Adverse Drug
  Reactions
Jalan Percetakan Negara No. 23
JAKARTA 10560
Indonesia

Ireland
Ms. Niamh Arthur
Senior Adverse Reactions Officer
Tel. +353-1-676 4971
Fax +353-1-676 7836
E-mail: imb@imb.ie

Irish Medicines Board
Adverse Reactions Section
Earlsfort Centre
Earlsfort Terrace
DUBLIN 2
Ireland

Israel
Dr. Dina Hemo
M.Sc. Pharm.
Tel. +972 2 782 508, 705 744
Fax +972-2-672 58 20

Ministry of Health
Clinical Pharmacology Department
Drug Monitoring Center
Horkania 8a street, P.O. Box 1176
JERUSALEM 91010
Israel

Italy
Dr. Dina De Stefano
Tel. +39-6-5994 32 12
Fax +39-6-5994 33 65

National Pharmacovigilance Center
Pharmacovigilance Department
Ministry of Health
Via Civiltà Romana 7
I-00144 ROMA
Italy

Japan
Mr. Koichi Ishii
Tel. +81-3-350 145 07
Fax +81-3-350 843 64

Ministry of Health and Welfare
Pharmaceutical Affairs Bureau
Safety Division
Office of Appropriate Use of Drugs
2-2-1-Chome, Kasumigaseki, Chiyoda-ku
TOKYO 100-45
Japan

Korea, Republic of
Dr. Soo-Yung Choi
Director
Tel. +82-2-503 7585, 500 3041
Fax +82-2-503 7591, 504 1456
E-mail:
bokji12@nownuri.nowcom.co.kr

Ministry of Health and Welfare
Pharmaceutical Affairs Bureau
Pharmaceutical Development Division
1, Chung-ang Dong, Government Complex II
KWACHON CITY, KYUNGKIDO 427-760
Republic of Korea

Malaysia
Dr. Anis bin Ahmad
Tel. +60-3-757 3611
Fax +60-3-756 2924

Ministry of Health Malaysia
National Pharmaceutical Control Bureau
National ADR Monitoring Center
Jalan Universiti, P.O. Box 319
MA-46730 PETALING JAYA
Malaysia

Morocco
Dr. Rachida Soulaymani-Bencheikh
Tel. +212-7-770 137
Fax +212-7-772 067

Institut National d'Hygiène
Centre Anti Poisons et de Pharmacovigilance
Avenue Ibn Batouta 27
B.P. 769, Agdal
M-11400 RABAT
Morocco

Netherlands
Dr. Arthur P. Meiners
Senior Drug Safety Officer
Tel. +31-70-340 7487, 340 7152
Fax +31-70-340 5155
E-mail: ameiners@pi.net

Medicines Evaluation Board
P.O. Box 5811
Sir Winston Churchillaan 362
NL-2280 HV RIJSWIJK
Netherlands

New Zealand
Dr. Peter Pillans
Medical Assessor
Tel. +64-3-479 7248, ext. 8345
Fax +64-3-477 0509
E-mail:
peter.pillans@stonebow-otago.ac.nz

University of Otago Medical School
National Toxicology Group
P.O. Box 913
DUNEDIN
New Zealand

Norway
Mrs. Krystyna Hviding
Tel. +47-22-897 700
Fax +47-22-897 700

Norwegian Medicines Control Authority
Statens Legemiddelkontroll (SLK)
Adverse Drug Reaction Section
Sven Oftedals vei 6
N-0950 OSLO 9
Norway

Oman
Dr. Ph. Sawsan Ahmad Jaffar
Tel. +968-602 177, 601 044
Fax +968-602 287, 604 684

Ministry of Health
Directorate General of Pharmaceutical Affairs and
    Drug Control
P.O. Box 393
113 MUSCAT
Oman

Philippines
Mrs. Nazarita T. Lanuza
Tel. +63-2-842 5606, 807 0731
Fax +63-2-842 4603

Bureau of Food and Drugs
Department of Health Compound
Alabang 1702, Muntinlupa
METRO MANILA
Philippines

Poland
Ms. Agata Maciejczyk
Tel. +48-22-416 742
Fax +48-22-651 4366

Institute for Drug Research and Control
Centre for Monitoring of Adverse Effects to Drugs
30/34 Chelmska Street
PL-00725 WARSAW
Poland

Portugal
Dr. António Faria Vaz
Tel. +351-1-795 6164, 6170
Fax +351-1-795 9069

Centro Nacional de Farmacovigilancia
Instituto Nacional da Farmácia e do Medicamento
  (INFARMED)
Parque de Saúde de Lisboa
Avenida do Brasil, no. 53
P-1700 LISBOA
Portugal

Romania
Dr. Rodica Badescu
Tel. +40-1-666 6035
Fax +40-1-312 9783

State Institute for Drug Control and Pharmaceutical
  Research
Str. Aviator Sanatescu no 48, Sector 1
R-71 324 BUCURESTI
Romania

Singapore
Ms. Amy Lim
Deputy Director
Tel. +65-325 5629
Fax +65-224 2352
E-mail: kbtoh@cs.gov.sg

Adverse Drug Reaction Monitoring Unit
Drug Administration Division (DAD)
No. 2 Jalan Bukit Merah
SINGAPORE 0316
Singapore

Slovakia
Dr. Pavol Gibala
Tel. +421-7-566 5075, 211 860
Fax +421-7-566 4127, 566 4029

National Centre for Monitoring Adverse Reactions to
  Drugs
State Institute for the Control of Drugs
Kvetná 11
852 08 BRATISLAVA
Slovakia

South Africa
Ms. Ushma Mehta
Tel. +27-21-471 618
Fax +27-21-448 6181
E-mail: umehta@uctgsh1.uct.ac.za

National Adverse Drug Event Monitoring Centre
c/o Department of Pharmacology
Faculty of Medicine
University of Cape Town
OBSERVATORY 7925
South Africa

Spain
Dr. Fransisco José de Abajo
Tel. +34-1-509 7947
Fax +34-1-509 7948

Centro Coordinador del Sistema Español de
    Farmacovigilancia
Instituto de Salud "Carlos III"
Centro Nacional de Farmacobiología
Carretera a Pozuelo, Km 2
E-28220 MAJADAHONDA (MADRID)
Spain

Sweden
Dr. Bengt-Erik Wiholm
Tel. +46-18-17 46 00
Fax +46-18-54 85 66

Medical Products Agency
Division of Drug Epidemiology,
Information and Inspection
Adverse Drug Reaction Section
P.O. Box 26, Husargatan 8
S-751 03 UPPSALA
Sweden

Switzerland
Dr. Rudolf Stoller
Tel. +41-31-322 0352, 322 0211
Fax +41-31-322 0418, 322 0212

Interkantonale Kontrollstelle für Heilmittel
Pharmacovigilance Centre
Erlachstraße 8
CH-3000 BERN
Switzerland

Tanzania
Mr. Henry Irunde
Tel. +255-51-262 11, ext. 2571
Fax +255-51-462 29

Tanzania Drug and Toxicology Information Service
P.O. Box 65088
DAR ES SALAAM
Tanzania

Thailand
Mrs. Suboonya Hutangkabodee
Tel. +66-2-591 8449, 591 8458
Fax +66-2-591 8457
E-mail:
suboonya@health.moph.go.th

Drug Information Center and NADRM, Technical
    Division
National ADR Monitoring Centre
Ministry of Public Health
Food and Drug Administration
Ti-wa-nondh Road
NONTHABUREE 11000
Thailand

Tunisia
Prof. Chelbi Belkahia
Tel. +216-1-264 763
Fax +216-1-571 390

Centre National de Pharmacovigilance
Sis Hôpital Charles Nicolle
TUNIS 1006
Tunisia

Turkey
Ms. Sevgi Oksuz
Chemist
Tel. +90-312-431 1446
Fax +90-312-434 4518
E-mail: saglik@servis.net.tr

Turkish ADR Monitoring Center (TADMER)
Türk Ilac Advers Etkilerini Izleme ve
Skolas str. 28
Saglik Bakanligi
Ilac ve Eczacilic Genel Müdürlügü
06434 Silihiye ANKARA
Turkey

United Kingdom
Dr. Susan Wood
Head
Tel. +44-171-273 0400
Fax +44-171-273 0282, 273 0675

Medicines Control Agency
Pharmacovigilance, Department of Health
Market Towers, 1 Nine Elms Lane
Vauxhall
LONDON SW8 5NQ
United Kingdom

United States of America
Dr. Richard M. Kapit
Tel. +1-301-594 5682
Fax +1-301-827 3529
E-mail: kapit@a1.cber.fda.gov

Food and Drug Administration
Center for Biologics Evaluation and Research
Adverse Event Section, HFM-225
1401 Rockville Pike
ROCKVILLE, MD 20852
United States of America

Dr. Robert O'Neill
Tel. +1-301-443 4227
Fax +1-301-443 5161

Food and Drug Administration
Center for Drug Evaluation and Research
Office of Epidemiology and Biostatics
Room 15B-31 (HFD-730), 5600 Fishers Lane
ROCKVILLE, MD 20857
United States of America

Venezuela
Dr. Carman Lozada A
Tel. +58-2-662 4797
Fax +58-2-662 4797, 662 5074

Instituto Nacional de Higiene "Rafael Rangel"
Sección de Farmacología Sanitaria
Centro Nacional de Vigilancia Farmacológia
Ciudad Universitaria
Apartado Postal 60.412 – Oficina del Este
CARACAS
Venezuela

WHO-HQ
Dr. Martijn ten Ham
Tel. +41-22-791 2111, 791 3638
Fax +41-22-791 0746
E-mail: tenhamm@who.ch

World Health Organization
Drug Safety Unit
10 Avenue Appia
CH-1211 GENEVA 27
Switzerland

Associate member countries

China, People's Republic of
Prof. Zhu Yonghong
Tel. +86-10-701 7755, ext. 339
Fax +86-10-701 3755

National Centre for ADR Monitoring
c/o National Institute for Drug Control
Temple of Heaven
BEIJING P.R.C. 100050
People's Republic of China

Cyprus
Dr. Eftychios Kkolos
Director
Tel. +357-2-302 001
Fax +357-2-302 721

Ministry of Health
Pharmaceutical Services
44 Kimonos Street
NICOSIA 138
Cyprus

Egypt
Dr. Gamila Mohamed Moussa
Tel. +20-2-354 9802
Fax +20-2-354 2627

Ministry of Health
Directorate General of Drug Control
CAIRO
Egypt

Islamic Republic of Iran
Dr. Mohammed Sharifzadeh
Fax +98-21-675 868

Iranian Drug Information Center
ADR unit
Under-secretary for Curative and Drug Affairs
Building no. 3
Fakhre Razi, Enghlab Avenue
TEHRAN 13145
Islamic Republic of Iran

Pakistan
Prof. M. Sultan Farooqui
President
Tel. +92-21-588 2997, 589 2801
Fax +92-21-589 3062, 588 7513
E-mail: whocpsp%paknetbbs@
sdnpk.undp.org

College of Physicians and Surgeons Pakistan
Department of Clinical Pharmacology
7th Central Street
Phase II, Defence Housing Authority
KARACHI 75500
Pakistan

Sri Lanka
Dr. U. Ajith Mendis
Director
Tel. +94-1-695 173
Fax +94-1-695 173

Ministry of Health
Medical Technology and Supplies Division
No. 120, Norris Canal Road
COLOMBO 10
Sri Lanka

Yugoslavia, Federal Republic of
Prof. Vaso Antunovic

Clinical Centre of Serbia
National Centre for Adverse Drug Effects
Visegradska 26
YU-11000 BELGRADE
Federal Republic of Yugoslavia

Zimbabwe
the Registrar
Tel. +263-4-792 165
Fax +263-4-736 980

Drugs Control Council
P.O. Box UA 599,106 Baines Avenue
Union Avenue
HARARE
Zimbabwe

Index of drugs

Page numbers in **bold** indicate where the given drug is discussed in detail.

Index of side effects

malignant hyperthermia
  chlorocresol, 138
  general anesthetics, 105
  neuromuscular blocking agents,
    140
  sevoflurane, 111
  suxamethonium, 138
mania
  clarithromycin, 242, 278
  corticosteroids, 369
  molgramostim, 339
  serotonin re-uptake
    inhibitors, 8
  sertraline, 8
mastalgia
  estradiol, 382
mastodynia
  cyproterone acetate, 386
Mazotti reaction
  ivermectin, 280
membranous nephropathy
  diclofenac, 89
  fenoprofen, 89
  griseofulvin, 255
  ibuprofen, 89
  nabumetone, 89
  naproxen, 89
  NSAIDs, 89
  tolmetin, 89
memory disorder
  aluminium, 207
  alpha interferon, 327
  lithium, 12
  topiramate, 66
memory loss
  see amnesia
meningeal irritation
  iopamidol, 418
meningism
  propofol, 115
meningitis
  baclofen, 140
  immunoglobulin, 301
  MMR vaccine, 291
  mumps vaccine, 291
menstruation disturbance
  cyclophosphamide, 342
  cyproterone acetate, 386
  oral contraceptives, 385
  progesterone, 384
  risperidone, 51
  spironolactone, 388
mental disturbance
  aluminium sulfate, 207
  amiodarone, 176
  neuroleptics, 41
  tetrahydrocannabinol, 27
  topiramate, 66
  vigabatrin, 70

mesothelioma
  thorium dioxide sol, 423
metabolic acidosis
  fructose, 311
  propylene glycol, 113
  topiramate, 66
  total parenteral nutrition, 310
methemoglobinemia
  EMLA, 127
  flutamide, 388
  prilocaine, 129
  primaquine, 259
microalbuminuria
  see proteinuria
micturition disturbance
  estradiol, 382
  thyrotrophin-releasing
    hormone, 404
  topiramate, 66
  tramadol, 82
migraine
  cabergoline, 389
  estradiol transdermal, 383
  losartan, 198
mitochondrion toxicity
  zidovudine, 274
mood disturbance
  danazol, 386
  alpha interferon, 327
  levodopa, 146
  remacemide, 65
mortality
  beta2 adrenoceptor agonists,
    165
  aprotinin, 314
  artemether, 259
  bronchodilators, 165
  calcium antagonists, 185, 186
  cocaine, 20, 128
  colloid volume expanders, 310
  contrast media, 422
  corticosteroids, 165
  cromoglycate disodium, 165
  desogestrel, 385
  dextran, 310
  diamorphine, 26
  diazepam, 26
  diethylene glycol, 438
  digitalis glycosides, 173
  digoxin, 173
  diltiazem, 185
  diuretics, 200
  encainide, 177
  ethanol, 26
  fenoterol, 165
  flecainide, 177
  gelatin, 310
  general anesthetics, 105
  gestodene, 385

  hetastarch, 310
  ipratropium bromide, 165
  levonorgestrel, 385
  3,4-methylenedioxymeth-
    amphetamine, 19
  neuromuscular blocking agents,
    310
  nifedipine, 185
  nimodipine, 188
  opioids, 20
  oral contraceptives, 384
  pyrimethamine, 263
  quinine, 259
  salbutamol, 165
  sulfonylureas, 398
  suxamethonium, 134
  temazepam, 26
  thyroxine, 393
  tolbutamide, 398
  verapamil, 185
  xanthines, 165
motor dysfunction
  aluminium, 207
  mercury, 213
  sodium valproate, 67, 68
  suramin, 284
motor neuron disease
  enflurane, 108
mouth cancer
  selenium, 215
mouth lesion
  erythromycin, 239
mouth ulcer
  see also stomatitis
  astemizole, 162
movement disorder
  see also involuntary movement
  ketamine, 103
  midazolam, 113
muscle cramp
  beta adrenoceptor blockers, 183
  amiodarone, 175
  aretinolol, 183
  carteolol, 183
  danazol, 386
  metoprolol, 183
  pindolol, 183
  propranolol, 183
muscle ischemia
  zidovudine, 274
muscle rigidity
  diamorphine, 26
  droperidol, 51
  halothane, 109
  neuroleptics, 38, 41, 42
  retinoids, 154
  risperidone, 52
muscle spasm
  mepivacaine, 125